THE SPINE E

*Everything You've Wanted to Know About Back and
Neck Pain but Were Too Afraid to Ask*

A Patient and Physician
Guide

YOSHIHIRO
KATSUURA, MD

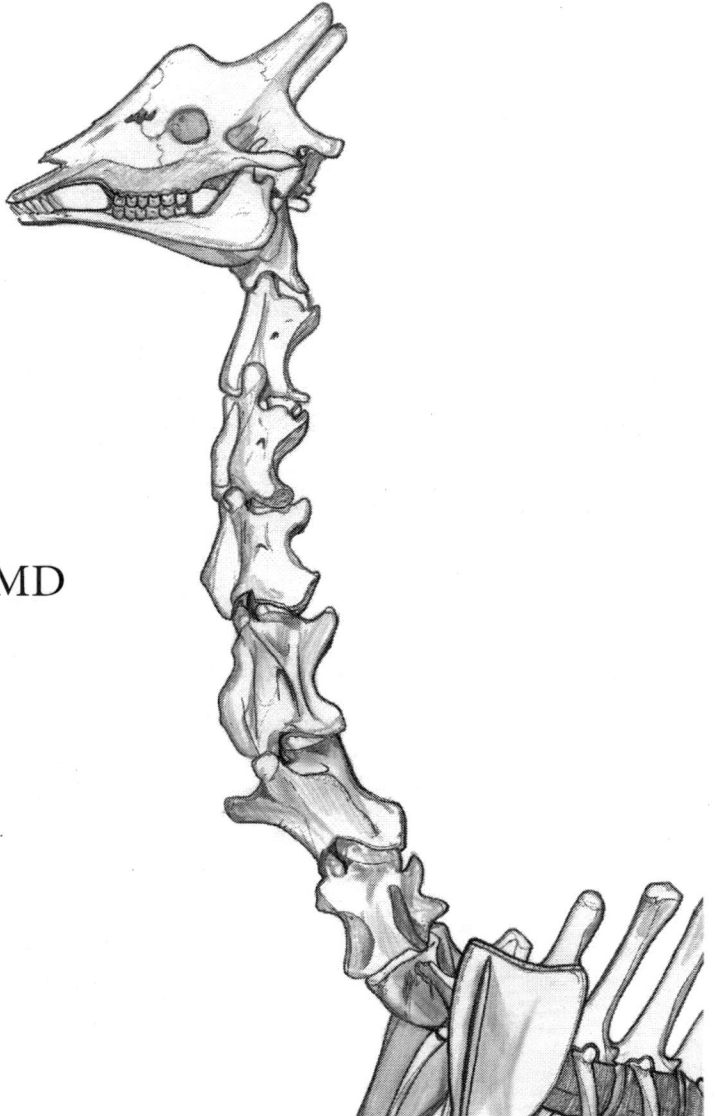

Copyright © 2022 by Yoshihiro Katsuura MD
All Rights Reserved

First Edition

Paperback ISBN: 979-8-9872441-0-4
Ebook ISBN: 979-8-9872441-1-1

Editor: Myrna Schlegel
Illustrations: Yoshihiro Katsuura MD

All rights reserved. This book was self-published by the author Yoshihiro Katsuura under Subtilitas Press. No part of this book may be reproduced in any form by any means without the express permission of the author. This includes reprints, excerpts, photocopying, recording or any future means of reproducing text.

If you would like to do any of the above, please seek permission first by contacting me at yoshi@katsuuramd.com

Published in the United States by Subtilitas Press

Version 1.994
Printed by Kindle Direct Publishing

Dedication:

To my wife Julia, who has always been my best cheerleader and our two boys Hiro and Hide.

To my parents Hidefumi and Frances and my brother Tak, who made me who I am.

To my Aunt Susan, who always pushed me to do more.

"There it is. Take it"

-William Mulholland, November 1913

Acknowledgements:

The path towards a career in spine surgery is only accomplished with the guidance of those who came before. The people who have helped me in this regard were instrumental in shaping my thought process, clinical practice and hence, this book. While there were many, those who taught me specifically in the field of spine surgery are listed in alphabetical order:

Todd Albert, MD
Dick Alvarez, MD
Peter Boehm Jr, MD
Peter Boehm Sr, MD
Jeremy Bruce, MD
Bill Bowen, MD
Garrick Cason, MD
Matthew Cunningham, MD
Jad Dorizas, MD
Jesse Doty, MD
Jim Farmer, MD
Mark Freeman, MD
Michael Gallagher, MD
Ren Gardner, MD
Alex Hughes, MD
Chevy Iyer, MD
Russel Huang, MD
Brian Kelly, MD
Han Jo Kim, MD

Daniel Kueter, MD
Virginie Lafage, PhD
Bruce McCormack, MD
Wendell Moses, MD
Jody Miller, MD
Patrick O'Leary, MD
Jim Osborn, MD
Rob Quigley, MD
Sheeraz Qureshi, MD
Andrew Sama, MD
Vin Sandhu, MD
Frank Schwab, MD
Michael Tew, MD

To my brothers in surgery from residency, thank you for caring for me unconditionally.

Joey Boaen, MD
Jason Fogleman, MD

To my brothers in surgery from fellowship, thank you for your past and future guidance.

Jeremy Steinberger, MD
Ravi Verma, MD
Sohrab Virk, MD
Phil York, MD

Also, a special thanks to the **Librarians of the Hospital for Special Surgery.**

About the Author

Yoshihiro Katsuura is a board-certified Orthopedic Surgeon who specializes in and is passionate about the care of the spine. He has been a faculty member at the world's most prestigious orthopedic hospital, The Hospital for Special Surgery, but now is in private practice in California, his home. This is his first book. He stretches his back and neck daily.

Preface

The medical body of knowledge is ever evolving. No one book can encompass every aspect of this body, nor can hope to reflect it with total accuracy. The spine is a nuanced organ system, and our understanding of it continues to grow. Use caution when applying the concepts in this book and understand that you should always make medical decisions with your physician. The author and publishers are not liable for errors or omissions in this book or any consequences of its application. The statements made in this book are for information only, and are not made to diagnose, prevent, treat or cure disease. Case discussions in this book have been modified to protect the identity of patients, while still attempting to portray real-life scenarios.

Contents

Introduction
How to Use This Book 1

SECTION 1
Getting to Know Your Back:
Chapter 1
Spine Basics 7
Chapter 2
What Causes Pain In the Spine 33
Chapter 3
Low Back Pain, Buttock Pain and Tail Bone Pain—When to Seek Care and Do I
Need Surgery? 49
Chapter 4
Neck Pain and Treatment 57
Chapter 5
What Causes Spinal Cord Compression and Myelopathy? 67
Chapter 6
Imaging of the Spine: X-RAY To MRI 77

SECTION 2
Common Spine Problems that Might Require Surgery
Chapter 7
What is a Herniated Disc and What Happens When It Occurs in the Neck
(Cervical) or Low Back (Lumbar) 93

Chapter 8
Lumbar Stenosis and Spondylolisthesis. **105**

Chapter 9
Thoracic Spinal Cord Compression **119**

Chapter 10
Scoliosis: Fact vs Fiction **125**

Chapter 11
Scheuermann's Kyphosis **145**

Chapter 12
Osteoporosis and the Spine **153**

Chapter 13
Fractures and Dislocations of the Spine **173**

Chapter 14
Infections of the Spine: Osteomyelitis, Discitis, Post-Surgical Infection **189**

Chapter 15
Cancer and Tumors in the Spine **201**

Chapter 16
Spinal Cord Injury **215**

Chapter 17
Injury to the Nerves Once they Leave the Spinal Canal (Peripheral Nerve Injury and Neuron Regeneration) **233**

Chapter 18
Nerve Problems Affecting the Extremities Aka Peripheral Nerve Entrapments . **243**

SECTION 3
Good Spine Habits and Treating Your Spine Without Surgery

Chapter 19
Medical Treatments for Back Pain. **269**

Chapter 20
Narcotic Pain Medicine. **295**

Chapter 21
Alternative Therapy: Ergonomics, Exercise, Physical Therapy, Acupuncture, Chiropractor and Others. **305**

Chapter 22
Sports and the Spine—Dos And Don'ts. **323**

Chapter 23
Calcium, Parathyroid Hormone, Vitamin D and the Spine. **335**

Chapter 24
Obesity, Diabetes, Smoking: Lifestyle Factors That Affect Spine Degeneration and Spine Surgery **345**

Chapter 25

Care of the Aging Spine: Keeping Your Back Working For You in Your Golden Years Instead of the Other Way Around. **363**

SECTION 4

What You Need to Know About the Different Types of Spine Surgery

Chapter 26

Finding the Right Spine Surgeon and Hospital **379**

Chapter 27

Preparing Yourself for Surgery **391**

Chapter 28

How Your Thoughts and Feelings Affect Pain and Outcomes in Spine Surgery . **423**

Chapter 29

The Bottom Line, Do I Need Surgery? **435**

Chapter 30

What Are the Risks of Spine Surgery? **445**

Chapter 31

The Changing Spine: Understanding Why Sometimes One Surgery to Fix the Spine Leads to Another Surgery—Revision Surgery and Spinal Deformity **461**

Chapter 32

Managing Bleeding in Spine Surgery: Anticoagulant and Coagulant Therapies . **473**

Chapter 33

A Brief Introduction to Anesthesia **489**

Chapter 34

Spine Surgery in the Elderly **497**

Chapter 35

Orthopedic Surgery in the Era of Covid 19: Protecting Yourself From Hospital-Acquired Infection **507**

Chapter 36

Spinal Decompression: Taking Pressure Off the Spinal Cord and Nerve Roots Directly (by Removing Tissue) or Indirectly (by Realigning the Spine)—Laminectomy and Foraminotomy. **517**

Chapter 37

Spinal Fusion, Bone Graft Technology and Bone Morphogenic Protein (BMP) . **525**

Chapter 38

How Surgeons Get to And Open The Spine to Fix the Problem: Open vs Minimally Invasive Spine Surgery, Lasers, and Other Spine Surgery Techniques **539**

Chapter 39

Removing a Spinal Disc Fragment That is Compressing a Nerve in The Low Back (Lumbar Discectomy) **551**

Chapter 40
How Surgeons Remove a Damaged Disc in the Neck and Restore the Cervical Spine to Good Function—Anterior Cervical Discectomy and Fusion (ACDF) **559**

Chapter 41
When Fixing the Spine in the Low Back Requires Fusing 2 Vertebrae: Lumbar Spinal Fusion **567**

Chapter 42
Scoliosis and Deformity Correction Surgery **583**

Chapter 43
Procedures to Fix Stenosis in the Neck: Laminectomy, Fusion With Laminectomy, and Laminoplasty **591**

Chapter 44
Fixing Disease in the Neck While Preserving Neck Movement: Cervical Disc Replacement and Cervical Foraminotomy **599**

Chapter 45
Replacing a Disc in the Low Back to Relieve Low Back Pain—How and Who it is for: Lumbar Disc Replacement/Arthroplasty **611**

Chapter 46
Treating Osteoporotic Fractures in the Spine With Bone Cement: Vertebral Augmentation—Kyphoplasty and Vertebroplasty **623**

Chapter 47
Minimally Invasive Procedures for Lumbar Stenosis: Interspinous Process Devices and Techniques **633**

Chapter 48
Sacroiliac (SI) Joint Pain and Treatment **643**

SECTION 5
What to Expect After Spine Surgery

Chapter 49
Wound Care During and After Spine Surgery **653**

Chapter 50
Aftercare—Taking Care of Yourself at Home Following Spine Surgery: Pain Control, Diet and Activity Recommendations **663**

Chapter 51
Conclusions and Further Reading **677**

A Glossary of Common Terms in Spine Surgery **681**

Common Abbreviations: **699**

Index **701**

Introduction

How to Use This Book

The spine is an amazing organ composed of 24 linked vertebrae that allows you to live your life upright. Most people fail to appreciate how it works and how to care for it and are daunted when it breaks down. To the extent of my knowledge as a spine surgeon, I endeavor to help people understand their backs, prevent injury, and treat problems when they arise. Luckily, the majority of what I do focuses on helping ease pain without surgery, but occasionally surgery is necessary.

The prospect of undergoing spine surgery is a scary, overwhelming concept. Part of my job is to attempt to unpackage this fear to help patients face challenging clinical problems. What I have found is that most of the fear is in the unknown and the more you understand about the process, the easier it is to make decisions that can improve your life or the life of a loved one.

While some anxiety is normal—spine surgery is serious—most people's understanding of spine surgery is based on anecdotes from friends (that is, they "had spine surgery and their backs never got better" stories), popular media such as sitcom TV, tabloid articles and podcasts (1). These forms of information tend to be inaccurate or highlight the most extreme cases in spine surgery. This book was written for one main purpose: to dispel misconceptions about the spine and its problems and to replace those wrong ideas with facts and the latest information that will help both you and your doctor achieve excellent results. Instead of exploring the vast and uncharted seas of the internet, I provide a curated review of the most critical information regarding the medical care of the spine.

This book is divided into sections:

- **Section I, Getting to Know Your Back**

- **Section ll, Common Spine Problems that May Require Surgery**

- **Section lll, Good Spine Habits and Treating Your Spine Without Surgery**

- **Section IV, What You Need to Know About the Different Types of Spine Surgery**

- **Section V, What to Expect After Surgery.**

In the first section I will help you understand what's wrong with you or your loved one's back and why it may –or may not—require surgery. I will also cover some basic principles of anatomy, physiology and surgery. In the second section I will give an overview for specific ailments of the back and neck. In the third section we will talk about how to maintain your back, but also about treating back pain without surgery. My belief is that the spine is a machine, and like any machine it can be tuned and taken care of to last longer. We will then take the plunge into the assortment of common spine surgeries that can be performed, including their risks and benefits and even compare treatments. In this section I'll discuss the specifics of different surgical procedures and what happens in the operating room. We go into more depth about the expected results of surgery and possible complications. Finally, in the last section I'll discuss your recovery following spine surgery, what progress can be expected and general aftercare. You will learn how to look out for early warning signs of a complication so you can alert your doctor.

This book is written based on scientific evidence, and the references are provided. Do not let this intimidate you if you are not used to it. These may be either ignored or used to "read deeper" into a topic based on your desire.

The practice of medicine is based on experience but also is guided by the available evidence or "literature" as physicians commonly refer to it. There is a hierarchy that exists within the body of medical evidence. At the top of the food chain is the prospective, randomized controlled trial or RCT. These are scientific studies where a group of patients with the same medical condition are split into two groups. The first group receives an experimental or selected treatment whereas the second group receives a placebo. Both the patients and doctors should be "blinded" to which group any patient is assigned to so there is reduced risk of bias. Randomized controlled trials are the ideal method of getting medical evidence but are far from perfect. First, these trials are incredibly expensive to run, require a dedicated team and can also be easily influenced by industry pressure to support the use of a certain treatment. Also, in orthopedic surgery most individual problems are just that— individual problems with significant nuances that are difficult to group. How do you ensure that each patient in each study is suffering from the same problem? Moreover, how do you ensure that two different surgeons provide the exact same surgical care? And how do you blind patients to the fact that they are getting surgery?

In this book I try to cite any randomized controlled studies that are available on a given topic, but I also cite studies which are not RCTs. I refer to studies which have impacted the way that I practice medicine and influence the decisions I make with patients. In orthopedic surgery, there are different ways an individual problem is experienced by different patients, but there are also similarities that do allow them to be grouped to a degree. I present surgical treatments as though every surgical technique will be performed the same by every surgeon, but this is usually not the case, and different surgeons will use techniques differently, even though the techniques will be given the same name.

Each section will explore the current state of the art and scientific understanding of the topic in plain language and review common questions patients frequently ask. As stated above, I list references which I think are notable or landmarks for those interested in learning more or understanding where the information comes from. It is my assumption that the book will be out of date the minute it is published, because science and surgery are continually advancing, and so I try to focus on concepts which have stood the test of time, and carefully introduce new ideas in surgery.

This book fills over 600 pages of sometimes dense, technical material. Not every chapter may be of interest to you, nor is it necessary to read every chapter. In fact, I designed each chapter to be read independently, if you want. Furthermore, you do not even need to read the whole chapter. Make use of the table of contents to find those topics you want to know more about. For example, if you are researching a cervical disorder, the chapters on the lumbar spine will not be of interest. Each chapter starts with a brief introduction giving you a fast overview. This is followed by a case example based loosely off situations I have encountered in real life. Although the case examples are influenced by my interactions with patients, they have been modified to protect privacy. At the end of each chapter there will be a summary of the important concepts followed by some frequently asked questions (FAQ). If you are like me, you will find it easier to digest information through repetition, which I build into each chapter. If you would rather read this book from front to back your understanding of the spine will be much stronger. I suggest you read the summary,

skim the chapter, and look at the figures/FAQ at the end. Then read the parts you find interesting.

And because there are times when a picture really is worth a thousand words, at the end of most chapters, following the references, are drawings (figures) that will help you better understand that chapter. I would recommend taking a quick look at those drawings before beginning to read each chapter so you are aware of these learning aids and can refer to them as you go through the chapter material.

Throughout the book I have tried to explain all the medical terms as I use them. There is also a glossary of common terms and a reference of abbreviations at the end of the book.

This book was born out of a hope to connect better with my patients. I believe spine surgery is a team effort whose success is partly based on education and communication. I hope this book will help guide you to a solid understanding of the basic concepts of the spine as well as surgery involving the spine and help you live a more active and pain free life.

References

1.   Globe TB. Clash in the name of care - A Boston Globe Spotlight Team Report [Internet]. BostonGlobe.com. [cited 2020 Apr 2]. Available from: http://bo.st/1MLW-mPp

SECTION 1

Getting to Know Your Back:

Build an Understanding of the Anatomy of the Spine and the Physiology of Pain

"Learning is the only thing the mind never exhausts, never regrets and never fears"
-Leonardo da Vinci

Chapter 1

Spine Basics

Summary

The spine is an amazing machine composed of bones, soft tissue and nerves. It allows you to stand erect and most importantly houses one of the most critical and sophisticated structures in your body—the spinal cord and nerves. In this section I give an overview of basic spine anatomy and how it works. This is a difficult topic to understand even for those who have studied it for many years so don't feel bad if it's confusing. I have tried to include drawings to make things easier to grasp. In brief, you have 4 main sections of your spine: your neck or cervical spine, your upper back or thoracic spine, your lower back or lumbar spine and in your pelvis the sacrum. Each section consists of interlinked vertebra bones that are connected by discs and ligaments to allow specific types of motion. Nerve impulses are transmitted from the brain through the spinal cord and then via nerves to the muscles of your body to control movement. Similarly, impulses (such as sensation) are transmitted from the extremities back up through the nerves and spinal cord to the brain.

Case

Mr. Red is a 35-year-old carpenter. One day he is installing an outdoor barbeque and throws his back out lifting the heavy object. He has severe back pain and leg pain which prevent him from standing. His pain is so severe he must go to the emergency room. The emergency room doctors suspect he has suffered from a lumbar disc herniation, a condition where there is a rupture of a structure known as an intervertebral disc that acts as a cushion between the vertebrae. The doctors explain that when a disc herniation occurs, the ruptured material can compress and irritate nerves in the spine resulting in pain that radiates down the leg. They give him some pain medications and he has enough improvement to return home. The continuing pain causes him to go see his primary care provider who obtains an MRI which confirms the diagnosis of an "L5-1 herniated disc causing compression of the thecal sac" and refers him to physical therapy after giving him an epidural steroid injection. Ultimately after several months he makes little improvement and seeks the counsel of a spine surgeon. The spine surgeon suggests a microdiscectomy, a procedure where a small opening is made in part of the vertebra (the bone of the lamina) through which the disc fragment may be removed to "un-pinch" the nerve. The surgeon says he will use a posterior approach to access the herniation. Mr. Red agrees to the procedure, and afterward has immediate relief of his leg and back pain.

Introduction

It is easier to make sense of body parts if you know where they are in relation to other body parts. Doctors are trained in a language to describe the relationship of body parts that can be very confusing to patients. You can look at the table below of anatomic terms that doctors use to make talking about the body easier. If you spend a few minutes learning these it will be easier to understand the discussions in this book and any discussions, you will have with your doctor. Let's just discuss a few basic terms that are used routinely in the spine surgery world.

The terms anterior, posterior and lateral are used very commonly in spine surgery because they describe from what direction the spine may be surgically accessed. The term anterior, for example, is used to describe accessing the spine from the front of the body. So, an anterior approach to the neck would be one that goes through the skin at the front of the neck. A posterior approach is used when you make an incision on the back of the neck. Lateral approaches are those that go through the side of the body, for example a lateral approach to the lumbar (low back) spine goes through the side of the abdomen.

There are many other terms which will commonly occur throughout this book and that doctors will routinely use but may be confusing to the average reader. I did my best to write this book so that anyone could understand it, but I am so used to medical writing some may have slipped through. There is a glossary of common terms at the end of this book, but below is a list of terms which are critical to understand from a spine surgery perspective, and that doctors use so much they may not even realize you don't know them.

Anatomic Terms Indicating Direction

Term	Meaning
Anterior	front (Your face is on the anterior part of your head.)
Posterior	back (Your buttocks are on the posterior part of your body.)
Cranial/ Cephalad	towards the head (The heart is cranial to the liver, meaning the heart is closer to the head than the liver is.)
Caudal	toward the sacrum (The liver is caudal to the heart, meaning the liver is closer to the sacrum than the heart is.)
Proximal	closer to the body (Your elbow is proximal to your hand.)
Distal	farther from the body (Your hand is distal to your elbow.)
Superficial	closer to the surface (The skin is superficial to the bone.)
Deep	closer to the interior (The bone is deep to the skin.)
Dorsal	being on the surface of the back
Ventral	being on the surface of the abdomen

The Bones

Most bones in the body act as a scaffold to hold up tissues and muscles. The spine, as a network of bones, serves as the suspension bridge from which the muscles of the torso and internal organs hang. But the spine is different from other bones in the body because it also protects the soft spinal cord and nerves, totally encasing them in a tunnel. Thus, the spine is not only responsible for allowing you to stand erect, but it protects one of your most sensitive organs, the information super-highway known as the spinal cord that allows your brain to control your body and receive input from your senses. As a spine surgeon I am constantly amazed by its elegance and complexity, but also have a healthy respect for how problems can occur. Small shifts in the bones can cause serious problems resulting in compression of the nerves. Masses the size of a pea or smaller can cause major problems in the spinal canal where real estate is minimal. Any of these issues in the spine can turn the elegant machine into a major source of pain and suffering.

The spinal column is formed from bones called the vertebrae. There are no two vertebrae in your spine which are identical, but each vertebra is composed of similar components that are common to all the vertebrae. The vertebrae are grouped into four main groups: cervical, thoracic, lumbar and sacral. They are divided this way because the vertebrae in each section have anatomic similarities.

In its most simple terms, **there are four main parts to each vertebra which form a ring shape: the vertebral body, the lamina, the facets and the pedicles.** The vertebral body, the pedicles and the lamina form the bony ring of the spinal canal, which protects and supports the spinal cord that runs through it.

- **The vertebral body is the large round part of the vertebra which is responsible for bearing most of the weight of your upper torso. The vertebral body has a hard outer layer (cortex bone) and a honeycomb inner structure (cancellous bone), which contains bone marrow.**

- **The lamina is the thin arch of bone that shelters the spinal canal on the back side of the vertebra. The lamina is flat in keeping with its name's meaning (lamina means a thin sheet of material in Latin). Extending from the lamina are several bony processes—a bony process is a part of the bone that projects or extends out. One of these, the spinous process, is the largest of the lamina's bony extensions and serves as an attachment for muscles and ligaments. It is the long, tapered bone extending off the spine and is the part of your spine you can feel when you touch your back. There are also paired extensions called articular processes (see below).**

- **The articular processes form facet joints. The articular processes are small seashell shaped bones that extend from the vertebra and form the joints that connect one vertebra to another. There are two facets on the top of a vertebra, one on each side, and two on the bottom, one on each side. The two processes at the top are called the superior articular processes and the two on the bottom are the inferior articular processes. Stated another way, each vertebra contains 4 articular processes, 2 going up (superior) and 2 going down (inferior). They are paired because the superior and inferior articular processes are mirror reflections of one another, allowing them to fit snugly into each other. When the superior articular process of one vertebra links with the inferior articular process of the vertebra above it, they form a facet joint. The facets are perhaps the most confusing part of the bony anatomy of the spine and so I suggest** looking at the pictures at the end of this chapter rather than trying to understand them by reading alone.

* The pedicles are simply the two tubes of bone, one on each side of the vertebra, that connect the lamina to the vertebral body.

Random Words Doctors Use So Much They Forget You Might Not Know Them:

Term	Meaning
Approach	The term approach is used to describe the procedure for getting to the spine (or whatever organ you are operating on) in surgery. So an anterior approach to the spine will expose the front of the spine to do surgery on it by entering the body from the front of the body.
Benign	This can have multiple meanings in orthopedic surgery. First, regarding tumors and cancer, benign means that the cancer will not spread to other areas of the body. Benign can also be used to indicate that the medical problem is not life or limb threatening or does not require surgical intervention.
Clinical	An adjective used to describe things that a doctor observes or discovers or learns on his or her own (so without diagnostic tests) at the bedside with the patient. For example, a clinical exam is a physical examination that the doctor performs on you with their own hands. Compare this to a radiological exam, which is done with an imaging machine. **Clinical signs** are observable features on your physical exam which point towards a certain diagnosis. **Clinical symptoms** are the symptoms you directly tell your doctor.
Decompression or Decompress	A surgical procedure where a spine surgeon removes structures or material that are pinching nerves or the spinal cord. A good majority of the work spine surgeons do are decompressions. Decompressions are usually accomplished by removing the lamina (the arch of the vertebra) in a procedure called a laminectomy, but also include removing other bones, tumors, abscesses, and disc fragments among other things.
Innervate	This is a verb that describes how a nerve carries signals between the brain and a body part and in this way controls that body part. For example, the C5 nerve root innervates the biceps; the vagus nerve innervates the stomach.
Open and Minimally invasive	Open surgery has been the traditional way of doing surgery, where a larger incision is used to completely expose the spine and allow procedures to be performed. Minimally invasive surgical (MIS) approaches are those which use small incisions to access the spine. An MIS approach typically includes technology that allows the surgeon to better visualize the spine such as arthroscopes, microscopes and CT-guided navigation. An important concept to remember is that just because it's done as a minimally invasive procedure, does not mean it's better or has better results.

To summarize, the vertebra consists of an anterior (front) part and a posterior (back) part. The anterior part is the cylindrical vertebral body which is the major weight bearing portion of the spine. Every vertebra is connected to the vertebra above and below it by an intervertebral disc. That disc sits between the two vertebrae's vertebral bodies. The posterior part consists of the lamina, facet joints, spinous processes (this is the part you can feel with your fingers), transverse processes and pedicles and contribute to spinal stability and motion. Thus, anterior surgical procedures focus on the vertebral body and discs, while posterior procedures focus primarily on the lamina, pedicles, and facets. This will be important to remember for the later sections of this book discussing specific anterior and posterior procedures.

Random Words Doctors Use So Much They Forget You Might Not Know Them: Continued

Term	Meaning
"Presents with"	This is a phrase physicians use to describe what problems the patient has on the first encounter. It can be used to describe symptoms (for example, the patient presents with symptoms of leg pain), or it can be used to describe findings on the physical exam or as relates to diagnostic imaging (for example, the patient presents with leg weakness and a large disc herniation was found on MRI).
Segment and level	Spine surgeons use the terms segment and level to refer to a specific location in the spine. Level is used to refer to a single vertebra or a single disc space between two vertebra. Segment describes the unit of two adjacent vertebrae and the disc space between them. For more on this see the last paragraph in the bone section of this chapter. Adjacent segment disease typically describes a problem at a spinal segment (disc space and vertebrae) above or below an operated segment. When discussing procedures, surgeons often refer to two adjacent vertebrae and the disc between them as a level. A one-level fusion joins 2 vertebrae; a 2-level fusion joins 3 consecutive vertebrae.
Stenosis	Stenosis just means narrowing. In the context of spine surgery, the narrowing usually occurs in the spinal canal, reducing the space available for nerves and the spinal cord (spinal stenosis). The terms stenosis and compression are often used interchangeably.
Thoracolumbar	A compound word joining thoracic (thoraco) and Lumbar to indicate the junction between the thoracic and lumbar vertebrae, or the vertebrae T10 through L2. It may also be used to reference the thoracic and lumbar spines in one word.

The spinal column is divided into five main sections or groups, based on the location and overarching shape of the vertebrae in each section: the lumbar spine, the thoracic spine, the cervical spine, the sacral spine and the coccyx. Your surgeon will be referring to these sections in your spine so it's very important to understand the naming process. Each vertebra is given a label based on two things: its group (Letter C for cervical, T for thoracic or L for lumbar) and its number, from top to bottom, within that group. For example, the first cervical vertebra is given the label C1 (C because it's cervical, that is, located in the neck, and 1 because it's the first one of 7, one being the closest to the head). The coccyx is rarely operated on and so is not typically given an abbreviation.

Most humans have 24 mobile vertebrae (5 lumbar, 12 thoracic, and 7 cervical). The sacrum consists of 5 fused and non-mobile vertebrae but each of those vertebrae are still referred to as if they were individual bones such as S1 and S2 etc). The most consistent section of the spine is the cervical spine —almost all mammals universally having 7 cervical vertebrae. The two exceptions to the rule are the manatee and the two-toed sloth which have 6 cervical vertebrae. However about 5% of humans have only 23 vertebrae and about 4% have 25. It is also common to have transitional vertebra which means that a lumbar vertebra looks like a sacral vertebra or vice versa (1).

The cervical spine is in your neck and consists of 7 bones, each with a diameter about that of the top of a soda can, **(commonly labeled C1-C7)**. These sit directly under your skull. They allow your neck to move up and down as well as bend and rotate from side to side. Most of the motion in your neck comes from the upper part of your cervical spine, namely C1 and C2, with 40% of your bending and rotating ability also coming from these levels (2). Most of your nodding motion comes from the joint formed at the junction of the occiput (the bone at the base of your skull) and the C1 vertebra. This joint is like a ball and socket joint (think of the range of motion of the shoulder joint). The remainder of your neck motion comes from the lower cervical spinal levels (C3-C7), with each segment contributing about 15% of your neck motion.

The thoracic spine is in your upper back and consists of 12 medium-sized bones (commonly labeled T1-T12) and are unique in that they are attached to your ribs. This is important because the rib cage is a rigid structure and thus these bones do not bend or twist as much as either the cervical or lumbar vertebrae (3). Hence only a fraction of your upper body motion comes from your thoracic spine and it is rare to develop arthritic conditions in this area.

The lumbar spine is in your low back and consists of 5 large-sized vertebrae (labeled L1-L5). The large size makes it possible for them to support the entire weight of your head, torso and spinal column (think of the Eiffel tower which is skinny at the top and broad at the bottom). They are also important because, unlike the thoracic spine, the lumbar vertebrae are not attached to the ribs and thus can generate quite a bit of your trunk motion.

Finally, there is the **sacrum** which is one of the three main bones in your pelvis. The sacrum is triangle-shaped and sits between your two hips. It is composed of five fused vertebrae (meaning they are not separated by discs like the rest of the vertebrae) and thus generally referred to as just the sacrum although surgeons may call the upper part of the sacrum S1. The sacrum is the platform on which your spine sits (again think of the wide base of the Eiffel tower). However, the sacrum also serves as the cornerstone of the pelvis and transmits load down to your legs and the ground (think of the cornerstone at the top of a masonry bridge which braces the entire load of the bridge). **The sacrum is one single bone, but we refer to its individual parts just as we do with the rest of the spine, with the top segment called S1, and the last S5.**

The overall shape of the spine is very important to its function, and you may hear your surgeon talking about this, using words like scoliosis (an abnormal curvature in the spine) kyphosis (a forward bend, moving that part of the torso forward) or lordosis (a backwards bend, moving that part of the torso backward). Put simply, the spine should be perfectly straight when looking from front to back; however, when looking at the spine from the side, it has three curves: cervical lordosis, thoracic kyphosis and lumbar lordosis. These three curves allow you stand erect without expending much energy.

When spine surgeons want to refer to a specific location in the spine they will often use the terms level and segment. Level is likely the most commonly used term. Level is used loosely to describe a single vertebra or the single disc space between two vertebrae. For example, the third vertebra in the lumbar (low back) spine (L3) will be referred to as the **L3 level**. If surgeons want to talk about the disc space between L3 and L4 they will say the **L3-4 level**.

When surgeons talk about two adjacent vertebrae and the disc space between them, they will frequently talk about that unit as a segment. For example, the unit of the vertebra L3 and vertebra L4, including the disc space between them is called **L3-4 segment**.

When surgeons talk about a 1-level or 2-level fusion or discectomy they are noting how extensive the surgery is. For example, a single level procedure involves a single vertebra;
a 1-level spine surgery involves two adjacent vertebrae; a 2-level vertebrae involves 3 consecutive vertebrae. Even though this sounds confusing, just remember level is used to describe a location in the spine, and can be used interchangeably with segment.

Sometimes segment and level are interchangeable terms, especially when your surgeon is discussing procedures. Just remember that when surgeons use the words level and segment they are talking about one or more vertebrae and

sometimes the discs between them. When in doubt, ask! Next let's discuss the soft tissues.

The Soft Tissues

The spinal column is supported by soft tissue structures that hold the bones together and provide cushioning between them. The three main kinds of soft tissue that support the spinal column's work are the intervertebral discs, the ligaments and muscles.

The intervertebral discs are puck like structures which are situated between every vertebra except the connection between your skull and your spine (C0 and C1) and between C1 and C2. The discs are designed to allow motion between vertebrae as well as act as shock absorbers between the bones. They are composed of a tough outer ring (annulus fibrosis), which allows motion to occur within a certain limit, and a soft gel center (nucleus pulposus), which absorbs the weight of the body. Interestingly, the disc is an avascular structure, meaning it has very little blood supply and thus limited capacity to repair itself—hence why degenerative disc disease occurs. I describe the disc to my patients as a jelly doughnut, an outer casing with a soft jelly center.

There are many ligaments in the spine. Ligaments are tough structures that bind and hold the bones together (think ACL—the Anterior Cruciate Ligament which connects the tibia and the femur at the knee). While there are several ligaments in the spine, the ligamentum flavum (colloquially called the yellow ligament because it is yellow-colored) is perhaps the ligament most frequently involved in spinal problems. This ligament connects the arch of the lamina of one vertebra to the one in the adjacent level.

Muscles: There are an intricate array of muscles which attach to the spine and help hold the bones erect. These principally include the so called "core muscles" which include the long paraspinal muscles which run up and down the back, and the flank and abdominal muscles. I describe these muscles in detail in a later chapter on rehabilitation of the spine. The muscles are important because they not only help the spine move but also help stabilize the spine. Weak muscles cause increased load to be borne by the ligaments and bones which increases wear.

Spinal Cord and Nerves

You can think of the spinal cord as a bundle of electrical wires which conduct signals to and from your brain. The nerves are the individual wires which supply your body's individual parts. The spinal cord starts around C1 in your cervical spine, is attached to the brainstem (in the skull) and ends at the top of your lumbar spine (around L1). At each segment, nerve roots branch off the spinal cord and exit. For example, the L1 nerve roots exits the spinal canal between the L1 and L2 vertebrae on each side (right and left) of your body. When you want to move your big toe your brain transmits this signal down through the spinal cord, then out of the spinal canal via the L5 nerve root which travels down your leg to the muscle which moves your toe. Similarly, when you stub your big toe, the signal is carried up through the L5 nerve root to the spinal cord and into your brain where you experience it as pain. Each nerve root is composed of rootlets which originate on either the dorsal or the ventral surface of the spinal cord, depending on their task. The dorsal rootlets carry sensory information *to* the brain and the ventral rootlets carry motor impulses *from* the brain.

The naming of the nerves corresponds to the naming of the vertebrae but follows an old and somewhat cumbersome system. In the cervical spine the nerve root is named for the vertebra *beneath* where it exits from the spinal canal. For example, the C3 nerve root is so named because it exits *above* the C3 vertebra. Oddly, there is a C8 nerve root that exits at the C7-T1 junction–although there is no C8 vertebra, which has confused many medical students and doctors over the years. However, each nerve root in the lumbar and thoracic spines is named after the vertebra that is *above* where it exits from the spinal canal. So, the L4 nerve root exits *under* the L4 vertebra. Though this information is not critical to understand as a patient, you may find it helpful in discussions about decompression of the spine. Those of you who are curious may be wondering, if the spinal cord ends at L1, then what is in the spinal canal between L1 and S1? The nerves drape down from the spinal cord and hang in this area which we call the cauda equina (horse's tail in Latin).

The spinal cord is more sophisticated and complicated than any computer system known to man and thus it is very sensitive to any kind of damage. Fortunately, it is housed within the protective bony ring of the spinal canal. Moreover, the spinal cord floats in a protective fluid called the **cerebrospinal fluid** (**CSF**—think of the fluid which is drawn during a spinal tap procedure) which is contained by a thin outer membrane called the **dura**. In a normal healthy person, the CSF is perfectly clear and there is about 150 CC total at any given point (about half of a soda can's worth). The CSF is constantly being circulated and reabsorbed back into the blood stream. About 450 cc is produced and circulated through the brain and spinal cord every day. The CSF is produced by the ventricles (hollow parts) in the brain which are essentially large cisterns. The CSF then flows down the spinal canal and reenters the blood stream through small ports called arachnoid granulations.

The Nervous System as a Whole

The nervous system is the electrical system that controls and regulates your body while also feeding back information to the brain. There are a lot of complex parts and the physiology is quite elaborate. To simplify things, we will break it down into two main components: the autonomic and somatic nervous systems. The autonomic nervous system is, well, automatic and controls parts of your body which run on autopilot (such as digestion and your heart). The somatic nervous system is responsible for conscious activities such as movement and sensation.

the autonomic nervous system

The autonomic nervous system is so-called because it is automatic and the organs it supplies nerves to are not under volitional control. You cannot tell your stomach to digest food faster or slower because your stomach, like many of the other visceral organs—heart, lungs, intestines, kidneys, to name a few—are under the control of the autonomic nervous system. The autonomic nervous system is regulated by a series of nerves that create either sympathetic or parasympathetic tone in the body (tone meaning activity). In general, sympathetic tone is created by the release of the neurotransmitter noradrenaline. (A neurotransmitter is a chemical messenger that helps move nerve impulses along nerve cells called neurons.) The neurotransmitter noradrenaline causes your heart rate to increase, your pupils to dilate, your blood pressure to go up because your blood vessels constrict. This is all in preparation for a fight or flight response when you need your body to respond to a threat. In contrast, parasympathetic tone is created by the release of the neurotransmitter acetylcholine which stimulates gastric secretions, salivation, intestinal motility, lowers your heart rate and constricts your pupils. Ever notice that you have a hard time digesting food when you are stressed? This is thanks to overactivity of the sympathetic autonomic nervous system.

The sympathetic system is formed from a chain of nerve clusters (or ganglia) which exit at each spinal level and then flow out into the body in a diffuse pattern. The parasympathetic system is mainly formed from your cranial nerves (nerves which emerge directly from the brain).

the somatic nervous system

Your body produces both conscious and unconscious movement which is extremely precise and well-coordinated. Similarly, your body receives both conscious and unconscious sensory input.

First let's discuss motion. Most of us take the motion of our bodies totally for granted until something in the nervous system goes haywire, causing a disturbance. Conscious movement arises when a thought produced in your cerebral cortex (part of the brain) is transmitted through the brain then down the brainstem and spinal cord, out through a specific nerve which synapses on a muscle which contracts and moves a joint. However, the regulation and processing of movement is extremely more complex than this. It requires a tight coordination between muscle groups to produce smooth motion (when you move your body in one direction certain muscles have to contract, and their opposing muscles must relax). Even the act of holding your hand up requires a tremendous amount of brain processing power to balance the muscles and hold your arm in a single position in space.

Also, some movements are preprogrammed. Notice how you don't need to think about every single muscle contraction to walk in a straight line. But a significant amount of brain and nerve power is devoted to ensuring one step after another is taken in a fluid motion seemingly effortlessly. This happens because sensory neurons that tell your body how tense muscles and ligaments are in your walking legs coordinate with other sensory neurons that let you know where in space those limbs are, and then this and other information is transmitted through your spinal cord into your cerebellum (a sort of mini brain devoted to motion and balance), which helps control precise movement. This entire process is of course governed by your cerebral cortex which wills the motion to occur.

The major motion centers of the nervous system (the basal ganglia, the cerebellum, the prefrontal motor cortex) all have tracts (long columns of neurons) which run down through the spinal cord in an area known as the white matter (called the white matter because it is literally a white tissue). Within the white matter are also connections between tracts (which help facilitate coordination between different limbs of the body (think arms swinging with the legs during running). Within the spinal cord there is also a gray matter which contains interneurons which serve as more connections between neurons. Interneurons help regulate the signals received and transmitted by the white matter.

Sensory input comes in many forms. When most people think of sensation they think about the various textures you can interpret with your skin, or hot and cold. These are all part of the conscious sensory system which is relayed though the spinal cord into the post central gyrus of your cerebral cortex. However, we do not commonly think about unconscious sensory inputs such as how much our muscles are stretching, how much force is being applied to the joints and bones and where limbs are in space. These, too, are sensory input regulated by the spinal cord and transmitted to the brain to help coordinate smooth motion of the limbs.

That's it in a nutshell! Now we can talk about how problems in the spine arise and why it causes pain.

Conclusion

The spine really is a miraculous machine which allows for an upright life. It protects the spinal cord, which powers your entire body from the neck down. It takes years of study to comprehend its function even partially, and this chapter only serves as a starting point. Next, we will start to discuss how things can go wrong in the spine.

Frequently asked Questions

• **What is the difference between lordosis and kyphosis?**

Both are names for normal curvatures in the spine. The cervical and lumbar spines are lordotic meaning they bend backward. An exaggerated example of lordosis would be the person who could paint a low ceiling without having to bend his back more than usual. The thoracic spine is kyphotic which means it bends forward. An exaggerated example of kyphosis would be the little old lady who is so bent over she can pick up a coin from the ground without even having to change how she is standing.

References

1.   Carrino JA, Campbell PD, Lin DC, Morrison WB, Schweitzer ME, Flanders AE, et al. Effect of Spinal Segment Variants on Numbering Vertebral Levels at Lumbar MR Imaging. Radiology. 2011 Apr;259(1):196–202.

2.   Panjabi MM, White AA. Basic biomechanics of the spine. Neurosurgery. 1980 Jul;7(1):76–93.

3.   Rahm MD, Brooks DM, Harris JA, Hart RA, Hughes JL, Ferrick BJ, et al. Stabilizing effect of the rib cage on adjacent segment motion following thoracolumbar posterior fixation of the human thoracic cadaveric spine: A biomechanical study. Clinical Biomechanics. 2019 Dec;70:217–22.

Figures:

The Spine

C1

Cervical Spine (C1-C7)

Cervical lordosis

C7

T1

Thoracic Spine (T1-T12)

Thoracic Kyphosis

T12

L1

Lumbar Spine (L1-L5)

Lumbar Lordosis

L5

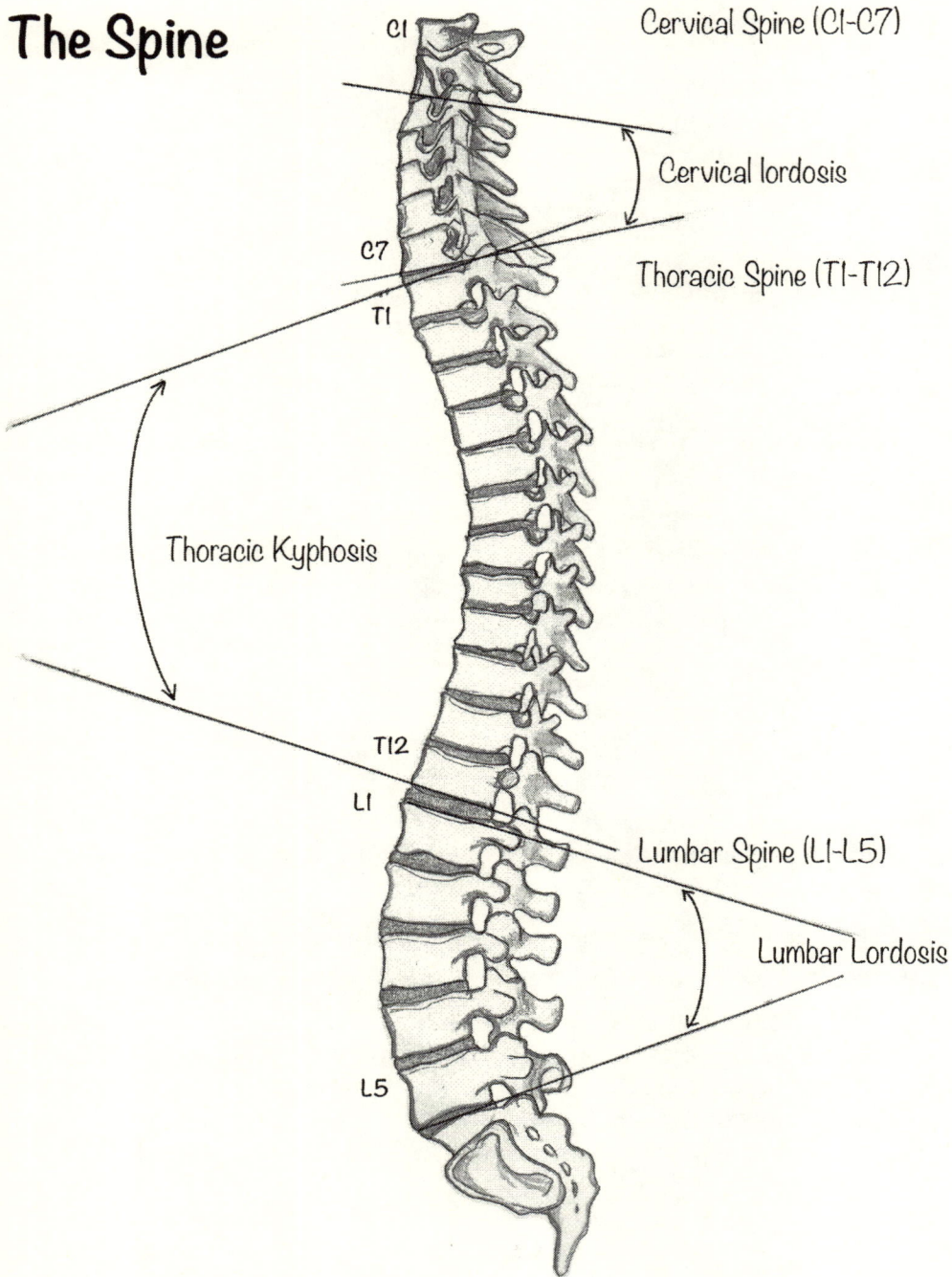

Lateral spine. The spine as viewed from the side (nose and toes would be on your left). There are three main sections: cervical, thoracic and lumbar, each which have a curve. The cervical and lumbar spines have lordotic curvatures meaning they bend backward, whereas the thoracic spine has a kyphotic curvature meaning it bends forward. There are 7 cervical, 12 lumbar and 5 lumbar vertebrae.

The Lumbar Spine (Viewed from the Back)

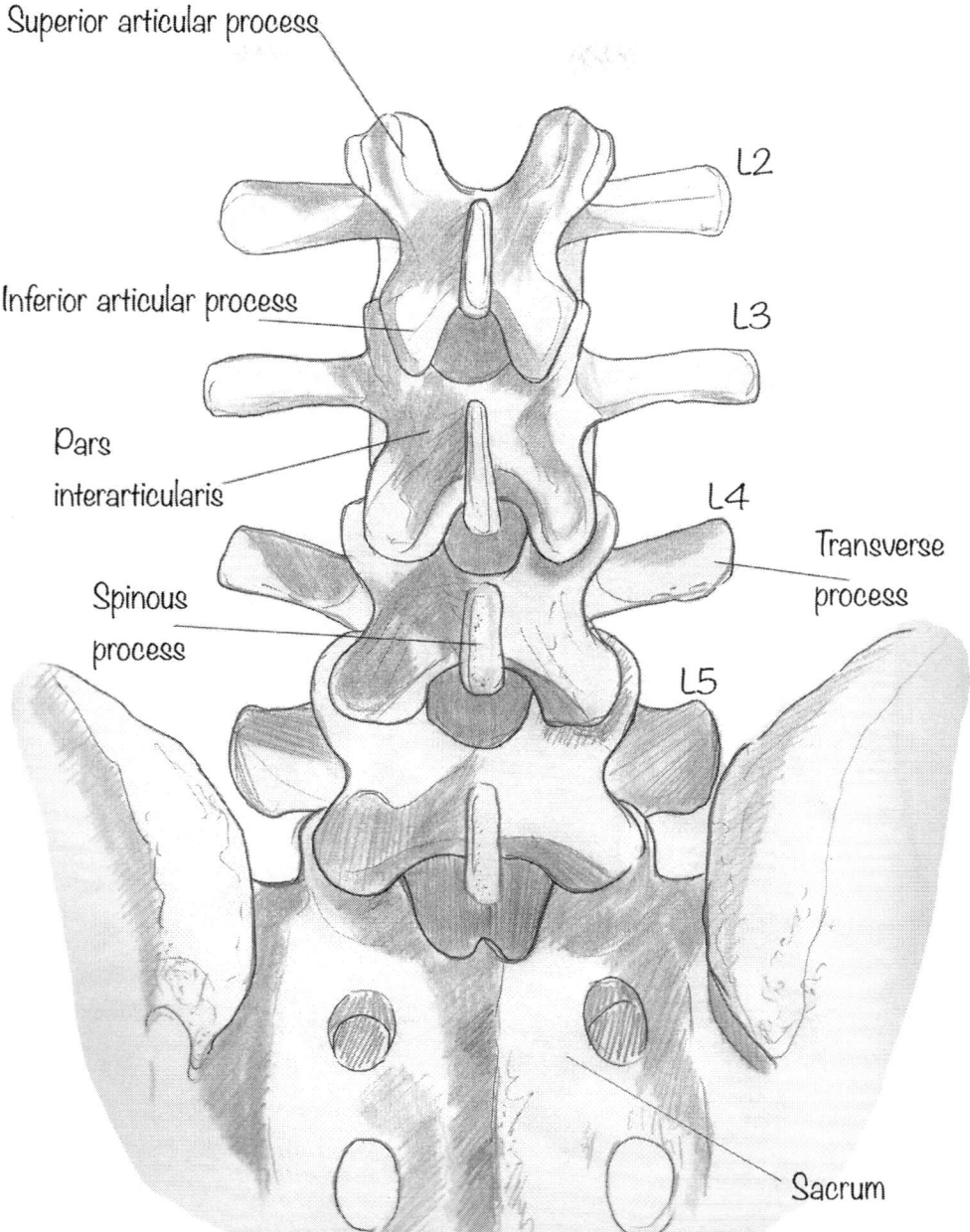

Superior articular process

Inferior articular process

Pars interarticularis

Spinous process

L2

L3

L4

Transverse process

L5

Sacrum

Posterior lumbar spine. Here four lumbar vertebrae are connected to the sacrum and the pelvis at the bottom of the figure. The vertebrae are interlocked by the facet joints that are composed of the superior articular processes and the inferior articular processes—bony protuberances that arise from the lamina on both sides. The pars interarticularis is the designation for the part (pars means "part" in latin) of the lamina that joins the superior and inferior articular process (hence: inter-articularis). Damage to the pars interarticulars can result in spondylolisthesis, which is discussed more in the upcoming chapters. The transverse processes stick out from the sides of the vertebrae and the spinous processes stick out from the backside.

The Cervical Vertebra

Posterior view:

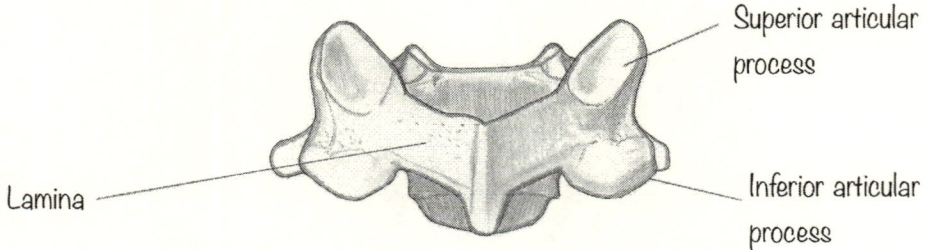

Superior articular process

Lamina

Inferior articular process

Lateral view:

Vertebral body

Lateral mass

Spinous process

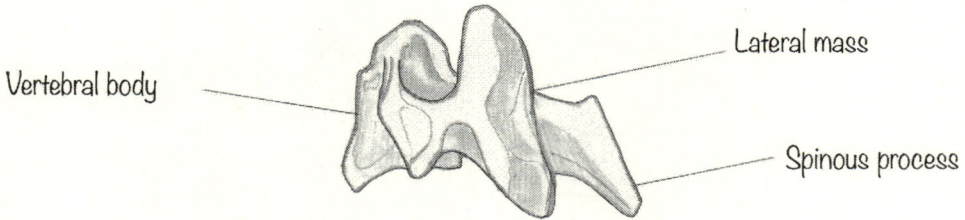

Anterior view:

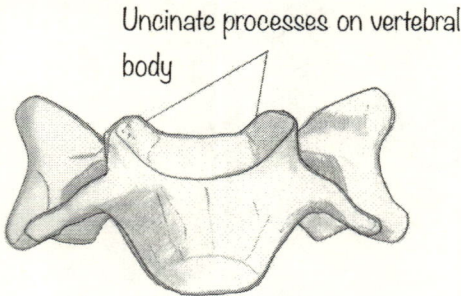

Uncinate processes on vertebral body

Superior view:

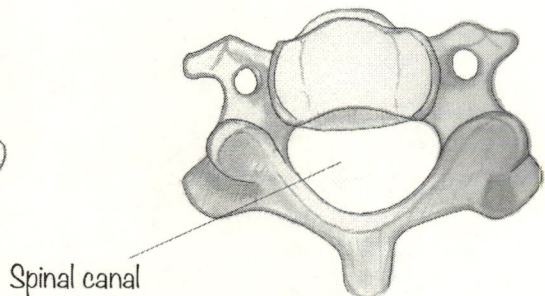

Spinal canal

Cervical vertebrae. All cervical vertebrae are slightly different, however C3 through C7 all have similar features and are known as the subaxial cervical vertebrae (because they are below the axis or C2). All have a vertebral body that is in the front connected to a lamina in the back. Cervical vertebrae have articular processes similar to the lumbar vertebrae, but they are attached to a piece of bone known as the lateral mass. Here a subaxial vertebrae is viewed from multiple directions.

The Motor System

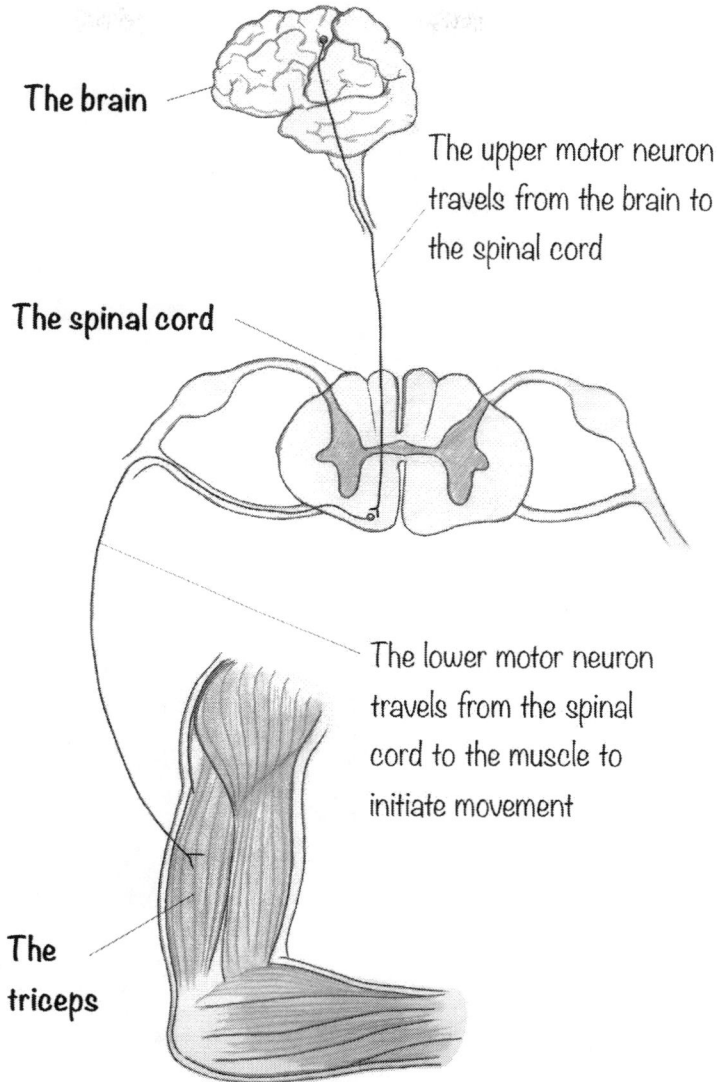

The brain

The upper motor neuron
travels from the brain to
the spinal cord

The spinal cord

The lower motor neuron
travels from the spinal
cord to the muscle to
initiate movement

The
triceps

The motor unit. The motor nervous system is responsible for motion and conscious muscular contraction. While the real motor system is quite complex, the essential parts can be broken down into a two-neuron schematic. The first neuron arises in the premotor cortex of the brain and travels down into the spinal cord where it connects (synapses) with a second motor neuron which travels out from the spinal cord into the body to innervate a muscle.

The Lumbar Facet Joints

Facet joints allow motion of the vertebrae

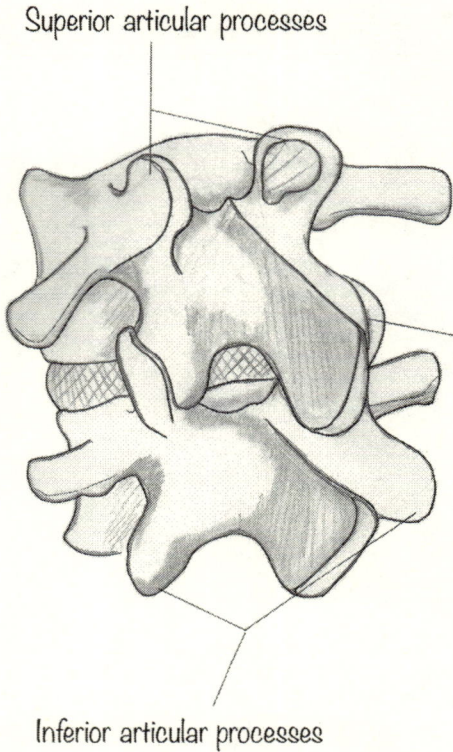

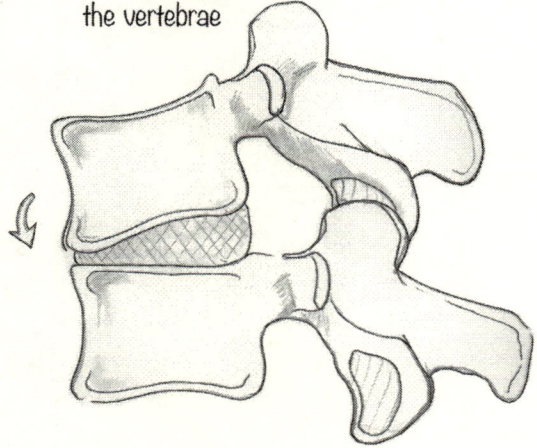

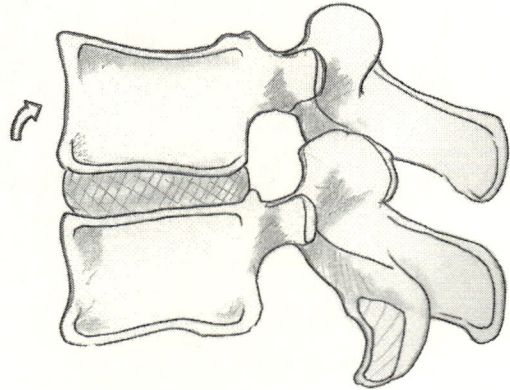

Superior articular processes

Facet joint

Inferior articular processes

lumbar facets. The facet joints allow motion between vertebrae in one direction while limiting it in others. In the lumbar spine the facets allow the vertebrae to angulate forward and backward but also twist to some degree.

C1 and C2: The Atlas and Axis

C1/Atlas

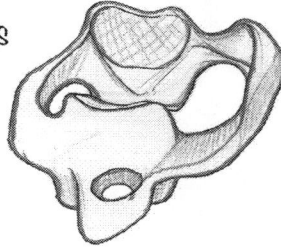

C2/Axis

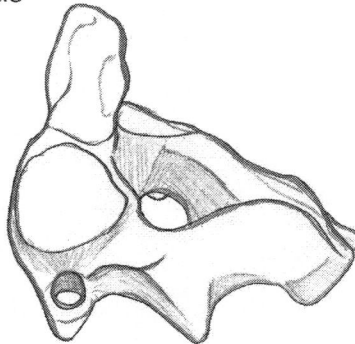

Atlantoaxis: C1 and C2 together

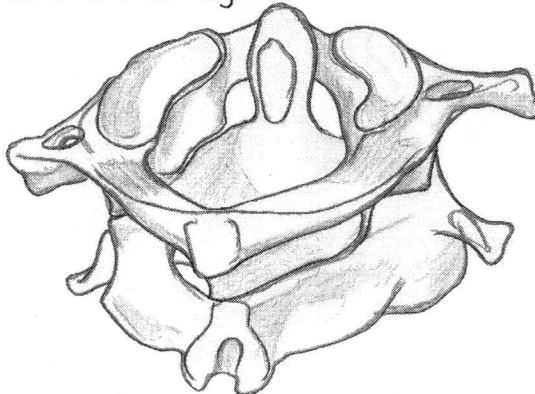

The Atlas and Axis. The atlas and axis are unique vertebra in the spine. Together they give the neck its rotatory function, allowing you to look from side to side. This is accomplished by the geometry of the axis C1 vertebra which rotates on the peg of the axis or C2.

The Brain and Spinal Cord

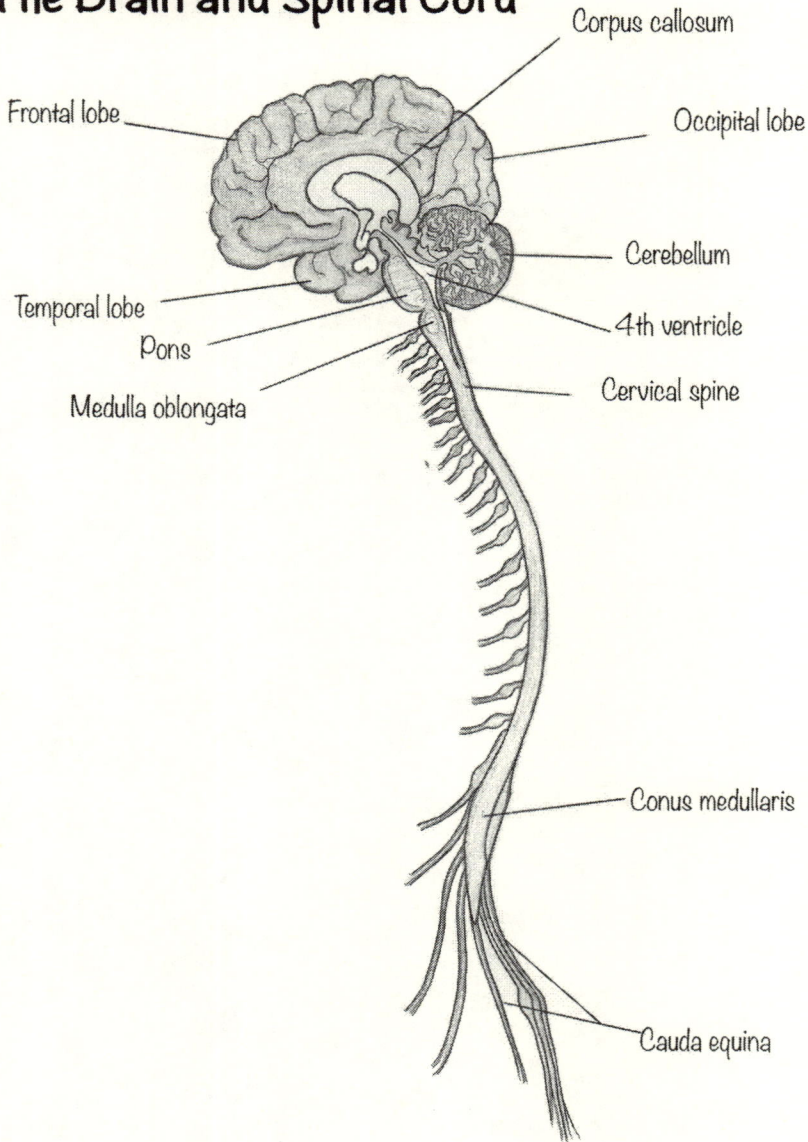

Corpus callosum

Frontal lobe

Occipital lobe

Cerebellum

Temporal lobe

4th ventricle

Pons

Cervical spine

Medulla oblongata

Conus medullaris

Cauda equina

The brain and spinal cord. The brain's cerebral cortex consists of four main lobes, the frontal, temporal, occipital and parietal, which are responsible for most executive cognitive function (thinking). Beneath the cerebral cortex are the more primitive processing centers known as the cerebellum and the brainstem (midbrain, pons, and medulla oblongata) which are attached to the spinal cord. Nerve roots branch off from the spinal cord at each segment. The spinal cord ends around L1 as the conus medullaris and the nerve roots beyond that form the cauda equina and lie in the spinal canal. These nerve roots also each exit at a specific segment.

The Cervical Spine (viewed from the side)

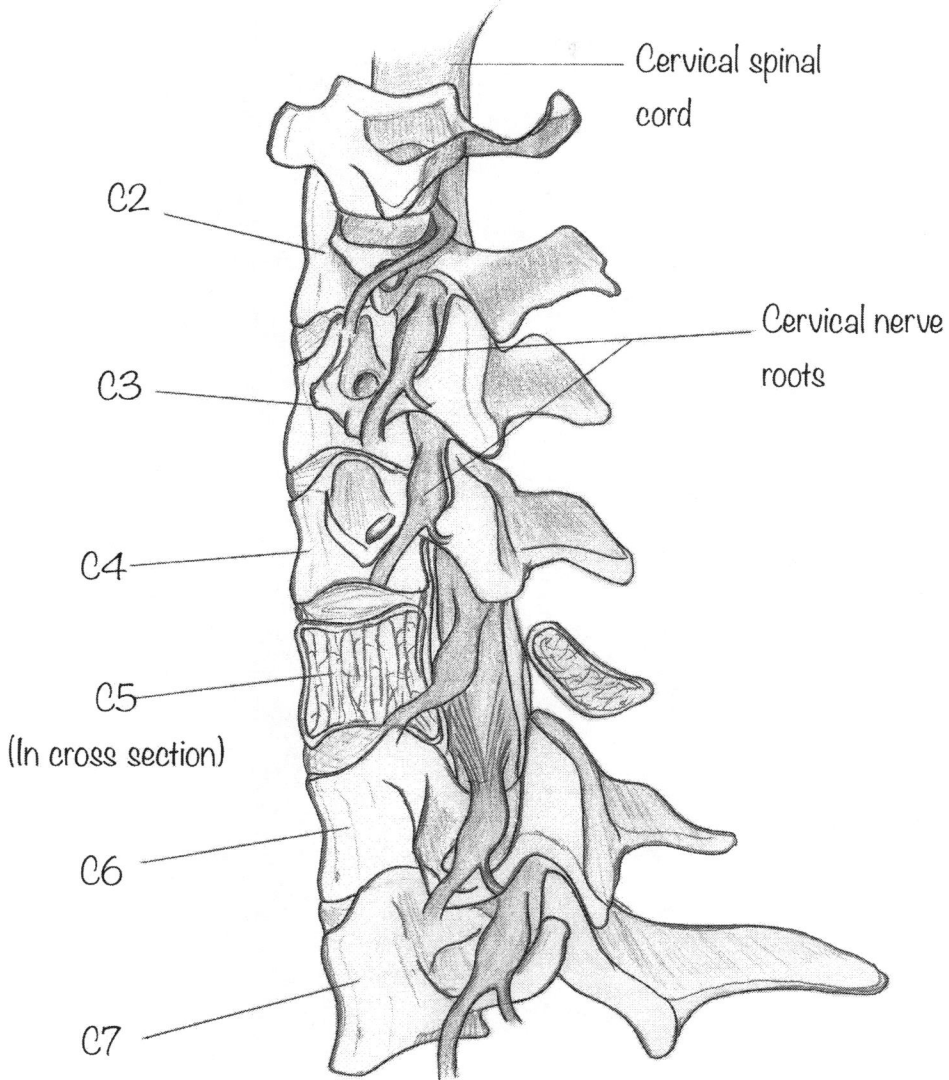

Cervical spinal cord

C2

Cervical nerve roots

C3

C4

C5

(In cross section)

C6

C7

Cervical spine lateral. The cervical spine as viewed from the side shows how nerve roots exit through the cervical foramen (opening in a bone). The spinal cord courses through the center of the spinal canal (visible in the cross section of C5).

Cross Section of the Lumbar Spine:

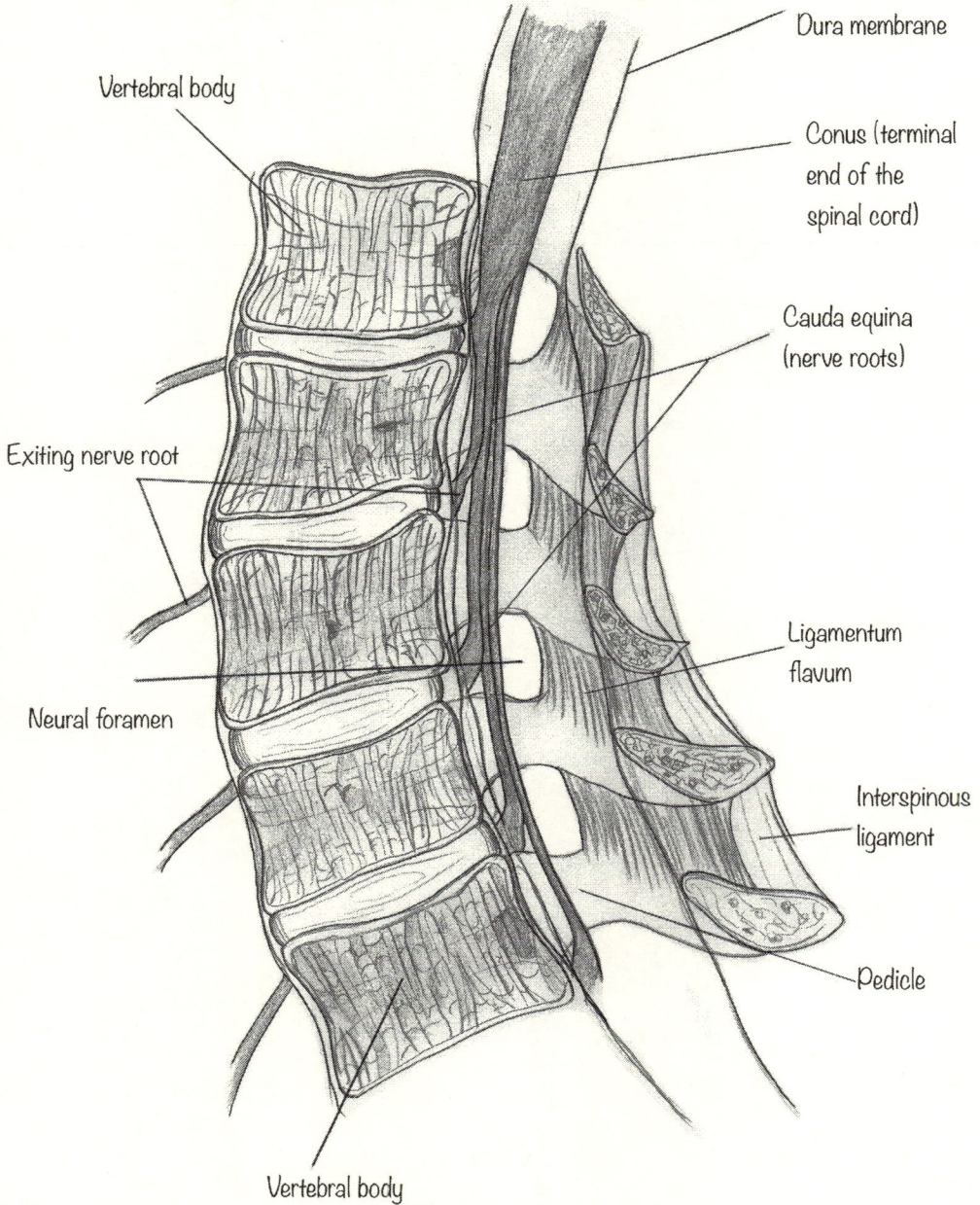

Vertebral body

Dura membrane

Conus (terminal end of the spinal cord)

Cauda equina (nerve roots)

Exiting nerve root

Ligamentum flavum

Neural foramen

Interspinous ligament

Pedicle

Vertebral body

Cross section of the Lumbar spine. In this cross section we can see how the lumbar spine differs from the cervical and thoracic spine as there is no spinal cord in the spinal canal, just nerve roots. These exit through the lumbar foramen (openings) beneath each pedicle.

The Sacrum and Pelvis

Sacrum

L5

Ilium (innominate bone)

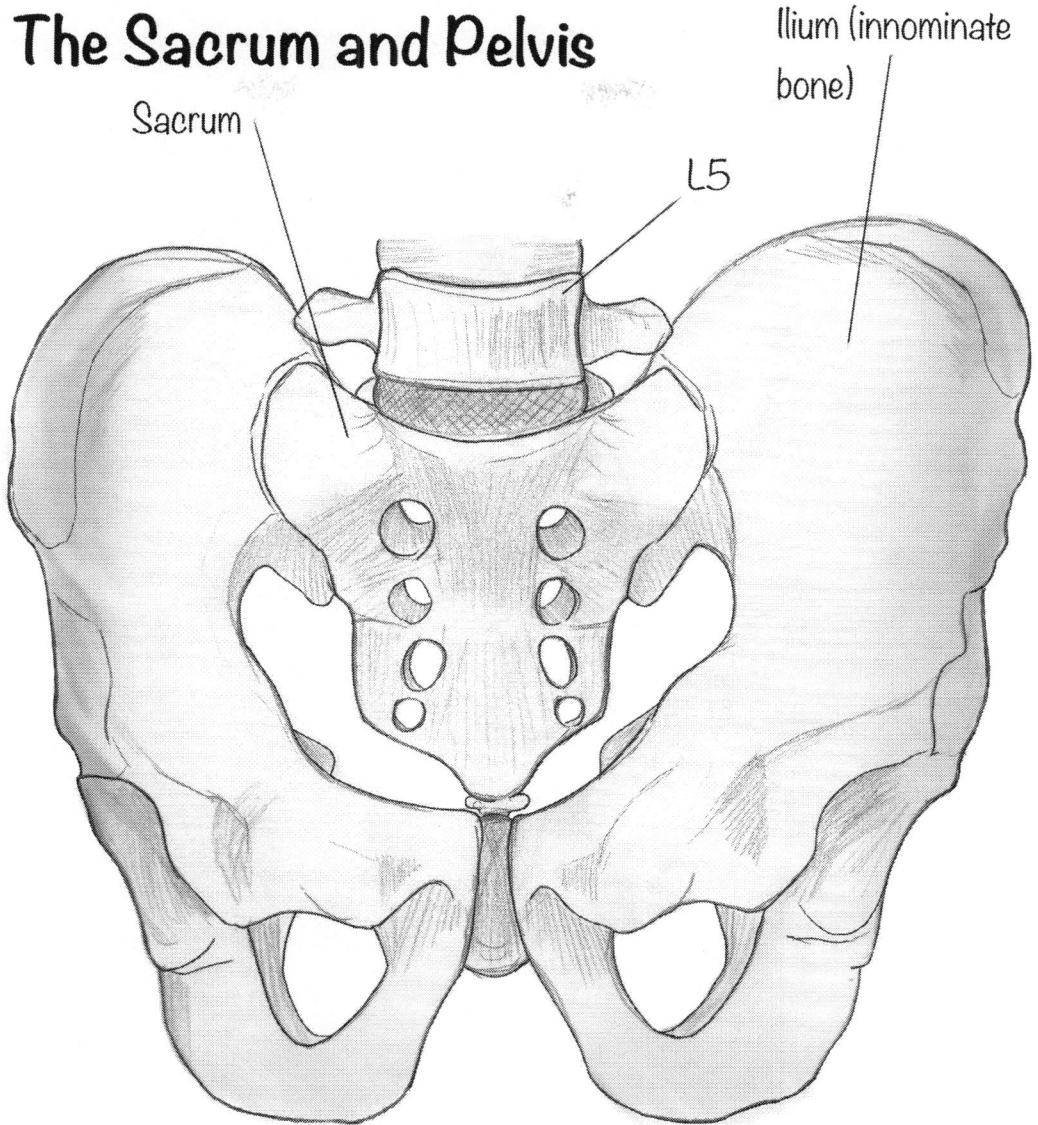

Sacrum and pelvis. The sacrum and pelvis as viewed from the front. The pelvis is made up of three large bones, the sacrum, and two iliac bones. Together they make a very rigid bony ring and serve as the base on which the spine sits.

Spinal Cord (Cross Section)

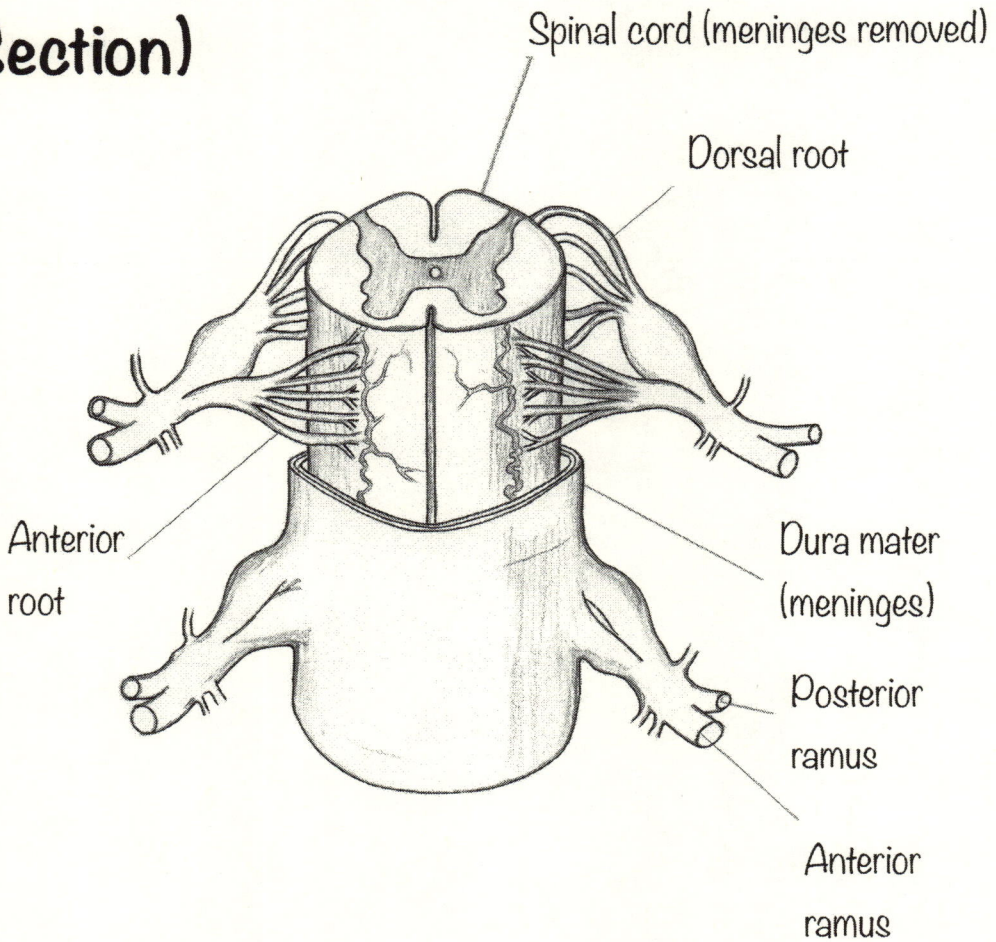

Spinal cord (meninges removed)

Dorsal root

Anterior root

Dura mater (meninges)

Posterior ramus

Anterior ramus

Spinal cord. A segment of the spinal cord viewed from the front in cross section. The nerve rootlets come off the dorsal and ventral portions of the spinal cord to form a nerve root which again branches to form the anterior and posterior rami. The spinal cord is covered by a protective triple layered membrane known as the dura mater.

Spinal Segmental Unit: 2 Vertebra and a Disc

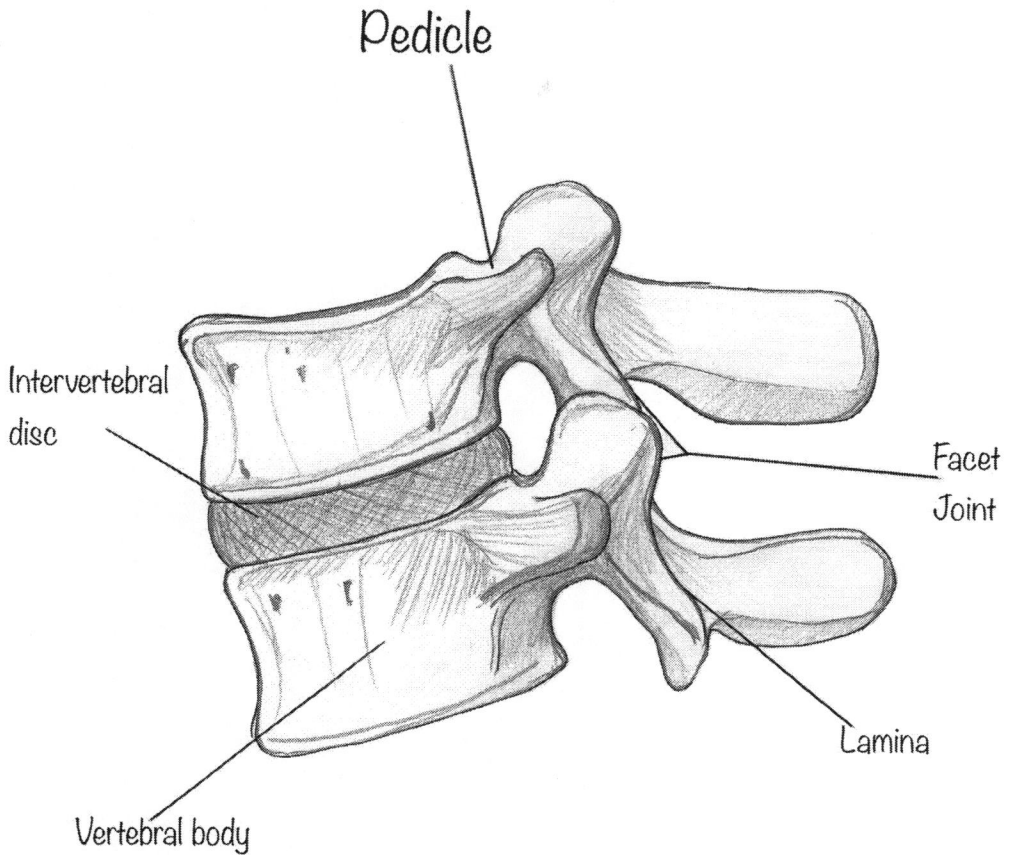

Pedicle

Intervertebral disc

Facet Joint

Lamina

Vertebral body

Spinal segmental unit. A functional unit of the lumbar spine viewed from side. The functional unit consists of two vertebrae separated by an intervertebral disc.

Chapter 2

What Causes Pain In the Spine

Summary

The sensation of pain is transmitted through long cells called neurons which function as the electrical wires of the body. Neurons are connected by synapses which serve as gateways where pain transmission can be modulated by the brain or pain medicines. The gate control theory of pain is an important concept in analgesia (pain relief) because pain can be modulated at the interconnections between neurons. How you interpret pain is dependent not just on the stimulus causing the pain but also on your mood, personality, and stress level. Past experiences of pain can sensitize you to (cause you to experience more easily) increasing pain in the future. Spine pain comes primarily in two forms: radicular pain (transmitted by a nerve) and mechanical pain experienced by the spinal joint/bone/muscle. Radicular pain describes pain which shoots down the arm or leg and originates from the spine. Radicular pain that affects the leg is commonly known as sciatica. Mechanical pain typically occurs localized in the back and in general is more common.

Case

Mr. Yellow is a 42-year-old construction worker. One day he lifts a heavy object at work and notices a "pop" in his back that causes excruciating low back and right leg pain. The pain seems to be traveling down his leg as if going down an electrical wire. He tries to rest, but the pain seems to just get worse. He is confused because there are no tender spots on his leg or back, but it seems like the pain is deep inside his body, yet still spreads to the surface. With any movement the pain sears down his leg. Pain pills won't touch the pain. He stops going to work and stays at home drinking alcohol to try and dull his nerves, but becomes depressed, only making the pain more intense. The confusion and uncertainty cause anxiety which makes the pain seem worse. He seeks treatment from his primary care physician and after a discussion feels he has a better idea of what is going on. Some basic treatments like nonsteroidal anti-inflammatories and physical therapy are prescribed, and in a few weeks, he is feeling much better.

Introduction to Pain

To understand pain, we must first describe the functional unit of the nervous system, the neuron. **The neuron is a very long cell that**, like a wire, **is able to convey an electrical signal**. On one end of the neuron are receptors, which are responsible for sensing a stimulus, and on the other end there is a synapse that allows the neurons to communicate with other neurons via chemical (neurotransmitter) release. **Nerves are composed of many of these neurons wrapped together and are responsible for carrying information to (afferent signal) and from (efferent signal) your brain.** Pain neurons generally have a small diameter (which decreases the transmission speed) compared to larger neurons (which is why there is a delay from when you get injured to when you experience pain). There are two types of pain sensing neurons: unmyelinated and myelinated (myelin is a coating that increases the speed at which nerves conduct). Unmyelinated neurons are responsible for sensing dull pain and myelinated neurons convey sharp pain (1).

While the science of spine pain transmission is complicated, it can be summarized in the following fashion: something irritates the nerve endings somewhere in your body (somatic pain) or irritates the nerves/nerve roots themselves (neuropathic pain) which then transmit an electrical signal through the spinal cord to the brain that is interpreted as pain. The irritating stimulus is typically either chemical (inflammation), extreme temperature (greater than 42°C or 107.6° F), or mechanical (something which exerts pressure, such as bony instability in the spine) or both (mechanical instability which causes inflammation).

The irritating stimulus sets off a response in small sensory neurons that is transmitted to the brain in the following fashion: Small neurons have chemical, pressure and temperature sensing receptors which are able to detect the irritating stimulus. These neurons course from the periphery (outside the spinal cord and brain) and convey the signal into the spinal cord via an area called the dorsal horn and from there connect with neurons which ascend the spinal cord and connect with a third set of neurons that then run to the brain. The pain (sense of danger) is transmitted up to the brain through the spinal cord where a neural map encodes the sensation of your entire body. Thus, the stimulus triggers your neural matrix (between the brain's thalamus, and its cortex), which evaluates input from all parts of your brain—including past experiences—to recognize pain in a specific area in the body. Between neurons are synapses or "gates" that can either turn up or turn down the transmission of pain into the brain. This is critical because at these gates the processing of pain can be modulated, which is the central theory of the gate control theory of pain.

The gate control theory, a popular theory about how pain is transmitted through the human body, states that the transmission of neural impulses can be amplified or silenced by special cells located in the dorsal horn (2). While the biology behind the gate control theory is somewhat complicated it is like the volume control on a CD player. There is a signal coming from the CD and if you turn the volume knob up, it makes the sound louder. The dorsal horn is a kind of relay station at every level of the spinal cord where this volume adjustment happens. How much modulation occurs here depends on how much transmission occurs through large fiber neurons and small fiber neurons. Large fibers that are responsible for transmission of signals other than pain, such as where your limb is in space, thus can decrease pain sensation at the gate. Moreover, descending nerves (efferents) can modulate the signal—thus it is theoretically possible to directly suppress or <u>increase</u> pain, based on your thoughts. This explains why some people may be more resistant to pain and others more sensitive to pain, depending on their personalities, mood, stress levels and past experiences/exposure to pain.

However, the concept of pain is not completely explained by the gate control theory. It is possible, for example, for paraplegics with complete transection (cutting across) of the spinal cord to experience severe phantom pain in the limbs (2). This happens because the brain can produce pain without a stimulus. This occurs when the area of the neural matrix in your brain that encodes pain, activates independently of stimulus. Longstanding pain or damage to a nerve structure can cause this to occur. The brain will adapt to this new "normal" by adapting its structure and assessment of the ongoing situation in a process called plasticity. **When a pain stimulus goes on for too long this can result in a feedback loop in the neural matrix of the central nervous system that can result in a chronic pain syndrome. That is, even if the noxious stimulus is removed, the brain continues to interpret the situation as dangerous and creates the sensation of pain.** In some other rare cases, in the presence of nerve damage, a second set of nerves that are responsible

for autonomic or involuntary function of your body (sweating, heart beating)—
nerves regulated by the autonomic nervous system—can try to repair the damaged
nerves, resulting in an interconnection between your motor and sensory nerves and
your autonomic nerves. This results in a syndrome known as complex regional pain
syndrome (CRPS).

To summarize: a pain stimulus (touching something sharp) is picked up by a neuron
that transmits the signal up the brain through the spinal cord. There is a volume knob
in the spinal cord that can either silence or amplify this signal. If there is damage
to the nerve, or the pain is continuous over a long period of time, the nerves in the
brain can become sensitized and continue to experience pain even in the absence of a
painful stimulus.

**Pain experienced in the back or spine is generally either radicular (pain
resulting from the compression or irritation of a nerve root), or mechanical
(pain from damage to the bones/ligaments of the spine itself).**

Radicular Pain

Radicular pain is pain related to an irritation of an individual nerve root and
thus can be experienced along the entire tract of the nerve root. When a nerve root
becomes pinched or inflamed radicular pain occurs. **Sciatica and radicular pain are
terms which are used interchangeably to explain pain in the legs.**

So how does this happen? Generally, this occurs when a nerve is pinched, or
inflamed. This is by far and away the most common cause of radicular pain. When
the spine wears out it tends to collapse causing the already small tunnels where
nerves travel to narrow. This can pinch or irritate the nerves resulting in radicular
pain or radiculopathy. Because your nerves are the wires responsible for conveying
information from the legs and arms back to the spine, when they are pinched it
can feel as though the pain is shooting down the whole extremity. **So even if the
problem is just in the spine, it can be experienced throughout the limb.** To
better understand how radicular pain occurs in the spine we must understand a little
about how the spine works and degenerates (wears out).

**The spine is an amazing machine, but just like any other machine, it
experiences wear and tear over time**. As you age the vertebrae in your body
become weaker from osteoporosis and can collapse (think of the wooden foundation
of a house slowly rotting, causing the house to sink). The intervertebral discs lose
their spongy centers and dry out, which causes them to collapse, shrink, tear and
rupture (think of the shocks on a car wearing down after a life on bumpy roads).
Eventually the disc disintegrates, and you are left with one vertebra rubbing on the
other or bone-on-bone contact. Over time the facet joints that connect two vertebrae

become arthritic and can wear out as well. It sounds scary, but degeneration of the spine is very common and, unfortunately, is part of the normal aging process for everyone (3).

Keep in mind bones are living structures and react to the forces that are exerted on them. Bones strengthen in reaction to moderate forces and tend to atrophy (waste away) and weaken if not used (think astronauts in space). Bones respond to external forces through their internal architecture, which is filled with pressure-sensing cells (discussed in the chapter on osteoporosis) and through the lining of the bone known as the periosteum (a soft covering layer that nourishes the bone). The periosteum is what allows the bone to heal if fractured. In cases of abnormal forces across the bone, the periosteum is stimulated to build more bone. Thus, when there is a problem with the joint, a bone will attempt to stabilize itself to redistribute forces in a more natural fashion. In spinal degeneration when the cartilage and discs of the spine wear out, bone-on-bone contact occurs, which causes the formation of bone spurs (or **osteophytes**) in an attempt to stabilize the vertebral levels via the periosteum.

Osteophytes tend to lock bones in place and increase the surface area over which forces are distributed—this is the body's natural way of stabilizing degenerative problems. However, the spine is a fine-tuned machine that is tasked with protecting and stabilizing the nerves and the spinal cord. There is little to no room for extra bone. Because of this, **in some people, when degeneration occurs it can result in the most common spine problem spine surgeons treat: stenosis**.

Stenosis means the narrowing of a passage. **Spinal stenosis simply means the space for the spinal cord and nerve roots has become constricted (imagine a clogged pipe, or a water hose that someone is stepping on).** In the Framingham Heart Study, the prevalence of anatomic lumbar spinal stenosis was as high as 47% in patients greater than 60 years of age (4). Moreover, the amount of spinal fusion surgeries performed for this reason increased from 122,697 cases in 2004 to almost 200,000 cases in 2015 in the United States (5).

One cause of stenosis is discs collapsing and bulging into the spinal canal and pinching the nerve roots or spinal cord. As the discs collapse the ligamentum flavum (the ligament which connects one vertebral lamina to the next) buckles inward, worsening the stenosis.

As degeneration progresses, the facets also wear out and instead of having a smooth ball-bearing surface, their surfaces become jagged and sloppy. This in turn allows one vertebra to shift onto another, resulting in **spondylolisthesis** (a fancy word for a slipped vertebra or slipped disc)(6). There are other causes of spondylolisthesis including tumor, infection, and stress fractures in the bone connecting the facets, called the pars. Regardless of cause, a slipped vertebra causes the stenosis to become even worse!

To understand spondylolisthesis, you must understand **spinal instability. The spine has a normal amount of motion between vertebrae, but when there is an excessive or** abnormal amount of motion between vertebrae it is called instability. Spinal instability occurs as the joints become slack, for example, as a result of the joints wearing out. As the degenerative process continues, the space available in the spinal canal for the nerve root and spinal cord decreases, the protective layer of cerebrospinal fluid (CSF) gets displaced and there is nothing stopping the discs and ligaments from directly pressing on these sensitive structures. Nerves do not like getting pinched and it is extremely painful when it occurs—generating radicular pain.

Damaged discs cause pain in other ways besides stenosis. You might have heard the term "slipped disc" before, which is not a very accurate term since it is used to cover many different problems. As stated in chapter 1, the disc contains two main parts, a tough outer ring (the annulus fibrosis), and an inner core (nucleus pulposus), which is jelly-like. Problems with the disc can range from a bulge in the annulus (a focal weak point in the ring) commonly known as a bulging disc (similar in concept to an abdominal hernia), to a small tear in the annulus, to a tear with extrusion (the pushing out) of disc nucleus to outside of the ring. Each of these conditions can potentially cause back pain as the disc and surrounding ligaments are all supplied by nerves capable of sensing pain. However, these conditions may also be completely asymptomatic (causing no pain). The main problem typically occurs when the damaged disc or surrounding bone causes compression of a nerve, causing radicular pain.

When a disc ruptures sometimes the jelly material in the center is herniated (protrudes) outside of the casing and can also pinch nerves—this is called an acute **disc herniation**. There are several subclassifying terms that physicians use to describe disc herniations. An extrusion occurs when the disc material has escaped out of the annular ring and is free in the spinal canal. This fragment may then become sequestered (isolated) if it completely disconnected from its disc of origin and lodges somewhere in the spinal canal.

When a disc herniation first occurs there is often a huge inflammatory reaction that also is very irritating to nerves. Inflammation or pressure on a nerve result in a condition known as **sciatica** or **radiculopathy** or simply **"nerve pain" as described above. When a nerve in your cervical spine or lumbar spine is pinched and inflamed, it gives the sensation of pain traveling down your arm or leg, respectively, in addition to local neck or low back pain.** For example, when the L5 nerve is pinched, you experience the pain traveling down the entire leg starting in the hip and typically down into the foot. It also causes local back pain. Everyone experiences this pain a little differently depending on how your body is wired and which nerve root is pinched. The spine unfortunately has certain weak spots which are inherently more prone to disc herniations. These are the L4-5 and L5-S1 discs in the lumbar (low back) spine and the C4-5, C5-6, and C6-7 discs in the cervical (neck) spine, which are the areas of the spine with a high degree of motion. As the thoracic (upper back) spine is very rigid it rarely has symptomatic disc herniations. Some disc herniations may be so catastrophic as to block off the entire lumbar spinal canal and choke off all the descending nerves resulting in a syndrome known as **cauda equina syndrome**. In this case there is profound weakness in the legs, bowel and bladder incontinence, as well as numbness of the groin. It is a medical emergency.

As discussed, radicular pain is typically perceived as originating from the back or neck and traveling to the extremities. However, compression of the nerve itself can result in localized pain. This is because the nerves themselves have mini nerves contained within the nerve itself called *nervi nervorum* which transmit pain locally.

One important concept to keep in mind is that radiculopathy is caused by compression of the nerves, not of the spinal cord. Compression of the spinal cord is much more serious and results in a syndrome known as myelopathy (discussed in a later chapter). Nerves branch off the spinal cord like exit off-ramps on a highway. So, when a nerve is compressed as it exits the spinal cord this is totally different from spinal cord compression.

Mechanical Pain

Mechanical pain refers to the pain experienced by a bone or joint when there is force or motion involved across a damaged or injured area. This is distinct from radicular pain which originates from the nerve. Mechanical pain occurs when there is something wrong in the bone or joint itself and can occur without nerve compression.

Back Pain

Spine pain can be broadly categorized as neck pain or upper or lower back pain. Upper back pain occurs in the thoracic spine and in general is more serious than low back pain. This is because the rib cage stabilizes the upper back making it more rigid and thus less prone to wear. Upper back pain should raise concern for problems involving the internal organs (aortic aneurysm, pancreatic disease, gastric ulcers which have ruptured, etc.). These problems typically present with other significant symptoms and signs, but back pain is often the presenting problem (the problem that gets you to go to the doctor). Other serious causes of spine pain must also be ruled out such as tumors, fractures, and infections.

Thankfully these serious conditions are very rare compared to the high incidence of simple low back pain. As discussed above, low back pain can result from nerve compression; however, there are a multitude of both serious and benign (not dangerous) causes which can often make the diagnosis difficult. In fact, low back pain is an extremely common problem with up to 70% of people experiencing it at some point in their lives (7). Theoretically it can originate from any of the diverse anatomic structures of the spine, including the intervertebral discs, the facet joints, the spinal ligaments, and the muscles around the spine (8).

While this list is not exhaustive, here are **some serious causes of low back pain** (things you should see a spine surgeon for):

- **Disc herniations**

- **Fractures**

- **Infection**

- **Tumor**

- **Spinal canal stenosis**

- **Spondylolisthesis/Spinal instability**

- **Visceral disease mimicking a spinal problem (such as an aortic aneurysm)**

Luckily these things are rare, and account for only 1% of total cases of back pain that lead to an appointment with a primary care physician (9). Most causes of low back pain are benign and much more common (10). Unfortunately, these remaining causes get categorized as "non-specific" or "idiopathic" (what we call a disease with no identifiable cause) because it is difficult to attribute a single source to the pain or make a conclusive diagnosis (8).

Here is a list of **the most common nonspecific causes of back pain**:

- **Degenerative disc disease of the spine (general wear and tear) that does not cause stenosis**

- **Facet degeneration, or capsular strain**

- **Sprains (injury to the ligament—the tough tissue connecting bones to each other)**

- **Strains (injury to muscles or the tendons that connect them to bones)**

You can see it is critical to work together with your physician to determine the cause. He/she will likely ask you specific questions to help rule out serious causes of back pain and perform an examination. Diagnostic tests such as X-rays, and MRI scans (more on this in chapter 4) may also be performed if appropriate.

Neck Pain

Your neck is supported by a series of muscular struts and allows a wide range of motion through a complex system of joints. Like any sophisticated machine, it is prone to damage if it becomes out of alignment. There are many small muscles in the neck which allow precise control of motion, however, if torn, can result in chronic neck pain. Moreover, the facet joints and joint capsules (the tissue which encapsulates or encloses the joint) may be torn which can also result in pain in the back of your neck or shoulder blades. Finally, compression of the nerves of the neck can result in headache, particularly when the C2 nerve root is compressed, which results in a characteristic pain in the back of your head. Neck pain is also very common, and I discuss it in its own chapter.

Why Did This Happen to Me?

Spinal disease has many causes and specific risk factors for each condition differ. However, for general degenerative disease of the spine the cause seems to be an interplay between genetics and environment. As stated above, almost everyone experiences degeneration to some degree over the course of a lifetime. However, some develop degeneration much earlier in life and there have been numerous genetic causes which are suspected to play a role (11–13). Moreover, the incidence of early degeneration is much higher in those with a family history of back problems and a person's hereditary predisposition seems to play a dominant role in early degeneration (14–16). Surprisingly physical loading and heavy lifting have not been shown to be significantly associated with early disc degeneration (16). Other causes such as smoking, obesity, diabetes have been implicated in early disc degeneration.

Conclusion

So, if that was a lot to digest, its ok. The spine is an incredibly complex organ system and, unfortunately, has a lot of different ways to cause pain and suffering. **The take home message from this chapter should be the following:**

- **Pain is transmitted to the spinal cord and brain from nerves which branch off the spinal cord and travel into the body. Nerves are the electrical wires of the body that convey information to and from the brain.**

- **Nerves can be stimulated to transmit pain signals if there is tissue damage which they are excellent at sensing, or if they themselves are damaged or compressed.**

- **The two main types of spine pain are from nerve compression (radicular pain) that results in pain shooting down the arm or leg. Mechanical pain occurs from physical damage to the spine itself (that is the bones, muscles or ligaments).**

- **Low back pain is very common and usually benign. There are many different potential causes.**

- **Because there is so much complexity, it's hard to "diagnose yourself." Really, if you are experiencing a problem in the spine, you should seek the advice of a spine surgeon or doctor who specializes in the musculoskeletal system.**

Frequently Asked Questions

- ### Could my buttocks pain be coming from my hip?

The short answer is yes. Distinguishing the difference between pain originating from the spine and pain originating from another source is at times very complicated. Your surgeon will help you make distinctions.

- ### What is sciatica?

Sciatica refers to pain that travels along the sciatic nerve and is experienced as pain shooting down the leg. Another term physicians use when discussing this nerve condition is radiculopathy or radiculitis. This results from nerve compression which occurs typically in the lumbar spine but the resulting pain is "referred" to the areas that are innervated by the sciatic nerve.

References

1.   Kandel, eric. Principles of Neuroscience. In Mcgraw-Hill Medical; 2013.

2.   Melzack R, Katz J. The gate control theory: Reaching for the brain. Pain Psychol Perspect. 2004;13–34.

3.   Boden SD, McCowin PR, Davis DO, Dina TS, Mark AS, Wiesel S. Abnormal magnetic-resonance scans of the cervical spine in asymptomatic subjects. A prospective investigation. J Bone Jt Surg. 1990;72(8):1178–84.

4.   Kalichman L, Cole R, Kim DH, Li L, Suri P, Guermazi A, et al. Spinal stenosis prevalence and association with symptoms: the Framingham Study. Spine J. 2009 Jul;9(7):545–50.

5.   Martin BI, Mirza SK, Comstock BA, Gray DT, Kreuter W, Deyo RA. Are Lumbar Spine Reoperation Rates Falling With Greater Use of Fusion Surgery and New Surgical Technology?: Spine. 2007 Sep;32(19):2119–26.

6.   Kirkaldy-Willis WH, Wedge JH, Yong-Hing K, Reilly J. Pathology and pathogenesis of lumbar spondylosis and stenosis. Spine. 1978 Dec;3(4):319–28.

7.   Papageorgiou AC, Croft PR, Ferry S, Jayson MI, Silman AJ. Estimating the prevalence of low back pain in the general population. Evidence from the South Manchester Back Pain Survey. Spine. 1995 Sep 1;20(17):1889–94.

8.   Deyo RA, Weinstein JN. Low back pain. N Engl J Med. 2001 Feb 1;344(5):363–70.

9.   Henschke N, Maher CG, Refshauge KM, Herbert RD, Cumming RG, Bleasel J, et al. Prevalence of and screening for serious spinal pathology in patients presenting to primary care settings with acute low back pain. Arthritis Rheum. 2009 Oct;60(10):3072–80.

10.   Maher C, Underwood M, Buchbinder R. Non-specific low back pain. The Lancet. 2017 Feb;389(10070):736–47.

11.   Seki S, Kawaguchi Y, Mori M, Mio F, Chiba K, Mikami Y, et al. Association study

of COL9A2 with lumbar disc disease in the Japanese population. J Hum Genet. 2006 Dec;51(12):1063–7.

12.   Rajasekaran S, Kanna RM, Senthil N, Raveendran M, Ranjani V, Cheung KMC, et al. Genetic susceptibility of lumbar degenerative disc disease in young Indian adults. Eur Spine J. 2015 Sep;24(9):1969–75.

13.   Rigal J, Léglise A, Barnetche T, Cogniet A, Aunoble S, Le Huec JC. Meta-analysis of the effects of genetic polymorphisms on intervertebral disc degeneration. Eur Spine J. 2017 Aug;26(8):2045–52.

14.   Varlotta GP, Brown MD, Kelsey JL, Golden AL. Familial predisposition for herniation of a lumbar disc in patients who are less than twenty-one years old.: J Bone Jt Surg. 1991 Jan;73(1):124–8.

15.   Battié MC, Haynor DR, Fisher LD, Gill K, Gibbons LE, Videman T. Similarities in degenerative findings on magnetic resonance images of the lumbar spines of identical twins. J Bone Joint Surg Am. 1995 Nov;77(11):1662–70.

16.   Battié MC, Videman T, Parent E. Lumbar Disc Degeneration: Epidemiology and Genetic Influences. Spine. 2004 Dec;29(23):2679–90. :

Figures:

Schematic of How Pain is Transmitted

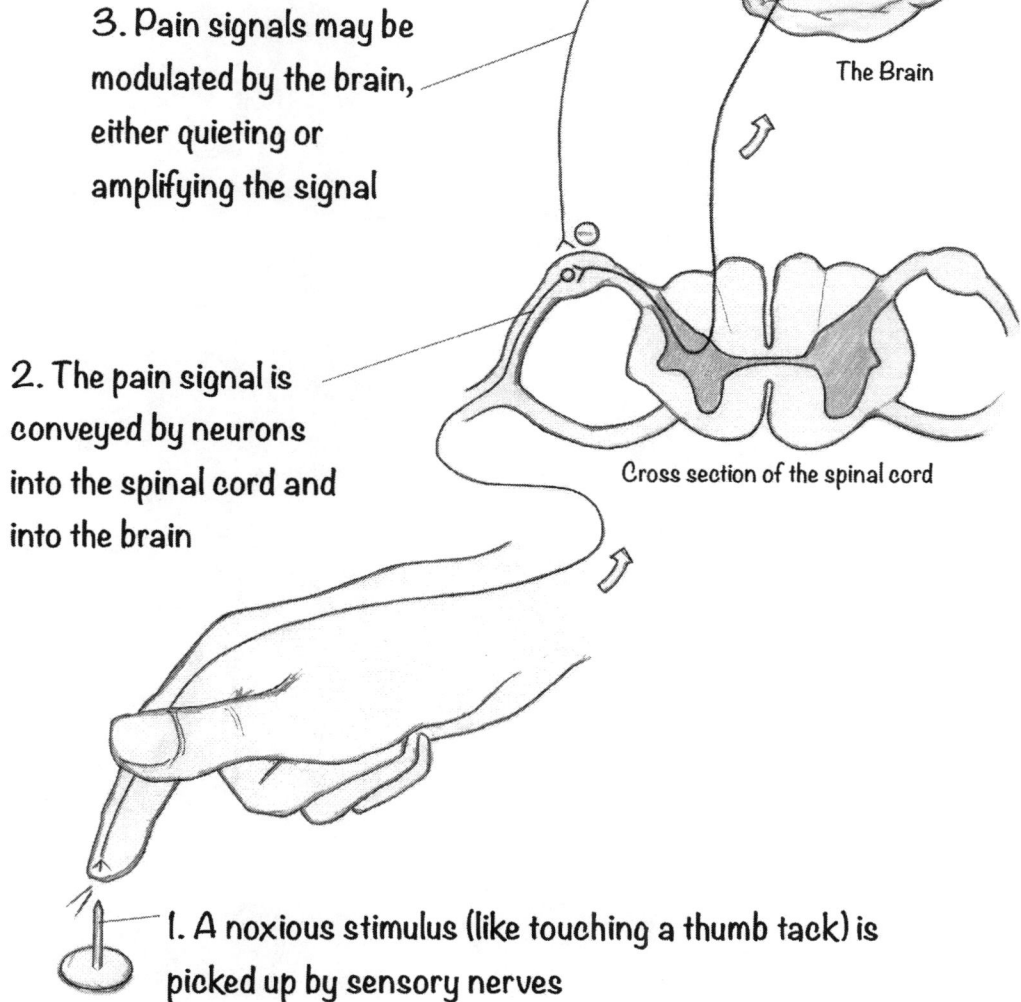

3. Pain signals may be modulated by the brain, either quieting or amplifying the signal

The Brain

2. The pain signal is conveyed by neurons into the spinal cord and into the brain

Cross section of the spinal cord

1. A noxious stimulus (like touching a thumb tack) is picked up by sensory nerves

Pain transmission. Pain is a sensation that is initiated by a stimulus such as touching something sharp. The sensation is transmitted to the brain by a "three-neuron" system. First, the pain signal is transmitted to the spinal cord. The signal then synapses (a connection between neurons) with the second neuron that ascends the spinal cord to the thalamus in the brain. Here there is a third synapse with a final sensory neuron that transmits the sensation to the sensory cortex in the brain where it is interpreted.

Sciatica/Radiculitis:

Pain that travels down the leg

The nerves are
pinched in the
lumbar spine

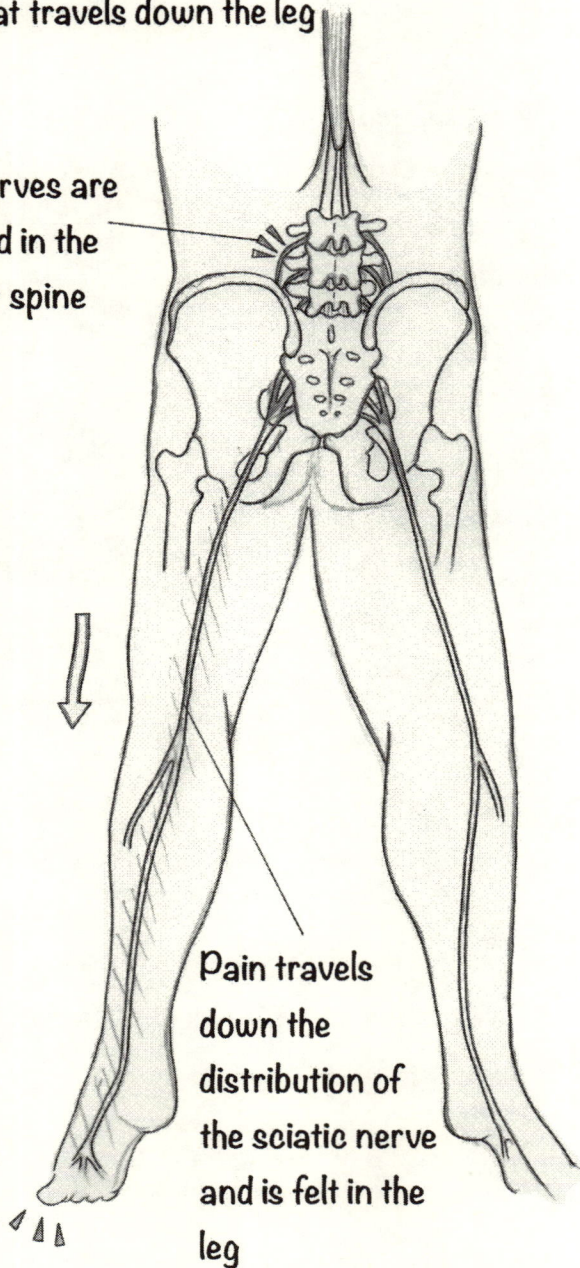

Pain travels
down the
distribution of
the sciatic nerve
and is felt in the
leg

Radiculopathy. Radiculopathy is the phenomena of a nerve
being pinched in the spine and transmitting pain either
down the leg or the arm (in this case the leg).

Lumbar Degeneration

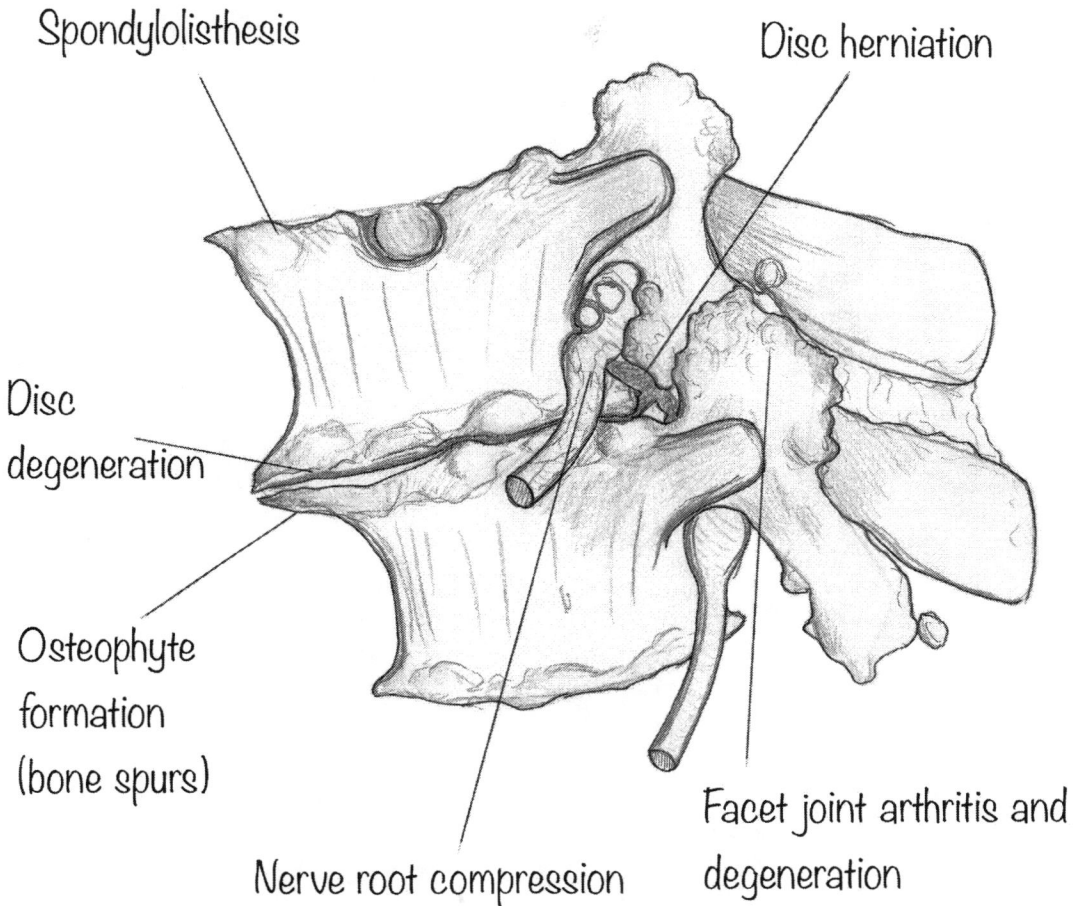

Spondylolisthesis

Disc herniation

Disc degeneration

Osteophyte formation (bone spurs)

Nerve root compression

Facet joint arthritis and degeneration

Lumbar degeneration. A schematic of characteristic changes that occur in lumbar spine with degeneration. The disc space erodes and causes the generation of osteophytes (bone spurs) from the endplates of the vertebral body that can encroach on the nerve roots. The facet joints become eroded and allow the superior vertebra to slip forward. As a response the facets grow more osteophytes that also encroach on the nerve roots.

Chapter 3

Low Back Pain, Buttock Pain and Tail Bone Pain—When to Seek Care and Do I Need Surgery?

Summary

Back pain is extremely common and almost all adults will experience it in some form at some time in their lives. For most, this is a temporary experience that does not persist and certainly does not require surgery. However, if your back pain persists for more than 6 weeks despite physical therapy, you should have it evaluated by a specialist—although serious causes of back pain are very rare, they need to be ruled out. Back pain should not be treated with bed rest. Keeping a strong muscular core is important for prevention of future episodes. Back pain may be associated with tail bone pain or buttock pain. These same pain patterns may also be associated with problems of the hips or coccyx (tail bone).

Case

Mr. Grey is a 45-year-old pilot who has had about a 2-year history of back pain. He has always had a "bad back" but it seems to have progressed significantly recently. He attributes it to sitting during long flights for much of his career. He comes to see me, and I order an MRI that shows some minor degeneration in his discs but nothing significant. Yet he continues to suffer from so much daily back pain, surgery is beginning to feel like a good idea. His MRI does not seem to explain his problem, and so we embark on a rigorous physical therapy program to work on strengthening the muscles and ligaments of the back. Overtime his pain subsides as his core strength and flexibility improves.

Introduction

When low back (lumbar) pain occurs, it can be a debilitating problem that can significantly decrease function and quality of life. Unfortunately, nearly two thirds of adults will suffer from low back pain in their lifetimes, and it is a major cause of visits to the doctor (1). Furthermore, back pain is a very common cause of disability, particularly for the young worker. Nonetheless, the majority of this back pain does not require surgery and is temporary. In fact, a year after the initial episode only about 10% of patients will still suffer from low back pain, though it may take at least several weeks to resolve (2). While back pain is pervasive in society it is interesting to note that the United States has a 40% higher rate of back surgery than other developed countries such as the United Kingdom (3). It is unclear why this is. It could be related to higher numbers of surgical providers than in other countries, making appropriate care more available, but it could also mean some people who do not strictly need back surgery are getting it.

What Causes Back Pain

Most back pain is initiated by a poorly timed or awkward movement and can send you reeling into back spasm. I remember a time when I did this to my back in college and could barely get out of bed because of the pain. Your body reacts in a serious way to any upset to the spine because it is such a core part of daily function. Luckily the great majority of causes are related to muscular strain. Muscle strain causes your back to go into severe spasm and clamp down, resulting in immense pain which symptomatically is much more dramatic than the actual problem because, whether you realize it or not, your back is critical for most types of motion. Thus, what seems like a catastrophic problem often is nothing more than a simple strain. However, for anyone who has experienced this, it is quite memorable.

The problem with diagnosing back pain is that there are so many different causes. It can range from benign muscle spasm to something far more sinister. There are multiple structures in the back that can generate pain, including discs, joints, ligaments, nerves and muscle. More serious problems include fractures, cancer, large disc herniations, and infections. Luckily these are very rare. There are even non-spine related problems such as bleeding gastric (stomach) ulcers which can mimic back pain. This makes the clinical diagnosis complicated and about 85% of patients with back pain will not be given a concrete diagnosis. Most problems are given the label of **back strain**, which generally refers to minor tears in the muscle or ligaments. These generally occur from twisting or bending awkwardly and are not the result of major trauma.

Incidence of Serious Problems in Patients Who Have Back Pain (1)
Spondylolisthesis (slipped disc) 10%
Disc Herniation 5-10%
Spondylolysis (stress fracture of the pars) 5%
Compression fracture 4%
Spinal Stenosis 3%
Visceral (internal organ) Disease 2%
Cancer/Tumor 0.7%
Infection 0.01%

Critical to differentiating serious causes of low back pain from the much more common benign conditions are so called **red flags**. These are symptoms which indicate diagnoses that need further work-up (tests). These symptoms include unexpected weight loss, nighttime pain, pain that does not get better lying down, bladder incontinence, loss of motor strength and severe numbness or sciatic pain (pain traveling down the leg). If your back pain does not immediately start getting better over several days or even continues to get worse over the next several weeks, you may have a more serious problem. If you are older than age 65 sudden onset of back pain is more likely to indicate a serious problem than for those in a younger age group. Pain in older individuals could be the result of disease that more commonly occurs in older age such as a fracture or cancer. **If you are suffering from any of these red flag symptoms, you should seek medical attention immediately.**

On the other hand, **if your pain seems related to movement and loading of the spine, for example, your pain gets worse when you stand, walk or strain, it's**

more likely your pain is caused by a musculoskeletal problem. If you think this is the case, and you are not having any major neurologic problems as described above, then it's ok to wait it out for a few days and see if things get better. Most doctors will not offer much in the way of treatment for a musculoskeletal issue that does not involve a fracture other than to reassure you there is nothing major going on. However, if your pain persists or is worsening, it is important to seek medical attention. Most insurance companies will not authorize the use of MRI unless there is a clinical indication such as a red flag, or your pain has persisted for at least 6 weeks.

Recovery

In most cases low back pain is a self-limiting condition (4). **The majority of back pain episodes will resolve within 2 weeks (5)**. Unfortunately, there is a high incidence of recurrence—as many as 40% of patients will have another episode within 6 months—indicating that in some patients back pain can be a chronic phenomenon (6). Keep in mind, though, that even if the pain recurs it is usually not as severe as the first episode. Low back pain is rarely disabling and most patients are readily able to return to work. Surgery is only rarely required to deal with back pain.

Tips for Treating Acute Back Pain
Take a short course (4-7 days) of a non-steroidal anti-inflammatory drug (NSAID) such as Ibuprofen (Advil) or acetaminophen (Tylenol) or both in combination as directed. Consult with your physician if you have liver, heart of kidney issues before using NSAIDS. Avoid strong narcotic medications if possible. Place ice on the inflamed area for 10-15 minutes per hour.
A short period of rest (1-2 days) can be helpful to prevent more injury: lie on your back with your knees and ankles elevated or on your side with a pillow between the knees. This will unload the spine. It's important to understand that prolonged bed rest is not good for your back, but a short period may be necessary to get over an initial flare. Even if you are taking a day to rest, lying down all day and night is not good for your body system. Get up every hour or so to try and stretch, but avoid any bending, lifting or twisting.
Gently massage the area of tenderness. You can use an over-the-counter liniment, a soothing medication such as Bengay® or Tiger Balm®, that is rubbed superficially on the skin to massage the tender area. Be careful not to apply to any open sores or areas where you are placing ice.
As your back starts to improve you should try walking and stretching more. You should discuss physical therapy with your primary care physician and learn a home back exercise program (see later chapters for basic spine exercises and stretches).

Non-steroidal anti-inflammatories and muscle relaxants may be used sparingly to help deal with acute (coming on suddenly and caused by something specific) back pain. Physical therapy and manipulation by a chiropractor are alternative treatments, but in general are unnecessary since most cases self-resolve (end with the passage of time). **The best treatment is to return to normal life as quickly**

as possible. Bed rest is not useful and can worsen back pain. From randomized controlled trials we have learned that bed rest is harmful in the treatment of back pain, and, even in the treatment of severe back pain, bed rest should be restricted to at most one or two days. Though exercise in the acute phase may also worsen your pain and should be avoided when the low back pain is intense, keeping your core fit and exercising regularly seems to be a good way to prevent future episodes (7). In other words, once you have experienced back pain and it has resolved, it's a good idea to find a good physical therapist so you can learn about exercises to prevent future episodes from occurring.

It should be noted that **some back pain has a psychological component**. Low back pain, even if diagnosed as benign low back pain, can cause great anxiety and can lead to depression and other issues if it persists. Also, in the same way that pain causes stress, stress may cause pain. Research shows that cognitive behavioral therapy to reduce stress can result in a reduction of back pain (8). In the past, narcotic pain medicines were used to treat low back pain but we know now that this practice is very flawed. Opioids lead to dependence and may actually sensitize you to pain (cause your brain to overreact to other uncomfortable stimuli in a way that makes you feel pain all the time) over the long term, leaving you stuck in a cycle of endless pain. It is possible for opioid withdrawal to actually cause back pain (9).

Buttock/ Groin Pain

Buttock and groin pain may also be non-specific (not clearly tied to a cause). They can be caused by problems of the spine but can also be caused by issues in many other muscular structures nearby. Since both an injured hip and an injured lumbar spine can result in buttock pain, it can be very difficult at times to determine the source of your pain.

If you have lumbar nerve roots that are compressed, they may cause pain radiating to the buttocks bilaterally (on both sides). This should be differentiated from pain running down the low back or pain above the buttocks as described above in the back pain section.

Groin pain is typically attributed to hip problems such as arthritis. Buttock and low back problems are more often associated with the spine.

If you have pain when putting on your shoes and getting in and out of a car, the hip is likely to be the culprit. If you have pain on the side of your hip, you may have bursitis—an inflammation of the membrane that covers the hip (10). Lumbar spine pain tends to get better with leaning forward and is also associated with sciatica and other neurological problems.

Coccydynia (Pain in the Tailbone)

The coccyx or tail bone derives its name from an ancient Greek word for cuckoo because the tailbone resembles the beak of that bird. It is the most southward portion of the spine and is attached to the sacrum. Unlike the rest of the spine bones, it does not have a letter abbreviation, and is not something most spine surgeons will offer treatment for. Many strong pelvic ligaments and muscles attach to the coccyx. The rectum is just anterior to (in front of) the coccyx. Pain in the tail bone, otherwise known as coccydynia, is like low back pain—it can be non-specific and difficult to attribute to a specific diagnosis. However, it can result in significant pain and discomfort.

There are many different causes of coccydynia. Trauma resulting from a fall onto the coccyx is a common cause. This can result in a fracture or dislocation of the coccyx. Childbirth is another cause. Coccydynia is also thought to be more common in the obese (11). It is commonly associated with low back problems. It may be more common in those with a hypermobile coccyx. This is because there are many pelvic muscles which attach to the coccyx and when they pull on the hypermobile coccyx this results in pain. For unknown reasons, it is also possible to form a membranous sac called a bursa around the coccyx which can become inflamed and painful.

Conservative management is successful in most cases of coccydynia. Common treatments include using a ring cushion while sitting, which unloads the coccyx, and massage and pelvic floor stretching When none of these measures help, injection of the coccyx may be attempted to ease the pain. Surgical removal is only reserved for those with prolonged pain which is not responsive to conservative measures.

Conclusion

Back pain is unfortunately a part of the lives of most human beings. Luckily most back pain is benign. If it happens to you, you should try to seek out a physical therapist who can help. If the pain does not go away, you may need to see a specialist. Look for serious "red flags" symptoms including weakness, numbness, incontinence, fevers, chills or unintentional weight loss. If any of these are occurring, it's important to seek treatment sooner rather than later.

Frequently Asked Questions

- **When should I see a doctor for my pain?**

    If your pain is the result of a significant trauma (fall from height or a car accident) or you have red flags as described above. If you have pain that persists after 6 weeks of conservative therapy. Begin with a general practitioner. If needed, you will be directed to a spine specialist. Keep in mind most back pain is a result of muscles strain that occurs from moving awkwardly or from lifting something too heavy or lifting with poor posture. (Always look up as you begin to lift—this will help keep your spine straight.)

- **My back pain has been ongoing for years—will I need surgery to fix it?**

  Most likely no. Spine surgery is only useful for certain problems in the back and will not be helpful in most cases of common back pain. In fact, it may even worsen some cases. However, if you feel better hearing that from a professional, then seek the care of a spine surgeon.

- **Why won't spine surgery help me?**

  Spine surgery is very good at treating mechanical problems in the back such as instability, or compression of nerves roots. If these are not what is causing you pain there is a very good chance that spine surgery will only make your back pain worse.

References

1.   Deyo RA, Weinstein JN. Low back pain. N Engl J Med. 2001 Feb 1;344(5):363–70.

2.   van den Hoogen HJ, Koes BW, van Eijk JT, Bouter LM, Devillé W. On the course of low back pain in general practice: a one year follow up study. Ann Rheum Dis. 1998 Jan;57(1):13–9.

3.   Cherkin DC, Deyo RA, Loeser JD, Bush T, Waddell G. An international comparison of back surgery rates. Spine. 1994 Jun 1;19(11):1201–6.

4.   Indahl A, Velund L, Reikeraas O. Good prognosis for low back pain when left untampered. A randomized clinical trial. Spine. 1995 Feb 15;20(4):473–7.

5.   Coste J, Delecoeuillerie G, Cohen de Lara A, Le Parc JM, Paolaggi JB. Clinical course and prognostic factors in acute low back pain: an inception cohort study in primary care practice. BMJ. 1994 Feb 26;308(6928):577–80.

6.   Carey TS, Garrett JM, Jackman A, Hadler N. Recurrence and care seeking after acute back pain: results of a long-term follow-up study. North Carolina Back Pain Project. Med Care. 1999 Feb;37(2):157–64.

7.   Lahad A, Malter AD, Berg AO, Deyo RA. The effectiveness of four interventions for the prevention of low back pain. JAMA. 1994 Oct 26;272(16):1286–91.

8.   Cherkin DC, Sherman KJ, Balderson BH, Cook AJ, Anderson ML, Hawkes RJ, et al. Effect of Mindfulness-Based Stress Reduction vs Cognitive Behavioral Therapy or Usual Care on Back Pain and Functional Limitations in Adults With Chronic Low Back Pain: A Randomized Clinical Trial. JAMA. 2016 Mar 22;315(12):1240.

9.   Farrell M. Opiate withdrawal. Addict Abingdon Engl. 1994 Nov;89(11):1471–5.

10.   Buckland AJ, Miyamoto R, Patel RD, Slover J, Razi AE. Differentiating Hip Pathology From Lumbar Spine Pathology: Key Points of Evaluation and Management. J Am Acad Orthop Surg. 2017 Feb;25(2):e23–34.

11.   Nathan ST, Fisher BE, Roberts CS. Coccydynia: A REVIEW OF PATHOANATOMY, AETIOL-OGY, TREATMENT AND OUTCOME. J Bone Joint Surg Br. 2010 Dec;92-B(12):1622–7.

Chapter 4

Neck Pain and Treatment

Summary

Like low back pain, most neck pain will not require surgical treatment. However, there are certain symptoms that you should look out for that could indicate a more serious condition. Most cases of neck pain can be treated with postural correction and gentle exercises. Manipulation of the neck (that is, having someone twist and turn it forcefully) is generally not recommended as the neck is delicate and this sort of therapy can cause serious problems. You should have your neck cleared by a spine specialist prior to having manual therapy. If your pain persists after physical therapy for 6 weeks, there are many noninvasive treatments that are available and can offer good relief such as medial branch blocks and radiofrequency ablation.

Case

Ms. Pink is a 56-year-old attorney who spends most of her time either on the phone or in front of a computer. She will type up reports for hours at a time, seldom moving her neck. Occasionally she will spend 30-40 minutes on the phone talking to a client with the handset pinned against her neck. When she

gets home, she is exhausted, and her neck is incredibly painful. Eventually she recognizes she needs to make some lifestyle changes. She starts seeing a physical therapist who works with her on gentle stretching and strength exercises. She starts using a hands-free handset for her phone and takes frequent breaks from the screen. Gradually her neck pain improves to the point where it is tolerable.

Introduction

Neck pain, like low back pain, is very prevalent, with almost two-thirds of the population experiencing it at some point in their lives. It is the fourth most common cause of disability worldwide (1). The neck has a difficult job: suspending your heavy skull in space and allowing you to turn your head to look around. It accomplishes this task through a complicated system of joints, ligaments and muscles that are perfectly in balance. It's easy for a small injury to a muscle to throw this system entirely off and cause significant pain. Furthermore, the neck contains 7 vertebrae known as the cervical spine that intricately fit together to allow this motion. Arthritis in these bones can also result in neck pain. In most people neck pain is caused by an acute injury such as whiplash and resolves with conservative treatment. However, in about 10% of people it can become chronic (2). It is critical to rule out serious causes of pain that may require surgical management.

Serious Causes of Neck Pain

With neck pain it is first important to rule out dangerous causes such as compression of the spinal cord, which may require surgery. If you are suffering from any neurologic symptoms, including weakness of the upper or lower extremities, numbness or tingling in the upper or lower extremities, difficulty with urination or incontinence (inability to control urination and bowel movement), loss of balance or dexterity, you may be suffering from a spine problem that requires a more comprehensive work-up (set of tests). These symptoms result from compression of the nerves and spinal cord. Absence of these symptoms does not necessarily rule out a serious problem, but it makes it less likely.

Like back pain, physicians look for specific **red flag** symptoms that could indicate other serious conditions. While most cases of neck pain are not serious, here are some signs of potentially more dangerous conditions:

- **Sudden unexpected weight loss, intractable night pain, history of cancer which could indicate a metastatic lesion (cancer cells that have spread to a second site)**

- **Fever, night sweats, sensitivity to light, rash which may indicate infection or meningitis (an infection of the spinal fluid)**

- **Generalized joint pain/swelling, which could indicate an inflammatory condition**

- **Difficulty with ambulation (walking), loss of manual dexterity (skill and ease in using hands), or weakness, which could indicate spinal cord compression**

- **Numbness in the arms or legs**

- **Vision changes, a tearing or ripping pain in neck, vertigo that could indicate an arterial problem like a vertebral artery dissection (a flaplike tear in the vertebral lining)**

- **History of acute trauma to the neck or other medical conditions that make you more susceptible to neck problems such as rheumatoid arthritis, ankylosing spondylitis (a form of spinal arthritis), diabetes, chronic steroid use**

- **Pain that fails to go away after 4-8 weeks of conservative medical therapy.**

Patients with red flags should be seen by a spine surgeon or orthopedic surgeon immediately. Evaluation by a neck expert with Imaging such as X-rays, CT scan and MRI scans should be performed to rule out these serious causes of neck pain.

Common Causes of Neck Pain

Now that the scary causes of neck pain are out of the way, let's talk about some more garden variety causes of neck pain. Neurogenic (related to the nervous system) pain occurs from irritation or compression of the nerves and spinal cord. The clinical condition resulting from compression of the nerves exiting from the spinal canal is known as **radiculopathy**, which typically manifests as pain shooting down the arm from the neck but can also cause isolated neck pain (3). **Mechanical pain** occurs from damage or degeneration to the facet joints, intervertebral discs, ligaments and muscles of the cervical spine. Findings of degeneration on X-rays are very common even in asymptomatic (without symptoms) populations and do not necessarily mean you need surgery (4). **Whiplash** is a common cause of mechanical pain where the neck undergoes a sudden acceleration and deceleration resulting in ligamentous damage or damage to the facet joints. **Only about 7% of cases of neck pain are due to purely neurologic compression with most cases being related to mechanical or mixed mechanical/neurogenic problems in the neck** (5).

The neck has a normal curvature called lordosis where the neck curves slightly toward the front. When this normal alignment of the neck is lost and becomes flattened as the head moves forward **(forward head posture)**, this can result in chronic tension and pain. You may think sitting in front of a computer and working at a desk are harmless activities, but this behavior can have a profound impact on your posture and can result in neck pain. When you sit at a desk it is very common to allow your shoulders to push the neck forward, allow the shoulders to lift slightly and round, which moves the shoulder blades forward, and at times causes you to hold your breath!

It is also possible for pain from other areas of the body, particularly the shoulders, to cause neck pain (6). In fact, **problems in the shoulder are a more common cause of neck pain than pain that originates from the neck**. This is because the shoulder and the cervical spine are interconnected not only by muscles but also by nerves. This can pose a diagnostic challenge for physicians (6). If you have an old shoulder injury it is important to mention this to your doctor as a possible source of neck pain.

Most patients with acute neck pain due to musculoskeletal injury or compression of a nerve root (radiculopathy) will improve over time (3,7). Neck pain can be very scary, and you may think that the degree of damage being done is significant. Be assured that most neck pain is benign and resolves with some form of non-operative care.

Treatment of Neck Pain

Once serious causes have been ruled out, neck pain can be managed with a host of treatment methods. The most common-sense treatments are the most effective at treating benign neck pain. These include getting enough sleep, maintaining good posture, committing to physical fitness and mental health. Obvious but not always easy!

Postural alignment is critical for the treatment of both acute and chronic neck pain. This is especially true for desk workers who may spend hours on end at a computer screen. It is important to realize that holding any position, even a proper one, for too long can cause muscle fatigue and strain. Moreover, bones and joints degenerate if not moved every so often. Get up and move around ever 30-40 minutes or so. Also, it is critical to optimize your ergonomic set up as well as following these common-sense practices:

- **Ensure your screens are at eye level to keep awkward neck tilts to a minimum.**

- **Make sure your elbows are at 90 degrees so that your shoulders can hang in a neutral position.**

- **Do not carry heavy backpacks or shoulder bags which put tension on the shoulder.**

Your neck may also get aggravated from sleeping in awkward positions. Having a comfortable pillow is essential. I recommend the use of a soft synthetic latex pillow, but really anything you find comfortable is acceptable (I like the Extra Soft Talalay Pillow from Organic Textiles that I bought from Amazon). The important concept to remember is to keep the neck aligned with the spine and body such that the neck is not craned. What this means is that your head is not bent at an angle compared to your body, such as tucking the chin, or resting your ear on your shoulder. Imagine if you spent several hours in this position while awake. If you sleep on your back, putting a pillow under the knees is a comfortable way to achieve proper neck alignment. The number of pillows under your head in this position will vary from person to person, but what you want is to have your chin in a neutral position—not tucked and not hyperextended (chin pointing up). If you sleep on your side, it may take several pillows underneath your head to keep the neck aligned with the body.

Contrary to age old beliefs, immobilizing the neck is not recommended in minor strains of neck muscles. Wearing collar braces may cause deconditioning of the neck muscles (a loss of strength, mass and supportive ability) and may increase your pain.

Exercises may be performed under the guidance of your physician or physical therapist. In cases of whiplash, early mobilization is encouraged to reduce the chances of chronic pain (1,2). It is best to warm up your neck prior to exercises either with a hot towel or even a heating pad.

Exercises for the neck include a gentle stretching regimen of rotating/tilting the head gently to the left and right and strengthening your neck muscles. Shoulder flexibility is also essential and can be achieved by rolling the shoulders and a few other exercises described below. After completing your exercises, you can apply some cold. If at any point your pain or symptoms becomes worse, you should stop the exercise or stretch and check in with your therapist.

Simple Neck and Shoulder Exercises—to be performed gently, slowly and mindfully:

- **Neck tilts: pull your head to one side, using your arm to grab the side of your head so that your ear moves closer to your shoulder**

- **Neck turns: twist your neck to look over one shoulder and then use your hand to push or pull on the chin to deepen the stretch.**

- **Neck strengthening: lie supine (on your back) and tuck your chin to your chest. Hold for 6 seconds.**

- **Shoulder stretching: 1) pull one arm across the body and hold with the other. 2) Roll your shoulders forward and backward. 3) Pull your shoulder blades together and stretch your pectorals out as when making a big chest.**

Each exercise may be performed 4-5 times per day.

Heat and cold may both be useful for treatment of neck pain. Avoid prolonged skin contact with the heat or cold source, no more than 15 minutes at a time (I commonly see burns from people falling asleep on a heating pad). If you have sensitive skin, you should spend even less time in contact with hot or cold and frequently check your skin. I personally have found the FlexiKold® neck pad to be a useful way to treat my own neck pain.

Common medicines used in short courses include non-steroidal anti-inflammatory medications such as ibuprofen, diclofenac and Mobic® (meloxicam). Oral steroids may also be used. Narcotics are effective for short-term pain control in the emergency room or in an inpatient setting but should not be used for more than 1-2 weeks because of their significant side-effects and addictive properties. In general, opioids should be totally avoided in the outpatient treatment setting for neck pain. Muscle relaxants such as cyclobenzaprine (Flexeril®) and methocarbamol (Robaxin®) may be used if there is a significant component of muscle spasm (7); however, these medicines can be sedating, particularly Flexeril®.

Many alternative treatments are available. Stretching and mobilization as performed by a physical therapist or chiropractor have some modest short-term benefits, but long-term data is lacking. Similarly, acupuncture has some short-term benefits and may be pursued in the absence of red flags. Caution must be used prior to initiating alternative therapies such as mobilization or stretching exercises to ensure they do not worsen neck conditions. Prior to seeing a chiropractor for your neck condition, you should be cleared by an orthopedic surgeon. The best practice is to use common sense and stop such treatments if they do not seem to be working.

Neck pain becomes "chronic" when it has been ongoing for longer than 12 weeks. Chronic neck pain may require some different more invasive types of treatment to improve. For example, a pain management doctor can administer medial branch blocks or radiofrequency ablation to treat chronic neck pain. In a **medial branch block** the pain is quieted by injecting the medial nerve that comes out of the spine to supply the facet joint and surrounding muscles. The injection stops pain signals coming from that nerve. One randomized controlled study found that corticosteroid injections around these nerves can give pain relief for up to 14 weeks (8). If these injections prove helpful, **radiofrequency ablation (RFA)** of the nerves may be performed. In radiofrequency ablation, the nerves suppling the back of the neck are burned such that they can no longer transmit pain. RFA may provide longer-term benefit than corticosteroid injections. In one randomized controlled study RFA provided relief of symptoms up to 260 days while a placebo only controlled pain for 8 days (9).

Many other treatments such as traction, TENS (transcutaneous electrical nerve stimulation), and soft collars/braces may be tried. They offer little chance of harm; however, their efficacy is unknown. Low level laser therapy is thought to work similarly to acupuncture; however, the method of action is unknown. These treatments are generally not recommended for the treatment of chronic neck pain.

Conclusion

Most neck pain is just that, a pain in the neck. Rarely there are more serious causes, but generally, neck pain can be treated with some life-style modifications. There is an assortment of untested treatments out there for neck pain ranging from braces to traction to manipulation. While most of these are safe, some can potentially make problems worse so these should be discussed with your physician before giving them a try. A pain management specialist may be able to offer invasive treatments such as medial branch blocks and radiofrequency ablation which deactivate the nerves transmitting pain signals. These should only be used in carefully selected patients after consultation with a physician.

Frequently Asked Questions

- ### Is traction useful for neck pain?

Traction is performed by pulling on the jaw and elongating the neck. It can be done manually either by a chiropractor/osteopathic doctor or by a device designed to lengthen your neck. The theory is that this can decompress nerves. It may be helpful in the short term, but the problem is your neck returns to a normal position once traction is released. You should discuss traction and manipulation with your surgeon prior to using it.

References

1.   Childress MA. Neck Pain: Initial Evaluation and Management. 2020;102(3):7.

2.   Binder AI. Neck pain. BMJ Clin Evid. 2008 Aug 4;2008.

3.   Radhakrishnan K, Litchy WJ, O'Fallon WM, Kurland LT. Epidemiology of cervical radiculopathy: A population-based study from Rochester, Minnesota, 1976 through 1990. Brain. 1994;117(2):325–35.

4.   Boden SD, McCowin PR, Davis DO, Dina TS, Mark AS, Wiesel S. Abnormal magnetic-resonance scans of the cervical spine in asymptomatic subjects. A prospective investigation. The Journal of Bone & Joint Surgery. 1990;72(8):1178–84.

5.   Liu R, Kurihara C, Tsai HT, Silvestri PJ, Bennett MI, Pasquina PF, et al. Classification and Treatment of Chronic Neck Pain: A Longitudinal Cohort Study. Reg Anesth Pain Med. 2017 Feb;42(1):52–61.

6.   Katsuura Y, Bruce J, Taylor S, Gullota L, Kim HJ. Overlapping, Masquerading, and Causative Cervical Spine and Shoulder Pathology: A Systematic Review. Global Spine Journal. 2019 Feb 17;219256821882253.

7.   Cohen SP. Epidemiology, diagnosis, and treatment of neck pain. Mayo Clin Proc. 2015 Feb;90(2):284–99.

8.   Manchikanti L, Singh V, Falco FJE, Cash KM, Fellows B. Cervical medial branch blocks for chronic cervical facet joint pain: a randomized, double-blind, controlled trial with one-year follow-up. Spine (Phila Pa 1976). 2008 Aug 1;33(17):1813–20.

9.   Lord SM, Barnsley L, Wallis BJ, McDonald GJ, Bogduk N. Percutaneous radio-frequency neurotomy for chronic cervical zygapophyseal-joint pain. New England Journal of Medicine. 1996;335(23):1721–6.

Figures:

Whiplash

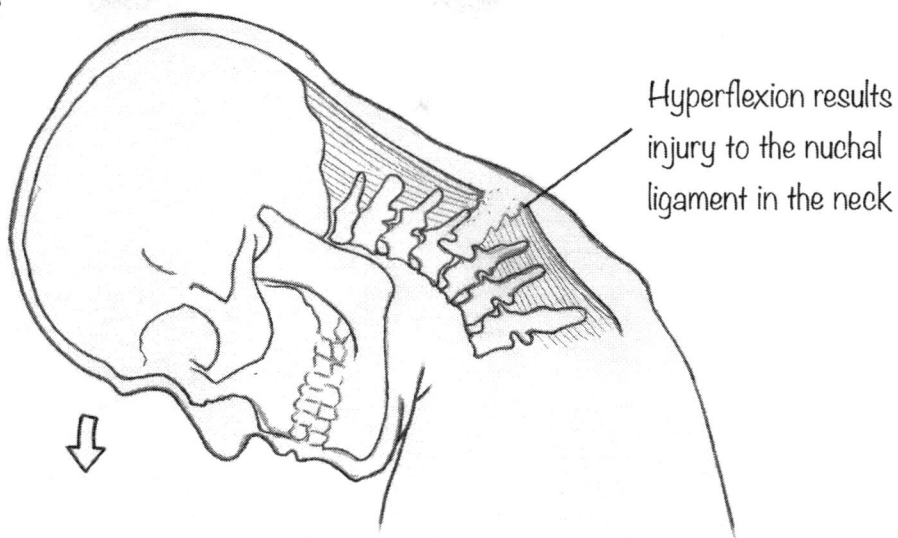

Hyperflexion results injury to the nuchal ligament in the neck

Whiplash. Whiplash occurs when the head is suddenly decelerated and the ligaments, joints and muscles of the back of the neck are strained. Whiplash is painful, but typically benign (not requiring surgical treatment), although it is possible for it to become a chronic condition.

Neck Exercises

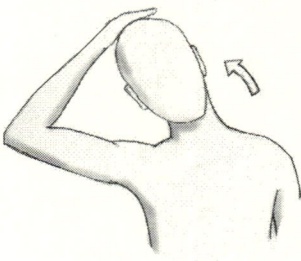

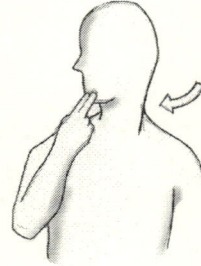

1. Neck side bend: gently pull the neck to the shoulder. Repeat on other side

2. Neck rotation: gently rotate the neck to each side. Repeat on other side.

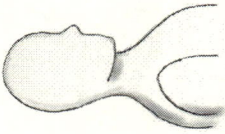

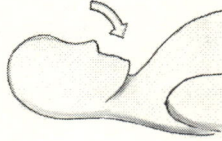

3. Chin tuck: gently retract the head and chin without bending the neck.

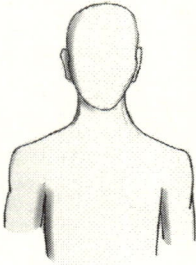

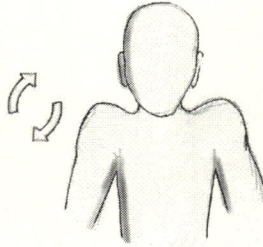

4. Shoulder rotation: gently rotate the shoulders forward and backwards.

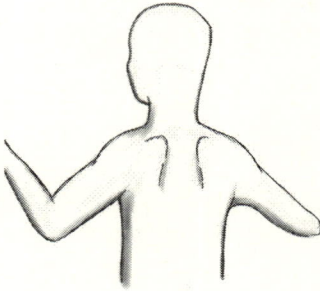

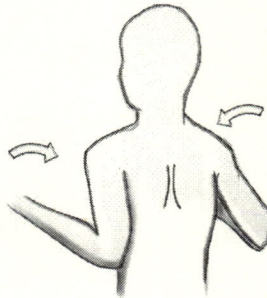

5. Shoulder retraction gently pull your shoulder blades together to stretch the chest

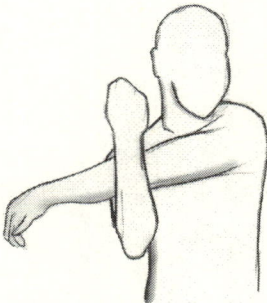

6. Upper back stretch: cross your arm over your torso and hold. Repeat on other side

Neck exercises. Different types of exercises you can use to improve neck pain. Try to do each exercise 2-5 times per day. Consult your physician if you are having pain.

Chapter 5

What Causes Spinal Cord Compression and Myelopathy?

Summary

Spinal cord compression occurs when the spinal canal becomes constricted—a condition known as stenosis. Stenosis usually results from a degenerative process in the spine. This chapter focuses on spinal cord compression in the cervical (neck) spine (another chapter will explore the thoracic spine.) The development of cervical stenosis and spinal cord compression can be hidden and only become a noticeable problem after the disease is far along in its course. When the spinal cord compression becomes bad enough it generally has symptoms of difficulty with balance, walking and fine motor coordination—a syndrome known as cervical myelopathy. The diagnosis is made based on imaging, looking for a damaged part (lesion) of the spine that is compressing the spinal cord. However, imaging alone is not enough; it must be combined with a careful neurological exam performed by your doctor. The treatment is almost always surgical decompression with or without a fusion. Treatment can halt the progression of the disease and may reverse some symptoms if performed early enough.

Case

Mr. Orange is a 65-year-old retired contractor who also suffers from chronic obstructive pulmonary disease (COPD) and high blood pressure. He is normally very steady with his hands but recently he has noticed he has started to drop things. Moreover, he has trouble walking long distances or climbing stairs where previously he had no trouble going for long walks. At first, he thinks it's just "getting old", but things continue to get worse. It gets to the point where he can barely keep his balance getting to the bathroom and he starts to suffer multiple falls. Ultimately, he sees his doctor who recommends an MRI which shows severe cervical stenosis with a slipped vertebra and severe spinal cord compression as a result. Mr. Orange is referred to see me. I perform a cervical fusion and decompression on him and immediately his symptoms start to fade. A year from surgery, although he has not regained his full strength, he is back to walking and working with his hands.

Introduction

Because it is so important, I devote this entire chapter to explaining degenerative problems (problems resulting from tissues losing their ability to do their jobs, usually as a result of aging, wear and tear and sometimes injury) affecting the spinal cord, particularly in the cervical spine. The reason we focus on the cervical spine or neck, is because that is the location where your spinal cord is most vulnerable.

The spinal cord is the relay conduit which transmits all information between your body and brain. It is composed of millions of neurons (small, extremely long cells) that run like wires from your brain to your muscles and organs and back. The spinal cord controls almost all of your body's functions, including your breathing, your muscles (including your bladder and rectum) and your sense of balance. The only senses that are not controlled by the spinal cord are those that arise from nerves coming directly off the brain called the cranial nerves, including vision, hearing, taste and the systems in the ear that also contribute to your sense of hearing, balance and position. The spinal cord runs from the base of your skull all the way to the top of the lumbar spine and is one of the most complicated structures known to man. It is extremely sensitive to any pressure, compression or damage.

Pathology of Spinal Cord Compression (How Compression Occurs and What It Does to the Spinal Cord)

When doctors talk about **spinal cord compression**, they are talking about the spinal cord being squeezed or compressed by adjoining tissues to the point of injury.

The spinal cord is housed within the spinal canal, a narrow tube created by the vertebrae that make up the spinal column. Vertebrae are shaped in a way that allow them to encircle and protect the spinal cord. However, the spinal canal is a small space to begin with and injury or wear and tear or aging can cause problems in the spine that make that narrow space still narrower or more constricted. **The medical term for that narrowing of the spinal canal is spinal stenosis**. When spinal stenosis occurs in the neck it is called **cervical spinal stenosis**. Stenosis just denotes narrowing of the tube of the spinal canal. You can have stenosis without spinal cord compression as there is a buffer zone of fluid surrounding the spinal cord (the cerebrospinal fluid or CSF). When cervical spinal stenosis becomes severe enough to displace all the fluid it often can result in spinal cord compression.

As with lumbar (low back) stenosis, several different factors can contribute to cervical spinal stenosis. Examples include buckling of ligamentum flavum (the yellow ligaments that connect vertebrae to each other), degenerative disc disease with protrusions, bone spur formation, and a disease process where the ligaments of the spine become calcified (**ossification of the posterior longitudinal ligament, or OPLL**). (See the glossary for more on these conditions).

Additionally, instability in the cervical spine can result in stenosis when the canal narrows because of one vertebra moving abnormally on another (a slipped disc). Disc herniations (discussed more in chapter 7 which covers disc herniations in detail) can also result in stenosis. Rarer causes of spinal canal stenosis include tumors, infections and fragments of bone caused by fractures.

As stated above, luckily there is a layer of fluid surrounding and protecting the spinal cord; however, if the stenosis becomes severe enough it results in **spinal cord compression** (where there is actual deformation of the spinal cord). In some patients the compression becomes severe enough to cause symptoms, which are discussed in the next section.

Eventually severe spinal cord compression can cause a progressive condition known as **myelopathy. Here we primarily focus on cervical myelopathy, but it can occur anywhere along the course of the spinal cord.**

Spinal cord compression is different from nerve/nerve root compression (radiculopathy) (discussed in chapter 2, What Causes Pain). **Unlike nerve root compression, which is painful, spinal cord compression is typically painless. Nerve root compression tends to only affect a single nerve and the discrete area of the body that that nerve supplies, while spinal cord compression affects the entire body. Nerve root compression has the possibility to improve with time, while spinal cord compression is progressively degenerative.**

It is important to note that not all patients with cervical stenosis have spinal cord compression, and not all patients with cervical spinal cord compression have cervical myelopathy. What this means is that cervical stenosis (narrowing) must get to a certain point to damage the spinal cord by compression. This in turn must be severe enough or go on for long enough to cause symptoms. Just because you have stenosis does not mean you need surgery immediately. Similarly, just because you have spinal cord compression does not mean you are clinically symptomatic. Moreover, it is possible for cervical myelopathy to coexist with cervical radiculopathy such that you have overlapping clinical syndromes and evidence of both diseases.

Everyone is familiar with the clinical scenario where an unfortunate patient involved in a car wreck, breaks his or her neck and becomes paralyzed. I tell patients that **cervical myelopathy** is the same process, but occurring in slow motion, often over months to years. How does this work? Spinal cord compression results in several changes. First, the spinal cord itself undergoes microtrauma, where each time you move your neck, the spinal cord is kinked and neurons (the cells that make up the spinal cord) die. Also, cervical stenosis chokes off the blood supply from the spinal cord which results in small vascular insults (think mini strokes) which also kill neurons (1).

The incidence of surgically treated cervical myelopathy is luckily relatively rare and is estimated to affect only about 2 to 4 persons per 100,000 people, although the true incidence is unknown (1,2). Similar to lumbar stenosis, it tends to affect mainly patients older than 60, particularly men older than 70 and women older than 80. For patients in this age group who have evidence of spinal cord compression on their MRI studies, about a quarter are estimated to become symptomatic in 4 years' time (3). Also, like lumbar stenosis, some people are at increased risk for developing cervical stenosis because they are genetically more likely to have a congenitally (born with) narrower spinal canal or are genetically more prone to early calcification of ligamentous structures (ossification of the posterior longitudinal ligament) (1). Either of these occurrences make you more prone to develop stenosis. Furthermore, certain physical activities may increase your risk of developing cervical stenosis such as bearing weight through your head, smoking, diabetes, excessive weight gain, and being exposed to high gravitational forces on your neck such as those experienced by military fighter pilots (1).

What are the Symptoms of Spinal Cord Compression?

The medical term for the group of symptoms that occur when the spinal cord is compressed over time is **myelopathy**. Myelopathy is insidious because you may not notice that you are developing it and the progression can be slow and incremental, taking place over many years. The clinical features can be subtle and easily missed.

In fact, the incidence of cervical myelopathy that is missed or that the diagnosis is delayed is quite high. In many instances it can take up to 5 trips to the doctor before the diagnosis is made (4). You might not even notice it is happening until you are far along in the disease process.

Typical symptoms of myelopathy are neck pain and stiffness, pain and numbness in the limbs, weakness in the limbs, loss of balance and bladder problems or incontinence. However, the symptoms may be subtler, such as increasing clumsiness using your fingers, resulting in difficulty with routine tasks such as writing, buttoning shirts, also difficulty with coordination, headaches, muscle cramps, and progressive loss of ambulatory capacity (hard time walking long distances). Some patients might just think they are "getting older." One important note is that in asymptomatic patients with cervical stenosis, even minor trauma to the neck (whiplash, slipping and falling, being struck by an object in the head), can commonly cause a rapid deterioration (in one study, 50% of patients) (5).

Diagnosis

Cervical myelopathy is a clinical diagnosis (based on signs and symptoms and the patient's history) that is made in conjunction with a compressive lesion (a damaged part of the spine that is compressing the spinal cord) that is visible on MRI or other imaging. In rare cases it is possible for myelopathy to occur without visible compression—this happens when there is a dynamic component to the compression. In dynamic compression, the damage is caused by some abnormal motion between vertebrae which may only occur during certain head positions and thus may not be visible on advanced imaging where your head is placed and kept in a certain position. An imaging technique known as diffusion tensor imaging (DTI) which tracks the movement of water up and down the spinal cord may be useful to detect problems with spinal cord function (6). Narrowing and/or signs of edema (swelling) in the cord diameter may also be evident (7). Spinal cord compression tends to occur around the discs which constrict like napkin rings around the cord. The swelling tends to occur above and below these points.

But imaging alone is not enough to confirm the diagnosis. Your surgeon needs to do a careful neurological exam (exam that evaluates how the nervous system is functioning) to make a formal diagnosis of myelopathy. As stated above, not all patients whose spinal cord compression shows up on imaging are myelopathic.

Prognosis—What Is Likely to Happen

Unless treated somewhat urgently, the spinal cord has limited capacity to regenerate and functional deficits caused by myelopathy can be irreversible. The rate of progression can be difficult to predict; however, as many as 37-75% of patients clinically worsen within 5 years. Typically, patients will report having stable symptoms followed by periods of decline in a so called "step wise" fashion. Because of this progression and the severe impact myelopathy can have on your quality of life, surgery is generally recommended either in the form of a decompression alone, or a decompression and fusion (8,9). Surgery typically can improve symptoms if done within a certain time frame; however, the primary goal of surgery is to halt progression of the disease (4,10). Recovery may take 6 months to a year, and some deficits may remain permanent and require further functional therapy (10). Nonetheless, in a large prospective study, the incidence of both motor deterioration and number of falls decreased following surgery (11). Moreover, those with milder impairment may experience improvement in grip strength and manual dexterity following decompression (12).

There are several different treatment strategies for cervical myelopathy which are discussed in later chapters. The important takeaway is that the compression must be removed, and the spine stabilized if it is unstable.

Conclusion

Spine surgeons take spinal cord compression and myelopathy very seriously because the consequences are irreversible if left untreated. The problem is many patients may not even realize they have it until they are examined. There is a fine balance deciding when to treat mildly symptomatic cervical cord compression because some patients will feel fine yet have ongoing disease.

When deciding whether to wait to treat mildly symptomatic cervical cord compression the surgeon must consider the risks of surgery and the recovery time as well as the likely rate of deterioration of the patient's spine and then weigh those factors against the eventual serious consequences of myelopathy if left untreated. Usually, it is better to intervene early in the disease while the patient's motor strength and coordination is still intact.

Frequently Asked Questions

- **I have been told that I will end up paralyzed if my cervical stenosis is not treated. Is this true?**

   Not necessarily. The decline from cervical stenosis can be drawn out and occurs over many years. If the disease is allowed to go on for long enough, you will have significant decline in your motor capacity and control, but you may not be strictly paralyzed. A common phrase in spinal surgery is "if you are involved in a fall or accident" you may expect to be paralyzed from your stenosis. This certainly can happen, but is very rare and not necessarily a reason to have surgery. The decision for surgery should be made carefully with your doctor to make sure it's the right path for you.

- **What is the drug Riluzole and can it help with outcomes from cervical myelopathy?**

   Riluzole is a drug that is used to treat amyotrophic lateral sclerosis (ALS) and works to block certain sodium channels in damaged neurons. In randomized controlled trials,it has not been shown to be beneficial for the treatment of cervical myelopathy (13).

References

1.   Nouri A, Tetreault L, Singh A, Karadimas SK, Fehlings MG. Degenerative Cervical Myelopathy: Epidemiology, Genetics, and Pathogenesis. Spine. 2015 Jun;40(12):E675–93.

2.   Boogaarts HD, Bartels RHMA. Prevalence of cervical spondylotic myelopathy. Eur Spine J. 2015 Apr;24(S2):139–41.

3.   Wilson JR, Barry S, Fischer DJ, Skelly AC, Arnold PM, Riew KD, et al. Frequency, Timing, and Predictors of Neurological Dysfunction in the Nonmyelopathic Patient With Cervical Spinal Cord Compression, Canal Stenosis, and/or Ossification of the Posterior Longitudinal Ligament: Spine. 2013 Oct;38:S37–54.

4.   Davies BM, Mowforth OD, Smith EK, Kotter MR. Degenerative cervical myelopathy. BMJ. 2018 Feb 22;k186.

5.   Yoo DS, Lee SB, Huh PW, Kang SG, Cho KS. Spinal cord injury in cervical spinal stenosis by minor trauma. World Neurosurgery. 2010 Jan;73(1):50–2.

6.   Wu W, Yang Z, Zhang T, Ru N, Zhang F, Wu B, et al. Microstructural Changes in Compressed Cervical Spinal Cord Are Consistent With Clinical Symptoms and Symptom Duration. Spine. 2020 Aug 15;45(16):E999–1005.

7.   Fukushima T, Ikata T, Taoka Y, Takata S. Magnetic resonance imaging study on spinal cord plasticity in patients with cervical compression myelopathy. Spine. 1991 Oct;16(10 Suppl):S534-538.

8.   Tetreault L, Ibrahim A, Côté P, Singh A, Fehlings MG. A systematic review of clinical and surgical predictors of complications following surgery for degenerative cervical myelopathy. Journal of Neurosurgery: Spine. 2016 Jan;24(1):77–99.

9.   Rhee JM, Shamji MF, Erwin WM, Bransford RJ, Yoon ST, Smith JS, et al. Non-operative Management of Cervical Myelopathy: A Systematic Review. Spine. 2013 Oct;38:S55–67.

10.   Fehlings MG, Wilson JR, Kopjar B, Yoon ST, Arnold PM, Massicotte EM, et al. Efficacy and Safety of Surgical Decompression in Patients with Cervical Spondylotic Myelopathy: Results of the AOSpine North America Prospective Multi-Center Study. The Journal of Bone and Joint Surgery (American). 2013 Sep 18;95(18):1651.

11.   Kimura A, Takeshita K, Shiraishi Y, Inose H, Yoshii T, Maekawa A, et al. Effectiveness of Surgical Treatment for Degenerative Cervical Myelopathy in Preventing Falls and Fall-related Neurological Deterioration: A Prospective Multi-institutional Study. SPINE. 2020 Jun;45(11):E631–8.

12.   Cole TS, Almefty KK, Godzik J, Muma AH, Hlubek RJ, Martinez-del-Campo E, et al. Functional improvement in hand strength and dexterity after surgical treatment of cervical spondylotic myelopathy: a prospective quantitative study. Journal of Neurosurgery: Spine. 2020 Jun;32(6):907–13.

13.   Fehlings MG, Badhiwala JH, Ahn H, Farhadi HF, Shaffrey CI, Nassr A, et al. Safety and efficacy of riluzole in patients undergoing decompressive surgery for degenerative cervical myelopathy (CSM-Protect): a multicentre, double-blind, placebo-controlled, randomised, phase 3 trial. Lancet Neurol. 2021 Feb;20(2):98–106.

Figures:

Cervical Stenosis

Cross section of the cervical spine showing a large disc herniation pinching the spinal cord

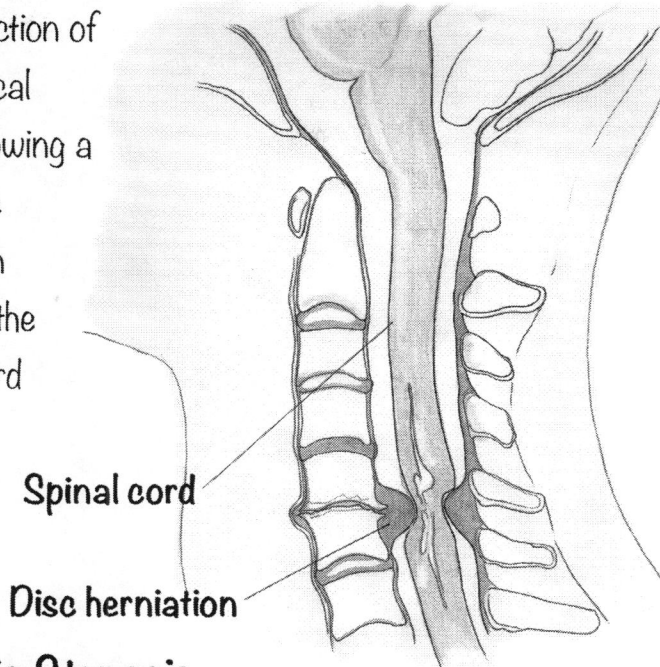

Spinal cord

Disc herniation

Dynamic Stenosis

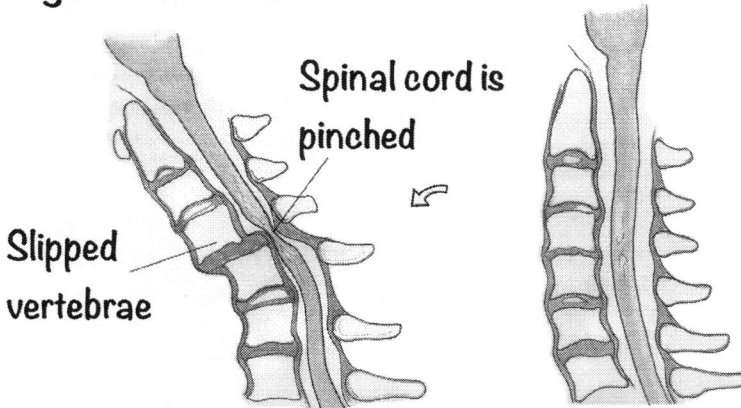

Spinal cord is pinched

Slipped vertebrae

Forward flexion of the cervical spine results in instability causing one vertebra to shift on another and pinch the spinal cord.

Cervical spinal cord compression. A cross section of how spinal cord compression occurs. A large disc herniation is compressing the spinal cord resulting in damage (top). A slipped disc (spondylolisthesis) occurs when the vertebra slides forward compressing the spinal cord (bottom). This is called dynamic stenosis because the narrowing occurs only when the patient moves in a certain way.

Chapter 6

Imaging of the Spine: X-RAY To MRI

Summary

Medical imaging of the spine ranges from X-rays to MRIs. X-rays acquire a single static image of the spine and are useful for looking at bones. Computer tomography scans (CT scans) are basically complex X-rays that can produce cross-sectional and 3D images. CT scans are useful for looking at the bones in high detail and for checking hardware and fusion status. It is important to know that both X-rays and CT scans work through the emission of ionizing radiation; however, the doses are low and should not have a major effect on you unless used repeatedly. Magnetic resonance imaging (MRI) recreates a highly detailed cross-sectional image of the spine that allows doctors to look at soft tissue and nerves. An MRI scan is generally required prior to spine surgery. Unlike CT, MRI scans do not emit ionizing radiation. Finally, CT myelograms, where dye is injected into the spinal canal, can be useful for patients who cannot have an MRI scan for one reason or another. Interpreting medical imaging is complicated and takes years of training and so it is important to review your images and radiology report with a surgeon who can help make sense of it.

Case

Ms. Fuchsia is a 45-year-old accountant who has been suffering from neck and arm pain. She comes to see me and I order an MRI to be performed. She is claustrophobic and has never had this type of test done, so there is a lot of anxiety about getting it. I explain to her that the test is totally safe and does not involve any ionizing radiation. On the day of the test she finds that the MRI tech is nice and is able to keep her calm. She is instructed to remove all metal and jewelry from her person before she enters the MRI suite. She is placed in the MRI scanner, which is a small tube, and feels anxious but the tech can communicate with her through a small speaker, and she is able to stay calm and still so that a nice image is produced (the tech notices that at first, she's moving too much and must repeat part of the scan). The machine emits a loud banging sound when its working, but she is given headphones with music of her choice to help block it out and the scan is done in roughly 25 minutes. When it's over, she wonders what she was so concerned about.

Introduction

Medical imaging is used to produce pictures of the inside of your body to aid the doctor in making a diagnosis and guiding treatment. It is especially important in spine care as there are so many possible sources for pain that the source of pain cannot always be pinpointed with a physical exam alone. In this chapter we will discuss different imaging modalities and how they are used. When you get an X-ray or some other kind of image it is typical for a radiologist (someone who specializes in reading an imaging study) to write a report—these are often very confusing and worrisome for patients. Your orthopedic surgeon will help interpret the images. It's important to keep in mind that just because something is abnormal on the image or called out in the radiology report, it does not mean it's a clinical problem. Once you are older than the age of 40 it is very rare to have a completely normal spine. Just because you have some mild disc degeneration, or some other abnormal finding does not mean you need surgery.

X-ray

In 1985 a German physicist named Wilhelm Röntgen (pronounced *rent*gen) produced the first X-ray when he exposed his own skeleton against a platinocyanide screen and saw the image of his bones! Since then, X-rays have been a major part of medical diagnostics and have helped countless patients.

X-rays are a form of high energy electromagnetic radiation that have a wavelength between ultraviolet radiation and gamma radiation. They are generated by a vacuum tube that accelerates electrons to a high speed and collides them with a metal plate. X-rays are released from the reaction and may be directed towards a target. Unlike lower energy electromagnetic radiation such as light, X-rays can pass through soft tissues but are blocked by dense structures such as metal and by the calcium in bone. Like photography, X-rays are detected on a plate and thus able to produce an image shaped by the number of X-rays the subject being X-rayed absorbs. X-rays are critical for the practice of orthopedics, which relies on evaluating the structure of bones and metal implants. Orthopedists often refer to X-rays as "plain films," "films" or "plain views."

X-rays are described in terms of the body part being X-rayed and the plane they are shot in. For example, an X-ray of the cervical spine shot from front to back is called an AP (anterior-posterior) cervical spine view. Similarly, if an X-ray of the neck is shot from the side it is called a lateral cervical view. Sometimes X-rays of the cervical spine are obtained through the open mouth to see the C2 vertebra. X-rays may also be obtained with the body held in a certain position. For example, for the cervical and lumbar spines, X-rays are commonly obtained in flexion (bending forward) and extension (bending backward). These are used to detect any abnormal motion of the vertebrae with the spine under stress. The radiology tech will have you bend your back or neck forward and then backward to obtain these views.

People often ask why you need to have X-rays since we already have a more advanced type of imaging such as an MRI or CT. The answer is simply that an **X-ray provides an excellent overview of the bones and spine**. CTs and MRIs are excellent at conveying fine detail, but they hold almost too much information for physicians to quickly process to get an overview of the problem. Also, since X-rays provide a snapshot in time of what the spine looks like, by taking a series of repeat images you can track the progress of healing or deterioration. For example, if you have a spinal fusion, X-rays can be used to follow the fusion process over time or progression of a spondylolisthesis (slipped disc). Orthopedic surgeons may use X-rays to monitor hardware and ensure it has not moved. Obtaining frequent CTs and MRIs to do this is not cost-effective, convenient, and, in some instances, not as safe for the patient. For example, obtaining multiple CT scans (that is, more than 3) can lead to high exposure of ionizing radiation.

fluoroscopy

Fluoroscopy is a form of X-rays that, in addition to taking static images, can produce a moving image. Fluoroscopy can do this by taking continuous X-rays that are directed towards an image-intensifier, which then transmits the enhanced image to a video screen. Fluoroscopy or simply "**fluoro**" is used commonly in orthopedics and spine surgery during procedures using a device known as a C-arm (because it is C-shaped). Fluoro is used to guide the insertion of hardware into the spine, do spinal injections and several other procedures. Interestingly fluoro was once used to fit shoes in department stores, but now is only used for medical purposes because of the X-ray exposure.

computer tomography

Computer tomography scan or CT (also CAT) uses X-rays to produce a cross-sectional image of your body. It does this by measuring how well an X-ray beam passes through the body (a property known as attenuation). X-rays are directed from multiple angles and then a computer program processes the values into a digital image. What this means is that, using the computer program, a CT scanner can produce an image which shows the inside of the body in a way quite different from a conventional X-ray beam. Computer tomography was originally invented by the South African physicist Allan M. Cormack and the British scientist Godfrey N. Hounsfield, who eventually won the Nobel prize for his discovery. Hounsfield, who worked for a record company at the time, took his idea of cross-sectional images to a leading neuro-radiologist in England. Incredibly, the idea was shot down by this doctor as "unnecessary" and Hounsfield was thrown out.

Unlike MRI, CT scans are fast to complete, and may be done in a matter of minutes. Typically, the patient lies on a table (also called a gantry) that conveys the patient through the CT doughnut—a circular device that contains X-ray generators and detectors. The **CT doughnut** rotates around the patient while shooting X-ray beams through the body from different angles. The detectors can tell how dense the tissue is based on the amount of penetration. This data is collected into a computer for each sequential cross-sectional slice of the body, each slice typically somewhere between 2-5 mm. Once the data is generated it is processed by a computer algorithm that turns it into a cross-sectional image. This image can then be reformatted in a way that allows the surgeon to assess it in different planes.

CT scans provide excellent imaging of the bones and are commonly used to assess the bone of the spine. They are also used to evaluate hardware and bony fusion following surgery and are superior to MRI and X-rays in this regard. There is a downside. Because CT scans require so many X- rays, they result in a considerably higher dose of radiation compared to a plain film. Although no study has directly shown this, CT scans are thought to increase the risk of cancer. It is estimated that 0.4% (4 out of a 1000) of all cancers in the United States are the result of radiation from CT scans (1). When talking about CT scans and X-rays, it's important to have a basic understanding of radiation safety.

radiation safety

Let's boil down an otherwise complicated subject to just the nuts and bolts: X-rays damage DNA, resulting in mutations that can cause cancer. How does this happen? X-rays are a form of radiation and thus have the potential to cause damage to biological tissue. This is primarily because ionizing radiation such as X-rays create free radicals when they interact with water contained in the body (think of free radicals as super charged molecules that can cause small chemical explosions). These free radicals cause damage to DNA (deoxyribonucleic acid—the molecule responsible for encoding your genes) by causing breaks in the long chemical strands. DNA damage can lead to mutations in genes. If these mutations deactivate genes that control cell growth, cancer can develop because the cell is allowed to grow unchecked. In most cases the lag between exposure to radiation and cancer is at least 10 years.

Radiation dosage is measured using two types of units. This is important to know because we use these measurements to compare how much radiation is delivered from different medical imaging techniques (see table 1). The Gray (Gy) is used to measure the absorbed dose of 1 joule of radiation per kilogram of matter. However, not all types of radiation produce the same effect, and some tissues are more susceptible to radiation damage than others. The Sievert (Sv) is used to measure the biologic dose of 1 joule of radiation per kilogram of matter and is dependent on both the type of energy and tissue, with higher energy radiation causing more damage to any tissue. Tissues that are more sensitive to radiation include bone marrow, colon, lungs, breasts and stomach. Radiation in medical imaging is measured using the millisievert (mSv).

Radiation Doses Associated with Various Medical Modalities, Air Travel, and the Natural Background (Environment)	
Exam and Other Sources of Radiation	**Radiation dose (mSv)**
Bone Density Scan (DEXA)	0.001
Chest X-ray	0.1
Fluoroscopy used in Intramedullary Nailing	0.08-0.1
Lumbar spine X-ray	0.7
Transcontinental US flight	0.03-1
Natural Background per year	3
CT Guided Spine Surgery (6)	6-7
CT Lumbar Spine	7.5
CT Abdomen and Pelvis	10

The average background annual radiation (radiation exposure just from living and breathing on earth) in the United States is around 3mSv (2). The life span study assessed the effects of the atomic bomb in Hiroshima and Nagasaki on approximately 120,000 survivors. From this study the Radiation Effects Research Foundation

(RERF) determined that for every 1 Sv (1000mSv) the risk of developing cancer increased 60% and the incidental risk of death increased 5% (3). The data from this environmental exposure is the most robust data available on radiation exposure. The risk from medical imaging which typically falls between 10-100mSV is less clear, but seems to suggest an increased cancer rate (2). Nonetheless the increased risk of a cancer-related death from any one medical scan is very low. One large study assessing the risks of CT scans on children and young adults found that in patients younger than 10 years, one excess case of leukemia and one excess case of brain cancer occurred per 10,000 head CT scans within 10 years of the study (4). Thus, while X-rays and CT scans should be used judiciously, imaging studies that can help figure out a best course of action have far more benefit than risk. Imaging may change the course of surgery or find a problem that may have been missed. Particularly the older you are, the less sensitive you are to the long-term effects of radiation and thus the less risk you have for radiation-induced cancer (2,5).

Radiation may be reduced with special leaded shielding and by limiting the number of studies performed to what is totally necessary.

Contrast

Contrast agents are substances that are used while performing X-ray, CT or MRI that **make it easier to see structures in the body** such as the arteries, veins and even the spinal canal. They do exactly what their name implies: create contrast between different tissue types to make it easier to make a diagnosis using medical imaging.

Contrast agents used in CT or X-ray typically contain iodine which is very radiopaque (good at blocking X-rays). Iodine contrast can be injected into the veins or directly into the desired structure such as the dural sac (as done in a myelogram, see below in the myelography section) or epidural space for an epidural steroid injection. Iohexol (Omnipaque®) is a common water-soluble (can dissolve in water) iodine-based contrast agent.

We haven't discussed MRI scans yet but since we are talking about contrast, it should also be noted that contrast can be used for MRI. MRI contrast agents are typically gadolinium (Gd-64) based as opposed to iodine. Gadolinium is used in MRI because of its magnetic properties that cause it to light up in an MRI scan, while iodine is used in X-ray studies because it is dense and capable of blocking X-ray beams. Gadolinium by itself is toxic, but it is attached to a binding molecule known as a chelator (diethylene triamine pentaacetic acid—DTPA), which effectively traps the gadolinium molecule, making it easily dissolvable in blood and very safe.

Both iodine and gadolinium-based contrast agents are very safe for general use. However, in rare cases anaphylaxis (a life-threatening allergic reaction) can occur in reaction to contrast. This is much more common with iodine-based contrasts than with gadolinium-based contrast agents. Anaphylaxis typically presents with wheezing, difficult breathing, mucosal swelling, and rash. Contrast agents are excreted renally (via the kidneys) and thus may be contraindicated in patients with renal failure or increased creatinine, which suggests kidney disease. Gadolinium and iodine contrast should be avoided in patients with a glomerular filtration rate (GFR) of less than 30ml/min per 1.73 m2, also an indication of poor kidney function. In patients with poor renal function, contrast may still be necessary and in such cases, protocols exist to limit the chances of worsening kidney damage. Gadolinium is contraindicated during pregnancy.

Magnetic Resonance Imaging (MRI)

Magnetic Resonance Imaging (MRI) is a marvel of modern technology that **allows tissues to be visualized with high resolution**. With MRI a doctor can peer into the deepest corners of the body without the need to make any incisions. As happened with the inventor of the CT scan, the inventor of the MRI, Paul Lauterbur, was also shunned initially because few thought there was much commercial value in an MRI scan. He later won the Nobel prize for his invention.

The physics behind MRI are complicated and beyond the scope of this chapter. What follows is a basic explanation of how an MRI works and if you are not interested in this, please feel free to skip to the next paragraph. Briefly, MRI technology is based on the fact that the protons in your body (protons are subatomic particles contained in all atoms) orient to a magnetic field. The most abundant source of protons in your body is in its water and fat, but all structures contain protons because they contain a lot of hydrogen (which is essentially just a proton). All protons have spin or angular momentum like a top in motion and all are oriented according to a magnetic field. At rest all the protons in your body are oriented randomly in different directions. An MRI scanner is basically a big magnet and comes in different strengths from 0.1 to 3 tesla (tesla is a measure of magnetic field intensity). When your body is placed inside an MRI scanner, the scanner's magnet forces all the protons in your body to orient along the same axis. You do not feel or even notice this. When scanning begins, an electromagnetic pulse is sent into your body which causes all the protons to flip. When the pulse is removed, the protons flip back to be in alignment with the magnet and in doing so release a small amount of radiofrequency energy which is picked up by the MRI machine antenna. This information is converted by software programs which use Fourier transformation to convert the signal to images. Different tissues have different relaxation rates which is how the different structures are identified.

MRI, unlike X-ray and CT, does not rely on ionizing radiation and thus is considered safer. Most potential ill-effects are related to the strong magnetic fields which are applied to the patient. Patients who have certain ferrous metals (iron and steel) implanted in their bodies for example, cannot have MRI scans because the metal would be pulled on by the magnetic field. All jewelry must be removed, and electronics left in a safe location. Other devices that contain complex circuitry may be permanently disabled by the MRI magnetic field—for example, pacemakers or medication pumps. Luckily, most modern orthopedic implants, pacemakers, and other medical devices are MRI compatible. An extensive list of medical and non-medical devices and implants that are MRI compatible can be found at www. mrisafety.com.

MRI is critical in the practice of spine surgery because it allows you to look at the soft tissues, particularly the nerves and spinal cord, with great clarity (CT scans are not as good at looking at the soft tissues). MRIs can tell you if there are disc herniations or compression of the nerves and thus, illuminate targets for surgery. In almost all cases, I use MRI scans to make surgical decisions. MRIs do have some shortcomings. Any metal in the body will severely distort the MRI image. Furthermore, MRI is not as good for depicting the structural quality of bone as either X-ray or CT scans.

Contraindication to MRI
Certain pacemakers/defibrillators
Spinal cord stimulators
Aneurysm Clips (many, not all, are ok—check the safety list)
Metallic implants with a high composition of cobalt or iron which heat up and move in a magnetic field
Metal in eye

open MRIs and claustrophobia

Many patients complain of claustrophobia when going into an MRI scanner because you must lie inside a long narrow tube. The study itself is also time intensive and can last several hours if scanning multiple body areas. Getting into an MRI scanner seems to be a part of deep-seated fear for some patients. So called "open" MRI machines that do not require a patient to get into a narrow tube have been developed as an alternative to standard MRI machines. These machines produce very poor-quality images compared to standard machines making them almost useless in my opinion. The open MRI may be used in cases where the weight of the patient prevents them from physically being placed inside a standard MRI machine but otherwise should be avoided. Spine surgery is a very precise discipline and requires precision imaging to make accurate decisions about exactly what kind of surgery you should have. Thus, I believe strongly all patients should have standard MRIs until the technology behind open MRI machines improves. This leads to another important point: not all MRI machines are created equal. Some have higher power (3 tesla vs 1.5 tesla) and, depending on how they are configured, will produce different quality images. Your surgeon may have a preference on where you go to get your MRI, or at least a list of places where you should not go.

To help with claustrophobia, your regular doctor may prescribe a light sedative prior to your scan to calm the nerves. MRIs are totally safe and can even be relaxing. You get headphones to listen to music and peace from the digital era (no cell phones, no tablets or laptops) for a short period of time.

Myelography

Myelography and CT myelography are older, invasive (injecting contrast) imaging techniques but are still useful today. Myelography is performed by injecting contrast dye into the dural sac—also known as the thecal sac. The dural sac is a membrane lining that holds the cerebrospinal fluid (CSF) and encases the spinal cord. The contrast dye is injected through a lumbar puncture, typically with fluoroscopic guidance. The contrast then coats the inside of the dural sac allowing doctors to see its outline on X-ray and see if there are any areas where the spinal cord is being compressed.

Myelograms are mainly indicated in patients who cannot have an MRI performed or in patients who have so much metal implanted that the distortion in the MRI makes the image useless (such as in spinal fusions). A myelogram is done by a surgeon or interventional radiologist who uses a long needle to perform a lumbar puncture. Contrast is then injected into the dural sac. After the injection of contrast, the imaging table is then tilted to allow the contrast to flow into the cervical spine. You may be asked to roll around a few times to allow the contrast to spread out. Once this is done you go straight to the CT scanner where usually a full spine scan is performed. The reason for this is that once you go through the trouble of injecting contrast into the spinal canal you won't want to have to repeat the process to look at the other areas (say the cervical spine, if only the lumbar spine is imaged). Thus, the entire spine is scanned to make sure the contrast is maximally utilized. The technique of injecting contrast directly into the dural sac is what distinguishes this technique from regular X-ray or CT scans.

At very high doses contrast can cause headaches so contrast is generally not allowed to pool in the brain. Once the contrast reaches the neck, the table is tilted back to prevent it from pooling in the brain.

When the lumbar puncture is performed, the spinal needle may come close to a nerve root and cause sciatica pain to shoot down the leg. If this occurs try not to jump, but let the doctor know so he can move the needle. It is also possible to develop a small cerebral spinal fluid (CSF) leak after the procedure, which can also give you a headache. Your doctor may have you rest for a few hours after the procedure to decrease the likelihood of a symptomatic headache. In the past, non-soluble contrast agents (those which did not dissolve in water) were injected into the spine. They caused a lot of nerve irritation and had to be sucked out of the spinal canal once they were injected. Luckily, with modern contrast agents this is no longer an issue.

Discography

Like myelograms, discography is an older style of imaging that is not used as commonly anymore. **In a discogram, a spinal needle is inserted into the disc space and a liquid is injected.** This liquid is typically contrast and a numbing agent. Injecting the contrast elicits pain and the numbing agent relieves it. The theory behind discograms is that when you inject the numbing medicine into the disc it can reduce pain coming from the disc if it was damaged or irritated (discogenic pain) which otherwise is almost impossible to diagnose. Many centers will require a discogram before performing a lumbar disc replacement to ensure the pain is in fact coming from the disc and thus the patient will benefit from surgical replacement.

Discography is used as an assessment tool and validation tool in the following ways (7):

- **analyzing the image for leaking of the contrast, which would indicate a tear in the disc**

- **stimulation of the disc by injecting a fluid such as contrast to recreate the patient's pain**

- **no pain recreated at an adjacent healthy disc, which acts as a "control" for the study.**

- **relief of pain with injection of a numbing agent such as lidocaine, which can help to pinpoint the source of pain.**

To put it mildly, discograms have many issues and can be easily misused. Discography is not used as commonly anymore because of fears that puncturing the disc space can result in early degeneration of the disc. Furthermore, injecting the disc can cause pain, and thus it is not always clear cut if the test was positive or negative. Discograms can be positive in patients with no history of disc disease or pain. Finally, discography will not always indicate that surgery will be successful (8,9).

Nuclear Imaging

In nuclear imaging, a small amount of radioactive substance (also known as a radiotracer or radionuclide) is placed inside the body. The radioactive substance is typically tagged to a molecule such as fluorodeoxyglucose-18 (FDG-18)—a radioactive fluoride molecule that is tagged to a regular glucose (sugar) molecule. The molecule is then ingested and in the case of FDG-18 becomes concentrated in areas of high metabolic activity (the cells are very active multiplying). Since tumors are very metabolically active (use a lot of sugar) they absorb a disproportionate amount of FDG-18. The radioactive tracer then emits radiation which can be picked up by a scanner such as in positron emission tomography (PET).

types of nuclear imaging

Bone Scan: bone scans or **bone scintigraphy** use the radionuclide technetium-99 (^{99m}Tc) which is used to label a diphosphonate—a molecule which is readily absorbed by bone. This radionuclide specifically accumulates in areas of high bone turnover (osteoblastic cells are making lots of new bone). These are three-phase studies because images are obtained immediately after injection (flow phase), 15 minutes following injection (pooling phase), and 4 hours after injection (bone phase). They are useful for examining for bone infections such as osteomyelitis. Unfortunately, many other conditions cause increased activity on bone scans (fracture, tumor, Paget's disease, and bone infarcts (dead bone tissue)). Do not confuse nuclear bone scans with a bone density scan or (DXA) described in another chapter. Bone scans produce a 2D silhouette image of the skeleton and areas with increased activity are very dark.

Positron emission tomography (PET): PET scans are like bone scans but tend to be much more expensive. They use fluorodeoxyglucose-18 (FDG-18) as described above and do have several advantages. They can incorporate a CT scan and thus have increased spatial resolution of the scan—meaning instead of just a 2D image like a bone scan, a PET scan is more like a CT where you can see the body in cross section. They are also faster to perform than a 3-phase bone scan. PET scans are commonly used in oncology for detecting tumors and metastases in the body.

A Note on The Radiology Report

Every image produced in the hospital typically will come with a radiology report—a summary of the findings as documented by a doctor who specializes in reading the images. Radiologists are highly trained doctors who spend years in school to learn how to interpret medical images and solely practice this art. They do not ask you about symptoms, or perform clinical exams, but just look at your images and tell you what they see in sometimes excruciating detail. Thus, radiology reports can feel scary, cold and puzzling at times. Things written like "severe disc degeneration at L5-S1" may cause patients to panic and worry that they may need immediate back surgery. The key to remember is that the reported findings are not necessarily relevant to you and your symptoms and often are not indications for surgery. Your surgeon will help make the connection between the report, the images and you as the patient.

Conclusion

In today's world, there are many different imaging modalities for doctors to choose from. It can be confusing to the patient as to why a doctor needs a certain scan, but ultimately the more information the doctor has, the better he/she can make a diagnosis and plan your surgery. From a surgeon's perspective, I like the saying "no stone left unturned" which means that it's better to have a complete understanding of the problem than to leave anything to chance. In my practice this means I make full use of not just MRI, but also X-ray and CT. Most tests are very safe and even invasive tests that require injection of contrast agents only rarely have complications. It takes years of study to be able to interpret the imaging and to know what is important and what is not, so try not to be alarmed if you happen to read a radiology report with a lengthy list of issues. Work with your surgeon to understand the report and what is clinically relevant.

Frequently Asked Questions

- **What are some common safety measures used in obtaining X-rays?**

    Patients are usually stood several yards away from the X-ray source, decreasing the dose. Lead shielding is commonly used to protect radiosensitive areas of the body such as the groin, breasts, and thyroid. X-ray machines now also have "rare-earth" screens which intensify the image while limiting the dose of radiation.

References

1.   Brenner DJ. Computed Tomography — An Increasing Source of Radiation Expo-sure. The New England Journal of Medicine. 2007;8.

2.   Lin EC. Radiation risk from medical imaging. Mayo Clin Proc. 2010 Dec;85(12):1142–6; quiz 1146.

3.   Pierce DA, Preston DL. Radiation-related cancer risks at low doses among atomic bomb survivors. Radiat Res. 2000 Aug;154(2):178–86.

4.   Pearce MS, Salotti JA, Little MP, McHugh K, Lee C, Kim KP, et al. Radiation expo-

sure from CT scans in childhood and subsequent risk of leukaemia and brain tumours: a retrospective cohort study. Lancet. 2012 Aug 4;380(9840):499–505.

5.   Ozasa K, Shimizu Y, Suyama A, Kasagi F, Soda M, Grant EJ, et al. Studies of the Mortality of Atomic Bomb Survivors, Report 14, 1950–2003: An Overview of Cancer and Noncancer Diseases. Radiation Research. 2012 Mar;177(3):229–43.

6.   Mendelsohn D, Strelzow J, Dea N, Ford NL, Batke J, Pennington A, et al. Patient and surgeon radiation exposure during spinal instrumentation using intraoperative computed tomography-based navigation. Spine J. 2016 Mar;16(3):343–54.

7.   Madigan L, Vaccaro AR, Spector LR, Milam AR. Management of Symptomatic Lumbar Degenerative Disk Disease: Journal of the American Academy of Orthopaedic Surgeons. 2009 Feb;17(2):102–11.

8.   Carragee EJ, Alamin TF, Carragee JM. Low-Pressure Positive Discography in Subjects Asymptomatic of Significant Low Back Pain Illness: Spine. 2006 Mar;31(5):505–9.

9.   Carragee EJ, Lincoln T, Parmar VS, Alamin T. A Gold Standard Evaluation of the "Discogenic Pain" Diagnosis as Determined by Provocative Discography: Spine. 2006 Aug;31(18):2115–23.

Figures:

Lumbar spine imaging

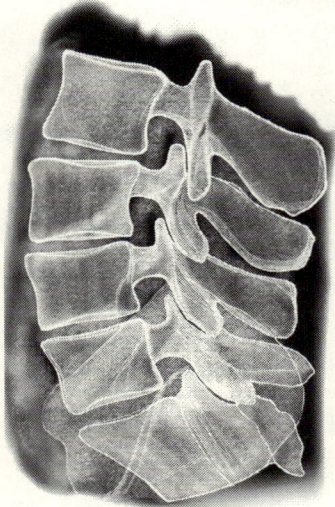

X-Ray

Shows a silhouette of the bone and some soft tissue

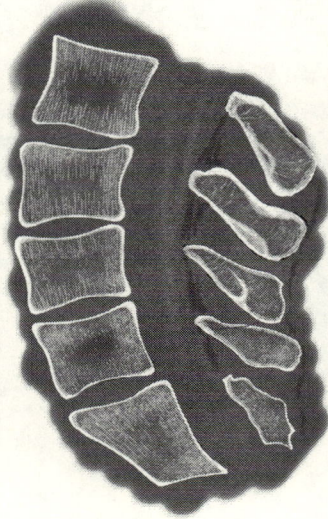

CT SCAN

Shows a cross section of bone in high definition

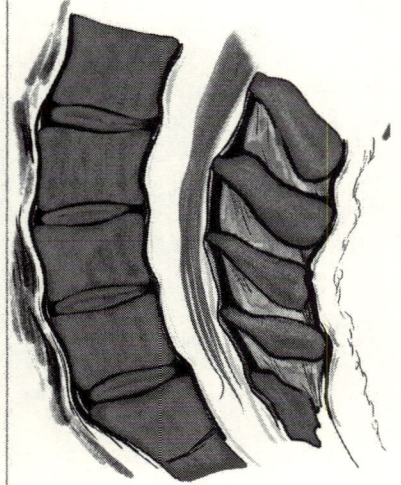

MRI SCAN

Shows soft tissue and bone

Lumbar Imaging. This figure depicts the lumbar spine using different imaging machines. On the far left is a plain X-ray of the spine that gives an overview of the bone. In the middle is a CT-Scan, which shows the bone in detail. Finally on the right is a MRI scan, that shows bone and soft tissues.

SECTION 2

Common Spine Problems that Might Require Surgery

"Be cheerful, the problems that worry us most are those that never arrive"
-Benjamin Franklin

Chapter 7

What is a Herniated Disc and What Happens When It Occurs in the Neck (Cervical) or Low Back (Lumbar)

Summary

A disc herniation is an extremely common reason to go visit the spine surgeon. Even though the symptoms can be severe and disabling, with supportive treatment and physical therapy, a disc herniation typically resolves (heals) on its own. When discussing disc herniations, many different terms get used; few are important for the patient to understand. Surgery is rarely indicated to treat a herniated disc unless you have severe pain that doesn't get better with time, or progressive numbness or weakness or bowel and bladder incontinence or severe spinal cord compression resulting in spinal cord damage. Surgery typically consists of a microdiscectomy in the lumbar spine or a foraminotomy/cervical disc replacement and fusion (ACDF) in the cervical spine.

Case

Mr. Blue is a 45-year-old city-worker who injured his back on the job about a year ago, suffering from a herniated disc. Ever since, he has had severe low back pain and right leg pain that seems focused in the buttock but shoots down the entire leg and into the foot. Moreover, he has numbness on the top of his foot, and it feels as if his foot is weak and dragging. He has an MRI performed which confirms the diagnosis of a herniated disc at L4-5 that is pinching on the L5 nerve root. He has tried epidurals in the past as well as physical therapy and, although helpful, nothing keeps the pain at bay for long. We decide that a microdiscectomy is the best option for him and after the surgery he notes immediate resolution in his pain. A year out from surgery he is doing great and is back to work and the activities he enjoys.

Introduction

Low back (lumbar) and neck (cervical) pain are extremely common disorders for which people seek medical care. Lumbar and cervical disc herniations are one of the most common ailments a spine surgeon treats. Lumbar disc herniations tend to cause severe pain that radiates down the leg called sciatica, because the disc fragments can pinch a nerve. Disc herniations in the neck (cervical disc herniations) cause neck pain and pain that radiates down the arm. Both can be associated with numbness and weakness.

What Is a Disc Herniation?

The intervertebral disc is somewhat like a jelly doughnut with an outer casing (known as the annulus fibrosis or just annulus) and a jelly-like core (nucleus pulposus). This design allows the disc to absorb force through the spine, so the spinal bones have some cushioning when you run, walk, and lift. A **disc herniation** occurs when there is a tear or weakening in the outer annulus casing of the disc and the nucleus pulposus jelly comes out. This can be benign and asymptomatic, but if the jelly touches or compresses a nerve it is generally extremely painful.

It is unclear exactly what causes a disc herniation, but in general it occurs when a force is exerted through the disc that results in a disruption of the outer annulus, which forces the nucleus pulposus to pop out. This can be due to a trauma such as a fall or intense twist but can also occur with seemingly no trauma.

There is likely a genetic predisposition to disc herniations that results in weakness of the annulus fibrosis (1). Studies of twins have shown that twins can have nearly identical disc herniations and disc degeneration (2). Recently, there has been growing evidence that disc degenerations and herniations are related to bacterial infections with slow growing organisms like P. acnes (the bacteria that causes acne), although this is still controversial (3). Small incidents of trauma may also play a role in disc degeneration (4). You might expect that disc herniations only occur in the elderly, but this is not the case. Even the young can have disc herniations.

Why Are Disc Herniations Painful?

The intervertebral (between the two vertebrae) discs have small nerve endings which allow them to sense pain, so the physical act of the annulus tearing, and herniating disc material can be painful and cause low back pain. However, it is when the disc gets close to a nerve that the real problem arises. Discs exert pressure on nearby nerves resulting in pain from that compression. Disc material can also be very inflammatory (causing an immune system response) and affect nearby nerves—also very painful.

When the nerve becomes compressed, irritated, or inflamed, it can result in a syndrome known as radiculopathy. **Radiculopathy** presents as searing pain that radiates down the extremity along the pathway that that nerve supplies. While each nerve follows a specific course, it is also interconnected with other nearby nerves and thus the pattern of pain is usually a little bit different for everyone. Generally, the pain consists of electrical sensation shooting down the arm or leg. You may also experience numbness and weakness of the extremity.

Disc herniations can occur anywhere in the spine where there are discs. The most common areas are in the lumbar (low back) and cervical (neck) areas because these are the mobile segments of the spine and subject to more force. Nonetheless it is also possible to have a herniation in the thoracic area. Depending on where the disc is herniated, the symptoms will be different. For example, lumbar disc herniations cause leg pain and sciatica, cervical disc herniations cause arm pain and thoracic herniations can cause chest pain.

Diagnosis

Your surgeon can usually diagnose a herniated disc based on classic signs and symptoms. One very common sign that a disc is herniating is pain radiating down your leg when you straighten it while raising it, known as a positive straight leg raise. This causes pain because that action places tension on the nerve lying against the herniation (5). Once your surgeon suspects a herniated disc, he/she may order tests such as an MRI scan. An MRI scan can show all kinds of socalled "problems" with your back and so it's important to remember that everyone has abnormal findings on MRI—having a perfect back is nearly impossible. Let your surgeon look at your MRI and work through what is important and what is not. Most herniations discovered on an MRI are asymptomatic. In fact, larger herniations that are impressive on MRI may actually resolve faster than smaller ones (6).

Terminology

There is a tremendous amount of jargon that doctors use to talk to each other about the specific shape and location of the herniated disc. The jargon can be confusing and is used to discuss information that is mostly more detailed than patients need to know.

The most important term to understand is **herniation**, which implies that disc material is displaced or pushes out beyond the intervertebral disc space (7). A disc herniation may also be referred to as a **disc fragment**. A disc "bulge" is different. Technically it is just "tissue extending beyond the vertebral ring" and is NOT a herniation, as all discs have a varying degree of bulging. A disc herniation tends to be focal (that is, occurring in one part of the circumference of the disc, changing its smooth contour) whereas a disc bulge is smooth. Disc herniations typically occur acutely (suddenly), whereas disc bulges are chronic (ongoing). Ultimately, even this distinction is not critical to understand. If it pushes on a nerve, whether it's a disc bulge or herniation it will still cause pain.

The outer layer of the disc, the annulus, is commonly described in MRI reports as "torn" or "fissured." This occurs when there is separation between annular fibers or between the annulus and the bone. The term "tear" is generally misleading as it suggests an acute trauma is the cause of the herniation when, in fact, that is commonly not the case. Tears can frequently be the result of degeneration.

Once the disc is herniated there are several descriptive terms to describe what the shape of the disc is. A **disc protrusion** just means the herniation is wider than it is tall, and a **disc extrusion** means the herniation is taller than it is wide. So, a disc extrusion extends more into the spinal canal than a protrusion. **Disc sequestration** occurs when the disc fragment is no longer attached to the original disc and exists on its own in the spinal canal. It is also possible for the disc to herniate directly into an adjacent vertebra (i.e., into the bone), instead of into the space between the vertebrae. A herniation that ends up in an adjacent vertebra instead of within the space between the vertebrae is known as a Schmorl's node. These nodes are common and are benign findings.

In the lumbar spine a disc herniation may also be described by its location. Central herniations occur directly in the center of the spinal canal, while paracentral disc herniations are off to the side (more lateral). The disc herniation may be so lateral as to occur in the neural foramen (where the nerve root exits the spine). Those are called appropriately far lateral disc herniations.

Treatment

The majority of disc herniations will resolve on their own, and thus treatment is primarily non-surgical and aimed at getting through the painful period and on to healing. Oral steroids are the first line treatment for acute disc herniations as they can reduce the inflammation caused by disc herniations. Epidural steroids can also be used which deliver a high dose of steroid directly into the area of herniation. These injections do not treat the disc herniation itself but do help reduce inflammation which can dramatically decrease your pain and at least allow you to think straight. Physical therapy in addition to steroids may be helpful, but a recent randomized, controlled trial showed it was no better than injection alone (8).

Advanced therapies such as platelet rich plasma, stem cells and gene therapy are all being studied, but at the time of this writing not clinically indicated for the treatment of disc herniations (3).

When is Surgery Indicated?

The only absolute indications for surgery are progressive motor function loss (steadily losing ability to control one's movements), and loss of control of the bowel and bladder. However, when the above-mentioned treatments fail, a discectomy surgery may be indicated for patients with severe pain after 6 weeks of symptoms. Typically, surgeons wait at least six weeks before considering surgery to ensure the disc isn't going to get better on its own and to give non-surgical treatment a fair shot. In the lumbar spine the most common procedure is called a microdiscectomy and in the cervical spine, a microforaminotomy. Both these procedures are minimally invasive, that is, disturb very little tissue, increasing the ease of recovery. You can read more about these procedures in other chapters, including chapter 39 which describes microdiscectomies and chapter 44 which discusses foraminotomies.

The SPORT trial was a randomized, controlled trial that looked at patients who had had 6 weeks of conservative care and were still in pain. The study compared those patients who went on to have surgery to those who simply continued their conservative therapy and found that those treated with surgery had a faster recovery with less disability (8). In some severe cases, earlier surgery may be indicated because the pain can be so extreme.

Conclusion

Disc herniations are perhaps one of the most common problems spine surgeons treat in their clinics. Herniated discs are striking not only for how much pain they can cause, but also for how they usually resolve with conservative care such as pain medication, anti-inflammatories, epidural injections, and physical therapy. Surgery may be necessary if you continue to experience symptoms after at least 6 weeks of non-operative treatment.

Frequently Asked Questions

- **Will I need surgery to deal with my disc herniation?**

    In almost 9 out of 10 cases cervical and lumbar disc herniations resolve on their own, requiring only non-operative treatment of the symptoms.

References

1.   Martirosyan NL, Patel AA, Carotenuto A, Kalani MYS, Belykh E, Walker CT, et al. Genetic Alterations in Intervertebral Disc Disease. Front Surg [Internet]. 2016 Nov 21 [cited 2021 Jun 4];3. Available from: http://journal.frontiersin.org/article/10.3389/fsurg.2016.00059/full

2.   Battié MC, Haynor DR, Fisher LD, Gill K, Gibbons LE, Videman T. Similarities in degenerative findings on magnetic resonance images of the lumbar spines of identical twins. J Bone Joint Surg Am. 1995 Nov;77(11):1662–70.

3.   Benzakour T, Igoumenou V, Mavrogenis AF, Benzakour A. Current concepts for lumbar disc herniation. Int Orthop. 2019 Apr;43(4):841–51.

4.   Sun Z, Zheng X, Li S, Zeng B, Yang J, Ling Z, et al. Single Impact Injury of Vertebral Endplates Without Structural Disruption, Initiates Disc Degeneration Through Piezo1 Mediated Inflammation and Metabolism Dysfunction. Spine. 2022 Mar 1;47(5):E203–13.

5.   Gregory DS, Seto CK, Wortley GC, Shugart CM. Acute lumbar disk pain: navigating evaluation and treatment choices. Am Fam Physician. 2008;78(7):835–42.

6.   Rhee JM, Schaufele M, Abdu WA. Radiculopathy and the herniated lumbar disc. Controversies regarding pathophysiology and management. J Bone Joint Surg Am. 2006 Sep;88(9):2070–80.

7.   Fardon DF, Williams AL, Dohring EJ, Murtagh FR, Gabriel Rothman SL, Sze GK. Lumbar disc nomenclature: version 2.0. Spine J. 2014 Nov;14(11):2525–45.

8.   Thackeray A, Fritz JM, Brennan GP, Zaman FM, Willick SE. A Pilot Study Examining the Effectiveness of Physical Therapy as an Adjunct to Selective Nerve Root Block in the Treatment of Lumbar Radicular Pain From Disk Herniation: A Randomized Controlled Trial. Phys Ther. 2010 Dec 1;90(12):1717–29.

Figures:

Types of Disc Herniations

Disc protrusion: disc herniation width is greater than depth into the spinal canal

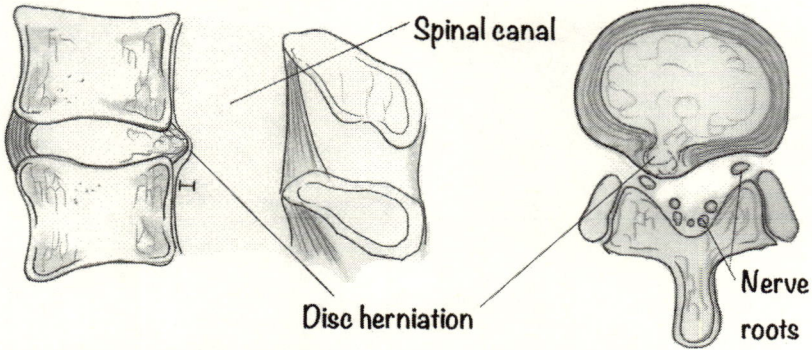

Spinal canal

Disc herniation

Nerve roots

Disc extrusion: disc herniation width is smaller than depth into the spinal canal

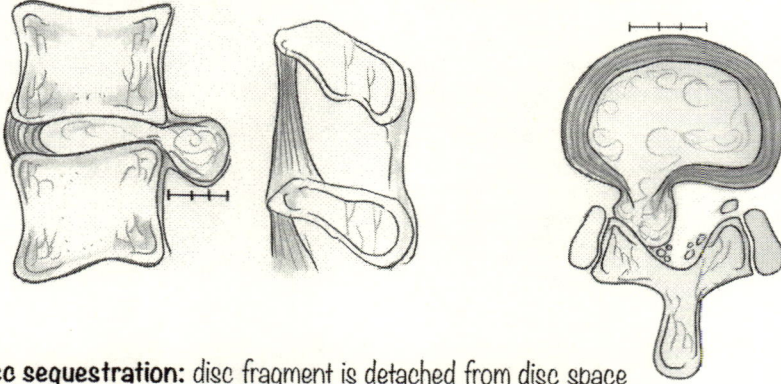

Disc sequestration: disc fragment is detached from disc space

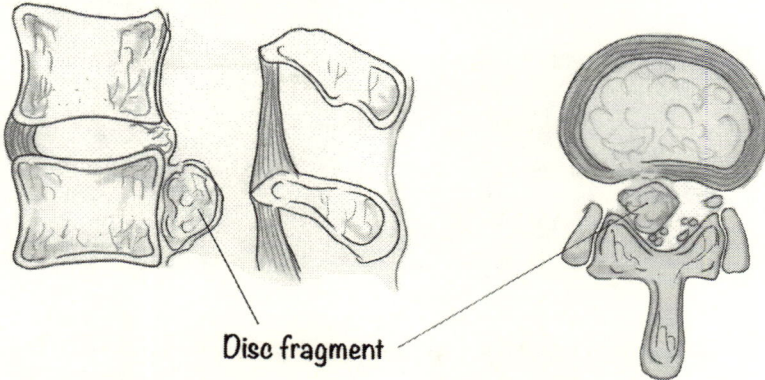

Disc fragment

Disc herniations. Disc herniations come in many shapes and sizes. On the left we have cross sections of the vertebrae and disc in the sagittal plane (front to back) and on the right cross sections in the axial plane (cutting across). We can see how the disc herniations can extend out of the intervertebral disc space in different ways. When the size of herniation from front to back is smaller than it is from side to side it is called a protrusion (top). When it is larger from front to back than side to side it is called an extrusion (middle). When the disc fragment becomes separated from the disc space itself it is known as a sequestration (bottom).

Disc Herniations

Normal Disc:

Annulus fibrosis: the tough outer casing of the disc

Nucleus pulposus: jelly-like inner core of the disc

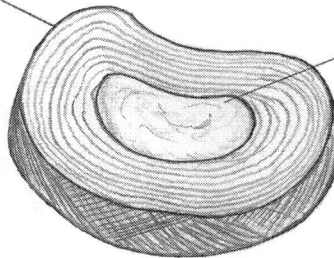

Herniated Disc:

A tear in the annulus fibrosis allows the nucleus pulposus to herniate out

Nucleus pulposus disc fragment

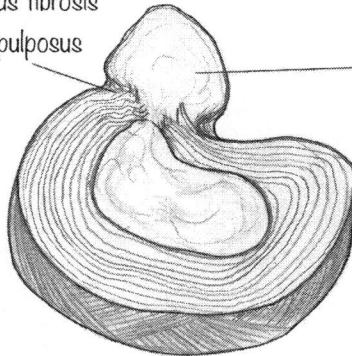

Normal Disc in Cross Section:

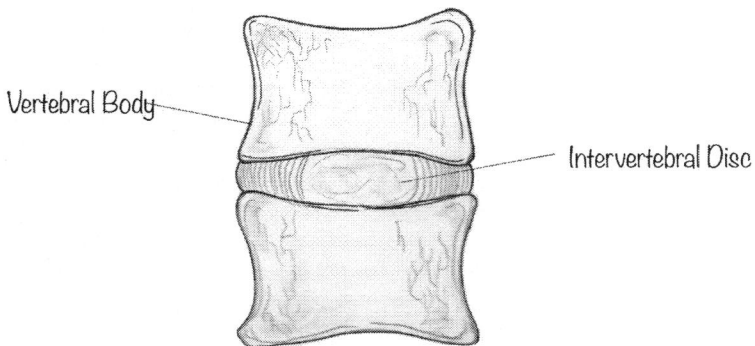

Vertebral Body

Intervertebral Disc

Lumbar Disc. A lumbar disc is composed of a tough outer ring called the annulus fibrosis and an inner jelly portion called the nucleus pulposus (top). When a fissure or tear occurs in the annulus, the nucleus material herniates outward (middle). The disc seen in cross section (bottom).

Spinal Radicular Pain Patterns

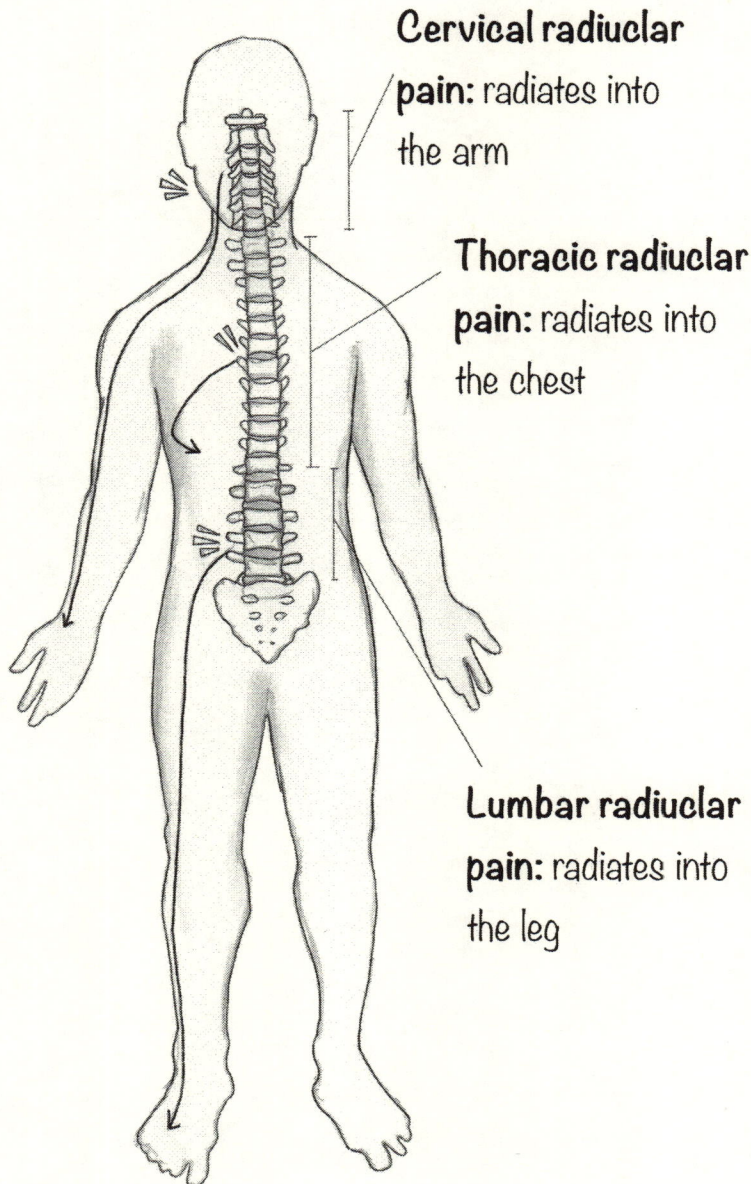

Cervical radiuclar pain: radiates into the arm

Thoracic radiuclar pain: radiates into the chest

Lumbar radiuclar pain: radiates into the leg

Spinal Radicular Pain Patterns. Disc herniations in different areas of the spine cause different symptoms. Cervical disc herniations tend to cause pain radiating into the arm, while lumbar disc herniations cause pain traveling into the leg.

Different Kinds of Stenosis

Foraminal Stenosis:

Central Stenosis:

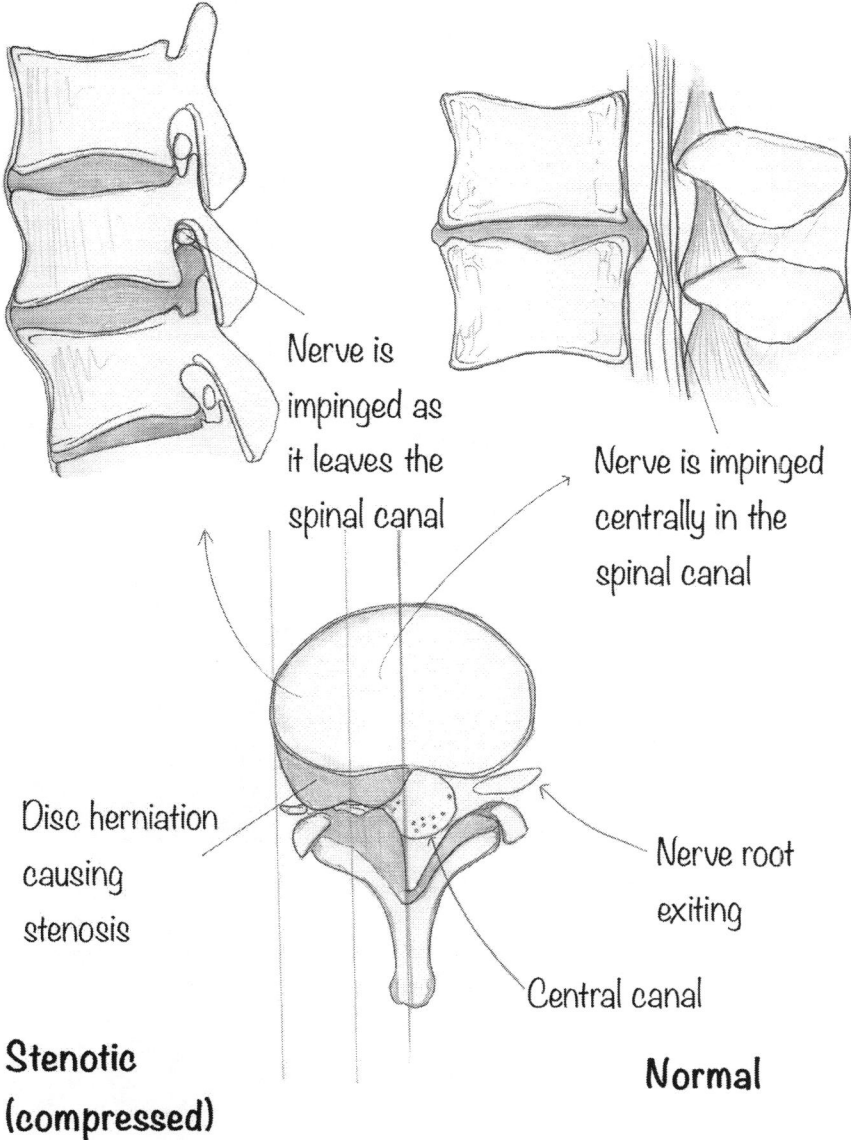

Nerve is impinged as it leaves the spinal canal

Nerve is impinged centrally in the spinal canal

Disc herniation causing stenosis

Nerve root exiting

Central canal

Stenotic (compressed)

Normal

Different Kinds of Stenosis. A disc herniation can pinch a nerve as it exits the spine through the foramen (foraminal stenosis) or inside the spinal canal (central stenosis). On the top left we see a sagittal (side view) cross section of the lumbar spine and a disc herniation pinching the nerve. On the top right we see a central cross section showing the lumbar spine with a disc causing central stenosis. The bottom image is an axial cross section (cutting across) showing how the spinal canal looks normally (on the right) and with a disc herniation (on the left).

Chapter 8

Lumbar Stenosis and Spondylolisthesis

Summary

Degenerative lumbar (low back) stenosis is a very common problem as we get older. Stenosis just means that the spinal canal is constricted and that the nerves are pinched. Stenosis may vary in degree from mild (not very tight) to severe or extreme (very tight and totally choking the nerves). Nonetheless, just because the spinal canal is stenotic does not mean the patient will have symptoms. Spinal stenosis goes hand in hand with spondylolisthesis (one vertebra slips over another), which can cause further narrowing of the spinal canal. Stenosis can be asymptomatic, but when it does act up generally causes pain shooting down the legs, leg tiredness, and cramping, collectively known as neurogenic claudication. When stenosis becomes symptomatic, surgery is generally superior to non-operative treatment and can be accomplished with a laminectomy decompression. Sometimes a spinal fusion may be necessary to treat stenosis caused by spondylolisthesis.

Case

Mrs. Plum is a 70-year-old gardener who just wants to enjoy her years of retirement. For the past year or so she notes that whenever she stands her legs go numb and become weak. Moreover, she has pain in her calves that seems to get worse with every step she takes. This significantly limits her walking capacity and the only relief she gets is when she lies down flat. Her primary care doctor recommends an MRI, which shows she has severe lumbar stenosis with a slipped vertebra (a spondylolisthesis) at L4-5. She comes to see me, and I examine her spondylolisthesis more closely. X-rays taken as she bends reveal the slipped vertebra gets worse when she moves. Based on all available information, I decide to perform a lumbar fusion and decompression. She does well with surgery and her leg pain and walking capacity are dramatically improved. Her back hurts for a while from the surgical pain, but this resolves within 6 weeks and now, a year from surgery, she is walking more than her husband who can no longer keep up.

Introduction

Lumbar stenosis is the medical term for a narrowing of the spinal canal in the low back region. This may or may not result in painful compression of the nerve roots. Think of it as having a clogged pipe where water can no longer flow because of an obstruction. In this case the water is the information flowing through the nerves to the extremities and back. Lumbar spondylolisthesis (a common cause of lumbar stenosis) occurs when one vertebra slips forward on another. As discussed in previous chapters (chapter 3 on low back pain) lumbar stenosis and spondylolisthesis are very common problems. Lumbar stenosis is the most common reason for spine surgery in adults greater than 65 years in age (1).

How Does Stenosis Occur?

Lumbar stenosis can occur in three areas in the spine: the central spinal canal (central stenosis), beneath the facet joints that connect adjacent vertebrae to each other (lateral recess stenosis) and in the neuroforamina, which are the holes where nerve roots exit from the spine (foraminal stenosis). All can result in symptomatic nerve impingement causing pain, numbness, and weakness down the leg (radiculopathy) or neurogenic claudication.

Degeneration is by far the most common cause of symptomatic stenosis.
To understand how degenerative stenosis can occur, keep in mind that the spine is composed of functional segments which consist of two vertebrae and an intervertebral (between two vertebrae) disc. Each functional segment is linked

together by three joints: the intervertebral disc (which is considered a special type of cartilaginous joint) and the two facet joints. Any instability or damage to one of these joints can alter the function of the other joints (think of a tricycle with a single flat tire—now the other two tires will function abnormally and be prone to damage). The degenerative process typically begins with some remote minor trauma and can take decades to become symptomatic. The intervertebral disc, which serves as the cushion between vertebral bones, is composed of a tough outer ring and a soft jelly-like center, which resists compressive loads.

As you age the disc becomes stiff, making it more prone to tears and herniations. Over time, because of cumulative trauma, the disc material herniates, gradually breaks down (resorbs) and the disc deflates, causing the vertebral bones to come into direct contact. This contact pressure, in turn, produces bone spurs that encroach on the spinal canal, causing it to narrow. Moreover, with the disc deflated, its casing can now push into the spinal canal and, additionally, the posterior ligamentum flavum (which connects the laminae of adjacent vertebrae) is likely to buckle into the canal, resulting in further narrowing. That is one way that a herniated disc can lead to stenosis over time.

Joint wear and tear in the vertebral segment can also lead to stenosis. The facet joints function like any other joint in the body and have articular cartilage to allow smooth gliding. This cartilage can degenerate, break, and lead to bone-on-bone wear which can generate bone spurs and loose fragments. As mentioned above, the bone spurs can crowd the spinal canal and cause stenosis.

Also, as the facet joints and intervertebral disc degenerate, the spinal segment loses its tautness, making it possible for one vertebra to slip on another (spondylolisthesis). Keep in mind that vertebrae are essentially bony rings which form a tunnel known as the spinal canal through which the nerves pass. Spondylolisthesis also results in a narrowing of the spinal canal since the rings that the nerves pass through are no longer in alignment. This shift or slip can be forward (anterolisthesis) or posterior (retrolisthesis). Anterolisthesis tends to be a common problem, while retrolisthesis is typically just an X-ray finding with no symptoms. As stated above, the most common cause of stenosis is the degenerative process described above; but it can also result from anything which takes up space in the spinal canal including bony fragments from trauma, abscess from infection and tumor.

Some patients also have so called congenitally narrow canals (meaning they were born with a narrower spinal canal) and thus can display symptoms of lumbar stenosis earlier in life compared to standard degenerative stenosis (2).

As the stenosis progresses, not only do nerves become pinched, but the arteries which supply the nerves become blocked and the veins which allow blood to drain from the area become engorged (3,4). Interestingly, not all patients who have stenosis have symptoms. Depending on how fast and severe the process of stenosis is, the nerves may become used to it.

Symptoms

A symptom called **neurogenic claudication**—or pain that radiates to the buttocks and legs bilaterally (on both sides)— is the most common problem that occurs with lumbar stenosis. The word claudication comes from the Latin *claudicare*, meaning "to limp." This pain typically gets worse with walking, and with any bending backwards and is relieved with sitting, bending forward and lying flat. Neurologic symptoms such as numbness and weakness in the lower extremities also commonly occurs. Many complain "my legs feel heavy" or "my legs feel dead." This can greatly limit your ability to walk long distances (5).

Back pain can also be a common complaint of lumbar stenosis and may be present in up to 20% of cases (6). Back pain occurs with standing and walking. This is often relieved with leaning forward, such as leaning over a grocery cart. This is because this motion opens the spinal canal, decreasing the severity of the stenosis. However, over time this can become unbearable because of the strain it places on the back muscles.

Treatment of Lumbar Stenosis

Unlike lumbar disc herniations, which may resolve on their own, lumbar stenosis generally does not improve with non-operative treatment. However, symptoms and neurologic function also do not generally worsen dramatically (7). Patients often ask, "If I don't do the surgery, are there any risks?" to which I usually answer no. The exception to this is when the stenosis is causing a problem that will worsen over time, for example, foot drop; then the sooner the nerve is decompressed, the better the chance of improvement (8). Thus, the decision to proceed with **surgery** is guided by the severity of symptoms and the patient's current lifestyle. While there is typically no urgency to do surgery, waiting for the symptoms to improve spontaneously is usually disappointing. Nonetheless, a trial of conservative therapy (physical therapy, injections, and non-steroidal anti-inflammatories) is the best first-line therapy.

Lumbar epidural steroid injections require a small needle to be placed—under X-ray guidance—into the spinal canal, typically either by a pain physician, a physiatrist, or a spine surgeon. Some patients say lumbar epidurals have helped them; however, in a small randomized, controlled trial of patients with lumbar stenosis, a steroid injection was compared to a placebo and no significant difference was found (9). I think this is primarily because there is less inflammation associated with lumbar stenosis than with a disc herniation, and thus the steroids are not as useful. However, injecting numbing medicine into the affected area can help confirm the diagnosis if there is temporary resolution of pain.

Should I Have Surgery to Treat Lumbar Stenosis?

Lumbar stenosis has been extremely well studied and there have been several large randomized, controlled trials (RCT) looking at how effective surgery is. Randomized studies in surgery are difficult, because you cannot blind a patient to the treatment they receive. They either get surgery or they don't, and both have psychological effects that could impact the ultimate outcome. Furthermore, the length of follow up is important after a study to see how long lasting the effects of surgery are. What follows below are what I think of as the best evidence we have comparing surgery to non-operative care in lumbar stenosis.

In the Maine Lumbar Spine Study surgical treatment of lumbar stenosis was compared to non-operative treatment and patients were followed for over 4 years. Going into the study, the surgical patients were worse off, being less mobile and experiencing more pain than their counterparts who, going into the study, had received only non-operative treatment for their lumbar stenoses. After 4 years, 70% of surgically treated patients reported improvement in their pain, while only 52% of non-op patients reported any improvement (10). In a 10-year follow-up, roughly 40% of the patients initially treated non-operatively later decided to undergo surgery. Although surgery was helpful it's important to keep in mind 23% in the operative group had undergone a second lumbar surgery during the first 4 years of follow-up—meaning that it may take more than one procedure to ensure success (11).

In the Finnish Lumbar Spinal Research Group's randomized, controlled trial comparing decompression surgery to non-operative management, surgery resulted in superior outcomes at 2 years (12).

Probably the best known RCT on this topic is the SPORT study (Spine Patient Outcomes Research Trial) which compared surgery to non-operative treatment. In the SPORT study, outcomes in the surgically treated group were significantly superior to non-operative treatment (13). Finally, an older study only tracking surgical patients reported a significant amount with low back pain (1/3) at 10 years of follow-up (14).

A common saying among spine surgeons is that you cannot use spine surgery to treat stenosis and expect the back pain to improve. This is probably because spine surgery hurts your back and gives you back pain, at least temporarily. It is thus thought that decompression surgery is generally effective to treat leg and buttock pain, but may worsen your back pain (again, at least temporarily). However, recently there is more evidence that decompression surgery is effective for the treatment of back pain resulting from stenosis and that it is possible for low back pain to improve after spine surgery. Several large studies such as the Canadian Spine Outcomes Research Network (CSORN) study, as well as the SPORT study, showed significant improvement in low back pain following decompression surgery (15,16). Walking capacity may also improve following decompression for lumbar stenosis (17,18). Patients who have been suffering with pain for a long time, who smoke cigarettes, and are experiencing a high level of medical comorbidities such as diabetes, may have worse surgical outcomes (19).

Other therapies for treating lumbar spinal stenosis are available (Koflex® and X-Stop®) and are discussed separately in the chapter on interspinous spacers, but long-term data are not available.

Treatment of Lumbar Stenosis with Spondylolisthesis

Armed with a basic knowledge of lumbar stenosis, let's discuss its close relative, **lumbar spondylolisthesis**. Again, as with lumbar stenosis, once you are experiencing symptoms with lumbar spondylolisthesis, non-operative treatment will generally not produce as favorable results as surgical treatment. In the SPORT study patient-reported outcome results of surgical treatments (decompression or decompression + fusion) were superior to continued non-operative treatment up to 8 years (20).

The main question, though, is not whether surgery should be used to treat spondylolisthesis, but should the spine be fused as part of the treatment or just decompressed. With fusion we surgically join two adjacent vertebrae with rods, screws, and bone graft (see the chapter 37 and 41 on spinal fusion). Decompression alone can provide symptom relief if the slipped vertebra remains stable (that is, one vertebra is not moving relative to one another). Degenerative spondylolisthesis is progressive (that is, the slip worsens over time) in only 30% of cases and thus the majority are stable (21). But if the slipped vertebra is not stable, a fusion can prevent progression from occurring, because fusion rigidly fixes the vertebrae together permanently. Determining the overall stability of the spinal segment is critical in making the decision. Your surgeon will use radiographs and MRIs, typically with you bending forward and backward looking for motion at the segment, to help her or him make this decision. There are also clinical signs of instability such as back pain that occurs with standing and loading of the spine. If the segment is unstable, fusion is usually a more reasonable choice (22).

However, in cases of low-grade stable spondylolisthesis (where the slippage is less than 50%), I usually tell patients that while a fusion provides a theoretical increase in durability compared to decompression alone (fusion stops further degeneration), there are increased short-term and long-term complications that can happen when you add a fusion surgery to a simple decompression (23). Decompression alone is also easier to perform than a decompression + fusion, is better tolerated by the patient, takes less time and has shorter hospital stays (24). As a result, some spine surgeons may favor decompression alone.

In the Swedish Spinal Study, a randomized controlled trial comparing decompression alone to decompression + fusion found no significant difference between the two procedures up to 5 years post op (25). However, instability of the spine was not accounted for in this study. In contrast, the later SLIP (Spinal Laminectomy versus Instrumented Pedicle Screw) trial, which compared fusion+ decompression to decompression alone, showed both greater improvement in outcomes scores and higher reoperation rates in the group undergoing decompression alone over 4 years. This was likely since about 1/3 of patients in the laminectomy group developed significant instability after a laminectomy and eventually required fusion surgery. However, when using minimally invasive techniques, decompression alone has been shown to give durable results with less reoperation than decompression + fusion up to 5 years after surgery (26).

Ultimately the decision to have a spinal fusion is one your spine surgeon must make. There are many technical nuances which will push a surgeon towards decompression + fusion versus decompression alone. Furthermore, some patients may not even be able to tolerate a fusion surgery. This chapter was designed to help you understand how this decision is made, but, regardless, both decompression and decompression + fusion are effective treatments for stenosis.

Conclusion

Degenerative lumbar stenosis and spondylolisthesis go hand in hand and differ significantly from lumbar disc herniations (although herniations can also cause stenosis). While herniations have a large inflammatory component that is acutely painful, degenerative stenosis primarily causes symptoms that result from mechanical pressure on the nerves that accumulates over time. In cases of symptomatic lumbar stenosis, surgery is generally recommended and typically results in superior outcomes compared to non-operative treatment. There is no medicine or treatment which can magically open the spinal canal once it has a certain degree of stenosis.

Frequently Asked Questions

- **Will a TENS (transcutaneous electrical nerve stimulation) unit be helpful?**

    There is not any scientific evidence that this is useful, but it's fairly harmless to try (27).

- **Will the timing of surgery affect my recovery?**

Studies show that in the case of lumbar stenosis and spondylolisthesis, the longer you have symptoms before you undergo surgery, the less your symptoms will be helped by the surgery. In fact, symptoms ongoing for greater than 1 year may diminish the improvement one experiences from surgery (28–30). Nonetheless, the decision for surgery should be made carefully and not be rushed.

- **I have multilevel stenosis—do I need every level decompressed?**

Not necessarily. Symptoms may be related to a single compressed segment. This is a complicated decision your surgeon will help you make (31).

- **Will my back pain improve after surgery?**

It's difficult to treat back pain because so many factors cause and influence it (32). Stenosis can cause back pain and this can improve with surgery; however, it can be unpredictable (16).

- **Will my age prevent me from having surgery?**

In a large study comparing patients older than 65 to those less than 65 years of age, patients in both age groups reported similar improvements following their fusion + decompression procedures. In fact, the older patients had more to gain from surgery and showed higher improvement in patient-reported outcome scores (33).

References

1.   Ciol MA, Deyo RA, Howell E, Kreif S. An assessment of surgery for spinal stenosis: time trends, geographic variations, complications, and reoperations. J Am Geriatr Soc. 1996 Mar;44(3):285–90.

2.   Kirkaldy-Willis WH, Wedge JH, Yong-Hing K, Reilly J. Pathology and pathogenesis of lumbar spondylosis and stenosis. Spine. 1978 Dec;3(4):319–28.

3.   Rydevik B, Brown MD, Lundborg G. Pathoanatomy and pathophysiology of nerve root compression. Spine. 1984 Feb;9(1):7–15.

4.   Rydevik B, Lundborg G, Bagge U. Effects of graded compression on intraneural blood flow. J Hand Surg. 1981 Jan;6(1):3–12.

5.   Tomkins CC, Battié MC, Rogers T, Jiang H, Petersen S. A Criterion Measure of Walking Capacity in Lumbar Spinal Stenosis and Its Comparison With a Treadmill Protocol: Spine. 2009 Oct;34(22):2444–9.

6.   Kalichman L, Cole R, Kim DH, Li L, Suri P, Guermazi A, et al. Spinal stenosis prevalence and association with symptoms: the Framingham Study. Spine J. 2009 Jul;9(7):545–50.

7.   Simotas AC, Dorey FJ, Hansraj KK, Cammisa F. Nonoperative Treatment for Lumbar Spinal Stenosis. :8.

8.   Guigui P, Benoist M, Delecourt C, Delhoume J, Deburge A. Motor deficit in lumbar spinal stenosis: a retrospective study of a series of 50 patients. J Spinal Disord. 1998 Aug;11(4):283–8.

9.   Cuckler JM, Bernini PA, Wiesel SW, Booth RE, Rothman RH, Pickens GT. The use of epidural steroids in the treatment of lumbar radicular pain. A prospective, randomized, double-blind study. J Bone Joint Surg Am. 1985 Jan;67(1):63–6.

10.   Atlas SJ, Keller RB, Robson D, Deyo RA, Singer DE. Surgical and nonsurgical management of lumbar spinal stenosis: four-year outcomes from the maine lumbar spine study. Spine. 2000 Mar 1;25(5):556–62.

11.   Atlas SJ, Keller RB, Wu YA, Deyo RA, Singer DE. Long-Term Outcomes of Surgical and Nonsurgical Management of Lumbar Spinal Stenosis: 8 to 10 Year Results from the Maine Lumbar Spine Study. :8.

12.   Malmivaara A, Slätis P, Heliövaara M, Sainio P, Kinnunen H, Kankare J, et al. Surgical or Nonoperative Treatment for Lumbar Spinal Stenosis?: A Randomized Controlled Trial. Spine. 2007 Jan;32(1):1–8.

13.   Weinstein JN, Tosteson TD, Lurie JD, Tosteson ANA, Blood E, Hanscom B, et al. Surgical versus nonsurgical therapy for lumbar spinal stenosis. N Engl J Med. 2008 Feb 21;358(8):794–810.

14.   Katz JN, Harris MB. Lumbar spinal stenosis. N Engl J Med. 2008;358(8):818–25.

15.   Lurie JD, Tosteson TD, Tosteson ANA, Zhao W, Morgan TS, Abdu WA, et al. Surgical Versus Nonoperative Treatment for Lumbar Disc Herniation: Eight-Year Results for the Spine Patient Outcomes Research Trial. Spine. 2014 Jan;39(1):3–16.

16.   Srinivas S, Paquet J, Bailey C, Nataraj A, Stratton A, Johnson M, et al. Effect of spinal decompression on back pain in lumbar spinal stenosis: a Canadian Spine Outcomes Research Network (CSORN) study. Spine J. 2019 Jun;19(6):1001–8.

17.   Deen HG, Zimmerman RS, Lyons MK, McPhee MC, Verheijde JL, Lemens SM. Use of the exercise treadmill to measure baseline functional status and surgical outcome in patients with severe lumbar spinal stenosis. Spine. 1998 Jan 15;23(2):244–8.

18.   Budithi S, Dhawan R, Cattell A, Balain B, Jaffray D. Only walking matters—assessment following lumbar stenosis decompression. Eur Spine J. 2017 Feb;26(2):481–7.

19.   Paulsen RT, Bouknaitir JB, Fruensgaard S, Carreon L, Andersen M. Prognostic

Factors for Satisfaction After Decompression Surgery for Lumbar Spinal Stenosis. Neurosurgery. 2018 May 1;82(5):645–51.

20.   Abdu WA, Sacks OA, Tosteson ANA, Zhao W, Tosteson TD, Morgan TS, et al. Long-Term Results of Surgery Compared With Nonoperative Treatment for Lumbar Degenerative Spondylolisthesis in the Spine Patient Outcomes Research Trial (SPORT). Spine. 2018 Dec 1;43(23):1619–30.

21.   Matsunaga S, Sakou T, Morizono Y, Masuda A, Demirtas AM. Natural history of degenerative spondylolisthesis. Pathogenesis and natural course of the slippage. Spine. 1990 Nov;15(11):1204–10.

22.   Yone K, Sakou T, Kawauchi Y, Yamaguchi M, Yanase M. Indication of fusion for lumbar spinal stenosis in elderly patients and its significance. Spine. 1996 Jan 15;21(2):242–8.

23.   Yavin D, Casha S, Wiebe S, Feasby TE, Clark C, Isaacs A, et al. Lumbar Fusion for Degenerative Disease: A Systematic Review and Meta-Analysis. Neurosurgery. 2017 May 1;80(5):701–15.

24.   Chen Z, Xie P, Feng F, Chhantyal K, Yang Y, Rong L. Decompression Alone Versus Decompression and Fusion for Lumbar Degenerative Spondylolisthesis: A Meta-Analysis. World Neurosurg. 2018 Mar;111:e165–77.

25.   Försth P, Ólafsson G, Carlsson T, Frost A, Borgström F, Fritzell P, et al. A Randomized, Controlled Trial of Fusion Surgery for Lumbar Spinal Stenosis. N Engl J Med. 2016 Apr 14;374(15):1413–23.

26.   Kuo CC, Merchant M, Kardile MP, Yacob A, Majid K, Bains RS. In Degenerative Spondylolisthesis, Unilateral Laminotomy for Bilateral Decompression Leads to Less Reoperations at 5 Years When Compared to Posterior Decompression With Instrumented Fusion: A Propensity-matched Retrospective Analysis. SPINE. 2019 Nov;44(21):1530–7.

27.   Kreiner DS, Shaffer WO, Baisden JL, Gilbert TJ, Summers JT, Toton JF, et al. An evidence-based clinical guideline for the diagnosis and treatment of degenerative lumbar spinal stenosis (update). Spine J. 2013 Jul;13(7):734–43.

28.   Cushnie D, Thomas K, Jacobs WB, Cho RKH, Soroceanu A, Ahn H, et al. Effect of preoperative symptom duration on outcome in lumbar spinal stenosis: a Canadian Spine Outcomes and Research Network registry study. Spine J. 2019 Sep;19(9):1470–7.

29.   Radcliff KE, Rihn J, Hilibrand A, DiIorio T, Tosteson T, Lurie JD, et al. Does the Duration of Symptoms in Patients With Spinal Stenosis and Degenerative Spondylolisthesis Affect Outcomes?: Analysis of the Spine Outcomes Research Trial. Spine. 2011 Dec;36(25):2197–210.

30.   Jönsson B, Annertz M, Sjöberg C, Strömqvist B. A prospective and consecutive study of surgically treated lumbar spinal stenosis. Part II: Five-year follow-up by an independent observer. Spine. 1997 Dec 15;22(24):2938–44.

31.   Ulrich NH, Burgstaller JM, Held U, Winklhofer S, Farshad M, Pichierri G, et al.

The Influence of Single-level Versus Multilevel Decompression on the Outcome in Multisegmental Lumbar Spinal Stenosis: Analysis of the Lumbar Spinal Outcome Study (LSOS) Data. Clin Spine Surg. 2017 Dec;30(10):E1367–75.

32.   Chou R, Baisden J, Carragee EJ, Resnick DK, Shaffer WO, Loeser JD. Surgery for Low Back Pain: A Review of the Evidence for an American Pain Society Clinical Practice Guideline. Spine. 2009 May;34(10):1094–109.

33.   Glassman SD, Carreon L, Dimar JR. Outcome of Lumbar Arthrodesis in Patients Sixty-five Years of Age or Older: J Bone Jt Surg-Am Vol. 2010 Mar;92(Suppl 1):77–84.

Figures:

Lumbar Stenosis

A normal cross section of a disc space:

Lumbar vertebra

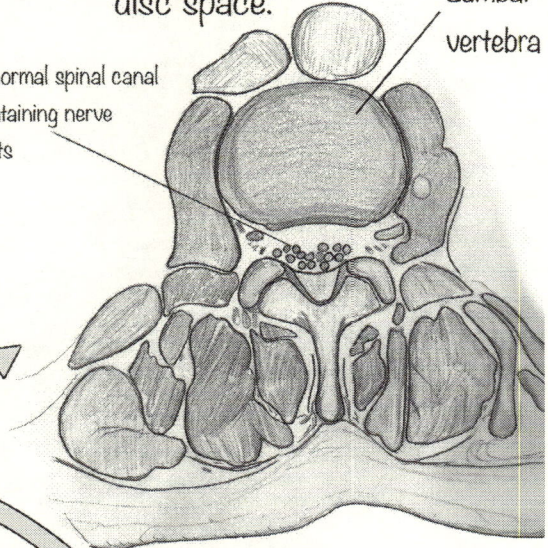

A normal spinal canal containing nerve roots

MRI Cross section of the lumbar spine:

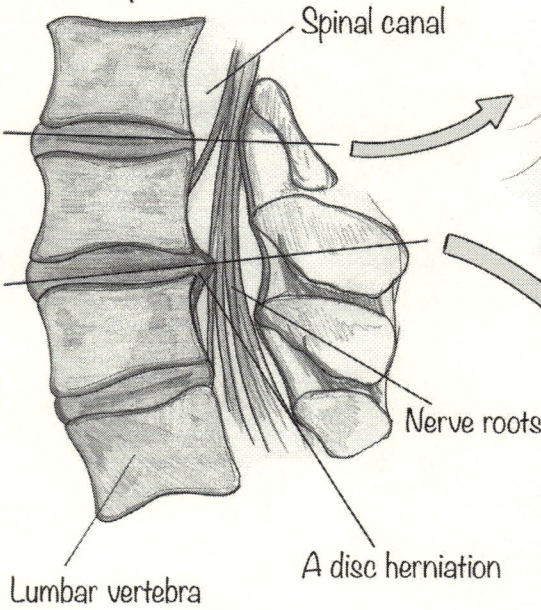

Spinal canal

Nerve roots

A disc herniation

Lumbar vertebra

A disc herniation causes stenosis:

A disc herniation compresses the nerve roots

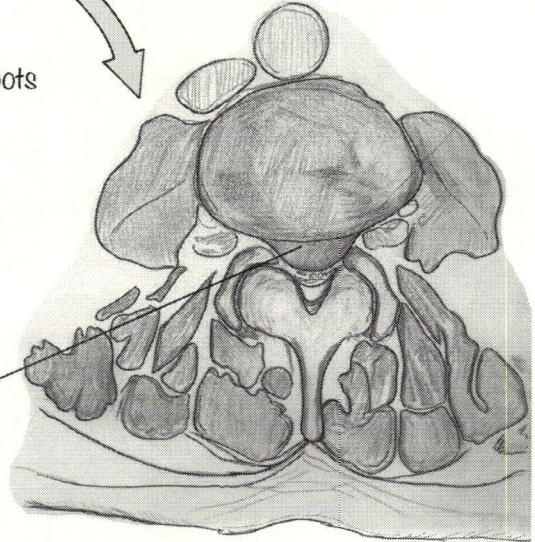

Lumbar stenosis MRI. A representative image of a normal lumbar MRI cross-sectional segment (top) and a segment that has stenosis because of a disc herniation (bottom) where we can see the nerves are being compressed.

Lumbar Degeneration and Spondylolisthesis

Normal: vertebra viewed from the side:

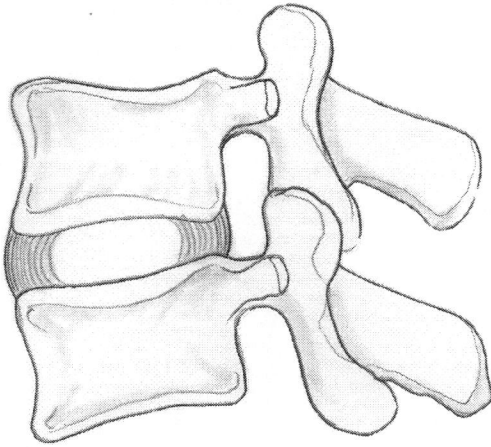

Vertebrae viewed from above:

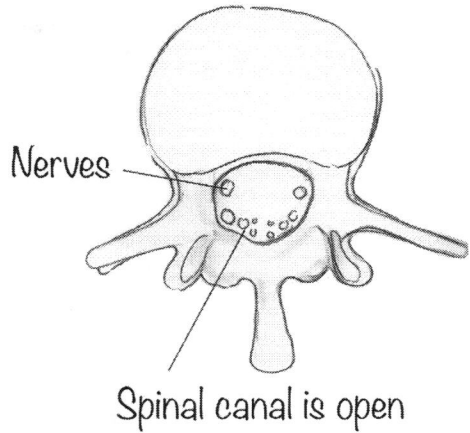

Nerves

Spinal canal is open

Disc degeneration results in a forward slip of the vertebra (called a spondylolisthesis, or slipped disc) that results in a narrowed canal

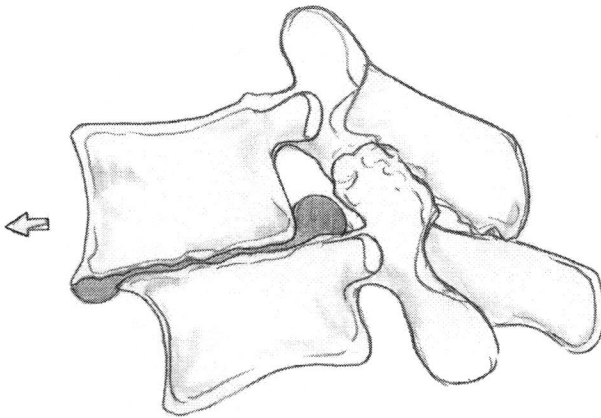

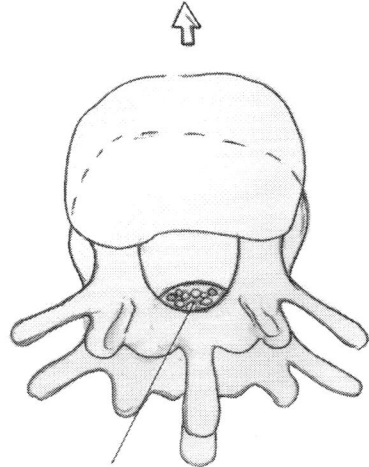

Spinal canal is narrowed causing compression of nerves

Spondylolisthesis dynamic. A normal lumbar segment (top). Spondylolisthesis occurs when the disc degenerates and loses its height causing the top vertebra to slide forward on the bottom vertebra, blocking the spinal canal and causing stenosis (bottom).

Chapter 9

Thoracic Spinal Cord Compression

Summary

Compression of the spinal cord in the thoracic region of the spine (upper back) is much less common than in the cervical spine because the thoracic spine is more rigid. Compression in the thoracic spine may be caused by disc herniations, calcifications, tumors, trauma, or infections. The symptoms of thoracic myelopathy (thoracic spinal cord compression) are like cervical myelopathy; however, the arms are typically spared. This is because the lesion causing the compression is downstream to the nerves of the arms. The legs can become weak and uncoordinated making falls common. Treatment is accomplished with decompression and fusion of the thoracic spine.

Case

Mr. Grey is a 75-year-old store owner who has had a long history of low back problems. He has had previous lumbar surgery. He has had weakness in his legs related to his lumbar spine problems in the past but recently he has noticed his legs just "do not seem to be working correctly." He feels as if "the connection

between his legs and his brains has been severed." A scan shows severe thoracic spinal cord compression around T10-11 literally cutting off neural supply to his legs. I perform a thoracic decompression and fusion, taking the pressure off the spinal cord. His symptoms improve to the point where he no longer needs walking aids.

Introduction

This chapter, which builds on the previous chapter on cervical spinal cord compression, discusses the specific issues associated with thoracic spinal cord compression. If you have not already done so, you will want to read chapter 5 before continuing here. Also, if you are interested in learning more about disc herniations check out chapter 7 which discusses disc herniations in some depth.

Thoracic spinal cord compression and thoracic myelopathy (the clinical syndrome resulting from thoracic spinal cord compression) are much less common than spinal cord compression of the cervical spine and account for less than 10% of spine surgery done for decompression. This is because the thoracic spinal cord is much more rigid than the cervical spine and thus is not as prone to wear and tear. Your cervical spine is mobile and allows you to look around in many planes. Your thoracic spine is lined by the ribs and provides a scaffold to hold the internal organs of the thorax.

Thoracic disc herniations are generally without symptoms (asymptomatic) and are often only discovered on MRI and CT scans. Because thoracic disc herniations are asymptomatic they rarely require surgical treatment. However, when the thoracic spinal cord becomes compressed because of a disc herniation, it can result in a myelopathic syndrome like cervical myelopathy and surgical treatment may be required. Since the nerves for your arms all exit from the neck, thoracic spinal cord myelopathy only affects the lower extremities.

What Causes Thoracic Spinal Cord Compression?

Obviously, tumors or major trauma causing bone fragments to invade the spinal canal can result in compression of the spinal cord. However, degenerative processes can also result in compression of the thoracic spinal cord. The most common causes are **ossification** (calcifying) of the two major ligaments around the thoracic spine—the ossification of the posterior longitudinal ligament (OPLL) and the ossification of the ligamentum flavum (OLF). Disc herniations may also cause thoracic spinal cord compression but this is much less common. Disc herniations in fact are a common normal finding in many people and rarely become symptomatic or require surgery (1).

Though the thoracic spinal cord is the largest portion of the spinal cord (1), this part of the spine does not move very much, so spinal compressions here are not as common.

Signs and Symptoms

Thoracic disc herniations are in most cases asymptomatic. If they do become symptomatic, they present with axial (mechanically related) back pain, that is, you feel the pain when you move in a certain way. Occasionally a thoracic disc herniation may cause pain to radiate across the ribs from compression of the intercostal nerves (the nerves supplying the spaces between the ribs). However, a nerve compression that causes pain but is without other symptoms usually doesn't require surgery and typically is managed conservatively. This is different from thoracic spinal cord compression which is described below.

Regardless of the causes of thoracic spinal cord compression, in most cases it takes years before the compression of the thoracic spinal cord becomes serious enough to cause symptoms and then the condition may resemble both cervical and lumbar compression. Most patients notice tingling and numbness of the lower extremities and even shooting pains. Because the spinal cord is affected, you may also notice that your gait is off or that you no longer have balance with your legs. It is possible to also have weakness of the legs. Unlike cervical myelopathy, your hands and upper extremities are spared, making the diagnosis sometimes more difficult. It is possible for myelopathy to occur rapidly. In that event severe gait disturbances and weakness are typically noted. In about 10-15% of cases, the bowel and bladder are affected and may result in incontinence. Because the symptoms of thoracic spinal cord compression are vague, they may not even be noticed by the patient until the symptoms become impossible to ignore.

The **diagnosis** is clinical (based on physical symptoms) but generally confirmed with advanced imaging of the spine including an MRI and a CT scan. CT scans are particularly useful in this part of the spine because many of the pathologies that cause thoracic compression occur due to calcification of the ligaments which are readily visible on CT scans.

Treatment

Thoracic disc degeneration alone rarely requires surgery and can be managed with physical therapy and pain medications. However, once the degeneration progresses to a point where there is significant spinal cord compression, the treatment is almost always surgical.

The standard treatment for thoracic myelopathy is surgical decompression and fusion. **Decompression** may consist of a laminectomy (removal of a lamina—the thin part of the vertebra on the backside of the vertebra) or hemilaminectomy (partial removal of a lamina) to remove the posterior portion of the vertebra and make space in the spinal canal. Unfortunately, there are no medical treatments for this problem, and it is imperative to relieve the pressure causing damage to the spinal cord.

Because the thoracic spine is rigid, **fusion** is used much more commonly than in the lumbar spine to prevent further break down and damage to the spinal cord. Spinal fusion uses surgery to attempt to get two bones to grow together by connecting them with metal rods and placing bone graft. Fusion is also more commonly used to protect the spinal cord from further damage or changes in alignment that may occur from laminectomy. This is because in a laminectomy, bone must be removed to make space in the spinal cord. Removing bone can have the effect of destabilizing that segment in the spine.

In some instances, such as when a thoracic disc herniation is causing the spinal compression, the safest way to access the spinal cord is with a side approach. In these cases where it is too dangerous to approach the spinal cord directly from the back, it may be necessary to either remove part of the rib and transverse process of the vertebra (a procedure known as a costotransversectomy) or to perform a thoracotomy (surgically creating a space in the rib area for viewing adjacent tissue). At other times the surgeon may need to approach the spine laterally (from the side) by moving the lung. Typically, a lateral approach to decompress the spinal cord is combined with a posterior (from the back) approach to place the screws used for fusion.

Outcomes

The results of surgery for thoracic spinal compression are good, with many patients experiencing improvement in their symptoms. However, results are typically not as good as those for decompression of the cervical spinal cord for unknown reasons. Patients whose thoracic myelopathy is treated sooner have a better chance of recovery than those whose myelopathy has been ongoing for some time as the damage may become permanent. Patients with ossification of the posterior longitudinal ligament also may have a worse outcome because it is difficult to remove all the compressive tissue (2).

The compressed thoracic spinal cord is also more likely to be further traumatized by surgery than both the lumbar and cervical spines. Sometimes even the smallest manipulation of the thoracic spinal cord during surgery can cause a worsening of symptoms. Temporary or permanent paralysis may result from surgery. This may be since the blood supply for the spinal cord is more tenuous in the thoracic spine than in either the lumbar or cervical spines such that even gentle motion may compromise the thoracic spine's blood supply. Unfortunately, in some cases this is unavoidable.

Conclusion

The spinal cord runs through the cervical and thoracic spines and may be compressed at either site (unlike in the lumbar spine where there are only nerve roots). Thoracic spinal cord compression is much less common, and thus may easily be overlooked. Pain affects the back and legs, and weakness/poor coordination can occur. Treatment when symptoms reach this point is surgical decompression and fusion.

Frequently Asked Questions

- **Why do I need to have a fusion treatment, and will it affect my mobility?**

Decompression is the primary treatment for thoracic spinal cord compression; however, it is often performed in conjunction with a thoracic fusion—a procedure to join the bones surgically. The reason is that decompressions have the possibility to destabilize the spine. The lumbar spine is quite mobile and so we spine surgeons like to avoid fusions here if possible. The thoracic spine is rigid, and so fusions are not as noticeable here, and can prevent spinal instability from occurring.

References

1.   Vanichkachorn JS, Vaccaro AR. Thoracic Disk Disease: Diagnosis and Treatment: Journal of the American Academy of Orthopaedic Surgeons. 2000 May;8(3):159–69.

2.   Aizawa T, Sato T, Sasaki H, Matsumoto F, Morozumi N, Kusakabe T, et al. Results of surgical treatment for thoracic myelopathy: minimum 2-year follow-up study in 132 patients. Journal of Neurosurgery: Spine. 2007 Jul;7(1):13–20.

Figures:

Thoracic Spinal Cord Compression

Posterior view of the thoracic spine:

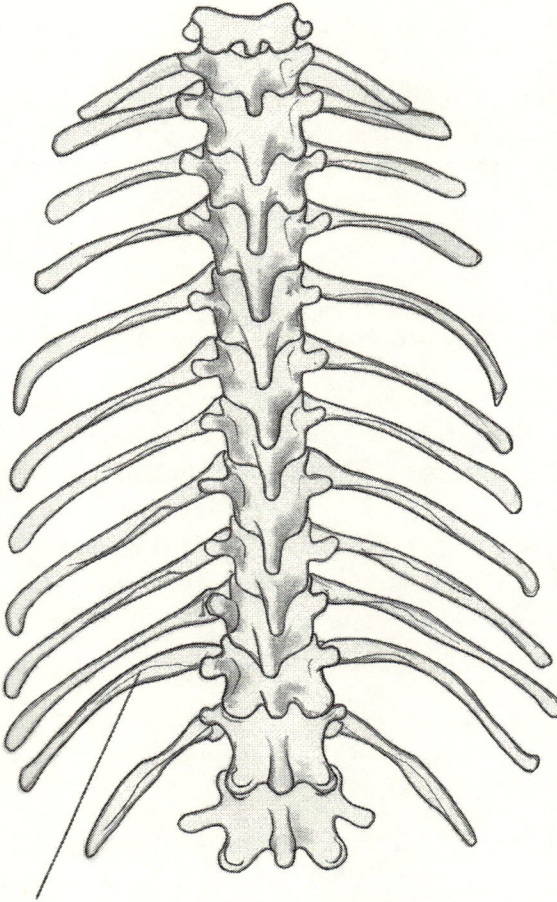

Cross section of the thoracic spine:

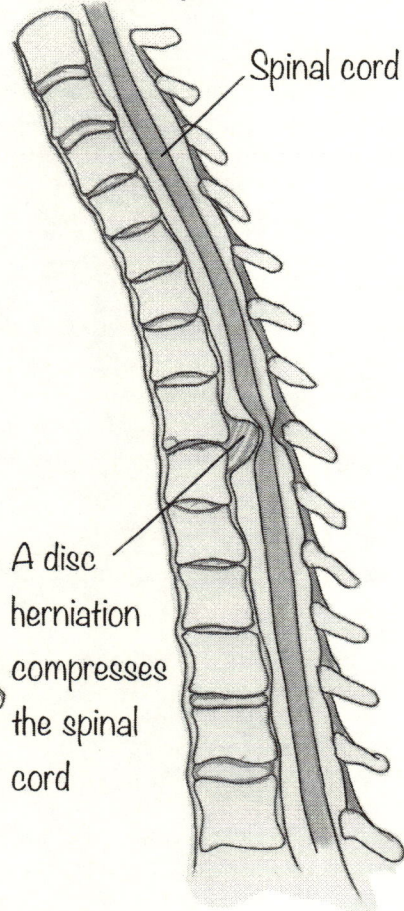

Spinal cord

A disc herniation compresses the spinal cord

The thoracic spine is rigid because the ribs are attached here

Thoracic spinal cord compression. The thoracic spine as viewed from behind. The ribcage stabilizes the thoracic spine making it much more rigid than either the cervical or lumbar spines (left). A thoracic disc herniation compressing the spinal cord (right) as seen in side view cross-section.

Chapter 10

Scoliosis: Fact vs Fiction

Summary

There are two main types of scoliosis: one which develops at a young age (adolescent) and one which develops at an older age (adult). Adolescent scoliosis may be benign and not require any treatment, or may require bracing or surgery, depending on the severity of the curve. If you have adolescent scoliosis, it is important to understand that it won't suddenly go away when you become an adult. Scoliosis continues into adult life and may progress, which is why it is screened for and treated if necessary. Adolescent scoliosis is usually painless but if left untreated can result in severe pain and disfiguration in adulthood.

Unlike adolescent scoliosis, which is due to a complex set of genetics, adult scoliosis occurs because of spinal degeneration and will affect a large proportion of adults at some point in their lives, particularly post-menopausal females. Treating the scoliosis of an adult is a much more complicated endeavor than treating a child's scoliosis because adult patients are usually not as healthy and the spine is not flexible anymore, making deformity corrections harder and riskier to achieve.

The treatment of adult scoliosis is aimed at treating pain whereas adolescent scoliosis treatment is aimed at preventing progression, that is, preventing it from getting worse.

Introduction

Scoliosis confuses patients and physicians alike, so let's try to make things simple. Scoliosis means you have a curve in the spine from side to side (remember curves in the spine from front to back, that is, lordosis and kyphosis, are typically normal). In reality the scoliosis deformity occurs in three dimensions, and includes rotation of the vertebrae, but for the sake of defining what scoliosis is, most doctors talk about scoliosis as occurring in a single plane (side to side). Spine surgeons do not consider a patient to have scoliosis unless the curve is larger than 10° in magnitude (smaller curves than this are typically considered inconsequential) (1). Spine surgeons also distinguish between scoliosis that develops in a child (idiopathic), and scoliosis that develops in an adult (degenerative). Because the treatment of the two is totally different we will talk about each separately. If you are specifically interested in adult scoliosis, please skip to the later section in this chapter. Adult scoliosis can develop from childhood scoliosis, but more commonly occurs independently.

Case

JR is a 16-year-old girl who had her scoliosis noted by her parents at age 14 when they found that her back looked asymmetric. She thinks she might have had school screening at age 12 but can't remember. JR's parents took her to an orthopedist at age 14. At that time her orthopedist said JR's curve was 40° and could be considered stable since her height had not changed in 6 months and it had been at least a year since she had had her first period. The orthopedist concluded the scoliosis wasn't big enough for surgery and bracing would not be effective anymore. All they could do was watch it. She didn't have any pain or disability but didn't like the way she looked. She returned for yearly visits and her curve progressed to 47° over this period. At this point surgery was recommended and she had a spinal fusion from T2 to L2 which she and her parents agreed to. She spent a week in the hospital and was back to school in 3 months' time. Today she participates in all the activities she wants to and denies having any limitations. She thinks her back looks great and is happy she had the procedure.

Scoliosis in the Young Person

The term adolescent idiopathic scoliosis is reserved for patients older than 10 years in age with a spinal curvature from side to side greater than 10°, as measured on an X-ray. Similar but younger patients (between three and ten years of age) are considered to have juvenile scoliosis, while patients under the age of three with that degree of side-to-side spinal curvature are classified as having infantile scoliosis.

Some scoliosis curves have a definite cause, such as a neuromuscular disorder like polio, or a congenital birth defect. Congenital scoliosis refers to abnormally formed vertebrae or extra vertebrae and are present from birth and often coincide with other problems present at birth such as kidney and cardiac issues (1). In contrast, the term idiopathic simply means there is no obvious cause, such as a fracture, tumor, neurological disease, or problem occurring at birth (congenital anomaly). Roughly 80% of scoliosis cases have no known cause and are thus idiopathic. Idiopathic scoliosis occurs in about 2-4 % of adolescents with only a small fraction requiring eventual surgical treatment (about 10 percent of these patients)(2,3). Thus, while having scoliosis is common, requiring surgical treatment is not.

Females are disproportionally affected by scoliosis, and are about 10 times more likely than males to have a curve which requires treatment (4). Scoliosis is believed to be a disorder caused by a number of different factors that originate from your genetics; however, there is no specific "scoliosis gene" that has been identified (5). Instead, there are multiple genetic abnormalities which are associated with the development of scoliosis. Melatonin (the sleep hormone) has also been implicated (6,7). So far genetic tests have not proven useful in either identifying or predicting the prognosis of scoliosis (8), though promising research continues in this field (9). There are so many different shapes/degrees of scoliosis, it's likely there are several types of genetic causes for scoliosis; we just don't know them yet.

Even though scoliosis is relatively common, there is disagreement regarding the need for schools to screen for scoliosis and so it may no longer be routinely performed in many schools (10). States that mandate school screening include Alabama, Arkansas, California, Connecticut, Delaware, Florida, Georgia, Indiana, Kentucky, Maine, Maryland, Massachusetts, Nevada, New Hampshire, New Jersey, New York, Pennsylvania, Rhode Island, Texas, Utah, Vermont, and Washington. The most typical scoliosis screening test is the Adams forward bend test, where the doctor will have the child bend down until their back is horizontal. The doctor will place a small gauge device called a scoliometer on the back and look for trunk rotation greater than 7°, which is the cut off for referral to get an X-ray. Most of the time taking this measurement is inconsequential as curves which require surgical treatment are obvious to pediatricians and clinicians who are paying attention (and even to parents and family members who notice significant changes in the child's posture and back).

But early detection of scoliosis definitely can help prevent the need for costly surgical interventions (11).

The reason early diagnosis of scoliosis is critical is that it allows for monitoring the disease and for non-operative treatment. Parents can look at their kids (who will try to avoid being scrutinized) for asymmetry in their backs, waists, or ribs. Historically screening was performed in schools, but this practice was halted in 2004 by the United States Preventative Services Task Force (USPSTF) leaving only those 15 states mandating screening as of 2019 (11). This was directly in conflict with the American Academy of Orthopedic Surgeons and the Scoliosis Research Society, which both recommended females be screened at 10 and 12 years of age and boys screened between ages of 13 and 14 years.

The most critical question with scoliosis is whether the curve will progress as the patient gets older, as most small curves are totally benign. The size of the curve is one of the most reliable ways to predict if the curve will continue to progress into skeletal maturity (when the skeleton has finished growing). Typically the larger the curve and the younger the patient (with a higher growth potential remaining) the more at risk the child is for curve progression (12,13). Curves less than 30° when a patient is skeletally mature are not likely to progress, while those greater than 50° will progress about 1° per year (14). If the curve threshold is greater than these thresholds and there is still significant growth remaining, progression is almost 100% guaranteed.

In most cases scoliosis is painless; however, roughly 30% of patients with scoliosis will complain of pain. In these cases it is important to rule out other causes of pain which may be occurring simultaneously with the scoliosis (15). While scoliosis typically does not pose significant functional limitations at younger ages, as patients get older, pain and degeneration may occur and is much more difficult to treat. In a long-term study following patients up to 50 years, it was shown that patients with scoliosis had an increased risk of chronic back pain compared to healthy volunteers (16). Importantly, progressive scoliosis can result in a significant cosmetic deformity of the spine. These factors explain why surgeons typically choose 50° as reasonable cut off in patients to suggest surgical correction and why we use 25-30° as an indication to start a patient on bracing. Braces which are properly constructed, fitted and worn for more than 13 hours a day may reduce the need for surgery by 56% (17).

diagnosis

The diagnosis of scoliosis in the adolescent begins with a clinical (looking for physical signs and symptoms) exam. Typically, the physician will have the patient bend forward to examine for abnormal curves in the back. The physician may even use a "scoliometer" which measures tilt in the back—readings greater than 7° warrant a referral and X-rays. A scoliometer cannot give an exact measure of the curvature, and hence X-rays are necessary.

Once scoliosis is suspected on a forward-bending test, the child is generally recommended to see a spine surgeon and referred for full body X-rays that show the entire spine from the neck to the pelvis. Radiation exposure is a concern for many parents as the diagnosis of scoliosis may consign a child to repeated X-rays for years until skeletal maturity is reached. Luckily new scanners are available which allow for less radiation than standard X-ray machines (18).

Knowing how mature the bones are is important to effective treatment so surgeons will look at the growth plates of the pelvis and may even get an X-ray of the hand to determine its "bone-age," using a reference called The Atlas of Greulich & Pyle. Using this book, the surgeon can compare the X-ray image of the patient's hand to the many hands of different ages recorded in that book.

curve types

Within idiopathic scoliosis there are many different patterns of curves. There are several complicated classification systems that surgeons sometimes use; however, for this chapter we will focus on several of the main types. The right thoracic curve is perhaps the most common—it curves to the right and has its apex (the place where the vertebra curves furthermost out to the side from the spine) in the thoracic spine. Thoracolumbar or lumbar curves occur slightly lower than a thoracic curve and involve the lumbar spine. Curves may be "structural" or "non-structural." A non-structural curve is one that bends out to the left or the right of the spine when you move, while a structural curve is rigid, that is, will not change with bending of the spine.

treatment

This section focuses on the treatment of adolescent scoliosis. Juvenile scoliosis and infantile scoliosis are very rare and generally only treated in specialty centers in the United States.

Bracing is the first line of therapy for adolescent scoliosis and consists of wearing a ThoracoLumbar Spinal Orthosis (TLSO) of some variety. There are many common types of TLSO braces for scoliosis (Milwaukee, Charleston, Providence, Wilmington) but the Boston style is perhaps the most common. It is not clear whether certain brace styles are superior to others so the brace which your provider is most comfortable with is the one you will likely get (19). The Boston brace is a custom brace that exerts force on the spine to mold it to a achieve a certain correction, like dental braces.

Bracing is indicated in skeletally immature patients with curves between 20-40°. This group of patients is typically between 10 and 15 years old, so still have sufficient growth remaining to provide an opportunity for change. As just mentioned, skeletal maturity is measured using X-rays of the pelvis and hands. Orthopedists also look at the amount of calcification in the top of the pelvis known as the Risser sign, which gives an excellent indication of how mature the spinal bone is.

There is a major study—The Bracing in Adolescent Idiopathic Scoliosis Trial (BRAIST)—that assessed how effective the use of bracing is as a treatment of scoliosis. That study determined that bracing significantly reduced the number of patients whose curves progressed to a degree requiring surgery (greater than 50°) (17). Bracing must be done for at least 13-18 hours a day to be effective (the more the brace is worn the more effective it is), although certain brace types are done at nighttime only (Charleston and Providence). Nighttime-only braces are not as effective as full-time braces but may be useful for children who frankly refuse to wear their braces during the day.

Currently a low-profile brace such as the Boston is used for adolescents, whereas bulkier braces such as the Milwaukee brace are mainly used for treatment of kyphosis in adults. Bracing is most effective for curves falling between T8 and L2 whereas curves occurring higher in the spine are more difficult to brace. Once the brace is fit, the patient is X-rayed to see how much correction has been achieved, aiming for somewhere between 30-70% correction. Bracing is continued until skeletal maturity is reached and the risk of further progression of the scoliosis is low or until the curve progresses beyond 50°, at which point surgery is recommended. If your height remains stable for 6 months this is likely a sign you are done growing, and your doctor may discontinue your brace. Ideally a brace will prevent worsening of the scoliosis—a brace can never completely straighten out a spine. Once your bracing period is complete, your body will need to be gradually weaned from the wearing of it. This will take several months because, believe it or not, after several years of use, your body will become accustomed to the brace. Although braces are uncomfortable at first, your body will quickly become used to wearing it and your muscles can even grow dependent on it.

Exercise is commonly recommended in the treatment of scoliosis, but it's important to know exercise will not do anything to reduce the curvature of scoliosis. It is just an adjunct to ensure you are fit, flexible and have good muscular tone. Exercise can also have the added benefit of decreasing pain you may experience in your back from muscle cramps.

Surgery for scoliosis is performed once the curve reaches at least 50˚ and is done to prevent further progression and correct deformity. Some patients also choose to have correction for cosmetic reasons. Patients who are treated surgically tend to have improved back pain, activity levels and self-images compared to those who do not undergo treatment (20). Scoliosis correction may also benefit lung and cardiac function as major curves (>50˚) can abnormally compress these organs resulting in pulmonary hypertension (9). There are many different surgical techniques for the treatment of adolescent scoliosis, but in general the main surgical treatment is posterior instrumented spinal fusion. This procedure fuses or causes the vertebrae to grow together in a way that corrects the spine. Screws placed in the spine connect to a rod that physically bends the spine back into a normal and correct shape. Determining the extent of the fusion (that is, deciding which levels should be included) is a debated topic even among orthopedic surgeons, but no more vertebrae should be fused than is needed to adequately address the deformity. I devote an entire chapter to the science of spinal fusion but in essence it is the use of bone graft to help adjacent vertebrae grow together such that they no longer move relative to one another. The screws and rods help hold the desired shape while this occurs. If the curve is inflexible (which surgeons will measure using bending X-ray films) special cuts in the bone known as osteotomies may be required to achieve full correction.

Scoliosis surgery is complex but can be done safely with minimal complications by those with adequate training. In a large multicenter data base study, the incidence of complication for adolescent scoliosis treated with surgery was 6.3 percent, with the majority of the complications being related to implants (21). Most adolescents (59%) who have surgery for scoliosis are able to return to sports at the same or higher level, depending on the extent of the fusion (22).

Newer techniques used in the surgical treatment of scoliosis include anterior tethering. Parents are very enthusiastic about this technique because it does not require a formal fusion and instead "guides" growth such that the spine can straighten out. In anterior tethering the screws are not directly placed from the back of the spine but are instead placed through the lung cavity and attached to an elastic rod which can expand to hold the correction as the skeleton grows. This is theoretically supposed to allow for guided correction of the curvature as the spine grows. Scoliosis tethering is only useful in those who have remaining growth and should not be used in skeletally mature patients. Many of these patients require a second surgery to correct or finish the work done in the first procedure and up to 40% of these patients end up with a traditional posterior spinal fusion (23). As of this writing, the tethering technique is still being pioneered and will likely improve in years to come.

If you are only interested in scoliosis in children, you can now skip to the conclusion, questions, references and drawings

Adult Scoliosis

Case

Ms. Clay had scoliosis as a child but never had it treated. She never had any pain so why would she want to undergo a huge surgery? She was fine for many years but around the age of 40 she started to have pains in her hips from an unbalanced gait. Her muscles in her back started to ache constantly and she had a hard time working in her office job. She noticed that her clothes didn't fit right anymore. Eventually she decided to come to see us, and we noted that her curve had progressed significantly until it was about 75°. By this time her pain was severe and incapacitating and she couldn't walk for any distance. She underwent a spinal fusion surgery extending from T10 to her pelvis which brought her curve back down to 20°. It took 8 hours. Recovery was long—she spent a week in the hospital, and it was about 3 months until she resumed her previous activity levels. She is doing well now with no issues but does note her back feels stiff.

Adult scoliosis is broken into two groups: those who had scoliosis as a child and were never treated or never required treatment (idiopathic) and those who initially had a normal spine and only developed scoliosis in their elderly years because of degeneration (de novo, meaning new). In the de novo group are those whose scoliosis progresses rapidly, typically from degeneration of the vertebrae, facet joints and discs, all of which causes the spine to tilt. Sometimes It's difficult to determine which type of scoliosis you are experiencing and what the exact cause is. Stable idiopathic scoliosis that has been without any symptoms for many years may progress suddenly (24). Adult scoliosis tends to affect the lumbar spine whereas childhood scoliosis affects the thoracic spine. Once the deformity starts to progress, it usually continues to get worse over time as asymmetric (uneven) forces on the spine lead to further degeneration.

Adult scoliosis is an incredibly common problem affecting anywhere from 32 to 68% of those older than 65 years (25,26). It can have a profound impact on health and the ability to get around, on par with some types of cancer (27). In women, this process of degeneration occurs rapidly around the time of menopause, at which time bones become osteopenic (lose mass) (see chapter 12 on osteoporosis). Just like adolescent curves, adult degenerative curves progress and actually do so at a faster rate of around 2° per year (24).

Back pain is the most common symptom with adult scoliosis (28). Pain may occur along the apex of the curve (the place where the vertebra curves furthermost out to the side from the spine), because of degenerated discs and facets, and because of strained muscles which are struggling to hold the spine erect. This pain is typically relieved when you lay down flat and allow the muscles to relax. While scoliosis itself can cause back pain, a greater problem occurs when the bones and discs start pressing on nerves (see the previous chapters on what causes pain in the spine) which is excruciating. Unlike in the child or adolescent, in the adult the bones and ligaments are much stiffer and thus the surgery is generally more difficult. (This is part of the reason spine surgeons like to correct scoliosis at a young age.) Thus, the decision to operate on a patient with an adult scoliosis is not guided by degree of curvature but rather the patient's level of disability and discomfort as well as the presence of any neurological abnormalities such as progressive weakness and bowel or bladder incontinence. Deciding whether to treat adult scoliosis with surgery can be difficult.

On the one hand, the surgeries to correct these problems are complex and have a high complication rate (discussed in chapter 42).

On the other hand, non-operative treatment of patients with significant disability from scoliosis at best maintains the patient's level of pain and disability and at worst allows her or him to decline further (29–31). In one study, 30% of patients reported an increase in pain over 2 years of non-operative treatment, 50% reported new back pain and 27% reported new leg pain (32). It's important to work with your surgeon to arrive at an informed decision about how best to deal with this issue. However, multiple studies have shown that surgery is effective at reducing pain and improving quality of life and can stabilize further deterioration (33,34).

diagnosis

Exactly like adolescent scoliosis, a patient is diagnosed as having adult scoliosis when there is a curve greater than 10°. Standard X-rays, like when diagnosing adolescent scoliosis, are used to evaluate the curvature; however, more advanced imaging (CTs, MRIs and CT myelograms) may be necessary to look for areas of stenosis (narrowing of spinal canal) and pinched nerves which are not present in adolescent scoliosis. In adult scoliosis there tend to be multiple areas of degeneration and pinpointing areas causing pain can be challenging. For this reason, painful segments may be better diagnosed with selective injections that numb the area and help the physician localize your pain.

treatment

Until recently, only childhood scoliosis was treated because surgery on adults with scoliosis was considered too risky. Hence the emphasis is on treating childhood scoliosis; as you get older you become less robust and have more medical problems. Your spine becomes stiffer, and treatments become more difficult. Better to correct major problems as a child. However, with modern spinal instruments and techniques, adult scoliosis has become something that can be more readily treated. As the population ages, adult scoliosis has become a much more common problem than childhood scoliosis. In fact, because adults find themselves unwilling to live with deformity and pain, treating adult scoliosis tends to be a large part of most spine surgeons' practices.

Despite advances in spinal surgery and anesthesia, the treatment of adult scoliosis is still a risky business. Conservative care such as physical therapy (PT), injections and oral medications should be exhausted before surgery is contemplated. Bracing can be used for temporary back pain but has absolutely no effect on reducing adult curves. This is because once you reach adulthood the spine becomes rigid and no longer responds as well to outside forces such as bracing. Once the decision for surgery is made, the decision for WHICH type of surgery can be just as complex. The extent of surgery depends not only on the surgical problem to be addressed but your overall health and bone quality. Some patients may not be fit enough to tolerate a major reconstruction.

In general, the two types of procedures offered for scoliosis in the adult are decompression and fusion. Decompression is done to relieve the pain caused from the scoliotic vertebrae narrowing the spinal canal and is accomplished by performing a laminectomy, that is, a removal of the thin part of the vertebra called the lamina. Fusion stabilizes the painful segment with rods and screws followed by bone graft. These two procedures are commonly performed in combination. Decompression alone is an attractive option because it is generally less invasive and requires less recovery. However, in scoliosis, the stenosis (narrowing of the spinal canal) that scoliosis causes is often accompanied by some form of instability of the vertebrae. If this is the case, a decompression alone, which removes some bone, may worsen the instability and the improvement from surgery can be short-lived (28). In these patients it may be necessary to perform a spinal fusion to stabilize the segment while also performing a decompression. There are many ways to perform a spinal fusion which are discussed in later chapters (Chapter 37 and 41).

It should be noted that the goal of spine surgery for adult scoliosis is to transition a patient from a painful state to a pain- free state if possible. The surgery generally does not enhance functional capacity, for example, it will not turn you into a marathon runner if you were not already one. There can be many complications from surgery, including implant failure, failure of the bony fusion to heal (pseudoarthrosis), infection, worsening of deformity, degeneration at adjacent segments requiring more extensive fusions (28). Thus, the decision about how best to treat your scoliosis should be made with care and include thoughtful discussion with your surgeon.

Conclusion

Scoliosis is a common problem both for children and adults and can commonly arise during adolescence for genetic reasons or during adulthood from break down of the discs and vertebrae. Once the curvature reaches a certain size (the bend goes from slight to great) the curve is destined to continue progressing. That is why scoliosis is treated early in childhood or adolescence, with bracing in mild cases or with surgery in severe cases. Bracing can prevent progression in children but has little use in adults. Moreover, performing surgical corrections for scoliosis on a young adult is much simpler than it is on someone 60 or 70 (when problems from untreated scoliosis will typically occur). Surgery is used to straighten the spine, stabilize parts that are unstable, and decompress areas of nerve compression.

Frequently Asked Questions about Adolescent (Idiopathic) Scoliosis

- **Will scoliosis interfere with my breathing ability?**

  Severe scoliosis with a curve measurement of greater than 80° interferes with a patient's breathing ability (16).

- **Will a brace help me?**

  Braces do not reverse scoliotic curves but can be helpful in halting progression of the curve in patients with remaining skeletal growth (35).

- **Will physical therapy such as the SCHROTH method prevent progression of my scoliosis?**

  While certainly not harmful, there is insufficient evidence that the Schroth method or any other form of physical therapy halts the progression of scoliosis and such treatment should only be used if combined with effective bracing or surgical strategy (36).

- **Is it better to shield my child from the knowledge of scoliosis?**

  While the parents ultimately will make the final decision on treatments for scoliosis, leaving children totally out of the loop is not necessarily beneficial. It can help a child psychologically to feel some ownership of the problem and be involved in the decision-making process. I believe this is especially true, because scoliosis is a long-term problem the patient will have to live with their whole life.

- **If I opt to do nothing to treat my child's scoliosis what are the future risks for my child?**

Children with curves in the surgical range (curves measuring 50° or greater) who go untreated are at risk for a progression of the curve, back pain, and cosmetic deformity in the future. It is more likely for children whose bones are still growing and have a scoliotic curve in the 20° to 40° range AND who go untreated to have the curvature of their spines progress further (worsen more) in the future compared to what similar children who undergo bracing are likely to experience.

- **As soon as I'm done growing, my curve will stop progressing, right?**

Not necessarily. Your curve can progress into adulthood. Curves 30-50 ° will progress 10-15° more while curves greater than 50° will progress 1 ° a year.

- **Can a brace help my symptoms or halt progression of adult scoliosis?**

There is not significant evidence to support bracing in adult scoliosis (37). In fact, it may lead to deconditioning, causing a further weakening of the spine.

- **What is non-operative treatment, and will it help my symptoms of adult scoliosis?**

Non operative treatment includes NSAIDS, bracing, physical therapy, and injections. Some patients will find relief from these and other alternative methods of treatment such as massage, acupuncture and chiropractics. To date there is no significant evidence that these treatments are effective in reducing pain, or improving pain and disability in adult scoliosis (33,37).

- **Who is a good candidate for non-operative therapy?**

Patients who have a low level of disability, and who for the most part are alreadysatisfied with their quality of life.

- **Will my period (menses) affect my surgery?**

No. A large study comparing patients who were having their period around the time of this surgery with those who were not found no significant difference in blood loss between the two groups (38).

- **Will pregnancy worsen the progression of my scoliosis?**

  Pregnancy has not been associated with worsening of scoliosis, nor has scoliosis been shown to cause problems with pregnancy (39).

- **Will my scoliosis surgery totally correct my curvature?**

  Even the best scoliosis curvature correction will leave some curve. In fact, it can be dangerous to fully correct a scoliosis curve.

- **Will my back pain totally go away after scoliosis surgery?**

  Back pain is complicated. Spine surgery is great at correcting some types of back pain but not others. When there is a structural cause of back pain (such as scoliosis), surgery can help relieve it. Your back pain may be improved but will likely not totally go away. The goal of surgery is to stabilize your spine and keep your functional, but some pain and achiness may remain.

References

1.   Basu PS, Elsebaie H, Noordeen MHH. Congenital spinal deformity: a comprehensive assessment at presentation. Spine. 2002;27(20):2255–9.

2.   Horne JP, Flannery R, Usman S. Adolescent Idiopathic Scoliosis: Diagnosis and Management. 2014;89(3):6.

3.   Lonstein JE, Carlson JM. The prediction of curve progression in untreated idiopathic scoliosis during growth. J Bone Joint Surg Am. 1984 Sep;66(7):1061–71.

4.   Bunnell WP. Selective Screening for Scoliosis: Clin Orthop. 2005 May;-NA;(434):40–5.

5.   Lowe TG, Edgar M, Margulies JY, Miller NH, Raso VJ, Reinker KA, et al. Etiology of idiopathic scoliosis: current trends in research. J Bone Joint Surg Am. 2000 Aug;82(8):1157–68.

6.   Miller NH, Justice CM, Marosy B, Doheny KF, Pugh E, Zhang J, et al. Identification of candidate regions for familial idiopathic scoliosis. Spine. 2005;30(10):1181–7.

7.   Moreau A, Wang DS, Forget S, Azeddine B, Angeloni D, Fraschini F, et al. Melatonin Signaling Dysfunction in Adolescent Idiopathic Scoliosis: Spine. 2004 Aug;29(16):1772–81.

8.   Tang QL, Julien C, Eveleigh R, Bourque G, Franco A, Labelle H, et al. A Replication Study for Association of 53 Single Nucleotide Polymorphisms in ScoliScore Test With Adolescent Idiopathic Scoliosis in French-Canadian Population: Spine. 2015

Apr;40(8):537–43.

9.   Sarwahi V, Galina J, Atlas A, Gecelter R, Hasan S, Amaral TD, et al. Scoliosis Surgery Normalizes Cardiac Function in Adolescent Idiopathic Scoliosis Patients. Spine. 2021 Nov 1;46(21):E1161–7.

10.   US Preventive Services Task Force, Grossman DC, Curry SJ, Owens DK, Barry MJ, Davidson KW, et al. Screening for Adolescent Idiopathic Scoliosis: US Preventive Services Task Force Recommendation Statement. JAMA. 2018 Jan 9;319(2):165.

11.   Oetgen ME, Heyer JH, Kelly SM. Scoliosis Screening. J Am Acad Orthop Surg. 2021 May 1;29(9):370–9.

12.   Tan KJ, Moe MM, Vaithinathan R, Wong HK. Curve Progression in Idiopathic Scoliosis. :4.

13.   Collis DK, Ponseti IV. Long-term follow-up of patients with idiopathic scoliosis not treated surgically. J Bone Joint Surg Am. 1969 Apr;51(3):425–45.

14.   Weinstein SL, Ponseti IV. Curve progression in idiopathic scoliosis. J Bone Joint Surg Am. 1983 Apr;65(4):447–55.

15.   Ramirez N, Johnston CE, Browne RH. The Prevalence of Back Pain in Children Who Have Idiopathic Scoliosis*: J Bone Jt Surg. 1997 Mar;79(3):364–8.

16.   Weinstein SL. The Natural History of Adolescent Idiopathic Scoliosis: J Pediatr Orthop. 2019 Jul;39:S44–6.

17.   Weinstein SL, Dolan LA, Wright JG, Dobbs MB. Effects of Bracing in Adolescents with Idiopathic Scoliosis. N Engl J Med. 2013 Oct 17;369(16):1512–21.

18.   Deschênes S, Charron G, Beaudoin G, Labelle H, Dubois J, Miron MC, et al. Diagnostic Imaging of Spinal Deformities: Reducing Patients Radiation Dose With a New Slot-Scanning X-ray Imager. Spine. 2010 Apr;35(9):989–94.

19.   Gomez JA, Hresko MT, Glotzbecker MP. Nonsurgical Management of Adolescent Idiopathic Scoliosis. J Am Acad Orthop Surg. 2016 Aug;24(8):555–64.

20.   Helenius L, Diarbakerli E, Grauers A, Lastikka M, Oksanen H, Pajulo O, et al. Back Pain and Quality of Life After Surgical Treatment for Adolescent Idiopathic Scoliosis at 5-Year Follow-up: Comparison with Healthy Controls and Patients with Untreated Idiopathic Scoliosis. J Bone Jt Surg. 2019 Aug;101(16):1460–6.

21.   Reames DL, Smith JS, Fu KMG, Polly DW, Ames CP, Berven SH, et al. Complications in the surgical treatment of 19,360 cases of pediatric scoliosis: a review of the Scoliosis Research Society Morbidity and Mortality database. Spine. 2011 Aug 15;36(18):1484–91.

22.   Fabricant PD, Admoni S har, Green DW, Ipp LS, Widmann RF. Return to Athletic Activity After Posterior Spinal Fusion for Adolescent Idiopathic Scoliosis: Analysis of Independent Predictors. J Pediatr Orthop. 2012;32(3):7.

23.   Parent S, Shen J. Anterior Vertebral Body Growth-Modulation Tethering in Idiopathic Scoliosis: Surgical Technique. J Am Acad Orthop Surg. 2020 Sep 1;28(17):693–9.

24.   Marty-Poumarat C, Scattin L, Marpeau M, Garreau de Loubresse C, Aegerter P. Natural History of Progressive Adult Scoliosis: Spine. 2007 May;32(11):1227–34.

25.   Schwab F, Dubey A, Gamez L, El Fegoun AB, Hwang K, Pagala M, et al. Adult Scoliosis: Prevalence, SF-36, and Nutritional Parameters in an Elderly Volunteer Population: Spine. 2005 May;30(9):1082–5.

26.   Diebo BG, Shah NV, Boachie-Adjei O, Zhu F, Rothenfluh DA, Paulino CB, et al. Adult spinal deformity. The Lancet. 2019 Jul;394(10193):160–72.

27.   Bess S, Line B, Fu KM, McCarthy I, Lafage V, Schwab F, et al. The Health Impact of Symptomatic Adult Spinal Deformity: Comparison of Deformity Types to United States Population Norms and Chronic Diseases. SPINE. 2016 Feb;41(3):224–33.

28.   Aebi M. The adult scoliosis. Eur Spine J. 2005 Dec;14(10):925–48.

29.   The Spinal Deformity Study Group, Smith JS, Shaffrey CI, Berven S, Glassman S, Hamill C, et al. IMPROVEMENT OF BACK PAIN WITH OPERATIVE AND NONOPERATIVE TREATMENT IN ADULTS WITH SCOLIOSIS. Neurosurgery. 2009 Jul 1;65(1):86–94.

30.   Smith JS, Shaffrey CI, Berven S, Glassman S, Hamill C, Horton W, et al. Operative Versus Nonoperative Treatment of Leg Pain in Adults With Scoliosis: A Retrospective Review of a Prospective Multicenter Database With Two-Year Follow-up. Spine. 2009 Jul;34(16):1693–8.

31.   Passias PG, Jalai CM, Line BG, Poorman GW, Scheer JK, Smith JS, et al. Patient profiling can identify patients with adult spinal deformity (ASD) at risk for conversion from nonoperative to surgical treatment: initial steps to reduce ineffective ASD management. Spine J. 2018 Feb;18(2):234–44.

32.   Scheer JK, Smith JS, Clark AJ, Lafage V, Kim HJ, Rolston JD, et al. Comprehensive study of back and leg pain improvements after adult spinal deformity surgery: analysis of 421 patients with 2-year follow-up and of the impact of the surgery on treatment satisfaction. J Neurosurg Spine. 2015 May;22(5):540–53.

33.   Teles AR, Mattei TA, Righesso O, Falavigna A. Effectiveness of Operative and Nonoperative Care for Adult Spinal Deformity: Systematic Review of the Literature. Glob Spine J. 2017 Apr;7(2):170–8.

34.   Liu S, Schwab F, Smith JS, Klineberg E, Ames CP, Mundis G, et al. Likelihood of Reaching Minimal Clinically Important Difference in Adult Spinal Deformity: A Comparison of Operative and Nonoperative Treatment. 2014;14(1):11.

35.   Nachemson AL, Peterson LE. Effectiveness of treatment with a brace in girls who have adolescent idiopathic scoliosis. A prospective, controlled study based on data from the Brace Study of the Scoliosis Research Society. J Bone Joint Surg Am. 1995 Jun;77(6):815–22.

36.   Day JM, Fletcher J, Coghlan M, Ravine T. Review of scoliosis-specific exercise methods used to correct adolescent idiopathic scoliosis. Arch Physiother. 2019 Dec;9(1):8.

37.   Schoutens C, Cushman DM, McCormick ZL, Conger A, van Royen BJ, Spiker WR.

Outcomes of Nonsurgical Treatments for Symptomatic Adult Degenerative Scoliosis: A Systematic Review. Pain Med Malden Mass. 2019 Oct 16;

38.   Chiu CK, Gani SMA, Chung WH, Mihara Y, Hasan MS, Chan CYW, et al. Does Menses Affect the Risk of Blood Loss in Adolescent Idiopathic Scoliosis Patients Undergoing Posterior Spinal Fusion Surgeries?: A Propensity-Score Matching Study. Spine. 2020 Aug 15;45(16):1128–34.

39.   Betz RR, Bunnell WP, Lambrecht-Mulier E, MacEwen GD. Scoliosis and pregnancy. J Bone Joint Surg Am. 1987 Jan;69(1):90–6.

Figures:

Idiopathic Scoliosis

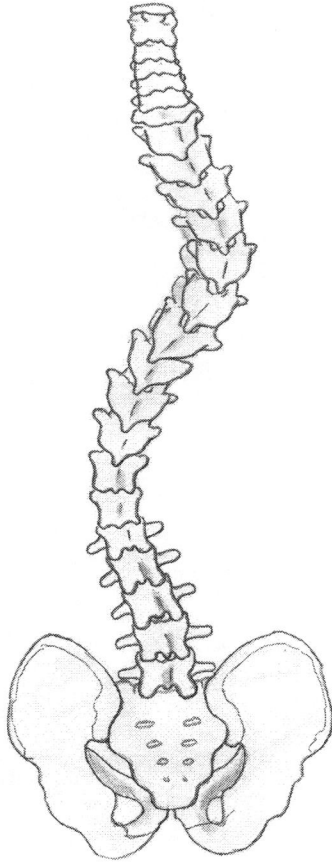

A scoliotic spine viewed from behind (posterior)

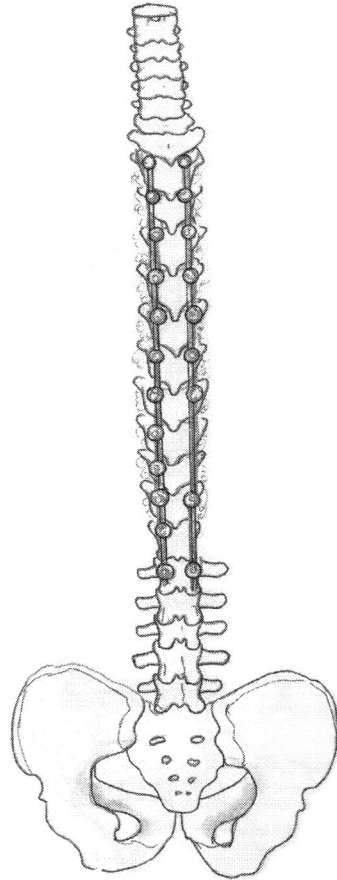

The scoliosis has been treated with a posterior instrumented spinal fusion (T2-L1)

Adolescent scoliosis. Adolescent scoliosis as viewed from behind with a characteristic major thoracic curve (left). Surgical fixation of scoliosis involves the use of screws and rods to straighten the spine and hold it in place. A spinal fusion acts as the glue to hold it in this position permanently.

Adult Degenerative Scoliosis

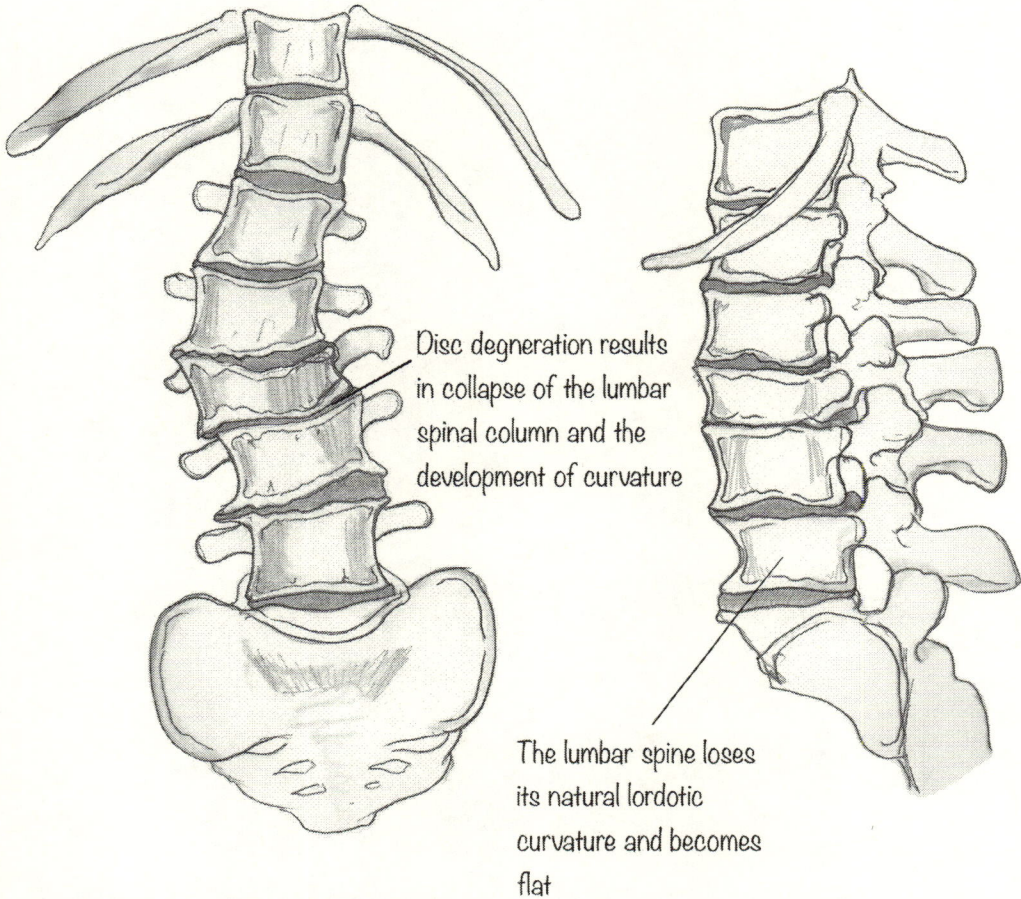

Disc degneration results in collapse of the lumbar spinal column and the development of curvature

The lumbar spine loses its natural lordotic curvature and becomes flat

Adult Scoliosis. Adult scoliosis differs from adolescent scoliosis in that it primarily affects the lumbar spine. The curve magnitude tends to be less, and the lumbar spine loses its characteristic curved shape becoming flat (left).

Examples of Braces for Scoliosis

Front: Back:

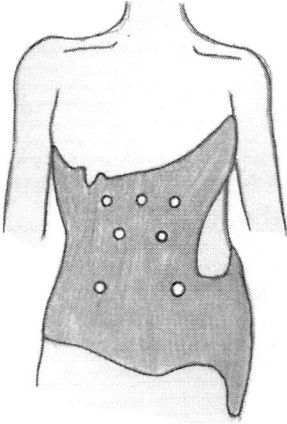
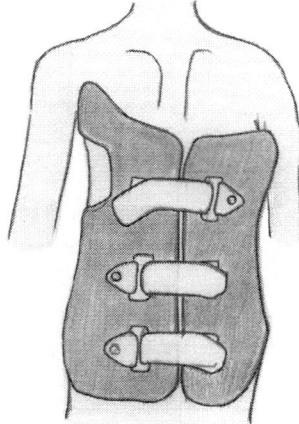

Boston
brace

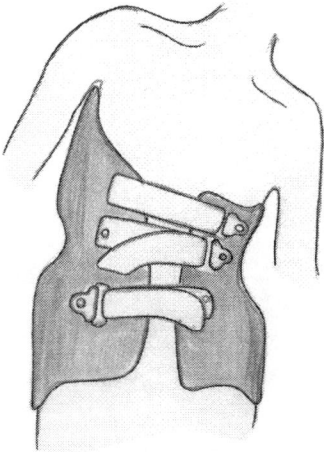
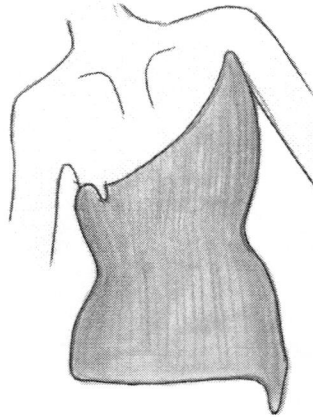

Charleston
nighttime
brace

Scoliosis braces. There are many different types of braces used to treat
adolescent scoliosis. The Boston and Charleston braces are commonly used
braces. The Charleston brace is worn at nighttime and is secured from the front
as opposed to the back (bottom).

Chapter 11

Scheuermann's Kyphosis

Summary

Scheuermann's kyphosis is a rare, likely genetic, disease where the thoracic spine slumps forward resulting in hunched back. Most cases are totally benign; however, in progressive cases, disfiguration, pain and cardiorespiratory/neurologic complications play a role in the decision for surgery. Surgery consists of a spinal fusion to correct the hunch back and prevent progression.

Case

Ms. Almond is a 14-year-old girl who comes to me with her parents to have her "slouched posture" evaluated. Her parents are concerned as she seems to progressively be becoming more hunch backed and is starting to complain of more pain. After X-rays, I can diagnose her with Scheuermann's kyphosis with a kyphosis angle of 90° (this means the curvature of her thoracic spine is 90° whereas a normal amount is around 40°). Her parents are concerned that this posture is somehow behavioral. I assure them that it is not, it is a structural problem with the spine. We try to put her in bracing and physical therapy

(PT) but her curve progresses. After several months of this approach and after learning more about the condition, the parents are interested in surgery as they do not want her posture to get worse or for her to have issues in old age. The patient herself is also self-conscious and wants to look more normal. We have a long conversation and ultimately when it becomes obvious PT and bracing are not working to treat her pain or deformity, decide to move forward with surgery which is a T2-L2 posterior spinal fusion. She spends a week in the hospital and afterwards makes a recovery over the next 3 months. After this period, she is a full 2 inches taller and feels great, returning to her normal school and athletic activities. She has a long scar, but the hunch back is gone, and she feels great about wearing tank tops. She has no limitations in activity and can play with others her own age.

Introduction

Scheuermann's kyphosis is a rigid deformity of the spine in which at least 3 consecutive vertebrae have wedging on their front sides (meaning they have a trapezoidal shape instead of the typical square) as well as other vertebral irregularities. Also common are **Schmorl's nodes**, a radiographic finding (unaccompanied by symptoms) where disc material is herniated into the vertebra itself (as opposed to a typical disc herniation where the herniation occurs into the spinal canal) (1). Unlike scoliosis, where the curve is side-to-side, Scheuermann's kyphosis is front-to-back. This means that the curve makes your back appear more arched or hunched.

The exact cause of Scheuermann's kyphosis is unknown but thought to result from a growth problem in the front of the vertebra making the back of vertebral ring disproportionate and asymmetric, creating the wedge shape. Successive vertebrae with a wedge shape (instead of a square shape) causes slouching (kyphosis) of the spine. Genetic causes for the disease have also been suspected as the condition tends to run in families.

Scheuermann's kyphosis can be either "typical" or "atypical." Typical Scheuermann's occurs in the thoracic spine with an apex (tip of the curvature) around T7-9. In an atypical Scheuermann's, the curve is lower in the thoracolumbar or lumbar region.

Does Scheuermann's Kyphosis Progress?

In most patients with Scheuermann's kyphosis, especially those with kyphosis less than 60°, there is little to no progression, and we expect no significant impact on their lives. Patients with Scheuermann's kyphosis typically report more back pain than healthy individuals but there is no significant difference in missed days from work, use of medication, social or recreational activity. Lung capacity may become restricted, but only at very high degrees of kyphosis that is greater than 100°(2). Overall, there typically is about 10-15° of expected progression over a patient's lifetime (3). Neurological complications such as paralysis or weakness of the extremities generally do not occur until there are very high degrees of kyphosis (greater than 100°).

Treatment

The degree of kyphosis necessitating surgery is still debated among spine surgeons. However, most agree that curves under 80° can be managed non-operatively. Bracing may be useful in children with flexible (40% correction on bending) small curves of less than 80° with remaining growth potential (4). Braces consist of a custom rigid ThoracoLumbar Sacral Orthosis (TLSO) worn for 16-23 hours a day until the patient is done growing. Physical therapy is also recommended if the curve is painful; however, there is no evidence that it will halt progression of the curve.

Surgery is recommended if there is persistent pain, nerve or spinal cord damage, progression of the curvature despite bracing, or a significant deformity in someone who has reached skeletal maturity. There is no agreed upon curve degree as an indication for surgery, but most surgeons would consider surgery for patients with curves greater than 80°. Pain and physical appearance dissatisfaction are important contributors to the decision to operate.

Surgical treatment generally consists of a long spinal fusion with pedicle screw instrumentation, as well as single or multiple osteotomies (cuts in the bones to make the spine more flexible). Please see chapter 42 on spinal deformity correction for more information on these treatments. The goal is typically to reduce the curvature into a normal range of around 40-50°.

Complications and Outcomes

The complication rate for a surgical correction of a Scheuermann's kyphosis is roughly 14% with the most common complication being a wound infection. It's important to note that kyphosis correction is more successful in children and adolescents who have more flexible spines than in adults, making the deformity easier to correct surgically. Complications in general are more common in adult patients compared to pediatric patients (5). Children in general heal from and tolerate spine surgery much better than adults, which is why most scoliosis and kyphosis correction is done in childhood.

Overcorrection is a common problem with surgical treatment of Scheuermann's kyphosis which can result in breakdown above or below the surgical fusion. This phenomenon is known as proximal or distal junctional kyphosis (explained in the chapter 42 on spinal deformity) and has been reported to occur in up to as high as 20-30% of cases (6). Spinal cord injury is another frightening complication which may occur at a rate up to 0.6% (6 in a thousand procedures).

Nonetheless, surgery is generally very successful at correcting the curvature, halting progression of the deformity and achieving good functional and quality of life outcomes (4,7).

Conclusion

Scheuermann's kyphosis can result in disfigurement, which is intolerable to some individuals. If you can live with your shape, surgery should only be considered if you are in pain, have neurologic symptoms, or your deformity is worsening, because there are significant risks to the operation. Nonetheless, with a thoracic curve greater than 80° at a young age, there is a high likelihood it will progress 10-15° which may impact quality of life as you get older. Surgery can be considered in these cases.

Frequently Asked Questions

- **I hate my slumped appearance and want surgery to correct it. I am not limited by pain or physical dysfunction, but I do not want to look hunched the rest of my life. Is it wrong to want surgery?**

Treating spinal deformity with surgery for cosmetic reasons is controversial. Surgery carries risk of complications and to undergo surgery for appearance some would argue is not worth that risk. Nonetheless, thousands of people undergo surgery for cosmetic reasons in the United States every year so what's the problem with having your spine done for those reasons? I think the issue lies in the risks of spinal surgery. If a problem arises during or because of surgery, a patient with previously totally normal neurologic function could become paralyzed. Correcting your back curvature may not be worth the risk of living with a neurologic deficit, no matter how uncommon the back curvature may be. While ultimately, I believe it's not wrong to want surgery to improve appearance from a major spinal deformity, especially if the deformity is only going to get worse, this decision must be made carefully with your spine surgeon, with a full understanding of the risks.

References

1.   Sardar ZM, Ames RJ, Lenke L. Scheuermann's Kyphosis: Diagnosis, Management, and Selecting Fusion Levels. Journal of the American Academy of Orthopaedic Surgeons. 2019 May;27(10):e462–72.

2.   Murray PM, Weinstein SL, Spratt KF. The natural history and long-term follow-up of Scheuermann kyphosis.: The Journal of Bone & Joint Surgery. 1993 Feb;75(2):236–48.

3.   Ristolainen L, Kettunen JA, Kujala UM, Heinonen A, Schlenzka D. Progression of untreated mild thoracic Scheuermann's kyphosis – Radiographic and functional assessment after mean follow-up of 46 years. Journal of Orthopaedic Science. 2017 Jul;22(4):652–7.

4.   Lowe TG, Line BG. Evidence Based Medicine: Analysis of Scheuermann Kyphosis. Spine. 2007 Sep;32(Supplement):S115–9.

5.   Coe JD, Smith JS, Berven S, Arlet V, Donaldson W, Hanson D, et al. Complications of Spinal Fusion for Scheuermann Kyphosis: A Report of the Scoliosis Research Society Morbidity and Mortality Committee. Spine. 2010 Jan;35(1):99–103.

6.   Lowe TG, Kasten MD. An analysis of sagittal curves and balance after Cotrel-Dubousset instrumentation for kyphosis secondary to Scheuermann's disease. A review of 32 patients. Spine. 1994 Aug 1;19(15):1680–5.

7.   Graat HCA, Schimmel JJP, Hoogendoorn RJW, van Hessem L, Hosman A, de Kleuver M. Poor Radiological and Good Functional Long-term Outcome of Surgically Treated Scheuermann Patients: SPINE. 2016 Jul;41(14):E869–78.

Figures:

Scheuermann's Kyphosis

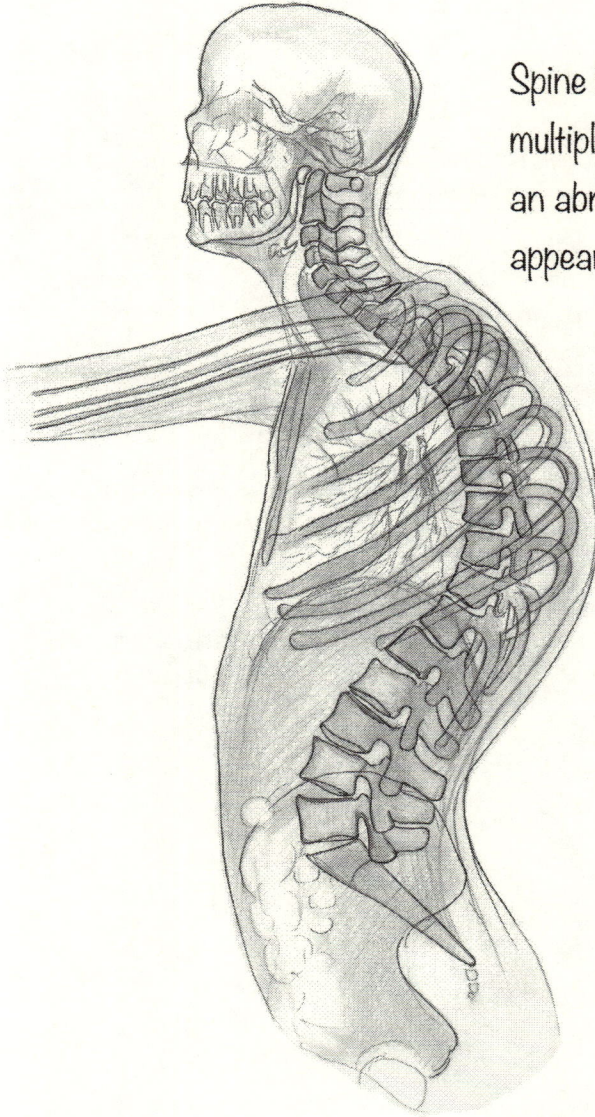

Spine is wedged at
multiple vertebrae giving
an abnormally curved
appearance

Scheuermann's kyphosis. Depiction of a lateral X-ray of a patient with
Scheuermann's kyphosis. The thoracic spine is abnormally curved
resulting in a hunch back appearance.

Normal Vertebral Segment

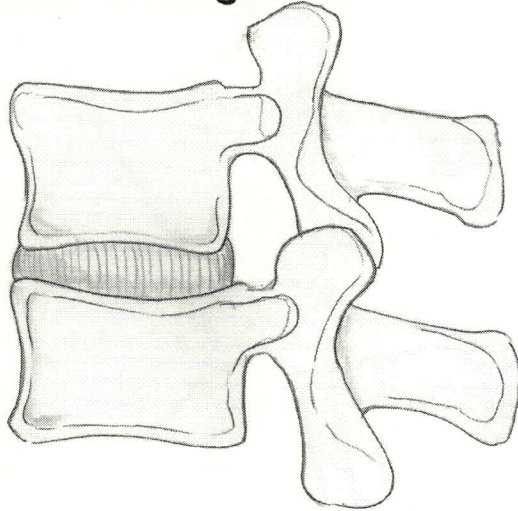

Scheuermann's Vertebral Segment

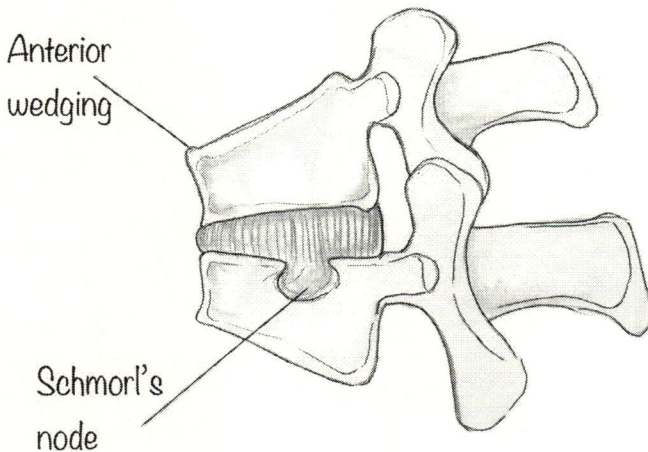

Anterior
wedging

Schmorl's
node

Scheuermann's vertebra. A normal vertebra viewed from the side (top). The change in shape of the vertebral body from a square to a wedge is what causes the abnormal curvature in Scheuermann's Kyphosis. Schmorl's nodes are abnormal disc herniations into the vertebral body (bottom).

Chapter 12

Osteoporosis and the Spine

Summary

Given enough time all bones degrade and become less dense and more brittle. This becomes a problem when you develop osteoporosis, that is, when your bones become so weak that they break under even small forces. Osteoporosis is important in spine surgery because it goes hand in hand with degeneration of the spine. We use rods and screws to fix problems in the back, but these work poorly in weak bone. For this reason, I recommend treatment for someone who has osteoporosis or has had a fragility fracture of the spine. Treatment generally consists of a combination of supplements such as vitamin D as well as a medicine. There are two main types of pharmacologic treatments: **antiresorptive therapy** with a drug such as alendronate (Fosamax®) that prevents bone breakdown or **anabolic therapy** with a drug such as Teriparatide (Forteo®) which helps build more bones.

Case

Ms. Gainsboro, is a 65-year-old waitress who has smoked a pack and a half of cigarettes for over 40 years. One day she is lifting a box of dishes at work and

notices a pop in her back. She immediately has severe pain but attributes it to a pulled muscle. However, the pain does not go away. She spends the next few days in bed unable to move. X-rays are ordered by an urgent care provider that reveal a compression fracture of her L3 vertebra. She is referred to me and we get a bone density study (DEXA Scan) that shows she has osteoporosis in her spine, and both hips. Her vitamin D levels are low and her parathyroid hormone levels are high. I treat her initially with a medicine called calcitonin that can help with pain from these fractures, but she is still in agony. Ultimately, we decide to perform a kyphoplasty procedure on her that immediately stops her pain. We then start the process of rebuilding her bones, by first starting her on high doses of vitamin D and then a bone-building medicine called Abalop-aratide. Within a year she is back to being a waitress and her bone scans show increasing bone mineral density.

Introduction

Your bones are living organs just like your heart, lungs, and brain; however, unlike the visceral organs, bones are mineralized to be strong and support your body. **Bones are composed primarily of special cells, proteins, and minerals: 1. cells called osteoblasts, osteoclasts and osteocytes** regulate the structure and mineral content of bones, **2. proteins such as collagen** provide bones with tensile strength, and **3. minerals such as calcium and phosphate** give bones compressive strength, making them hard. Just like the rest of the organs in your body, bones undergo changes related to age and disease. In the case of bones, typically there is mineral loss and thus reduced strength as you age. This is especially true for your spine and can result in fractures and complications with spinal surgery. In this chapter we will take an in-depth look into how the strength of your bones affect your spine and your spine surgery.

Your Bones Over Your Lifetime

You achieve your peak bone mass around the age of 30, which means that at this time, this is the strongest they will ever be (1). After this, whether you are male or female, your skeleton slowly undergoes age-related decline in bone mass. Both the rate of decline and the height of your peak bone mass are determined by many factors, including genetics, mechanical forces (that is, how you use your skeleton), exposure to drugs that are toxic to your bones (such as steroids and diuretics), and illnesses (such as diabetes). Additionally, in females, there is a dramatic decline in bone mineral density around the time of menopause (approaching 30%!) related to a decrease in their estrogen levels (2,3). Men also experience age-related decline in bone mass, but it doesn't show up until a later age because men have a higher peak bone mass and because men do not undergo the hormonal changes of menopause that increase low bone density (4,5).

What is Osteoporosis?

Simply stated, **osteoporosis is a state of increased fragility of the skeleton**. It is caused by loss of bone mineral density (thinning of the bones) as well as changes to the overall structure of the bone. Medically it is defined as occurring in a patient who has a certain measurement from a bone density scan (**DXA** or Dual X-ray Absorptiometry, also known as DEXA) which gives you two scores: a T-score and a Z-score. A bone density scan generates a **T-score** which is calculated based on the difference between your bone mineral density and that of a healthy sex-matched 20- to 30-year-old. A T-score of less than -2.5 is indicative of osteoporosis while a T-score between -1.5 and -2.4 is indicative of osteopenia. Alternatively, if you suffer from a "fragility fracture" you also technically have osteoporosis. A **fragility fracture** is a break in some of the typically strongest bones in your body (hip and spine) that occurs from a very minor injury (such as a fall, bending over or twisting). The **Z-score** is mainly used to compare your bone mineral density (BMD) to that of someone the same age and sex and is mainly used to assess the BMD of younger patients and children and thus is not as widely used.

 The lifetime risk for a hip fracture in a 50-year-old Caucasian woman approaches 15-20%, and the risk for any fragility fracture is 50%. This means that on average 15-20 women out of 100 aged 50 or older are going to fracture a hip some time before they die. And that one out of two women as they age are likely to break something just by bending, twisting wrong or falling or even sneezing/coughing hard. The lifetime risk of a vertebral fracture is about 16% in a 50-year-old Caucasian woman. Unfortunately, the risk of suffering a second vertebral fracture goes up four-fold once a patient has sustained a single one (6). Spinal fragility fractures may be inconsequential, but can also result in serious disability, chronic pain, loss of self-esteem and deformity. Osteoporosis affects all races and ethnicity but seems less prevalent in Hispanics and African Americans—although this does not mean these groups should forgo screening. It is projected that there will be a 2.7 fold increase in fragility fractures in Hispanics and other ethnic groups in the future (4).

When you get a DXA scan your report may come with a **FRAX score (short for Fracture Risk Assessment Tool)**. FRAX is a clinical calculator that estimates the probability of sustaining an insufficiency fracture (a fracture that occurs with "low energy" or very little trauma, for example a crack in the bone that occurs with only a minor injury such as a fall from standing or even lifting something heavy) over the next 10 years based on your bone mineral density and your risk factors. Patients with a 10-year risk of insufficiency fracture that is greater than 20% or a 10-year risk of sustaining a hip fracture that is greater than 3% are generally recommended to start osteoporosis treatment.

Osteopenia is a "pre-osteoporotic state" that is defined based on your T-score falling between -1.5 and -2.5. Patients with osteopenia are at risk for developing osteoporosis, but osteopenia is not a benign condition. Actually, a large portion of insufficiency fractures occur in patients with osteopenia and many more people suffer from osteopenia than osteoporosis. 82% of women with an insufficiency fracture have T-scores better than -2.5. Osteopenia is less commonly treated by physicians because osteoporosis drugs have mainly been tested to treat patients with T scores less than -2.5. For this reason osteopenia is generally only treated if the patient is at very high risk for a fracture (high FRAX score) or has already suffered an insufficiency fracture (5).

Risk Factors for Developing Osteoporosis

There are many risk factors for the development of osteoporosis: low physical activity, heavy alcohol and caffeine intake, smoking, taking certain drugs (steroids, serotonin reuptake inhibitors, antiseizure medications, thiazide diuretics, heparin), a family history of osteoporosis, nutritional deficiencies, including those caused by gastric bypass, early menopause, diabetes and other endocrine disorders, low vitamin D and low calcium (7).

Steroid use (common drugs such as prednisone and fluticasone) is the most common cause of secondary osteoporosis (osteoporosis that is not age-related)(8). Several studies have shown an increased risk of fracture in patients taking long-term steroids (8,9). Taking prednisone 10mg a day for more than 90 days can increase your risk of fracture in the hip or spine by 17 times (9)!

Diagnosis

Osteoporosis and osteopenia are both on the spectrum of declining bone mineral density. Women over the age of 65 and men over the age of 70 should have routine bone density assessment every 2 years. It is likely a good idea to get this checked prior to having spine surgery, especially if you are going to have a lumbar fusion. This is typically done with a DXA scan (Dual energy X-ray Absorptiometry scan); however, there are other methods such as quantitative computer tomography and plain computer tomography. DXA scans are safe, use very low dose radiation and are inexpensive. A DXA scan generates a score based on how dense your bones are. This is then converted to a T-score which is a comparison of your bones to a healthy 30-year-old (not fair!). T-scores that are positive (+) generally indicate good bone quality, while negative (-) numbers represent declining bone quality. Patients with a T score less than -2.5 on DXA scans are considered osteoporotic. As described above, you may also be considered osteoporotic regardless of your T-score if you suffer from a fragility fracture. A T-score between -2.5 and -1.5 indicates osteopenia.

The Problem with Osteoporosis and with Osteoporosis in Spine Surgery

As stated, osteoporosis represents a deterioration in the strength of the bone. It is painless and most people do not know they have it. So why should it be treated, you may ask. The problem with osteoporosis is that it increases your risk of suffering from a fracture of the spine or the hip. If you suffer a hip or spine fracture, it can dramatically impact your quality of life and increase your chances of dying (like other painless conditions doctors typically treat like hypertension). In fact, your risk of mortality (dying) one year after a spine insufficiency fracture is 23% for all age groups (10).

Spine surgery frequently involves instrumentation such as pedicle screws, hooks, and rods. Metal cages may also be used as disc spacers between vertebrae. And in spine surgery, just like in regular carpentry, if the "wood" is weak, brittle, or rotten, you will have a hard time getting metal screws to stay in place. Patients with untreated osteoporosis who need to undergo spine surgery are at increased risk for fractures, screw loosening, adjacent segment degeneration, cage subsidence and collapse, pseudoarthrosis (failure of vertebrae to fuse) and even progressive deformity (11,12). In general, osteoporosis increases the risk of complication from spine surgery significantly (10). For this reason your surgeon may want to obtain a DXA scan prior to surgery to ensure your bones will be able to handle it (13).

Treatment

non pharmacologic treatment

The primary non pharmacologic treatment of osteoporosis focuses on **weight-bearing exercises** that put stress on the bones (14). This works because bones are reactive tissues, which degenerate with lack of use. Vigorous activity of greater than 2 hours a week (either of exercise or chores) has been to shown to decrease the risk of fractures. On the other hand, those who are sedentary for long periods per day are at increased risk for osteoporosis and fragility fracture (15).

Another key component of an exercise program is working on balance to decrease the risk of falls and thus exercises such as yoga and tai chi may be beneficial. You should evaluate your home for tripping hazards to further decrease the risk of falls.

Cigarettes are associated with the development of low bone density and should be stopped. Alcohol should also be limited as it can contribute to balance problems and increase falls and worsen osteoporosis. Finally, you should have your medications reviewed by your general practitioner for anything which may contribute to low bone mineral density and discuss with your doctor about switching or stopping those medications if able (16,17).

Antioxidants: Antioxidants are chemical compounds which neutralize destructive chemicals known as free radicals which are produced by metabolic processes of the body and can damage cells and DNA in high enough concentrations (so called oxidative stress). Free radicals are also produced by exposure to smoke, alcohol, anxiety, lack of sleep, dehydration, refined sugars, saturated fat, and radiation. There is growing evidence that oxidative stress increases the risk of osteoporosis by inhibiting the cells which build bone, the osteoblast. Thus, a diet rich in antioxidants, such as one found from eating whole fruits and vegetables, vitamin C 500 mg a day and greater than 50mg isoflavones (see below) is recommended to prevent osteoporosis. A lifestyle aimed at preventing oxidative stress such as getting enough sleep, staying well hydrated, exercising, and avoiding alcohol, drugs and sugar may also be helpful (18).

Calcium (1200mg daily) and **vitamin D** (1000-2000 IU/daily) supplementation have been shown to decrease fracture risk and currently are recommended by the American Association of Clinical Endocrinologists (17,19).

supplements

Vitamin D deficiency treatment: Vitamin D is essential for bone health, muscle strength and the strength of your immune system. It is responsible in assisting the intestines to absorb calcium, ensuring you have the adequate building blocks for strong bones. Vitamin D is obtained through the diet, especially fish and cheese, or by exposure to sunlight and through supplementation. There are two main forms— Ergocalciferol (Vitamin D2) and Cholecalciferol (Vitamin D3)—which are both produced in the skin on exposure to UV light. When your vitamin D levels decrease, your parathyroid hormone increases, and your bones are broken down to maintain calcium in your blood stream. Thus, when your body is low on vitamin D your bones are constantly being degraded.

Vitamin D deficiency is measured through a blood test which looks at your 25-OH Vitamin D level, which is a precursor to 1,25 OH Vitamin D (the active form).   A level less than 20 ng/ml is considered **deficient,** and a level less than 30 ng/ml is considered **insufficient**. Vitamin D deficiency is an extremely prevalent problem and is estimated to affect 1 billion people worldwide and as many as 20-100% of elderly men living in North America. If you live at higher latitudes, such as in the northern part of the United States, you are more likely to have a Vitamin D deficiency.

While a maintenance dose of 1000-2000 IU Vitamin D daily is acceptable, those who are deficient in vitamin D may require higher doses up to 10,000-50,000 IU per week for several months to correct levels. Vitamin D is safe, and a toxic level of ingestion is very rare, but possible with ingestion of greater than 50,000 IU daily. Vitamin D can reduce the risk of cancer, and other chronic disease, prevent falls, as well as help you maintain your bone health (20,21).

Calcium: In general, most calcium is obtained from the diet and supplementation is not necessary. However, common supplements of vitamin D also contain calcium which is fine. Please see the chapter on calcium metabolism for more information. As stated above the daily recommended dose of calcium is 1200mg.

Soy isoflavones: As mentioned earlier, estrogen plays a crucial role in the maintenance of bone mineral density, and when estrogen levels drop during menopause, the result is a great decrease in bone mineral density. While hormone replacement therapy (HRT) can blunt the effects of post-menopausal bone loss, HRT is associated with other side-effects such as an increased risk of gynecological cancer. Soy Isoflavones, or so-called phytoestrogens, have a similar chemical compound to estrogen. They are found in soy products and have been associated with increased bone mineral density (22). Randomized controlled studies with **Genistein**, a particular soy isoflavone, was shown to increase bone mineral density. Whether this translates into reduced fracture risk is unknown; however, soy products are relatively safe and may be a reasonable part of the post-menopausal diet (23).

Resveratrol: Resveratrol is a chemical compound which is found on the skin of red grapes and has been shown to have a beneficial effect on bone as well as cerebrovascular function. A randomized, controlled double-blind trial comparing 75mg of resveratrol twice daily to placebo, showed that bone mineral density was significantly improved with resveratrol and chemical markers of bone breakdown were decreased (24).

medical management

There are two classes of medicine used to manage osteoporosis: **antiresorptive therapy** (medicines which block the breakdown of bone) and **anabolic therapy** (medicines which encourage new bone growth).

Antiresorptive therapy include treatment with bisphosphonate drugs such as **alendronate** or **zoledronic acid**, **denosumab** and **estrogens**. **Anabolic therapy** includes treatments with newer drugs such as **teriparatide** and **abaloparatide** which build bone!

bisphosphonates

Bisphosphonates are a large class of drugs which block bone degradation (breakdown). They are the first line of therapy for osteoporosis and multiple types have been shown to be reduce the risk of both hip and vertebral fractures. These drugs are generally well tolerated; however, two rare but serious side-effects warrant further discussion as they cause a lot of anxiety in patients.

Atypical femur fractures are breaks in the bone that occur just below the hip with very minor or low-energy trauma. This kind of fracture can occur in women who have been on long-term bisphosphonate (more than three years) at a rate of about 3-50 per 100,000 people treated every year. This means that in 100,0000 persons taking bisphosphonates, only about 3 will develop one of these fractures per year. This risk is microscopic compared to the risk of an ordinary osteoporotic or vertebral fracture, which is why bisphosphonates are still widely used and recommended (25). Bisphosphonates have not been found to interfere with normal bone healing in humans (26).

Osteonecrosis of the jaw is another anxiety-provoking side-effect I often get asked about by my patients. Osteonecrosis of the jaw occurs in even fewer patients taking bisphosphonates than the femur fracture just discussed. Osteonecrosis is defined as an area of exposed bone in the maxillofacial (jaw) region that does not heal within 8 weeks of identification by a health care worker. This complication typically only occurs in cancer patients receiving very high dosages of bisphosphonate drugs and denosumab. The risk of this occurring in those receiving bisphosphonates for osteoporosis is not significantly different from just being part of the general population and that risk is estimated to be about 0.001%. In other words, it occurs in about 1 out of 100,000 patients taking the medicine, which is not significantly different from the risk if you are not taking any medicine. Patients should have any dental or oral surgery work completed prior to starting a bisphosphonate as well as maintain excellent oral hygiene, which can prevent the occurrence. If you have dentures make sure they are well-fitting (23).

Bisphosphonates are excreted from the body through the kidneys, and thus **patients with renal (kidney) disease should not use them**. Another common side-effect of bisphosphonates is hypocalcemia (too little calcium in the blood), which can cause muscle aches and pains. That is why Vitamin D and calcium supplementation is always prescribed along with a bisphosphonate. Oral bisphosphonates can cause gastrointestinal (GI) upset and thus must be taken according to instructions and should not be taken by patients with esophageal disease (such as achalasia).

Gastroesophageal reflux is not a strict contraindication but should be discussed with your physician. Let's discuss some specific bisphosphonates.

Alendronate or **Fosamax**® is a 10mg tablet taken daily or a 70mg tablet taken once weekly and costs about $1 for a 1-month supply. In the Fracture Intervention Trial (FIT) which was a placebo-controlled, randomized trial, alendronate was compared to a placebo. The trial showed a reduction in vertebral and non-vertebral fractures by about 50% in the group taking alendronate. There were no significant differences in GI symptoms between the groups and adverse events were more common in the placebo group. Oral bisphosphonates like alendronate must be taken in the morning, 30 minutes or more before any food or beverage other than water. You should sit upright following ingestion of the pill to prevent any esophageal irritation (27,28). Alendronate can be taken continuously for up to 5 years, after which a "drug holiday" should be considered to prevent an atypical femur fracture. During this period a different drug such as teriparatide (see below) may be used (17).

Zoledronic acid or **Reclast**® is a 5mg infusion (a medicine given through an IV) given once a year at your hospital's infusion center and costs about $87 per month. It is one of the most effective bisphosphonates at preventing fractures and is useful for patients who cannot tolerate oral bisphosphonates (such as those who have esophageal irritation) (29). The Health Outcomes and Reduced Incidence with Zoledronic Acid Once Yearly (HORIZON) trial was a randomized, controlled trial comparing zoledronic acid to a placebo. That trial showed a reduction in vertebral fractures by about 70% over a 3-year period in patients taking zoledronic acid. Overall serious adverse events did not differ significantly between groups in this trial; however, a cardiac complication known as atrial fibrillation occurred more frequently in the zoledronic acid group (1.3% vs 0.5%). There were no cases of osteonecrosis of the jaw. Common side-effects were flu-like symptoms with fever, headache and joint pain which occurs in about 30% of patients and lasts for about 3 days after each administration of the drug (30)placebo-controlled trial, 3889 patients (mean age, 73 years. Taking Tylenol with the first infusion of zoledronic acid can help reduce this by about 50% (31).

denosumab (Prolia®)

Denosumab is an antiresorptive drug but differs significantly from the bisphosphonates. It is an antibody—a protein which blocks the action of other molecules in the body. Denosumab blocks the action of the receptor activator of nuclear factor-κβ ligand or RANKL, a molecule which stimulates bone resorption by activating the cells that break down bone called osteoclasts. Thus, denosumab blocks this molecule (RANKL) from activating osteoclasts and in this way prevents bone from breaking down. Denosumab is a 60mg injection given to you by a healthcare worker every 6 months. Its cost is about $196 per month. Unlike bisphosphonates it can be given to patients with kidney problems.

In the Fracture Reduction Evaluation of Denosumab in Osteoporosis every six Months (FREEDOM) trial, vertebral fractures were reduced by approximately 68% and hip fractures by 40% in the denosumab group compared to the placebo group. There were no significant differences in adverse events between denosumab and placebo. No cases of osteonecrosis of the jaw or atypical femur fractures were reported (32). You can take denosumab for many years (up to 10); however, when you stop you should typically be transitioned to another antiresorptive drug since there are reports of rebound fractures occurring when coming off denosumab (33). Typically, zoledronic acid is used following denosumab but expect some loss of bone mineral following discontinuation of the denosumab. See the FAQ below for more information on the duration of therapy.

estrogens

Estrogen has a potent effect on maintaining the strength of your bones. When menopause occurs, there is a significant drop in estrogen levels and thus a correlating drop in your bone health. However, the use of pure estrogen to treat osteoporosis is not recommended because of side-effects such as increased risk of blood clots, heart attacks and breast cancer. Nonetheless, a drug called **Raloxifene** which is a **selective estrogen receptor modulator** (or SERM), has been approved by the FDA for the treatment of osteoporosis. What this means is that it has similar chemical effects to estrogen but is not the full-blown estrogen. **Raloxifene** or **Evista**® is a 60mg pill taken orally daily and costs about $17 per month (27). This drug was designed to act specifically on bone tissue and thus does not have the same side-effect profile as regular estrogen.

The MORE (Multiple Outcomes of Raloxifene Evaluation) randomized, placebo-controlled trial showed that Raloxifene reduced vertebral fractures by about 30% compared to placebo but does not have the same effect on hip or extremity fractures. Long-term use was associated with increased risk of blood clots (about 1% of patients) and with a decreased risk of breast cancer. Thus, this drug should not be used in patients with a history of blood-clotting conditions, for example, deep venous thrombosis (DVT) or pulmonary embolism (PE). Other potential side-effects with Raloxifene included flu-like symptoms, hot flashes, and leg cramps (34). It is reserved primarily for younger patients who would benefit from reducing their chances of breast cancer or who have mainly spine osteoporosis (27).

anabolic therapy

Anabolic therapy differs from antiresorptive therapy in that it increases the strength of your bones. The two main drugs in this class are **teriparatide** or **Forteo®** and **Abaloparatide** or **Tymlos®.**

teriparatide

Teriparatide is a **synthetic version of parathyroid hormone**, which is a naturally occurring hormone in your body produced by the parathyroid glands. Teriparatide comes in an injector pen which you self-administer daily in your abdomen or thighs for up to 2 years. It is quite expensive—the current cost is currently at around $3,179 a month—but will likely become more affordable as it is no longer under patent. Injecting yourself daily sounds daunting, but once you learn how to do the injection, it's very manageable. In the Fracture Prevention Trial, teriparatide was compared to placebo and reduced the occurrence of vertebral fractures by 65% but did not reduce the occurrence of hip fractures. Teriparatide has been shown to be superior to bisphosphonates in multiple trials in the reduction of vertebral fractures (35,36). Teriparatide is generally reserved as a second-line medicine for those who cannot tolerate or have failed bisphosphonates but, as we will discuss later, has some off-label applications in spine surgery (27).

abaloparatide

Abaloparatide is like teriparatide but is a **synthetic version of a parathyroid-related peptide** (instead of parathyroid hormone) that is also a daily injection. It was approved by the FDA in 2017. Abaloparatide was evaluated in the ACTIVE trial which compared it in a randomized, blinded fashion to placebo and to teriparatide. In this trial abaloparatide reduced vertebral fractures by about 80% compared to placebo but was like teriparatide. Abaloparatide, unlike teriparatide, also reduced fractures in other areas besides the spine and increased bone mineral density more than teriparatide.

Abaloparatide is theorized to have a higher net anabolic (bone-strengthening) effect compared to teriparatide, but to determine the actual difference between the drugs would take a trial of almost 22,000 people, making proof very difficult. Abaloparatide has less of an incidence of hypercalcemia (too much calcium in the blood) compared to teriparatide but otherwise there were no significant differences in adverse events between the groups. The most common side- effects were nausea, headache, fatigue and palpitations (37).

Teriparatide and Abaloparatide both previously came with an FDA black box warning because at high doses can cause a rare bone cancer called osteosarcoma. However, in the 1 million individuals who have taken the medicine, there has only been one case of this reported, and thus, for the average patient the risk is not significant. This warning was removed in 2020(38). Teriparatide and abaloparatide are contraindicated in patients with a risk of developing osteosarcoma, such as patients with Paget's disease, or patients who have had large doses of radiation to the skeleton. Teriparatide should also not be used in patients with high serum levels of parathyroid hormone or calcium as it can cause calcium levels in the blood to increase. Common side-effects include orthostatic hypotension (a drop in blood pressure when you stand up), particularly the first time you use it. Thus, it may be best to take in the doctor's office for the first time or in a setting where you can sit down easily. It may also cause nausea, and high calcium in the blood. Like denosumab, once you stop teriparatide or abaloparatide you rapidly lose bone mass and thus treatment is generally followed with the use of a bisphosphonate.

romosozumab

A final agent is called romosozumab (Evenity®). Like denosumab, it is another antibody—this one binds a molecule called sclerostin, which is responsible for bone breakdown. In the placebo-controlled FRAME (fracture study in post-menopausal women with osteoporosis) trial, romosozumab use resulted in a 75% reduction in vertebral fractures and a 23% reduction in non-vertebral fractures. In this study the adverse-event profile in both groups was similar. One case of atypical femur fracture and two cases of osteonecrosis of the jaw occurred in the romosozumab group (39).

A second clinical trial, the ARCH (Active-Controlled Fracture Study in Post-menopausal Women with Osteoporosis at High Risk) trial showed a 48% reduction of vertebral fractures and a 19% reduction in non-vertebral fractures in patients taking romosozumab compared to those taking the bisphosphonate, alendronate. However, in the ARCH trial more serious cardiovascular adverse events were seen with romosozumab than with alendronate (40). As of the writing of this book, the FDA granted approval for romosozumab in the United States in 2019; however, there are black box warnings against the use of this medicine in any patient who **has sustained a heart attack or stroke** in the preceding year (41). The most common side-effects noted with romosozumab are joint pains and headaches.

Osteoporosis Treatment Prior to or After Spine Surgery

Osteoporosis medicines can be helpful in spine patients both to prevent future fractures and to make the surgery more successful. However, it is important to note that as of the writing of this chapter no drug is FDA approved specifically for use in spine surgery, and thus all are considered off-label. Nonetheless, there is considerable preclinical (testing the drugs on animals) evidence that both antiresorptives and anabolic agents can increase the success of spinal fusion and help prevent complications (42).

Bisphosphonates such as zoledronic acid can help prevent fractures adjacent to fusion constructs and can help prevent fusion cages from subsiding into the bone, and screws from loosening.

Teriparatide has been shown to decrease the rate of failure of spinal fusion surgery and improve fusion rates (42,43). It has also been shown to decrease the incidence of screw loosening with spinal hardware (44). Teriparatide has been shown to strengthen the bones above and below a spinal fusion construct and decrease the rate of breakdown and proximal junctional kyphosis (forward bending of the spine just above the fusion) or collapse of the vertebra above a fusion (45).

Other techniques exist to help prevent hardware failure in the osteoporotic spine. Longer fusion constructs (a fusion incorporating more levels (vertebrae)) may be used to decrease the chance of hardware failure. Alternative fixation devices such as hooks may also be employed. Newer technology such as fenestrated cement-augmented screws may also be used. Fenestrated screws are hollow and have small pores at the end. Bone cement can be injected through the screw's pores such that cement bonds the screw better to the vertebral body. There is growing evidence that this technique is useful in patients who have osteoporosis yet require spinal instrumentation (46).

Conclusion

There is an abundance of medications used to treat osteoporosis, so there is a great chance that one can be found that you are comfortable with and seems reasonable to you should you need one. Osteoporosis is a common finding in patients who need spine surgery and often can make having surgery more difficult because the instruments we use to hold the spine together will not hold in bad bone. For this reason, screening of bone density prior to surgery is common, and you may need treatment before or after your surgery.

Frequently Asked Questions About Osteoporosis

- **How often should I have a DXA Scan?**

  Every 2 years after age 65 in women and age 75 in men.

- **I have heard horror stories about Fosamax® (alendronate) and is it really for me?**

  The side effects from Fosamax are very rare but do warrant consideration. If you take the drug for too long (more than 3-5 years) the risk increases. If you are afraid of Fosamax®, then there are many other options available.

- **How long should I be on osteoporosis medication; can I take it forever?**

  The ideal time to stop medication for osteoporosis therapy is a clinical decision that is different for every patient and medication. Some higher-risk patients (such as those who have suffered from insufficiency fracture) may benefit from prolonged therapy. In low-risk cases, sometimes side-effects cause patients to stop taking the medication, and other times, the bone mineral density improves sufficiently where your doctor may feel comfortable taking you off the medicine.

  Bisphosphonates such as alendronate may be used up to 5 years and zoledronic acid up to 3 years. Bone density may decrease after discontinuation, but typically remains higher than baseline (47). Stopping after 5 years may be a reasonable choice for low-risk patients. Bisphosphonates may be restarted again after a 5-year holiday.

  Denosumab may be used for up to 10 years.

  Anabolic therapies may be used for 2 years.

References

1.   Bonjour JP, Theintz G, Law F, Slosman D, Rizzoli R. Peak bone mass. Osteoporos Int J Establ Result Coop Eur Found Osteoporos Natl Osteoporos Found USA. 1994;4 Suppl 1:7–13.

2.   Greendale GA, Sowers M, Han W, Huang MH, Finkelstein JS, Crandall CJ, et al. Bone mineral density loss in relation to the final menstrual period in a multiethnic cohort: Results from the Study of Women's Health Across the Nation (SWAN). J Bone Miner Res. 2012;27(1):111–8.

3.   Lupsa BC, Insogna K. Bone Health and Osteoporosis. Endocrinol Metab Clin North Am. 2015 Sep;44(3):517–30.

4.   Burge R, Dawson-Hughes B, Solomon DH, Wong JB, King A, Tosteson A. Incidence and Economic Burden of Osteoporosis-Related Fractures in the United States, 2005–2025. J Bone Miner Res. 2007;22(3):465–75.

5.   Eriksen EF. Treatment of osteopenia. Rev Endocr Metab Disord. 2012 Sep;13(3):209–23.

6.   Cummings SR, Melton LJ. Epidemiology and outcomes of osteoporotic fractures. The Lancet. 2002 May;359(9319):1761–7.

7.   Ross PD. RISK FACTORS FOR OSTEOPOROTIC FRACTURE. Endocrinol Metab Clin North Am. 1998 Jun;27(2):289–301.

8.   Weinstein RS. Glucocorticoid-Induced Bone Disease. N Engl J Med. 2011;9.

9.   Van Staa TP, Laan RF, Barton IP, Cohen S, Reid DM, Cooper C. Bone density threshold and other predictors of vertebral fracture in patients receiving oral glucocorticoid therapy. Arthritis Rheum. 2003 Nov;48(11):3224–9.

10.   Anderson PA, Freedman BA, Brox WT, Shaffer WO. Osteoporosis: Recent Recommendations and Positions of the American Society for Bone and Mineral Research and the International Society for Clinical Densitometry. J Bone Jt Surg. 2021 Apr 21;103(8):741–7.

11.   DeWald CJ, Stanley T. Instrumentation-related complications of multilevel fusions for adult spinal deformity patients over age 65: surgical considerations and treatment options in patients with poor bone quality. Spine. 2006 Sep 1;31(19 Suppl):S144-151.

12.   Formby PM, Kang DG, Helgeson MD, Wagner SC. Clinical and Radiographic Outcomes of Transforaminal Lumbar Interbody Fusion in Patients with Osteoporosis. Glob Spine J. 2016 Nov;6(7):660–4.

13.   Anderson PA, Morgan SL, Krueger D, Zapalowski C, Tanner B, Jeray KJ, et al. Use of Bone Health Evaluation in Orthopedic Surgery: 2019 ISCD Official Position. J Clin Densitom Off J Int Soc Clin Densitom. 2019 Dec;22(4):517–43.

14.   Evans RK, Negus CH, Centi AJ, Spiering BA, Kraemer WJ, Nindl BC. Peripheral QCT sector analysis reveals early exercise-induced increases in tibial bone mineral density. :10.

15.   Pfeifer M, Sinaki M, Geusens P, Boonen S, Preisinger E, Minne HW, et al. Musculoskeletal Rehabilitation in Osteoporosis: A Review. J Bone Miner Res. 2004 Aug;19(8):1208–14.

16.   Black DM, Rosen CJ. Postmenopausal Osteoporosis. Solomon CG, editor. N Engl J Med. 2016 Jan 21;374(3):254–62.

17.   Camacho PM, Petak SM, Binkley N, Clarke BL, Harris ST, Hurley DL, et al. AMERICAN ASSOCIATION OF CLINICAL ENDOCRINOLOGISTS AND AMERICAN COLLEGE OF ENDOCRINOLOGY CLINICAL PRACTICE GUIDELINES FOR THE DIAGNOSIS AND TREAT-

MENT OF POSTMENOPAUSAL OSTEOPOROSIS — 2016-- *EXECUTIVE SUMMARY*. Endocr Pract. 2016 Sep;22(9):1111–8.

18.   Kimball JS, Johnson JP, Carlson DA. Oxidative Stress and Osteoporosis. J Bone Jt Surg. 2021 Aug 4;103(15):1451–61.

19.   Bischoff-Ferrari HA, Willett WC, Wong JB, Giovannucci E, Dietrich T, Dawson-Hughes B. Fracture Prevention With Vitamin D Supplementation: A Meta-analysis of Randomized Controlled Trials. JAMA. 2005 May 11;293(18):2257.

20.   Holick MF. Vitamin D Deficiency. N Engl J Med. 2007;16.

21.   Holick MF, Binkley NC, Bischoff-Ferrari HA, Gordon CM, Hanley DA, Heaney RP, et al. Evaluation, Treatment, and Prevention of Vitamin D Deficiency: an Endocrine Society Clinical Practice Guideline. J Clin Endocrinol Metab. 2011 Jul;96(7):1911–30.

22.   Adlercreutz H, Mazur W. Phyto-oestrogens and Western diseases. Ann Med. 1997 Apr;29(2):95–120.

23.   Marini H, Minutoli L, Polito F, Bitto A, Altavilla D, Atteritano M, et al. Effects of the Phytoestrogen Genistein on Bone Metabolism in Osteopenic Postmenopausal Women: A Randomized Trial. Ann Intern Med. 2007 Jun 19;146(12):839.

24.   Wong RH, Zaw JJT, Xian CJ, Howe PR. Regular supplementation with resveratrol improves bone mineral density in postmenopausal women: a randomised, placebo-controlled trial. J Bone Miner Res [Internet]. [cited 2020 Jun 25];n/a(n/a). Available from: https://asbmr.onlinelibrary.wiley.com/doi/abs/10.1002/jbmr.4115

25.   Shane E, Burr D, Abrahamsen B, Adler RA, Brown TD, Cheung AM, et al. Atypical Subtrochanteric and Diaphyseal Femoral Fractures: Second Report of a Task Force of the American Society for Bone and Mineral Research: AFF TASK FORCE REPORT. J Bone Miner Res. 2014 Jan;29(1):1–23.

26.   Kates SL, Ackert-Bicknell CL. How do bisphosphonates affect fracture healing? Injury. 2016 Jan;47 Suppl 1:S65-68.

27.   Matzkin EG, DeMaio M, Charles JF, Franklin CC. Diagnosis and Treatment of Osteoporosis: What Orthopaedic Surgeons Need to Know. J Am Acad Orthop Surg. 2019 Oct;27(20):e902–12.

28.   Black DM, Cummings SR, Karpf DB, Cauley JA, Thompson DE, Nevitt MC, et al. Randomised trial of effect of alendronate on risk of fracture in women with existing vertebral fractures. The Lancet. 1996 Dec;348(9041):1535–41.

29.   Migliore A, Broccoli S, Massafra U, Cassol M, Frediani B. Ranking antireabsorptive agents to prevent vertebral fractures in postmenopausal osteoporosis by mixed treatment comparison meta-analysis. :13.

30.   Black DM, Boonen S, Leung PC, Caminis J, Sellmeyer D. Once-Yearly Zoledronic Acid for Treatment of Postmenopausal Osteoporosis. N Engl J Med. 2007;14.

31.   Wark JD, Bensen W, Recknor C, Ryabitseva O, Chiodo J, Mesenbrink P, et al. Treatment with acetaminophen/paracetamol or ibuprofen alleviates post-dose symptoms related to intravenous infusion with zoledronic acid 5 mg. Osteoporos Int. 2012

Feb;23(2):503–12.

32.   Cummings SR, Martin JS, McClung MR, Siris ES, Eastell R, Reid IR, et al. Deno-sumab for Prevention of Fractures in Postmenopausal Women with Osteoporosis. N Engl J Med. 2009 Aug 20;361(8):756–65.

33.   Cummings SR, Ferrari S, Eastell R, Gilchrist N, Jensen JEB, McClung M, et al. Vertebral Fractures After Discontinuation of Denosumab: A Post Hoc Analysis of the Randomized Placebo-Controlled FREEDOM Trial and Its Extension. J Bone Miner Res. 2018;33(2):190–8.

34.   Ettinger B, Black DM, Mitlak BH, Knickerbocker RK, Nickelsen T, Genant HK, et al. Reduction of vertebral fracture risk in postmenopausal women with osteoporosis treated with raloxifene: results from a 3-year randomized clinical trial. Multiple Out-comes of Raloxifene Evaluation (MORE) Investigators. JAMA. 1999 Aug 18;282(7):637–45.

35.   Liu CL, Lee HC, Chen CC, Cho DY. Head-to-head comparisons of bisphospho-nates and teriparatide in osteoporosis: a meta-analysis. Clin Invest Med. 2017 Jun 26;E146–57.

36.   Kendler DL, Marin F, Zerbini CAF, Russo LA, Greenspan SL, Zikan V, et al. Effects of teriparatide and risedronate on new fractures in post-menopausal women with severe osteoporosis (VERO): a multicentre, double-blind, double-dummy, randomised controlled trial. The Lancet. 2018 Jan;391(10117):230–40.

37.   Miller PD, Hattersley G, Riis BJ, Williams GC, Lau E, Russo LA, et al. Effect of Ab-aloparatide vs Placebo on New Vertebral Fractures in Postmenopausal Women With Osteoporosis: A Randomized Clinical Trial. JAMA. 2016 Aug 16;316(7):722.

38.   BlackBoxRX • Teriparatide (Boxed Warning removed 11/16/2020) [Internet]. [cited 2022 Jun 4]. Available from: https://blackboxrx.com/app/display/247?dir=black-box&whichpage=247

39.   Cosman F, Crittenden DB, Adachi JD, Binkley N, Czerwinski E, Ferrari S, et al. Romosozumab Treatment in Postmenopausal Women with Osteoporosis. N Engl J Med. 2016 Oct 20;375(16):1532–43.

40.   Saag KG, Petersen J, Brandi ML, Karaplis AC, Lorentzon M, Thomas T, et al. Romosozumab or Alendronate for Fracture Prevention in Women with Osteoporosis. N Engl J Med. 2017 Oct 12;377(15):1417–27.

41.   McClung MR. Romosozumab for the treatment of osteoporosis. Osteoporos Sarcopenia. 2018 Mar;4(1):11–5.

42.   Yolcu Y, Alvi M, Wanderman N, Carlson B, Sebastian A, Bydon M, et al. Effect of teriparatide use on bone mineral density and spinal fusion: a narrative review of animal models. Int J Neurosci. 2019 Aug 3;129(8):814–20.

43.   Black DM, Schwartz AV, Ensrud KE, Cauley JA, Levis S, Quandt SA, et al. Ef-fects of continuing or stopping alendronate after 5 years of treatment: the Fracture Intervention Trial Long-term Extension (FLEX): a randomized trial. JAMA. 2006 Dec 27;296(24):2927–38.

44.   Ohtori S, Inoue G, Orita S, Yamauchi K, Eguchi Y, Ochiai N, et al. Comparison of Teriparatide and Bisphosphonate Treatment to Reduce Pedicle Screw Loosening After Lumbar Spinal Fusion Surgery in Postmenopausal Women With Osteoporosis From a Bone Quality Perspective: Spine. 2013 Apr;38(8):E487–92.

45.   Yagi M, Ohne H, Konomi T, Fujiyoshi K, Kaneko S, Komiyama T, et al. Teriparatide improves volumetric bone mineral density and fine bone structure in the UIV+1 vertebra, and reduces bone failure type PJK after surgery for adult spinal deformity. Osteoporos Int. 2016 Dec;27(12):3495–502.

46.   Son H, Choi SH, Heo DR, Kook I, Lee MK, Ahn HS, et al. Outcomes of the Use of Cement-Augmented Cannulated Pedicle Screws in Lumbar Spinal Fusion. Spine J. 2021 May;S1529943021002369.

47.   Oba H, Takahashi J, Yokomichi H, Hasegawa T, Ebata S, Mukaiyama K, et al. Weekly Teriparatide Versus Bisphosphonate for Bone Union During 6 Months After Multi-Level Lumbar Interbody Fusion for Osteoporotic Patients: A Multicenter, Prospective, Randomized Study. Spine. 2020 Jul 1;45(13):863–71.

Figures:

Osteoporosis: Cross Section of Vertebrae

A normal vertebra with dense bony internal struts:

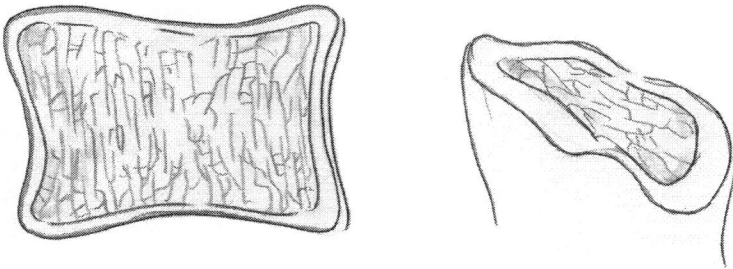

A osteoporotic collapsed vertebra with sparse bony internal struts:

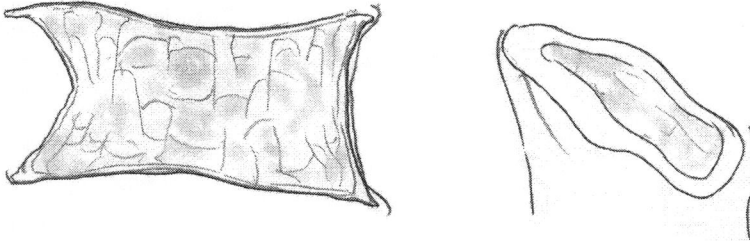

Osteoporosis cortex. A normal vertebra cross section (top). An osteoporotic vertebra cross section where there are microfractures resulting in collapse of the cortical bone and flattening of the box shape as well as loss of trabecular struts (sheets of bone inside the vertebra which act to support it) internally (bottom).

Chapter 13

Fractures and Dislocations of the Spine

Summary

Fractures of the spine are common in high energy trauma such as motor vehicle accidents and can result in serious injury. How you are treated depends on where in the spine you are injured and how bad the fracture is. The cervical spine and thoracolumbar spine (the junction between the thoracic and lumbar sections) are both mobile and are prone to injury. Luckily, treatment for spinal fractures is mostly non-operative with braces and collars. If your spine is unstable after the injury or you have neurologic injury you may need surgery both to stabilize and decompress the spine. Surgery for fractures typically consists of placement of rods and screws to hold things together while everything heals— known as spinal instrumentation. Formal spinal fusion may also be performed where bone graft is used to help the bones grow together.

Case

Ms. Coral is a 40-year-old pediatrician who is involved in a head-on motor vehicle collision on a family vacation. She is knocked unconscious but luckily

was wearing her seat belt, which prevented her from being ejected from the car. She is brought by ambulance to my hospital where a complete diagnostic work-up is performed. A CT scan reveals she has a burst fracture of her L1 vertebra. Luckily, she is neurologically intact and my first instinct is that she will be fine in a brace. However, an MRI shows that all her ligaments in the back of her spine are destroyed making this fracture very unstable. Furthermore, even with an external brace she is unable to walk because of pain. To protect her spinal cord, and to stabilize her spine we decide to place rods and screws from T12 to L2 (known as a short construct, versus a long construct which would go up and down two levels (two vertebrae) from the injury). The screws are meant to act as an internal brace to stabilize the spine and allow her bones to heal in the proper position. She spends another week in the hospital after the surgery but within 4 weeks has no more back pain. A year after her surgery, we remove the rods and screws and her back returns to normal without any loss of motion.

Introduction

Fractures can occur anywhere in the spine from the base of the skull to the pelvis. **A fracture** (or break—these terms can be used interchangeably) **occurs when a force applied to the bone surpasses its strength**. With the diversity of different vertebrae in your body it should come as no surprise that fractures in different areas of the spine require vastly different treatments ranging from doing nothing to surgery. While most fractures of the spine are benign (will heal uneventfully without requiring surgery), all should be evaluated by a spine surgeon or an expert in non-operative spinal care. Here we will explore the world of spine fractures and dislocations from the top (the skull) down (the sacrum). There may be more in this chapter than you want to know so feel free to pick the topics that are appropriate for you and use them as a quick reference to help you get your footing in an otherwise complex subject.

Fracture Healing

It is worth briefly reviewing the basics of fracture healing. Surgeons talk about two kinds of healing of fractures: primary healing, which involves holding the break in place with internal hardware, and secondary healing, which requires less rigidity and usually involves an external brace or casting.

In **primary healing**, bone-weaving osteoblastic cells fix the fracture gap directly, spanning it with newly formed mature bone. To accomplish this there must be very little motion across the fracture site and small fracture gaps. (Comminution or small bony fragmentation, where the bone is smashed into many pieces, will not heal by primary healing because the osteoblastic cells cannot "jump" the gap between those small pieces—they are too large). Primary healing can occur when a clean fracture has been rigidly fixed with internal hardware so the bone cannot move. In other words, a surgeon fixes the fracture back to "how god made it" and holds it in place with metal hardware. This is typically only possible in fractures that have simple configurations, that is, the bone is split, not shattered.

In fact, **most fracture healing occurs via secondary healing**, where a cartilage "soft callus" is first formed around the break (before mature bone is formed) to stabilize it. Secondary healing can occur in breaks that are less severe and require less-rigid types of immobilization, such as bracing or casting. It also occurs in the setting of high comminution, or shattered bone. Even if the surgeon fixes the fracture with hardware because there are so many fracture edges it will only heal by secondary healing. This cartilage that forms around the break is slowly converted to calcified bone by bone-forming osteoblast cells. Most fracture healing occurs this way (remember primary healing only occurs via a surgeon's hands) and secondary healing is the mode of healing which occurs in the spine when fractures are treated with a brace instead of internal hardware.

There are **three main phases to secondary fracture healing: inflammatory, reparative and remodeling**. The **inflammatory phase** occurs immediately after a fracture and lasts for about 1 week. During this phase a hematoma (blood clot) forms from ruptured bleeding vessels. At the same time, drawn by chemicals in the hematoma, macrophages (pac man-type cells which clean up debris), as well as other inflammatory cells, migrate to the location of the fracture and remove necrotic (dead) or damaged tissue. Following this, primitive mesenchymal stem cells (cells which can grow into many different types of tissue) migrate to the fracture to begin the work of repair.

During the **reparative phase** these stem cells differentiate into cartilage, bone, and fibrous tissue cells (chondrocytes, osteoblasts, and fibroblasts, respectively) which begin knitting the fracture back together. This process occurs over the next 2-12 weeks. This produces the soft callus that forms around the break and which is gradually converted to hard callus. The soft callus gradually restores the stiffness and strength of the bone not only by creating a tissue scaffold, but also by expanding the radius of the bone (1). It is critical to this biological process that the fracture be somewhat stable. Therefore, some fractures may not heal without intervention. Thus, fractures are braced, splinted, or fixed surgically to give the bone enough stability to allow healing.

During the final phase of secondary fracture healing **remodeling** occurs. At this stage, the hard callus, which is disorganized woven bone, begins to remodel according to the forces applied to the bone and, in time, becomes normal organized bone. This process can take anywhere from 6 weeks to over a year depending on the location of the fracture, and the patient's age and comorbidities (other medical conditions).

Non-operative Treatment of Spine Fractures

The overarching goal of all treatment of fractures is to restore or maintain alignment, and to stabilize the fracture to allow the patient to mobilize. Gone are the days of using prolonged bed rest to treat spinal fractures. Many of these fractures are stable on their own, and thus require no treatment at all other than some pain medication and physical therapy. For example, fractures occurring on the thoracic or lumbar spine are often stable and require very little treatment.

Sometimes fractures do require some additional stability to allow them to heal in the proper position. Non-operative treatment for fractures in the spine consists of the use of a rigid collar or brace. These come in many styles but all essentially perform the same function, which is to hold the spine in a certain position and prevent as much motion as possible. Non-operative treatment requires that the fracture pattern has some inherent stability. Bracing will not work on fractures that have no stability (that is, fractures that are significantly displaced).

An older but sometimes still-used form of bracing is called a halo vest. A halo vest consists of pins which screw into your skull and an outer frame that sits on your shoulder which prevents your head from moving (sounds awesome, right?). Thankfully these devices are not used as commonly anymore since they are associated with increased mortality especially in the elderly (2).

Operative Treatment of Spine Fractures

Fractures that are displaced or are unstable often required an intervention to put them back in the correct location. This maneuver is called a **"reduction"** and may be performed **closed** (without an incision) or **open** (with an incision). The spine is a series of bones which act like links in a chain. Thus, when one is fractured the chain is broken. To restore this, orthopedic surgeons sometimes also use hardware (called **instrumentation)** to span the broken segment and stabilize the spine. This is typically done with pedicle screws, which go into the vertebrae, and rods that connect them. Instrumentation can be done "minimally invasively" where screws are inserted through small incisions through the skin, or, if necessary, through a formal open midline incision. The screws act as a very rigid brace to allow the facture to heal and can be removed at a later date.

A fusion procedure may or may not be performed to turn several vertebrae into one vertebra with the use of bone graft. This is a more traditional method of fixing fractures. The number of levels (vertebrae) fused or instrumented (held together with screws or rods) depends on the area of the spine injured and the degree of the injury, but typically fixing a spinal fracture requires involving 3 vertebrae at a minimum (the fractured one, and the one above and below). If there are bony fragments which are impinging on the nerves or spinal cord, the fragments may need to be removed by a procedure called a decompression.

Overview of Cervical (Neck) Spine Trauma: Base of the Skull to C7

Injuries to the cervical spine are broadly categorized as upper and lower cervical spine injuries. Upper cervical spine injuries include injuries to the base of the skull (the occipital condyles), and the C1 and C2 vertebrae. Lower cervical spine injuries include everything from C3 to C7. Injuries commonly occur from motor vehicle accidents but can also occur from falls or in other ways.

In the upper cervical spine, ligaments are critical for the stability of the base of your skull; the bones here are less stable and thus primarily rely on the ligaments to keep them in place. The transverse atlantal ligament located in C1 is one such critical structure. It is critical because, if injured, it may render the spine unstable. Avoiding this situation is a guiding principle in the treatment of these injuries.

In the lower cervical spine, the bony structures contribute more to stability than do the ligamentous structures (meaning that the bones fit together better), and thus surgery is generally required to restore stability if there is significant disruption of the bony structures.

The cervical spine protects the spinal cord and nerve roots and thus injuries to this area of the body can result in profound neurologic deficits including paralysis, numbness and dysfunction of the bowel and bladder. Spinal cord injuries will be covered in another chapter 16.

occipital condyle fractures

The occipital condyles are a paired set of bony round mounds that are the part of the base of the skull that connects with the top cervical vertebra—the atlas (C1). The condyles sit on either side of the foramen magnum (the hole where the spinal cord exits from the skull).

It typically takes tremendous force to injure the occipital condyles which are strong. The usual injury is an axial loading force (a downward force) on the spine such as a heavy object landing on your head or falling on your head/neck from height. Any of these types of injuries should be evaluated immediately by an orthopedic surgeon.

Fractures of the occipital condyles range from bony crush injuries to ligament avulsions (tears). Typically, if only the bone is injured these fractures may be managed in a brace for 6-8 weeks. However, if there is a ligamentous injury, the junction between your skull and your cervical spine may become unstable, necessitating surgical instrumentation and fusion. Even following bracing, patients may expect mild neck disability following this type of injury (3).

occipital-cervical dislocation

Occipital-cervical dislocations (OCD), or so-called "internal decapitations" where the skull becomes detached from the cervical spine, are devastating injuries which are usually fatal. They are very rare injuries, typically requiring significant force to occur such as in a major motor vehicle collision. The resultant spinal instability can easily lead to secondary spinal cord damage or even sudden death. In those who are lucky enough to survive, surgery is almost always required. Occipital-cervical dislocations are associated with a high level of cervical spine trauma as well as injuries to the brain (4).

atlas (C1) fractures and transverse atlantal ligament rupture

The atlas is the first cervical vertebra and is the pedestal upon which the skull rests. It is ring-shaped and so a downward force can cause the bone to literally burst into pieces. This is called a Jefferson's fracture. Luckily most of these fractures can be managed conservatively as neurological complications are rare and the bone has excellent chances of healing in a collar. However, if there is disruption of the ligaments of the neck, the spine becomes unstable, and surgery is necessary. This is typically done with a C1-2 posterior spinal fusion.

The atlas (C1) is where much of your neck rotation occurs—it pivots on the peg known as the odontoid bone of the C2 vertebra. Connecting these two vertebrae is a ligament known as the transverse atlantal ligament, which acts as a sling, traveling behind the odontoid and keeping the atlas in place. As stated above, if this ligament becomes injured or divided your head becomes grossly unstable on your spine and this can result in serious neurological injury. If the ligament is injured, it generally does not heal, and a cervical fusion will be required to stabilize the spine (5).

odontoid fractures

The odontoid is a peg of bone which juts up from C2 and is the axis on which the C1 ring rotates. Odontoid fractures are one of the most common cervical spine injuries. There are several types of odontoid fractures. They can occur at the tip or at the waist of the odontoid process, or in the vertebral body of C2. By far the most common type of fracture occurs through the waist of the odontoid and is unfortunately the least likely to heal without surgical fixation. This is because the blood supply to this area of bone is limited and thus it's hard for this part of the body to heal on its own. As many as 77% of these fractures, left untended, may fail to heal (non-union/pseudoarthrosis), leaving the patient with significant cranial-cervical (head and neck) instability (6). Thus, surgeons typically fix these fractures. This is possible either with a posterior C1-2 fusion or with a technique called an odontoid screw. It has been shown that patients who have surgery have a trend towards a longer life span (7). Pseudoarthrosis or non-union (failure to heal) is more common in fractures with greater displacement and/or angulation, or in cases of chronic fracture or in patients who are older (8). These fractures tend to affect the very elderly who may not be able to tolerate surgery. In these cases, non-operative treatment may be used to avoid surgery, but the fracture can still be painful and never heal (9).

In the procedure known as an **odontoid screw**, the fracture is approached through the front of the neck and one or two screws are placed across the fracture. This may be an excellent way to treat the injury as it preserves much of your neck motion. However, the success of this surgery depends on many factors and will not work for every patient. Thus, all odontoid fractures should be evaluated by an orthopedic spine surgeon. Anterior odontoid screws have a high success rate and 80-100% of patients will heal using this method (10). Odontoid screws have been shown to decrease both the non-union and mortality rates (11).

Hangman's fractures: traumatic spondylolisthesis (slipping) of the axis (C2)

Hangman's fractures, named after the injury sustained from hangings in the old days, are fractures of the axis (C2) through a part of the bone called the "pars." Nowadays they most commonly occur because of motor vehicle accidents or falls from significant height. In this fracture the axis is split in half and may or may not be displaced. This can occur simultaneously with dislocations of the facet joints between C2 and C3. Most hangman's fractures can be treated with a rigid cervical collar. However, fractures which are severely angulated, displaced, or unstable, (such as with a fracture of the facet) require halo immobilization or surgical fixation (fusion). The prognosis of this fracture type is typically good with 90%-95% going on to union (healing together) (12).

lower cervical spine trauma: C3-7 injuries

The lower cervical spine (also known as the **subaxial cervical spine**) includes everything from C3 to C7. These vertebrae share a more similar shape compared to the upper cervical vertebrae. Unfortunately, there is less agreement among surgeons regarding when to operate on subaxial cervical spine injuries. Many complex classification systems have been developed to try and reconcile this disagreement. To simplify things, we will focus on 3 factors which are common to most classification systems: the morphology (shape) of the fracture, the integrity of the posterior ligaments and the disc (are they intact), and, finally, the presence of neurologic (nerve) injury.

In cases where there are ongoing or progressive neurologic deficits (meaning you are developing some form of paralysis) surgery is generally warranted. Symptoms associated with nerves that are not functioning properly, for example weakness or numbness in a limb, typically imply there is compression or instability which is compromising the spinal cord, or nerves. Thus, rigid surgical fixation with hardware is necessary to stabilize the injury, prevent further damage, and, hopefully, reverse the deficit.

Compared to the upper cervical spine, the vertebrae of the lower cervical spine are more stable and consequently are less mobile. What this means is that the bones are more directly interlinked than in the upper cervical spine. The shape of the fracture thus also helps guide surgical treatment as some fracture types are by their nature more unstable than others. Fractures where large portions of the anterior vertebral bodies are broken off, so called tear drop fractures, are inherently unstable and require surgery. In addition, fractures where there is significant damage to the facets and lateral mass of the vertebrae are also unstable and should be treated. In certain cases, the force to the spine causing the injury may be so severe it causes the facet joints to dislocate, requiring the surgeon to set the bones back into place, either with surgery or gentle traction.

As with the upper cervical spine, although perhaps less so, the discs and ligaments provide stability to the lower cervical spine. If there is significant damage to the disc and the posterior ligament, instability of the spine may occur which requires surgical stabilization.

whiplash

Whiplash is a very common injury seen in the spine clinic. The most common scenario occurs when you are rear-ended in a motor vehicle collision at low speeds (less than 14 mph) which causes a sudden acceleration and deceleration of your car that whips your neck forward. This motion can cause a sprain in the soft tissues and ligaments of the spine. The most affected structure is the membranous capsule around the facet joint; that capsule can rupture from whiplash, causing pain. These injuries typically heal on their own and do not require surgery.

Whiplash can have symptoms of neck pain, headaches, neck stiffness, paresthesia (tingling, burning) or pain in the upper limbs which, unfortunately, can persist for long periods of times, sometimes even years after the initial injury. Nonetheless,

66% of patients make a full recovery with only 2% ending up with permanent disability (13). There may be a substantial psychological component to these injuries, particularly if there is a possibility of financial compensation from insurance claims. This can be a major factor in symptoms which last for greater than 1 week (14). In fact, patients with whiplash can have greater pain than even those who sustain serious life-threatening fractures of the spine which, at least in part, shows there is some psychological component to the pain associated with these injuries (13).

Whiplash is treated effectively with physical therapy and nonsteroidal anti-inflammatories in the acute care setting. A soft collar may also be used for short periods. In chronic cases, medial facet blocks (in which nearby medial nerves are anesthetized) and radiofrequency ablation (which uses electrical current to block pain) are effective treatments for pain. Surgery is not indicated.

Thoracolumbar Fractures (Fractures of the Upper and Lower Back)

The transition from the rigid thoracic spine to the mobile lumbar spine creates a good environment for fractures (T12 to L2). This area is known as the thoracolumbar junction and is the most common location for a fracture in the spine below the neck (15). These fractures typically occur because of high-energy trauma and thus must be assessed in an emergency department as they can be associated with other critical injuries. They may also be associated with injury to the spinal cord or nerve roots, which may require emergency treatment. However, luckily most of these injuries are stable and do not require surgery.

Like subaxial cervical trauma, there are many different classification systems for thoracolumbar trauma but perhaps the most important distinction is determining which fractures are "stable" and which are "unstable." Fractures may be unstable biomechanically (that is, the spine can no longer hold itself up in a meaningful way) or unstable neurologically (the fracture impinges on the nerve roots or spinal cord).

Biomechanically, stability is determined by the type and shape of the fracture. The most common shapes are the burst and compression fractures, which for the most part are stable injuries. A simple way to think about mechanical stability is to organize the vertebra into three columns: anterior (the front of the vertebral body), middle (the back of the vertebral body) and posterior (the pedicles and facets). Fractures that involve only two of the three columns are so called stable and many of these generally require only conservative treatment.

Fractures of the transverse processes and the spinous processes, which do not affect the weight-bearing portion of the spine, are considered "minor," and do not typically require any treatment other than pain control.

Fractures that involve three columns—meaning all three parts of the vertebra are affected—are classified as unstable. Important to note is that this classification does not necessarily mean all three parts are fractured—some injuries affect the ligaments and spare the bones but can still be unstable. The ligamentous structure that is particularly important in the thoracolumbar spine is called the **posterior ligamentous complex (PLC)**, and disruption here can mean your fracture is unstable.

Fractures are typically evaluated using X-ray, CT scans and MRI scans. The reason all three of these imaging modalities are used is that each looks at a particular type of tissue in the body (please see chapter 6 on imaging). To evaluate bone injury both X-rays and CT scans are useful. MRI scans are particularly good at looking at the soft tissues like the ligaments, nerves, and spinal cord. If you just use one of these modalities, it is possible to miss significant injuries and, consequently, a comprehensive approach is best.

specific fractures that you will commonly hear about

Compression fractures: These are fractures that only affect the anterior column (the front of the vertebral body) and are typically stable. An MRI may be ordered to ensure your PLC is still intact. Most of these fractures can be treated conservatively.

Burst fractures: These involve both the anterior and posterior aspect of the vertebral body (so the anterior and middle columns). They are distinct from compression fractures because in the case of the burst fracture the bone from the posterior vertebral body can push back into the spinal canal and thus potentially cause damage to the spinal cord or nerves. The more severe and high energy the fracture the more likely bone can be pushed into the spinal canal and cause neurologic injury. In the past, burst fractures were often treated with surgery; however, a famous study done by Dr. Wood showed that the majority of burst fractures can be treated with conservative care so long as the PLC is intact and there is no damage to the spinal cord (16). However, if there is angulation in the spine greater than 25° or if there is compression of the vertebral height greater than 50%, this is likely to represent an unstable injury and, thus, may ultimately require surgery if conservative treatment fails (that is, your pain is not controlled, or you develop neurologic issues). Even if there is significant canal compromise, as long as there is no neurologic injury, these fractures may be safely treated in a brace without surgery as the bone heals itself (15).

Chance fractures/Three-column injuries: Chance fractures, sometimes called flexion distraction injures, involve all three columns of the spine. They can either involve all three columns of bone or may involve a soft tissue injury occurring through the disc or the PLC as described above. These injuries are very serious, generally requiring surgery and evaluation in the hospital setting.

treatment overview

Luckily most thoracolumbar fractures can be managed conservatively. Due to our advanced understanding of which fractures are stable and which are not, most patients can be braced with an off-the-shelf orthosis and mobilized quickly. The days of prolonged bedrest are over, and few injuries require surgical intervention. Some compression fractures may even be treated without an orthosis.

Surgery is reserved for fractures that result in mechanical instability or neurological compromise. If you are initially found to have a stable fracture, but due to the fracture settling you develop kyphosis (forward angulation of the spine), or if you have unremitting pain, you may require a surgery. Most unstable fractures are treated with a pedicle screw and rod construct spanning the injured segment. This can be done with a fusion (bone graft placed such that the segments heal together as one piece) or as instrumentation only (the screws and rods serve as an internal brace to allow the broken segment to heal). These two approaches have been shown to be essentially equal in long-term outcomes (17). If the anterior and middle columns are totally crushed, an anterior support graft may also be required to restore shape to the spine. This means the vertebra that is fractured is removed (called a corpectomy) and a synthetic cage is put in its place, which allows the spine to heal. This can essentially be thought of as vertebral replacement, where the cage and bone graft heal and form a new vertebral body.

Overall, the outcome for thoracolumbar fractures is good. Even patients who require surgery have an excellent chance of returning to work (18).

Osteoporotic Fractures

Fractures that occur under low energy such as a fall from standing, or simply bending, or twisting, or sneezing hard, are known as **insufficiency fractures,** and are treated totally differently from the high energy fractures described in this chapter. Insufficiency fractures occur primarily in the setting of osteoporosis which is a condition where your bones are very weak. These fractures are described in detail in a subsequent chapter 46.

In brief, most insufficiency fractures heal on their own; however, chronic low back pain may occur if they fail to heal (non-union) and because these fractures often result in a kyphotic deformity of the spine (19). Kyphotic deformities are painful because they cause you to become hunched over. The non-union rate may be as high as 18%, which can dramatically increase pain while decreasing function (20). Because the traditional ways to surgically repair fractures generally do not work well with osteoporotic fractures, a separate process to treat them has been developed. More on this in chapter 46 on cement augmentation.

Conclusion

Fractures of the spine are diverse and thus there are many kinds of treatment, depending exactly on which type you have. Surgery is reserved for the most severe cases where there is instability of the spine or where there is serious neurologic injury. In general, most spine fractures should be managed by an orthopedic surgeon or someone who is comfortable with the spine, because delayed or missed diagnoses can be harmful.

Frequently Asked Questions

• **How long do I need to wear the brace for?**

Most fractures are 90% healed by 12 weeks and thus bracing is generally recommended for this period or shorter.

• **What do I do if bracing treatment fails, and I am still having pain?**

Sometimes fractures fail to heal or heal in a bad position. In these cases, surgery is generally required to correct the problem. You should have a discussion with your surgeon about the potential benefits.

References

1.   Wozniczka J. Chapter 5 - Biomechanics of Fractures. General Principles. :28.

2.   Tashjian RZ, Majercik S, Biffl WL, Palumbo MA, Cioffi WG. Halo-Vest Immobilization Increases Early Morbidity and Mortality in Elderly Odontoid Fractures: The Journal of Trauma: Injury, Infection, and Critical Care. 2006 Jan;60(1):199–203.

3.   Maddox JJ, Rodriguez-Feo JA, Maddox GE, Gullung G, McGwin G, Theiss SM. Nonoperative Treatment of Occipital Condyle Fractures: An Outcomes Review of 32 Fractures. Spine. 2012 Jul;37(16):E964–8.

4.   Chang DG, Park JB, Song KJ, Park HJ, Kim WJ, Heu JY. Traumatic Atlanto-occipital Dislocation: Analysis of 15 Survival Cases With Emphasis on Associated Upper Cervical Spine Injuries. Spine. 2020 Jul 1;45(13):884–94.

5.   Dickman CA, Greene KA, Sonntag VK. Injuries involving the transverse atlantal ligament: classification and treatment guidelines based upon experience with 39 injuries. Neurosurgery. 1996 Jan;38(1):44–50.

6.   Jackson RS, Banit DM, Iii ALR, Ii BVD. Upper Cervical Spine Injuries. Journal of the American Academy of Orthopaedic Surgeons. 2002;10(4):10.

7.   Chapman J, Smith JS, Kopjar B, Vaccaro AR, Arnold P, Shaffrey CI, et al. The AOSpine North America Geriatric Odontoid Fracture Mortality Study: a retrospective review of mortality outcomes for operative versus nonoperative treatment of 322 patients with long-term follow-up. Spine (Phila Pa 1976). 2013 Jun 1;38(13):1098–104.

8.   Koivikko MP, Kiuru MJ, Koskinen SK, Myllynen P, Santavirta S, Kivisaari L. Factors associated with nonunion in conservatively-treated type-II fractures of the odontoid process. J Bone Joint Surg Br. 2004 Nov;86(8):1146–51.

9.   Koech F, Ackland HM, Varma DK, Williamson OD, Malham GM. Nonoperative management of type II odontoid fractures in the elderly. Spine. 2008 Dec 15;33(26):2881–6.

10. Montesano PX, Anderson PA, Schlehr FM++;, Thalgott JSM, Lowrey GM. Odontoid Fractures Treated by Anterior Odontoid Screw Fixation. Spine. 1991 Mar;16(3).

11. Vaccaro AR, Kepler CK, Kopjar B, Chapman J, Shaffrey C, Arnold P, et al. Functional and Quality-of-Life Outcomes in Geriatric Patients with Type-II Dens Fracture: The Journal of Bone and Joint Surgery. 2013 Apr;95(8):729–35.

12. Levine AM, Edwards CC. The management of traumatic spondylolisthesis of the axis. J Bone Joint Surg Am. 1985 Feb;67(2):217–26.

13. Bannister G, Amirfeyz R, Kelley S, Gargan M. Whiplash injury. J Bone Joint Surg Br. 2009 Jul;91(7):845–50.

14. Pobereskin LH. Whiplash following rear end collisions: a prospective cohort study. J Neurol Neurosurg Psychiatry. 2005 Aug;76(8):1146–51.

15. Wood KB, Li W, Lebl DS, Ploumis A. Management of thoracolumbar spine fractures. Spine J. 2014 Jan;14(1):145–64.

16. Wood KB, Buttermann GR, Phukan R, Harrod CC, Mehbod A, Shannon B, et al. Operative Compared with Nonoperative Treatment of a Thoracolumbar Burst Fracture without Neurological Deficit: A Prospective Randomized Study with Follow-up at Sixteen to Twenty-Two Years*. The Journal of Bone and Joint Surgery-American Volume. 2014 Jan;97(1):3–9.

17. Wild MH, Glees M, Plieschnegger C, Wenda K. Five-year follow-up examination after purely minimally invasive posterior stabilization of thoracolumbar fractures: a comparison of minimally invasive percutaneously and conventionally open treated patients. Archives of Orthopaedic and Trauma Surgery. 2007 Jun 11;127(5):335–43.

18. McLain RF. Functional outcomes after surgery for spinal fractures: return to work and activity. Spine (Phila Pa 1976). 2004 Feb 15;29(4):470–7; discussion Z6.

19. Iwata A, Kanayama M, Oha F, Shimamura Y, Hashimoto T, Takahata M, et al. Is Bone Nonunion, Vertebral Deformity, or Spinopelvic Malalignment the Best Therapeutic Target for Amelioration of Low Back Pain After Osteoporotic Vertebral Fracture? Spine. 2020 Jul 1;45(13):E760–7.

20. Inose H, Kato T, Ichimura S, Nakamura H, Hoshino M, Togawa D, et al. Risk Factors of Nonunion After Acute Osteoporotic Vertebral Fractures: A Prospective Multicenter

Cohort Study. Spine. 2020 Jul 1;45(13):895–902.

Figures:

Compression Fracture Fixation

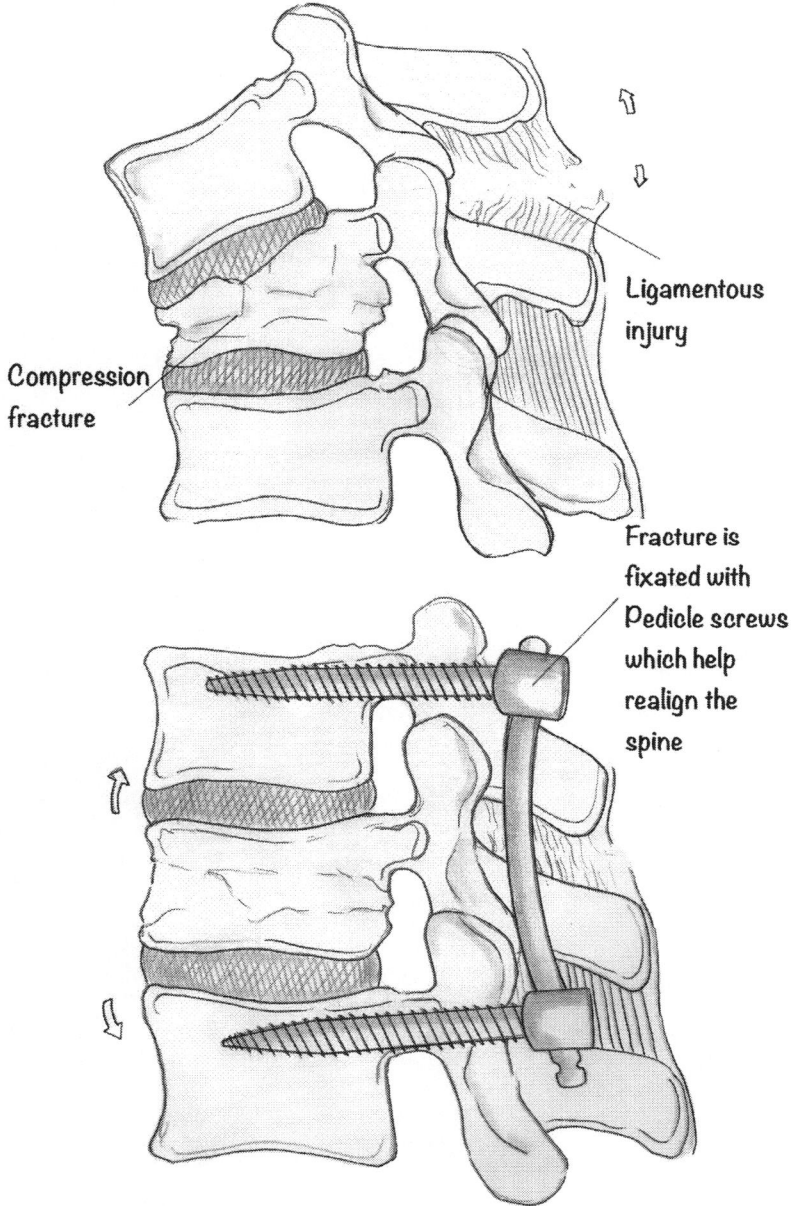

Ligamentous injury

Compression fracture

Fracture is fixated with Pedicle screws which help realign the spine

Fracture fixation. A burst fracture and tear of the posterior ligaments of the spine (top). The spine is stabilized, and the overall shape of the fracture is restored using screws and rods which hold the fracture in place allowing it to heal properly (bottom).

Fracture Healing

Normal Vertebra:

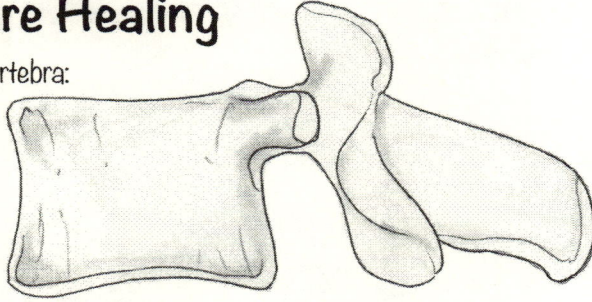

Acute: Fracture causes loss of
height and a hematoma

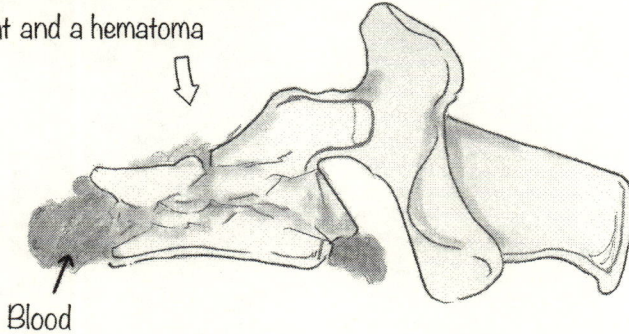

⇩

Blood

Repair: immature bone called
callus forms around the hematoma
and starts to solidify

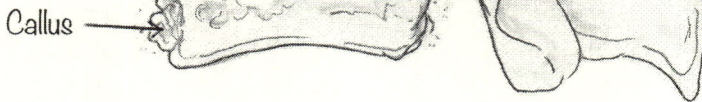

Callus →

Remodeling: the immature callus
consolidates into solid bone

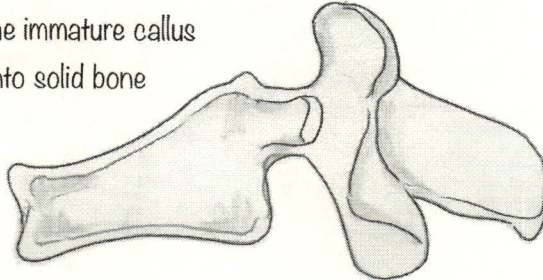

Fracture healing. Fracture healing occurs in several steps. The first step is hematoma formation where blood collects bringing in inflammatory cells (second from top). The hematoma turns into soft callus which is immature bone (second from bottom). Finally, the callus remodels to resemble normal bone more closely, however the shape of the vertebra is permanently changed (bottom).

Chapter 14

Infections of the Spine: Osteomyelitis, Discitis, Post-Surgical Infection

Summary

Spine infections are complicated problems that often mimic other diseases, resulting in a delay in diagnosis. These infections typically present with back or neck pain, fever, chills, and even neurologic dysfunction like numbness or weakness. The infections that occur in spines that have not had surgery are called primary spine infections. These infections usually start in some other part of the body, for example, the mouth or urinary tract, but can travel to the disc (discitis) or bone (osteomyelitis). They are treated with antibiotics and possibly surgery to debride (remove) infected tissue. Infections can also occur in spines that have had surgery. These are classified as secondary infections and tend to be much more complicated problems because infection is harder to eradicate when there are retained spinal implants. Unlike other areas of orthopedics, removing hardware from the spine can be very problematic and so is only done if necessary. However, with modern techniques, it is still possible to treat infections while leaving the hardware in place.

Case

Mr. Azure is a 70-year-old alcoholic who has bad teeth. Recently he has been having more pain in his mouth and a trip to the dentist reveals that he has a major tooth infection. The tooth is extracted but several days later he starts to have incredible back pain. Moreover, he becomes feverish and starts to develop chills and is sent to the hospital by ambulance. In the hospital an MRI is performed which shows osteomyelitis and discitis around L2 with an epidural abscess that is severely compressing his spinal canal. I come to see the patient and find that he has weakness in his lower extremities from compression of the nerves. He is brought to the operating room for an emergency decompression of his spine and the pus pocket is evacuated and biopsied. The biopsy is sent to the lab to see if there is microbial growth (that is, cultured) and the patient is started on IV antibiotics. Immediately he is clinically improved and regains strength in his legs. Within a day the cultures come back as Methicillin Resistant Staphylococcus Aureus (MRSA) a common bacterium and the patient is placed on an antibiotic known as vancomycin. Because he will need long term antibiotics for 6 weeks a special IV line known as a PICC line (peripherally inserted central catheter) is placed so he can receive daily infusions. He slowly recovers and is feeling well within a few weeks of antibiotic treatment.

Introduction

Infections of the spine may be incredibly frustrating to both patient and physician because they have the potential to mimic common benign spinal conditions like degenerative disc disease. I have seen several patients who have been told repeatedly that their back pain was related to simple degeneration when in fact the pain was related to a smoldering infection. The reason for this is that **spinal infections** are very rare, and there is no sure-fire way to diagnose them. They can occur **in the disc (known as discitis), in the bone (osteomyelitis)**, or **in the spinal canal (epidural abscess)**. (Note: the suffix "itis" means "inflammation of." Sometimes an inflammation is caused by something other than infection, but in this chapter, we are referring to infections.)

Infections can also, of course, occur after surgery. This is frustrating because it is so difficult to clear an infection when there are metallic implants in the spine. This is because the bacteria like to cling to the metal implants. Post-operative spinal infections can become big ordeals for both the patient and surgeon, often involving very deep emotional and physical setbacks. Just when you were expecting to be on the path to recovery, you are stricken with a new difficult problem. In this chapter we will discuss both primary infections (occurring where no surgery has been performed) and secondary infections (occurring after a surgery to the spine).

Discitis/Osteomyelitis (Infection of the Disc, of the Bone)

The intervertebral disc has a very limited blood supply which makes it susceptible to bacterial infection. This is because your blood contains many powerful chemicals and cells that fight infection. Areas with good blood supply (such as the scalp) generally have a very limited potential for infection. The disc, however, receives little blood and thus is a great natural host for bacterial infection.

Infection in the disc typically occurs by a process called **hematogenous seeding**. This is where bacteria travels from another site in the body, through the blood stream and lodges in the vertebrae (the bones have excellent blood supply) and then extends to the disc. The vertebrae are also predisposed to infection, but for the opposite reason of discs—vertebrae have many redundant vascular channels (extra arteries and veins, just in case), which allow pooling of blood, which, in turn, gives the chance for bacteria to latch onto the bone (think of dirty water pooling in a slow stream). Commonly bacteria can travel from other sources of infection such as from a urinary tract infection, a heart valve infection (endocarditis), joint space infection (septic arthritis) or IV lines which have become infected. Bacteria from the mouth can be dislodged from tooth extractions and dental work and is a known cause of discitis and osteomyelitis. Intravenous drug abuse is also a common cause of spinal infection.

Hematogenous seeding can allow the spread of infection from one area of the body to another, but direct contamination may also occur following an invasive spinal procedure. Spinal infections have been known to occur after even minimally invasive procedures such as epidural injections, discography or lumbar puncture.

Unfortunately, in most cases the presumed origin of the bacteria is only speculative and cannot be determined with full accuracy.

The lumbar spine is the most involved area, but infections may also occur in the thoracic and cervical regions. The infection can start in the bone and progress to the disc or vice versa. Bone infection can cause destruction and collapse, leading to deformity of the spine. The infection may also spread to the soft tissues surrounding the spine and may even seed other areas of the body, such as the heart, blood vessels, brain, spinal canal, or other joints, such as the hips and shoulders.

The most common culprit of spinal infections is the bacterial species *Staphylococcus aureus (abbreviated S. aureus).* You may have heard about MRSA before which stands for methicillin resistant Staphylococcus Aureus— (S. aureus that is resistant to methicillin antibiotics). However, there are other bacterial species, for example, tuberculosis, and other organisms, such as fungus, which may also cause infections of the spine. There are certain patient groups who are at higher risk for infection, such as diabetics, intravenous drug abusers, alcoholics, and those who are immunocompromised such as HIV patients or the elderly (1).

Infections are challenging for many reasons, but perhaps mainly because of the difficulty at times of making a correct diagnosis. In fact, only 30-40% of spinal infections are diagnosed within the first month of the start of symptoms (1,2). **Infections are the great mimickers of degenerative disc disease,** and the symptoms may be limited to vague back pain. Infections of the spine may mimic degenerative disc disease or disc herniations, metastatic disease (a disease spreading from another part of the body), or even routine fractures. Furthermore, even with advanced imaging many experienced radiologists and surgeons alike cannot differentiate normal degeneration changes from an infection.

diagnosis

Diagnosing spinal infection is an imperfect science that relies heavily on clinical suspicion. The methods we have are not sensitive to detecting infection in mild cases and in many cases an infection can be written off as just common back pain.

Most discitis and spinal osteomyelitis have symptoms of new or worsening back/neck pain accompanied by fever. However, fever may be absent in half of all patients with a spinal infection or masked by antipyretics (medicines which reduce fever) such as Tylenol (2). Muscle spasms or pain with movement are also very common. Notably the pain is often worse at night. Occasionally it may also present as new neurologic symptoms such as radiculopathy (pain in the legs or arms, weakness/numbness of the extremities).

Laboratory investigations typically include a complete blood count (CBC), erythrocyte sedimentation rates (ESR) and c-reactive protein (CRP). These tests all look for general inflammation in the blood. However, these tests may be negative in a quarter of all spinal infection patients or positive for other reasons other than infection (3). Cultures of the urine and blood are also routinely taken which can show if there are bacteria swimming in the bodily fluids. A positive blood culture eliminates the need for an image-guided biopsy. A test for tuberculosis (either a purified protein derivative PPD test or an interferon-γ test) is typically also performed.

Following this an **MRI** is the test of choice for investigating infection. MRIs are great for looking at the soft tissues and can show inflammation of the disc. Typically a physician asks for an MRI of the entire spine to rule out areas of infection occurring elsewhere in the spine, which sometimes occurs. Initial MRIs may easily be non-diagnostic and interpreted as noninfectious standard degeneration. In borderline cases, your physician may elect to reimage with MRI in 1-3 weeks to look for progression. Other imaging studies which may be used include computer tomography (CT), positron emission tomography (PET), and technetium bone scans. An echocardiogram may also be necessary in those who are elderly with positive blood cultures and a predisposing heart condition, to look for infection coexisting in the heart.

In patients in which there is a high clinical suspicion for infection (based on history, exam and labs, an **image-guided biopsy** may be performed. This can be done by your surgeon or by an interventional radiologist (see glossary). A biopsy is a procedure where the tissue is sampled. It is then sent to the lab where technicians try to get the bacteria to grow in a petri dish. However, image-guided biopsy may only be positive in 60-70% of patients (1)—making the diagnostic threshold very low. In cases where an image-guided biopsy is not obtained, a **surgical open biopsy** may be performed. These have a higher sensitivity because some actual tissue can be collected. The difference is an image-guided biopsy is performed only with a small needle where you try to collect a small sample. In a surgical biopsy an open incision is performed and the tissue is sampled directly. Because you can obtain a larger sample, surgical biopsy is more likely to give accurate information and increase the chances of collecting bacteria to grow in the lab.

Once a bacterium is isolated (that is, positive cultures are obtained), the lab will test a battery of antibiotics on the growing culture to see which ones will be effective in treatment. Not all antibiotics will work on certain bacteria and so this is a critical process in a successful treatment.

treatment

Most cases of discitis and osteomyelitis can be managed with **6 weeks of intravenous (IV) antibiotics** alone. Antibiotics are administered IV to increase the concentration in the blood stream and allow the antibiotic to penetrate the spine at sufficient concentrations (low concentrations of antibiotic may not penetrate the disc which, as stated above. does not have a good blood supply). If you are very sick, you will be started immediately on empiric antibiotics, which means you are given very powerful antibiotics capable of treating a range of infections in a shotgun method. However, in a stable patient, antibiotics may be held until the organism causing the infection can be identified. If you are given antibiotics before a biopsy is done, the chances of discovering what antibiotic will work go down greatly.

Antibiotic therapy is typically monitored by following inflammatory markers (ESR and CRP) over time. Usually you start to feel much better once the treatment is started.

In cases where there are progressive neurologic deficits, and or deformity or instability of the spine, surgery is generally recommended. Also, in cases where the infection cannot be controlled without a debridement (medically removing dead, damaged or infected tissue), surgery is recommended. Surgery of some kind is required in about 40-50% of patients with an infectious discitis (1). Many patients with epidural abscesses fail medical treatment alone and require surgery for definitive cure (4). In most cases surgery consists of a decompression that removes the abscess from the spinal canal but may also include reconstruction and stabilization of bones that have collapsed with rot from infection. Surgery is always done in conjunction with medical treatment with antibiotics.

prognosis

With appropriate antibiotic treatment the prognosis in most primary infection cases (roughly 60-70%) is good. However residual neurologic deficits or chronic low back pain may occur in up to 30% of patients. Relapse may occur in up to 10-20% of patients. The mortality rate may be as high as 10-15% (1,3).

Post-operative Infection

Post-operative infections can range in severity from nuisances which require antibiotics to major life-threatening ordeals. In almost all cases, they represent a significant challenge for both the surgeon and the patient that can have a negative psychological impact. Surgeons and patients, both expecting a good recovery, will be frustrated with the set back of an infection and will wonder where it came from. In many cases, the answer is never known.

 The rates of infection following spinal surgery range from 0.7-16%, depending on the type of surgery. Obviously, surgeries with larger wounds, and more non-native spinal implants have an increased risk of infection, as there is a greater opportunity for bacteria to lodge on the implants and proliferate in the body. Following surgery there is some tissue destruction and seroma formation (fluid build-up after surgery), both of which also provide excellent breeding grounds for bacteria. A single level decompression surgery has a significantly different risk than a multilevel spinal fusion for deformity correction. Similarly, larger cases with increased blood loss, and cases with longer operative times also increase the risk for post-operative infection (5,6).

Certain patient factors also increase the risk of infection, including older age, obesity, cardiovascular disease, previous spine surgery, chronic steroid use, immunologic compromise, lung disease such as chronic bronchitis or chronic obstructive pulmonary disease (COPD), smoking, diabetes, dependent functional status (needs help in daily activities), and cancer (5).

pathogenesis (how the disease develops)

Like primary spine infections, *Staphylococcus aureus* is the most isolated bacteria in post-operative infections. Post-operative spinal infections may be superficial and limited to the skin or subcutaneous tissue—these require only antibiotic therapy—or they may be complex deep wound infections, involving the bone and muscle—and require more extensive treatment. When spinal hardware is in place, it provides bacteria a scaffold on which the bacteria can form a film that coats the spinal implants. The immune system/antibiotics cannot readily penetrate this film, known as a **glycocalyx,** and once this occurs the only way to eradicate the infection is either to remove and replace the hardware or to debride the glycocalyx that covers the hardware. Neither is easy.

diagnosis

The same principles used to diagnose a primary infection of the spine described above are used in the diagnosis of post-operative spinal infections. As with primary infections of the spine, fever and increased pain are often present. Different from the primary infections discussed above, post-op infections commonly present with wound breakdown and drainage. Any wound issues should be discussed immediately with your surgeon.

Inflammatory markers such as ESR and CRP may not be as useful in the case of post-operative infections because these markers are non-specific and will be elevated from the inflammation caused by surgery, especially within the first 6 weeks. Similarly, MRI may also be difficult to interpret because many of the typical tissue abnormalities (swelling, edema, inflammation) on MRI may be normal occurrences in the post-operative spine. Thus, the diagnosis requires a high degree of suspicion on the part of the surgeon. In cases that are unclear, your surgeon may elect to biopsy the tissue or simply to start antibiotic treatment.

prevention

Luckily many protocols and interventions have been developed to reduce the number of post-operative infections. The likely most powerful of these interventions is the administration of IV antibiotics prior to the incision in surgery, which has been shown to reduce infection rates across all surgical fields. Typical antibiotics used for this purpose include cefazolin (a penicillin derivative), vancomycin, and clindamycin. It takes a substantial number of bacteria to cause an infection in surgery (as many as 10^5 organisms). Thus, orthopedic surgeons accustomed to implanting hardware are trained in meticulous sterile technique to ensure wound beds are kept as clean as humanly possible during surgery. Other techniques such as the application of topical antibiotics, and antiseptics may also be used to help keep the wound clean.

treatment

Superficial infections and those caught very early in the disease process may be treated with antibiotics alone (7). However, the treatment of most deep wound infections requires a second trip to the operating room to perform an **irrigation and debridement (I&D)**. During this procedure, all infected material is removed and the healthy tissue is irrigated with sterile saline to decrease the bacterial burden as much as possible. In most cases of spinal fusion, the hardware is left in place following the surgery because to remove it would be to risk spinal instability. Alternatively, it may be exchanged for new hardware that is clean of bacteria—but this can be a complex process if the hardware is ingrown. If there is a solid arthrodesis (fusion of the bones/joints) the hardware may be removed safely. Multiple debridements may be necessary depending on the severity of your infection. During the surgery, the surgeon will take samples and biopsies of the infected tissue, which are sent to the lab for culture to identify the species of bacteria. Once the bacteria are grown, the lab will also try to find out what types of antibiotics the bacteria are susceptible to in a process known as obtaining sensitivities.

Following the debridement surgery, the surgeon may apply a **vacuum-assisted closure (VAC) device** which can aid in the drainage of the wound and prevent infected material from reaccumulating. A VAC is essentially a sterile sponge connected to a suction hose that allows the area to drain. The suction is connected to a sealed canister. VAC sponges have been shown to help with wound healing (8).

Following all the surgical irrigation, biopsies and debridement, another type of doctor may step in to help manage your antibiotics. This is an infectious disease specialist trained in how to deal with all sorts of nasty infections. Infectious disease doctors (or ID doctors) use the cultures and sensitivities to help determine appropriate selection and dosing of antibiotics. They typically recommend the duration of antibiotics as well and may recommend you get a special IV line such as a **PICC (peripherally inserted central catheter)** which can be used for many weeks. Antibiotic therapy duration may range from 6 to 12 weeks to life. Life-time antibiotics (also called suppressive therapy) is sometimes required in patients in whom the infection is never expected to be fully cleared. This could be due to their underlying health issues or to the complexity of surgery performed on their spine; both require daily antibiotics for life to prevent a relapse of infection.

Prognosis

In cases where there are no retained implants, prognosis of the infection is generally good and antibiotics have a high rate of cure. Even in cases where there are retained hardware there is a good chance of cure of the disease with debridement and antibiotics but, ultimately, as many as 25% have treatment failure. Treatment failure seems to be related to the extent of spinal surgery with those with larger fusions being at more risk. Certain bacterial infections tend also to be more difficult to eradicate such as infections with the bacteria *P. Acnes (9)*.

Conclusion

Spine infections are scary and can easily be missed. They are rare but if they happen to you statistics go out the window. With modern techniques it is possible to eradicate them, but the treatment can be lengthy and require multiple trips to the operating room. If you suspect you have a spinal infection it is important to seek medical attention immediately.

Frequently Asked Questions

- **Will I have to stay in the hospital to receive my antibiotic treatment? How long will I have to be there?**

    The treatment of spinal infections is typically a lengthy process. You must have lots of labs and imaging done, and then possibly undergo a biopsy of the infected tissue. Following the biopsy, you need to wait for the bacteria to grow out in the lab during which time you are given empiric antibiotics (powerful antibiotics that can treat a range of bacteria). Finally, when cultures come back, the lab will perform sensitivities to guide antibiotic treatment, which can usually be done by day 3 after the biopsy. This is when your long-term antibiotics can be determined. Because it takes at least 6-8 weeks of intravenous antibiotic treatment you may require the placement of a special IV line that can last more than a few days (regular IV lines must be replaced after several days of use because they too become infected). You can usually have a home health nurse come to your house to administer these long-term antibiotics, but you may need to be in a care facility for this duration, depending on what the local resources are for this service. Some cases may be treated with oral antibiotics, but this depends on the species of bacteria. In summary, depending on your circumstances, you may need to be in a medical facility for many weeks.

References

1.   McHenry MC, Easley KA, Locker GA. Vertebral Osteomyelitis: Long-Term Outcome for 253 Patients from 7 Cleveland-Area Hospitals. :9.

2.   Berbari EF, Kanj SS, Kowalski TJ, Darouiche RO, Widmer AF, Schmitt SK, et al. 2015 Infectious Diseases Society of America (IDSA) Clinical Practice Guidelines for the Diagnosis and Treatment of Native Vertebral Osteomyelitis in Adults. Clin Infect Dis. 2015 Sep 15;61(6):e26–46.

3.   Gupta A, Kowalski TJ, Osmon DR, Enzler M, Steckelberg JM, Huddleston PM, et al. Long-Term Outcome of Pyogenic Vertebral Osteomyelitis: A Cohort Study of 260 Patients. :8.

4.   Patel AR, Alton TB, Bransford RJ, Lee MJ, Bellabarba CB, Chapman JR. Spinal epidural abscesses: risk factors, medical versus surgical management, a retrospective review of 128 cases. The Spine Journal. 2014 Feb;14(2):326–30.

5.   Veeravagu A, Cole T, Jiang B, Ratliff JK. Revision rates and complication incidence in single- and multilevel anterior cervical discectomy and fusion procedures: an administrative database study. Spine J. 2013 Oct 11;

6.   Pawar AY, Biswas SK. Postoperative Spine Infections. Asian Spine Journal. :8.

7.   Hong HS, Chang MC, Liu CL, Chen TH. Is Aggressive Surgery Necessary for Acute Postoperative Deep Spinal Wound Infection?: Spine. 2008 Oct;33(22):2473–8.

8.   Brown MD, Brookfield KFW. A Randomized Study of Closed Wound Suction Drainage for Extensive Lumbar Spine Surgery: Spine. 2004 May;29(10):1066–8.

9.   Maruo K, Berven SH. Outcome and treatment of postoperative spine surgical site infections: predictors of treatment success and failure. J Orthop Sci. 2014 May;19(3):398–404.

Figures:

MRI Representation of a Lumbar Infection

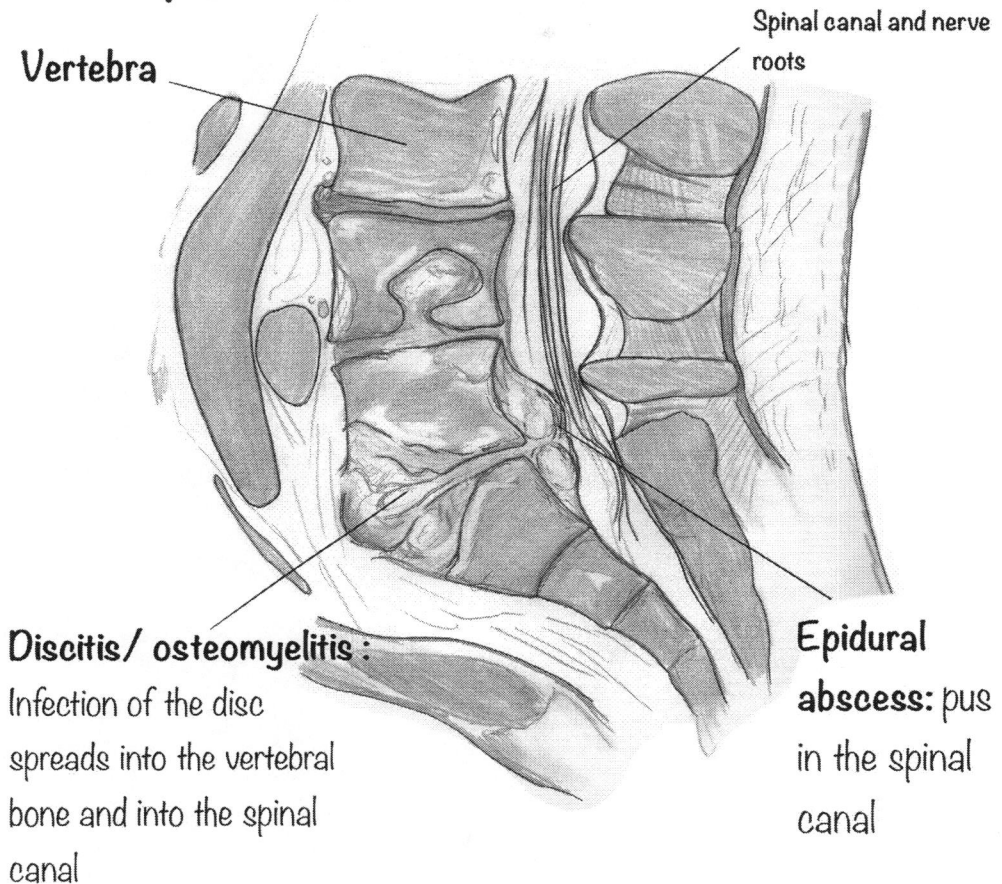

Vertebra

Spinal canal and nerve roots

Discitis/ osteomyelitis : Infection of the disc spreads into the vertebral bone and into the spinal canal

Epidural abscess: pus in the spinal canal

Discitis osteomyelitis. A cross section of an MRI image showing infection at the L5-S1 disc space. Discitis is infection of the disc itself, whereas osteomyelitis is infection of the adjacent bone. The infection can spread into the spinal canal resulting in an epidural abscess.

Chapter 15

Cancer and Tumors in the Spine

Summary

Spine tumors are diverse and can affect many different areas ranging from the bone, to the nerves, and even to the spinal cord. The most common type of spinal tumor is a metastatic tumor that has originated from another area in the body, but tumors may also arise directly from the spine (so called primary tumors of the spine). The treatment is different for each tumor but may consist of a combination of resection surgery, radiation and even chemotherapy. Nowadays there are many new less invasive techniques which makes the treatment of tumors more tolerable with less complications. Many tumors may be treated without surgery at all. Surgery is generally required to stabilize collapse of the spinal column or to decompress the spinal cord, which has been compressed by tumor invading into the spinal canal. The treatment of cancers is a continually evolving field and this chapter is meant as an introduction to the basic principles of diagnosis and treatment.

Case

Mr. Slate is a 65-year-old retired city worker who one day when working in his garden suddenly develops severe back pain and calls an ambulance. In the emergency room a CT and MRI scan of his back show that he has a pathologic fracture of his L2 vertebra, meaning that the fracture was caused by erosion of the bone from a tumor. He has never been diagnosed with cancer before, but the lesion looks like it is metastatic. We biopsied the lesion and also performed a kyphoplasty which greatly relieved his pain. The pathology report comes back as metastatic hepatocellular carcinoma (liver cancer). He gets connected with a radiation oncologist who performs targeted radiation treatment to the area of tumor and also with an oncologist who starts chemotherapy to treat the primary tumor. Within a few weeks he is walking again and feels much improved. His spine is stable and a year after surgery he is still enjoying life.

Introduction

The topic of spinal tumors and oncology (the study and treatment of tumors) is vast, and this chapter is intended only to give you a working framework. Spinal tumors may be classified several ways but the most common is to divide them into those which are **primary** (arising from the spine itself) and **metastatic** (spreading to the spine from another primary tumor site in the body). Primary tumors are further divided into a primary malignant tumor (which is a malignant tumor that arises from the spine itself and can spread to other areas) and a primary benign tumor (a spine tumor which will not spread to other areas of the body). The location of the tumor also helps classify them. Tumors can arise from the bone, nerves, and even the spinal cord. Tumors can arise from within the membranous lining of the spinal canal; those are called intradural tumors. As you can see, with all the different places a tumor can occur, there can be a lot of variation.

Not all tumors that occur in the spine are covered here, as some are very rare, but the basic principles may still apply. Because some spinal tumors are so rare, a spine surgeon working in the community may go his entire career without seeing a certain variety. That is why many primary tumors of the spine are dealt with at cancer and tumor centers that have a higher volume of those cases such as Memorial Sloan Kettering Hospital in New York or the Dana Farber Cancer Center in Boston.

Unfortunately, metastatic tumors to the spine, which typically can be managed but not cured, are much more common than primary tumors. All spinal tumors are scary, but luckily, the treatments for all spinal tumors have undergone a major revolution—today many can be successfully controlled and, in some cases, even cured. Spinal surgery can stabilize the spinal column that may be collapsing from the tumor and can even prevent paralysis resulting from a tumor encroaching into the spinal column. Some tumors may be completely resected, meaning they are totally removed/excised, from the body (aka enbloc removal), while other tumors are debulked (also known as curettage), meaning the tumor is made smaller but cannot be totally removed.

When surgeons talk about removing tumors there are several common terms we use. Excision and **resection** are essentially interchangeable terms used to describe the removal of a tumor. When a tumor is removed in its entirety it is called an **enbloc resection**. When it is removed partially it is "**partially resected or excised**" or **debulked or curetted**.

Primary Spinal Tumors

Primary tumors are tumors that arise directly from the tissue of the spine (that is, the bones, nerves, or spinal cord). They are further classified as benign, intermediate/ aggressive or malignant—those with the potential to metastasize (spread). Whether or not the tumor is likely to be benign or malignant is related to how old the patient is when the tumor is first discovered. Tumors presenting in younger age patients (younger than 18 years) are more likely to be benign, while those presenting in older age (older than 18 years) are more likely to be malignant. Where the tumor occurs also influences the chance that it is malignant or benign. Tumors which occur in the posterior aspect of the spine (pedicles, lamina, spinous process—remember the spinous process is the part of the spine you can feel running your fingers down someone's spine) are more likely benign, whereas those tumors which occur anteriorly in the vertebral body are more likely to be malignant.

Intradural Tumors of the Spinal Canal (Tumors Occurring within the Dura— the Membranous Lining of the Spinal Canal)

Remember that the spinal cord runs through the spinal canal. The spinal cord is bathed in cerebrospinal fluid (CSF). Both the spinal cord and the CSF, as well as nerve roots before they exit the spine, are encased in a thick membrane called the dura mater. Tumors of the spinal canal are classified in part by where they occur compared to that membrane.

Also, keep in mind the prefix "intra" means within (like intramural sports—within the school) and the prefix "extra" means outside (for example extracurricular activities occur outside the classroom). Tumors occurring within the spinal canal are referred to as **intracanal tumors**.

Extradural tumors occur within the spinal canal but outside the dura mater. Extradural tumors are more common than ones that occur within the dura mater.

As you might guess, tumors occurring inside the dura mater are called **intradural tumors**. If a tumor occurs inside the dura mater but outside the spinal cord it is called an **intradural extramedullary tumor** (medullary in this case referring to the spinal cord). If the tumor occurs within the spinal cord, it is called an **intradural intramedullary tumor.**

Primary Benign Tumors: notes on different tumors occurring in the spine. You can look at the ones that interest you, otherwise skip.	
Aneurysmal Bone Cyst (ABC)	Benign expansive tumors that are filled with blood channels. Mostly occur in patients younger than 18 years. May be treated with curettage and adjuvant therapies.
Chondroblastoma	Rare. Benign cartilage tumor which occurs in young patients under 18 years age. Treated with curettage.
Chondroma	Benign cartilage tumor. Treated with curettage
Chondromyxoid fibroma	Benign cartilage tumor, rare in the spine but common in hands and feet. May be aggressive and destroy cortex (outer layer) of bone.
Giant Cell Tumor	Rare. Benign aggressive tumor, typically located in the sacrum. Even though benign in most cases, can metastasize to the lungs in 2% of cases. Treated with enbloc resection but has a high recurrent rate.
Hemangioma	Benign vascular (blood vessel) tumor of the spine, very common in the spine. Most are incidental and do not require treatment. Rarely can be aggressive.
Lipoma	Benign fatty tumor
Osteoblastoma	Benign bone-forming tumor. Very painful, especially at night.
Osteoid Osteoma	Benign bone-forming tumor. Very painful, especially at night. Pain goes away with use of NSAIDS.
Primary Intermediate Tumors	
Chordoma	Most common primary tumor of the spine. Commonly occurs in the sacrum. Treated with wide resection. Intermediate because chordomas tend to be very locally aggressive and not easily eradicated with simple excision.
Primary Malignant Tumor	
Angiosarcoma	Rare. Malignant and aggressive tumor of blood vessels. Occurs in the elderly. Requires wide surgical resection.
Chondrosarcoma	Rare. Malignant cartilage tumor. Treated with wide surgical resection
Ewing's Sarcoma	Malignant neuroectodermal tumor affecting the bones. Occurs in patients younger than 18 years. Treated with chemotherapy and wide resection surgery.
Liposarcoma	Malignant tumor of fat origin. Treated with wide surgical therapy and radiation. Occurs in older adults.
Lymphoma	A blood-borne cancer that arises from white blood cells. Can be treated with chemotherapy and radiation.
Myeloma	Considered a systemic (affecting entire body) disease but may occur solitarily in the spine as a plasmacytoma.
Osteosarcoma	Second most common primary tumor of the spine. Typically requires a combination of chemotherapy and surgical treatment.

Intradural tumors are more rare than extradural tumors but the resection can be more challenging as it requires the dura casing to be opened. Typically, surgeons avoid cutting the dura mater because this can lead to CSF leakage, but in the case of intradural tumors, the dura mater is deliberately opened and, after the tumor is removed, the membrane is repaired, usually without problems. However, you may be required to be flat on your back on bed rest for several days after the resection.

Intramedullary tumors account for about 5-10% of tumors which occur in the spinal canal (1). The most common intramedullary tumors are ependymomas and astrocytomas. Resection of these tumors are often fraught with complications as it is difficult to preserve the spinal cord while still removing the tumor. These tumors are generally treated at specialty centers.

Intradural and Intramedullary tumors	
Astrocytoma	Extremely rare. Benign Intramedullary (tumor inside the spinal cord) tumor of the spine. Occurs more commonly in males in their 30's. Gross total resection is the goal, particularly if the tumor seems aggressive, but is often difficult(2). Those that are only mildly symptomatic may be observed.
Ependymoma	Most common intramedullary tumor (tumor inside the spinal cord). Commonly occurs in the cervical spine. Treated with total resection if symptomatic. Most are benign but has the potential for recurrence.
Meningioma	Most common intradural tumor. Arises from the arachnoid cap cells of the dura mater. Most occur in thoracic area and are much more common in females. It is possible for meningiomas to calcify (become bone-like). Treatment is resection if symptomatic
Neurofibroma	Benign intermediate tumor of fibrous cells. May occur in patients with neurofibromatosis. May be intradural. Removal may require the sacrifice of a nerve rootlet but is generally well tolerated. Treated with excision if symptomatic.
Schwannoma	Benign nerve sheath tumor that does not typically involve the nerve. Treated with excision.

Tarlov Cysts

Tarlov cysts are very common small cysts that arise in the spine when cerebral spinal fluid collects between a nerve fiber and its outer membrane coating. They are famous for causing panic in patents but typically are only incidental findings (meaning they are reported out on the MRI report by the radiologist but have no clinical significance and do not require any treatment). Tarlov cysts occur in around 8% of the population and out of these only 1% of all cysts are symptomatic. Only rarely do they can cause compression on adjacent nerves. Surgery to treat Tarlov cysts is typically very technically demanding, fraught with complication and may not offer significant relief (3).

Metastatic Tumors of the Spine

Unfortunately, **metastatic tumors** that have spread from other parts of the body **account for more than 90% of all spine tumors**. The spine is a very common site for bony metastasis. This is because the spine is surrounded by a rich network of blood vessels which allow cancer cells to spread to it easily. It is estimated that in the United States there are at least 100,000 new metastatic tumors of the spine each year requiring treatment (4). Metastatic tumors can have serious consequences for the spine. They can result in destabilization of the spinal column because the tumors eat away at the bones or cause spinal canal compression. Common malignancies which spread to the spine include breast, gastrointestinal, lung, prostate, renal and thyroid cancers.

Symptoms of Tumors of the Spine

The pain from primary tumors of the spine is usually different from the pain experienced by simple mechanical injury or degeneration. While the pain may differ from tumor to tumor, tumor pain is usually unrelenting and not activity-dependent, meaning it is painful whether you move the spine or not and can be present at rest (although it can still be worsened by movement). It may get much worse at night, which is the classic sign for spinal tumors. Because tumor can weaken the bone, fractures are more likely. If the tumor invades the spinal canal there may be symptoms of radiating leg or arm pain, weakness and numbness. If the tumor compresses the spinal cord there may also be loss of balance, bowel or bladder incontinence or loss of spatial awareness of the limbs.

Figuring Out If You Have a Tumor, What Type it Is

After a patient presents with symptoms, it's up to the doctor to determine what type of tumor is causing the problem. It's not always obvious and may require several tests before a final diagnosis is made. Management begins with imaging, usually an X-ray, CT scan and MRI scan. MRI scans are typically done with contrast (an intravenous fluid which helps to enhance the lesion). Nuclear bone scans and Positron Emission Tomography (PET) CT may also be used to help **stage the tumor** (determine how advanced it is), because these assessment tools are full body scans that can detect lesions elsewhere. Laboratory tests are generally also performed to check for signs of specific malignancies, including thyroid function tests, prostate specific antigen to test for possible prostate cancer, serum electrophoresis to look for multiple myelomas (a type of blood cancer).

Following imaging and labs, a biopsy may be performed. This can be done under X-ray or CT guidance where a small needle is used to sample the tumor and is generally an outpatient procedure. Open surgical biopsies may also be performed in some situations where a surgeon formally removes some tissue from the tumor during a surgical procedure.

Some tumors that are grow blood vessels (aneurysmal bone cyst, renal cell carcinoma, angiosarcoma) should be examined with arteriography and embolization prior to biopsy to prevent bleeding (studies to look at blood flow through the tumor). During arteriography an embolization procedure may be performed where the blood supply to the tumor is cut off prior to biopsy to prevent bleeding. A renal ultrasound may be used specifically in cases where renal cell carcinoma is suspected.

Staging Tumors and Treatment

Primary tumors are treated based on the principles of **orthopedic oncology** (treatment of bone cancer) which states the degree of resection must be sufficient to "cure" the problem. Primary tumors of the spine are graded on how biologically aggressive they are. Some benign tumors may simply be scraped out in a process called **curettage**, in which the tumor margins (edges of the tumor) are of little concern. Intermediate tumors may require curettage plus the use of an **adjuvant** (additional therapy, usually to help prevent secondary tumors) such as radiation therapy. Primary malignant tumors must be excised "enbloc" removing a portion of surrounding tissue to ensure that the tumor cannot spread again. Many malignant tumors are also treated with adjuvant radiation to help prevent recurrence.

Generally, the goal of treatment of metastatic tumors of the spine (tumors that started somewhere else) is to help with the symptoms of the tumor. Treatment of these tumors are different from the treatment of primary tumors. Achieving a cure is usually difficult, but not to despair, long-term "control" of the cancer may be possible meaning in some cases the cancer can be put into remission. Decreasing pain, obtaining local control of the tumor, relieving or preventing neurologic decline are important considerations. Thus, the goal is not necessarily "cure" but rather maintaining quality of life. The three main pillars of treatment are radiation, chemotherapy and surgery and so the treatment is generally coordinated with both a medical oncologist and a radiation oncologist. Metastatic cancer is a systemic problem affecting the entire body and will not resolve with surgery alone. Despite that, with modern advances in chemotherapy and radiation therapy, long-term survival may span for decades.

radiation therapy

Radiation therapy is the use of high energy beams to penetrate the body and kill tumor cells by destroying their DNA. This may seem counterintuitive to many people because doesn't radiation cause cancer to begin with? While it is true that radiation is harmful to the body and indeed can cause cancer, because tumor cells replicate so fast it is generally much more harmful to the cancer than it is to your healthy cells. This fact is what the field of radiation oncology —using carefully dosed and targeted radiation to kill tumors—is based on.

Radiation therapy has become so sophisticated that many tumors may simply be irradiated and surgery may be unnecessary. I have seen tumors disappear on MRI scans after a radiation treatment. Conventional radiation therapy involves sending a beam of radiation at a large area of tissue (typically including both tumor and healthy tissue). Depending on the tumor the radiation can be delivered by certain doses and schedules. **Radiation doses** are measured by **the unit Gray (Gy)** and range from 8Gy to 30Gy delivered in 1 to 10 sessions or "fractions." Only certain tumor types are "radiosensitive" and will respond to conventional radiation therapy. These include lymphoma, myeloma, breast, lung, and prostate cancer. Gastrointestinal cancers, melanoma, renal cell carcinoma, thyroid carcinoma are "radioresistant" and do not respond well to traditional radiation alone. With conventional radiation, tumor recurrence can be as high as 70% in these types of cancer (4). Many primary bone cancers are not sensitive to radiation and thus must be treated with surgery. Enter more advanced forms of radiation treatment.

Radiation obviously is harmful to the body and so trying to kill radioresistant tumors can be difficult with unfocused beams of radiation. However smart doctors and engineers have figured a way around this. With modern radiation machines, radiation can be delivered in high concentrations to the tumor from multiple different angles. This allows radiation oncologists to concentrate the dose in tumor tissue while limiting the dose to, or avoiding entirely, the surrounding critical healthy structures. This technique is known as **intensity modulated radiation therapy (IMRT) or stereotactic body radiation therapy (SBRT)** and works by directing beams of radiation through the tumor from different angles such that the dose to healthy tissue is very low and the dose to tumor is very high. IMRT can deliver such a high radiation dose, it can kill tumor cells regardless of whether they are radioresistant or not and thus provides much lower recurrence rates. Radiation oncology is a specialized field of medicine and doctors are trained to wield this power safely and to plan radiation doses in a way that makes it safe to give very high doses.

There are side-effects from radiation including difficulty with wound healing from surgery, bone marrow depletion, spinal cord injury, and even inducing new cancers of the bone. Spinal fusions that are followed by radiation therapy often heal poorly.

chemotherapy and medical treatment of cancer

Chemotherapy is a cancer treatment that uses medicines to kill or slow the growth of tumor cells. These medicines are generally administered by a medical oncologist. Like radiation therapy, certain cancers are more susceptible to chemotherapy than others. Cancers which are particularly susceptible to chemotherapy include breast carcinoma, certain bone cancers like osteosarcoma and Ewing's sarcoma, lymphoma, small-cell carcinoma of the lung, thyroid carcinoma. Those which are resistant to chemotherapy are melanoma, renal cell carcinoma, squamous cell carcinoma of lung. There are many different available medicines used in chemotherapy in different combinations, which is why they are directed by oncologists who specialize in their administration.

Unfortunately, many chemotherapy agents are also toxic to heathy cells and can interfere with post-operative healing.

Immunotherapy is a relatively new branch of medical oncology which activates the patient's own immune system to attack cancers. This is done by using proteins called **monoclonal antibodies** which are like your body's own antibody proteins in your immune system. In cancer, your own cells go haywire and start rapidly growing on their own. Your body's immune system sometimes has difficulty recognizing that these cells are bad because they are your own cells. In immunotherapy, synthetic antibodies are programmed to target the bad cells and help your immune system. The antibodies are injected into the body, which activates your immune system to help mop up the cancer. Immunotherapy has side effects but has one huge advantage, which is that it does not interfere with post-op wound healing, should you need surgery.

Cancer is in general an osteoporosis-inducing condition which can weaken the bones and result in fracture. Thus, treatment of osteoporosis with a **bisphosphonate** drug is generally also recommended.

surgery for cancer

In the case of metastatic cancer of the spine, surgery may be necessary to obtain a biopsy sample to get a diagnosis, but surgery is used principally to stabilize a collapsing spine and to decompress the spinal canal to preserve neurologic function. The goals are to ease pain and help keep your quality of life good while you undergo treatment with radiation and chemotherapy. Obviously, cancer patients are sensitive and have a higher risk of complications than healthy individuals so surgical approaches need to be tailored to the individual and kept as minimally invasive as possible. Some individuals may be too sick to undergo surgical treatment, and the risk may be greater than the benefit.

Because tumor can destroy the spinal column, reconstruction to stabilize the spine is one of the main surgical techniques to treat tumors. This can involve a procedure as relatively simple as **cement augmentation/kyphoplasty**, which can shore up the vertebral body bone and has been shown to dramatically reduce pain in cancer-related vertebral compression fractures (see chapter 46 on cement augmentation) (5). Augmentation works by injecting bone cement—polymethyl methacrylate (PMMA)—into the vertebra through a small percutaneous (through the skin) incision. It is a minimally invasive procedure with little recovery required. The cement augments the bone (increases its mass and fills in cracks) and stabilizes it, thus decreasing pain. Cement augmentation cannot be used in all patients and certain tumor types, such as those which have invaded the spinal canal, may not be good candidates for cement augmentation.

Sometimes surgery performed to stabilize the spinal column may require the use of screws, rods and cages. This is done at times when the spinal column has become unstable either from the tumor or because of the surgery used to resect (cut out) the tumor. **Instrumentation** of the spine can also be done in a percutaneous fashion to keep it minimally invasive. Because the bone in cancer patients is generally very porous and osteoporotic, new techniques have been developed such as integrating bone cement into the screws to make them less likely to loosen in the weak bone (6).

Spinal cord decompression is another critical aspect of spinal cancer treatment. When tumor invades the spinal canal, it can compress the spinal cord resulting in profound neurologic deficits such as weakness and numbness in those parts of the body innervated by spinal nerves that the tumor affects. These cases are considered emergencies in most instances and are treated with steroids and urgent surgery. There are many approaches to decompress the spinal canal; generally, decompression is accompanied by a fusion to prevent worsening of the neurologic deficit following surgery. In the landmark study performed by Dr. Roy Patchell surgical spinal cord decompression with radiation was shown to be superior to radiation alone for preserving walking capacity (7).

If the compression is severe (for example, the tumor is large), surgery must be performed before radiating the tumor. This is because the spinal cord is very sensitive to radiation damage so tumor tissue close to the spinal cord cannot receive radiation. The solution is to perform so-called "separation surgery" where the part of the tumor that is too close to the spinal cord is cut out (de-bulked), creating a safe margin between the tumor and the spinal cord. Then the remaining tumor can be targeted with stereotactic radiosurgery such as IMRT. Thus, what would once require extensive resection of the tumor can now be done in a simple minimally invasive way and allow radiation therapy to do the rest of the work. This technique has expanded the role of radiation therapy, converting many cancers that could not be treated to those that can.

For patients who are too sick to tolerate traditional surgery, other percutaneous methods are still available such as cement augmentation, minimally invasive spine surgery, radiofrequency ablation (RFA) laser interstitial thermal therapy (LITT) and cryoablation. RFA uses electricity at high frequency to destroy tumor cells. This may be done prior to a percutaneous cement augmentation to decrease tumor burden and pain (4). Even in patients with a limited predicted survival, these treatments may still be beneficial to decrease pain and increase function. Obviously, you will want to include your doctor and your family to help you decide what types of surgery, if any, is best for you.

Conclusion

Tumors of the spine can be frightening, painful and disabling. Your spine surgeon is equipped not only to help make an accurate diagnosis, but to use modern technology to dramatically improve your pain levels, neurologic function, and overall quality of life. Some tumors can be cured; others can be put into remission. Treatment of tumors can be a long road, and so it's critical you have a trusted surgeon who will help guide you along the path of healing.

Frequently Asked Questions

- **Once cancer has spread to the spine, what is the prognosis?**

That depends on many factors such as the type of cancer, the extent of the spread and your general health or condition. Some cancers that have spread to the spine can be controlled with surgery and radiation and long-term survival may be possible.

References

1. Abd-El-Barr MM, Huang KT, Moses ZB, Iorgulescu JB, Chi JH. Recent advances in intradural spinal tumors. Neuro-Oncol. 2018 May 18;20(6):729–42.

2. Kretzer RM. Intradural Spinal Cord Tumors. Spine. 2017 Apr 1;42(7):S22.

3. Lucantoni C, Than KD, Wang AC, Valdivia-Valdivia JM, Maher CO, La Marca F, et al. Tarlov cysts: a controversial lesion of the sacral spine. Neurosurg Focus. 2011 Dec;31(6):E14.

4. Sciubba DM, Pennington Z, Colman MW, Goodwin CR, Laufer I, Patt JC, et al. Spnal metastases 2021: a review of the current state of the art and future directions.

Spine J. 2021 Apr;S1529943021001959.

5.   Boonen S, Van Meirhaeghe J, Bastian L, Cummings SR, Ranstam J, Tillman JB, et al. Balloon kyphoplasty for the treatment of acute vertebral compression fractures: 2-year results from a randomized trial. J Bone Miner Res Off J Am Soc Bone Miner Res. 2011 Jul;26(7):1627–37.

6.   Son H, Choi SH, Heo DR, Kook I, Lee MK, Ahn HS, et al. Outcomes of the Use of Cement-Augmented Cannulated Pedicle Screws in Lumbar Spinal Fusion. Spine J. 2021 May;S1529943021002369.

7.   Patchell RA, Tibbs PA, Regine WF, Payne R, Saris S, Kryscio RJ, et al. Direct de-compressive surgical resection in the treatment of spinal cord compression caused by metastatic cancer: a randomised trial. The Lancet. 2005 Aug;366(9486):643–8.

Figures:

TUMORS OF THE SPINE
(Cross section lumbar spine)

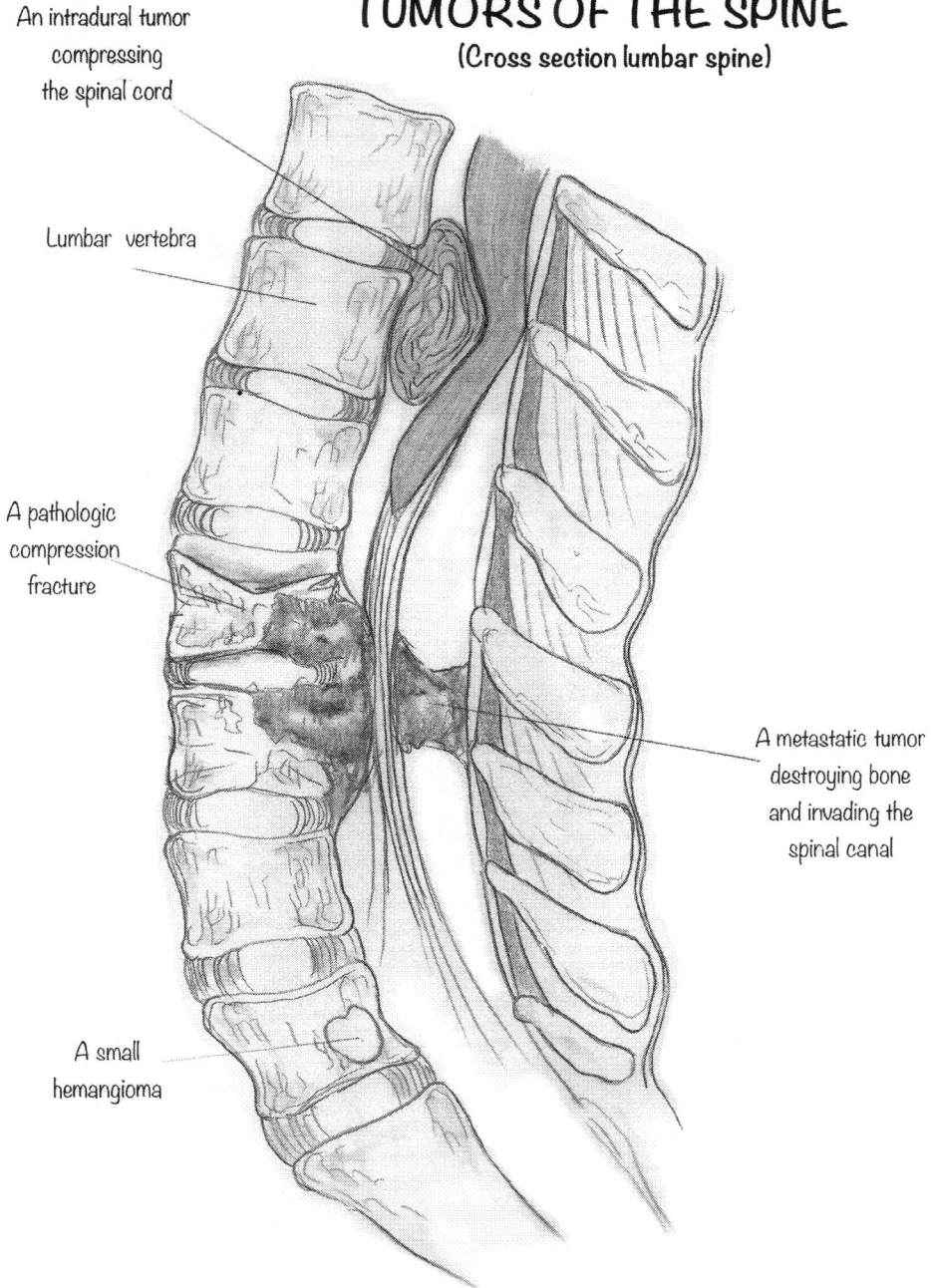

An intradural tumor
compressing
the spinal cord

Lumbar vertebra

A pathologic
compression
fracture

A metastatic tumor
destroying bone
and invading the
spinal canal

A small
hemangioma

Spine tumors. A cross section of the lumbar and lower thoracic spine
showing a representative intradural tumor compressing the spinal
cord (top of the image). In the lower lumbar spine, a metastatic tumor
breaks down the bone, resulting in fractures as well as central stenosis
(narrowing of the spinal canal) (bottom of image).

Chapter 16

Spinal Cord Injury

Summary

Spinal cord injuries typically occur because of a sudden trauma to the spine. Currently, there is no medicine or surgery that can reverse the damage of a spinal cord injury, and thus treatments consist of measures for damage control. Maintaining blood pressure, using steroids and surgery to decompress and stabilize the spinal column are the mainstays for treatment. The spinal cord has limited capacity for regeneration but usually some recovery is still possible. After the acute phase of the spinal cord injury, it is important to assemble an entire team of health care workers to help maximize recovery and prevent complications that can occur from paralysis. Spinal cord injuries are without question very serious injuries where the damage can be irreversible, but in some cases it may be possible to walk and regain normal function again.

Case 1

Mr. Lime is a 45-year-old telemarketer who suffered from a spinal cord injury in his 20s. He accidentally dove into a shallow portion of a lake severing his spi-

nal cord completely at C6-7. He underwent emergency surgery at a spinal cord injury center but, unfortunately, did not regain any significant motor or sensory function below the level of his injury. Currently he has some use of his arms, but his hands and manual dexterity are poor, and he has no use of his legs and is dependent on a customized wheelchair. The accident has caused him to lose function of his bowel and bladder so he must regularly self-catheterize. For this reason, he is checked for UTIs regularly by a urologist. Because he is unable to use his legs, his bones have become weak and brittle and he has suffered from fractures. However, despite all these setbacks and limitations, he maintains a positive attitude and is still determined to live as healthy and productive a life as possible. He has therapists who work with him weekly to keep his upper arms strong and he is part of a very supportive community of other quadriplegics. His home is configured so that he is nearly independent and can transfer using hand holds. He goes to work every day and drives a customized van fitted so that he can get in and out independently. His strength in the face of such disability is truly an inspiration and he has helped others who have suffered similar fates.

Case 2

Mr. Redwood is a 70-year-old retired plumber who sustains a fall in the bathroom after a slip. He is unable to move the left side of his body after the injury. He can't get up under his own power let alone walk. He is taken to a local hospital where doctors are initially unsure what the cause of his injury is. Did he have a stroke? Is he suffering from some neurologic disorder? An orthopedic specialist is consulted and spinal cord injury is considered. An MRI scan reveals significant—but not complete—injury to the spinal cord with severe degenerative compression. In essence he unknowingly had been suffering from spinal cord compression all along, and the impact of the fall has caused the spinal canal to narrow still further, resulting in increased compression and causing major damage to his cord. He has some motor function on the right side but has near paralysis of his left side. He undergoes urgent decompressive surgery at the local hospital. After surgery doctors are unsure if he will recover but he is so determined to beat his injury that he constantly works with his muscles forcing them to move. Within a day his arm and leg start to flicker again with life. Within a week he can get up with a walker. Within a month he can walk independently. Within a year he is back to normal, the memory of the event is a distant nightmare.

Introduction

Despite both the extensive research and scientific publications devoted to the physiology of neurons (the subunit of the spinal cord) and the spinal cord, it is a current fact that once injured, the neuron and the spinal cord have very limited healing potential. Nerves are incredibly sophisticated structures that are the biological equivalent of electrical wires. But unlike a damaged wire that can simply be replaced or reconnected, a neuron is a much more intricate structure that relies on the fine-tuned modulation of electrolytes (such as potassium and sodium ions) to convey a bioelectric signal. Modern medicine has yet to find a holy grail for nerve or spinal cord repair. Thus, once neuron damage starts to occur, the best most surgeons can do is remove the offending problem, such as a pinching disc or tumor, and hope that the damage is not permanent. To begin to understand the challenges of a spinal cord injury, it's important to talk a little about neuron biology.

Neuron Structure

Neurons are the functional subunit of the nervous system. Your entire nervous system consists of billions of neurons. The brain, spinal cord and nerves are all made from many neurons.

A **neuron is a long cell that contains three main parts: a cell body, an axon and an axon terminal.**

The **cell body**, which contains the nucleus, is where most of the metabolism occurs. The cell body has small processes which extend from it called dendrites.

The **dendrites** are the parts of the neuron that **receive signals from other neurons**. They are small processes or branches that extend from and surround the cell body.

The **axon is an elongated tubular structure which transmits the signal from the cell body to the axon terminal.** The axon joins to the cell body at a location called the axon hillock (where depolarization takes place, see next paragraph). The axon is a longer process than the dendrites and it ends in the axon terminal).

The **axon terminal** (or just terminus) is the final part of the neuron where the electrochemical signal is transmitted from one neuron to the next at a junction called the synapse.

Neuron function

The brain sends signals to all parts of your body via neurons (such as motor neurons that control movement) and other neurons (sensory neurons) carry information from all parts of your body to the brain—here is a very basic description of how those neurons do that job.

Basically, a neuron functions like an electrical wire, but instead of an electrical current it produces a biochemical current. The neuron does this by first receiving a chemical signal near the cell body at the dendrites. If the signal is strong enough, it triggers an electrical reaction known as depolarization, where sodium ions influx into the cell through specific sodium ion channels. Once the neuron is triggered, the signal is then transmitted by an electrochemical chain reaction that takes place all the way down the neuron's axon. At the terminal end of the axon the electrical impulse triggers the release of neurotransmitters (chemical messengers) that either cause the next nerve to depolarize and continue the messaging, or delivers the message to the targeted organ.

It is important to understand that although similar in concept, this process is different from how electricity is conducted in a wire which relays the flow of electrons in metal. For example, a cut wire can still be reattached together and transmit a signal. Neurons are more like tubes containing protein and fluid. They are tiny machines which if damaged are unable to simply reconnect and continue as normal.

For chemical impulses to be transmitted at a high speed, neurons are encased in an insulating protein called **myelin** which allow the chemical signal to travel at a much faster rate. If this myelin insulation is lost, the nerve will stop functioning properly. Myelination of a neuron plays an important role in the overall structure of the spinal cord (see below).

It takes a lot of energy for the neuron cell to function. Because of their great energy requirements, neurons are vulnerable metabolically (meaning any changes in the chemical environment around the nerve can negatively impact its function). Neurons are also vulnerable because of their elongated structure which makes them susceptible to injury. They are by far the largest cells in the body.

Damage to neural structures is dependent on both the degree of pressure exerted on them and on the amount of time the pressure is exerted. Pressure disrupts chemical flow, stops blood from nourishing the nerve and causes damage to the myelin sheath. Low pressure applied over long periods of time can result in significant neural degeneration similar to high pressure applied over short periods of time (1). Nerves can be severed, crushed or damaged in any other number of ways.

The Spinal Cord

The spinal cord is a complex organ that's major function is as the **information highway for your body**. Impulses from the brain travel down the spinal cord to control your body and all information from the extremities and torso travel up the spinal cord back to the brain (There are some functions which do not travel through the spinal cord, such as vision). The spinal cord is organized into two main sections: gray and white matter. The white matter is located on the periphery of the spinal cord and gray matter centrally. White matter consists of myelinated neurons which are organized into "tracts" that are generally responsible for discrete functions, such as movement of the hand or sensation of the foot. The gray matter consists of unmyelinated support cells (such as astrocytes), cell bodies and interneurons which act to interconnect the other cells. The spinal cord starts in your cervical spine beneath the brain stem and terminates at the conus medullaris, which in most individuals is in the lumbar spine around L1 or L2. As you move down the spinal cord, neuron clusters known as nerve roots break off to travel to different areas of the body. Nerve roots exit the spinal cord just like exits on a highway, and do so at each vertebral segment.

Spinal Cord Injury (SCI)

Spinal cord injuries are devastating injuries that have a profound impact on patients and their families. This section is devoted to acute spinal cord injury (rather than subacute or chronic which are discussed in the chapter on cervical myelopathy (chapter 5) and have different symptoms. Approximately 12,000 spinal cord injuries (SCI) occur in the United States per year with about 260,000 Americans living with an existing spinal cord injury.

There are several categories of spinal cord injury but they are broadly categorized as **quadriplegia** (an injury to the cervical spine affecting both the arms and legs) and **Paraplegia** (an injury occurring below the cervical spine affecting just the legs). Spinal cord injury may also be defined as a **complete injury** with total loss of motor and sensory function or an **incomplete injury** where some function/neural tracts are preserved (either motor or sensory or both). It is important to understand that not only are the motor and sensory systems affected by SCI, but also the autonomic systems that regulate your bowel, bladder, blood pressure, breathing and sexual function.

A common question is why spinal cord injuries can't heal themselves. Spinal cord injury is much more complex than peripheral nerve injury (see the next chapter) and healing capacity is limited. This is ultimately related to the complexity of the architecture of the spinal cord which is less a "wire" than a "mainframe" for relaying signals to and from the brain to all aspects of your body. As described above, the spinal cord consists of two main types of tissue: gray matter and white matter. The gray matter consists of many small nerve bodies that help regulate and interconnect neurons. If the gray matter is damaged it is extremely difficult for the body to rebuild. The white matter consists of long tracts of the neurons that transmit signals and do have potential to regrow, but because of the disruption of the gray matter and scarring caused by the inflammatory response, the white matter doesn't work very well after spinal cord injury. The nerves of your body will regenerate to some extent but when the complex circuitry of the spinal cord is disrupted, it is difficult for neurons to try to heal and reform this architecture. Try to imagine rebuilding the collapsed Twin Towers in New York City but using only the rubble as material and no original blueprints. To date, direct surgical repair of spinal cord injuries is not possible and would likely result in greater damage if attempted.

How Do Spinal Cord Injuries Occur?

Car collisions are the most common way to sustain a spinal cord injury and incomplete quadriplegia is the most common symptom. Typically, SCI begins with a blunt trauma that results in direct tissue damage. This can occur in varying degrees of intensity from a "stun" commonly referred to as "a stinger" where no actual physical damage is done, all the way to complete transection (severing) of the spinal cord. Following significant initial trauma to the spinal cord, the body reacts to the injury with a robust inflammatory response. This inflammation triggers the release of several neurotoxic chemicals that can cause a secondary injury that worsens the neurologic damage. The inflammatory response results in the formation of a scar which physically blocks the regeneration of the long neuron tracts of the spinal cord. Thus, the more robust this inflammatory response is, the more profound the neurologic deficit can be. Preventing this scar from forming is the focus of much research in the treatment of spinal cord injuries.

A Word about Navigating the Medical System in a Complicated Acute Situation

Spinal cord injuries are acute problems that should be dealt with immediately and as such many patients may feel at the mercy of the medical system. Patients may wonder, am I at the right institution? Do I have the right doctor? When under the stress of trying to deal with a serious injury to a family member or yourself, trying to navigate the medical system is daunting. Trying to sort out the complicated medical, scientific and social information on the web is even more difficult.

In these situations, I think it's best to trust your doctors and let them help you make good decisions. Making decisions under serious stress is challenging, which is why medical doctors are trained under stress. Take comfort in the fact that doctors choose a career in medicine to help people, are trained to win at all costs, and get satisfaction from making the "right choices" for their patients. In the setting of a serious injury like a spinal cord injury the most important thing is getting treatment and doctor shopping or trying to master the science of spinal cord injury in a short period of time is not really in your best interest. It is possible to seriously undermine your medical treatment wasting time trying to make complicated decisions best left to professionals.

How is SCI treated?

Treatment of SCI is controversial but aimed at stabilizing the spinal column, maintaining blood flow and reducing the secondary inflammatory reaction, thus decreasing scar formation. The uninjured spinal cord can normally regulate its own blood flow. However, with SCI, the spinal cord becomes vulnerable to changes in blood pressure. A critical part of the care of SCI is to maintain the blood pressure above a threshold level. In the intensive care unit, intravenous catheters are used to monitor blood pressure invasively and the patient may be given drugs that keep the blood pressure up. If there is active pressure on the vertebrae from fracture, the spinal cord is typically decompressed as soon as possible and possibly stabilized with hardware to prevent further destruction from occurring. The Surgical Timing in Acute Spinal Cord Injury Study (STASCIS) trial evaluated early surgical intervention versus late surgical intervention and found that early treatment resulted in better outcomes (2). Thus, **timely surgery is typically recommended in suitable candidates to maximize the chance for the best possible outcome**. Nonetheless, it is always in your best interest for the surgical team to be well rested and to do the procedure in as controlled fashion as possible.

Medical management is aimed at preventing the inflammatory response that leads to secondary damage. Starting in 1984, the National Acute Spinal Cord Injury Study (NASCIS) conducted a series of trials evaluating the efficacy of treating spinal cord injuries with a steroid drug called methylprednisolone since steroids reduce inflammation. Overall, the trials showed some improvement with steroid administration within an 8-hour window; however, the studies were highly controversial because of some design flaws. Furthermore, use of high dose methylprednisolone can result in serious complications such as sepsis (infection), wound breakdown, pulmonary embolism, gastrointestinal hemorrhage, and even death. Because of these complications, steroid treatment remains controversial and the decision to give the medicine should be made on a case-by-case basis by the physician. Steroids are still typically given in some form to patients with spinal cord injury (but maybe not in a similar fashion to how it was given in the NASCIS trial). Other compounds which can reduce secondary injury to the spinal cord, such as erythropoietin, opiate blockers, GM1 Ganglioside and Thyrotropin-releasing hormone, are all candidates for treatment of spinal cord injury but to date remain experimental.

In my practice we use medications like the steroid dexamethasone to decrease inflammation/ swelling and drugs like norepinephrine to keep the blood pressure up.

The Future of SCI Treatment

Another hopeful possibility to cure SCI is cellular-based transplantation. This group of therapies are aimed at either regenerating damaged spinal cord tissue or replacing them outright. One example of this, peripheral nerve grafts, uses tissue obtained from other nerves in the body such as from the olfactory bulb (the nerves involved in the sense of smell), but has not been terribly successful. Another biological implant uses activated macrophages, which are small "clean up" type cells that eat up cellular debris as the result of trauma. They have been injected into the spinal cord and have shown some effectiveness at reducing secondary damage. However, the company that produced them failed to complete the clinical trials necessary to bring the product to market so it is not available.

Stem cell therapy is a buzzword heard in all areas of medicine. This is mainly because stems cells, which are cells that have the potential to become any cell in the body, seem to offer the holy grail of treatments for many degenerative diseases, including spinal cord injury. In the early 2000s stem cell therapy was banned in the United States which significantly reduced research in this area. This ban was lifted in 2009 and so hopefully more research will emerge in the coming years (3).

Biotechnology offers another hopeful area where treatments for SCI may emerge. A promising form of treatment is the concept of "neural-bypass." In neural bypass, artificial intelligence and machine learning are used to decode the complex signals from the brain, which can be picked up from the surface of the scalp using electrodes. These signals are then converted to signals that neurons can recognize and are transmitted to the body through use of high-resolution electrical stimulation systems. In this way the injured section of the spinal cord is bypassed and brain signals can travel to the body (4). Although not currently available to the masses, the technology is progressing rapidly and could become a potential therapy.

Will I Walk Again?

After a spinal cord injury one of the most common questions the spine surgeon gets asked is "will I walk again?" Over time many ways to evaluate and try to predict the outcome of spinal cord injuries have been developed. There are complicated scales used to calculate the severity of injury and thus the chances of recovery. One of the most popular methods is the ASIA scale (American Spinal Injury Association). The ASIA scale divides SCI into complete injury and 4 stages of incomplete injury. The patient diagnosed with complete SCI has neither sensation in the body nor ability to move. The 4 stages of incomplete SCI describe various degrees of sensation and ability to move.

It is not important to memorize this scale, but rather to understand the concept that SCI may be complete (no function remains) or incomplete (some function remains). Most spinal cord injuries improve to some degree from the initial injury. The hope is that there is some structural integrity remaining in the damaged spinal cord and that it simply needs to recover from the initial trauma. The degree of improvement depends on the location and severity of the initial injury as well as the age of the patient. Twenty percent of ASIA A patients convert to ASIA B or some form of incomplete SCI, half regaining only sensation (ASIA B) and the other half regaining some motor function (ASIA C) (5).

Furthermore, the location of the injury can impact walking ability—the higher on the spine the injury occurs, the less likelihood of walking at 1 year after surgery (6). Those who have incomplete paraplegia (ASIA C or D) have a 50% chance of being able to walk at 1 year. Those with complete injuries (ASIA A) at T9 or higher have a 0% chance of walking at 1 year. However, patients with cervical injuries classified as ASIA D have a high likelihood of walking at 1 year.

ASIA Classification Scale for SCI		
ASIA SCORE	Type	DEFICIT: motor deficits are measured using the manual muscle testing scale (MMT) that grades muscle strength out 5 points.
ASIA A	Complete SCI	No motor or sensory function
ASIA B	Sensory Incomplete SCI	Sensory function only
ASIA C	Motor Incomplete SCI	More than 1/2 of key muscle groups have a strength of less than 3/5 on the MMT scale. Sensation may or may not be intact.
ASIA D	Motor Incomplete SCI	More than 1/2 of key muscle groups have a strength of greater than 3/5 on the MMT scale. Sensation may or may not be intact.
ASIA E	Normal	No motor or sensory deficit

In general, patients with incomplete injuries—even if just sensation is spared, particularly around the groin area—have a higher likelihood of walking again compared to those with complete injuries (7). What this means is that if some function remains there is a chance you may walk again, but only time will tell. Unfortunately, this still leaves many patients with permanent disability. Good motor function at the L3 nerve root (which innervates the quadriceps) and sensation at the

S1 nerve root (which innervates the lateral heel) are excellent indicators of ultimate ambulation (eventually walking). Finally, younger patients (younger than 65 years) have a higher chance of recovery than older patients (8).

Caring for the SCI Patient After the Initial Injury

After treatment of the initial SCI there is still a long road ahead for the SCI patient. Treating the SCI patient in the subacute (shortly after the initial injury) and chronic phase (after the disease has stabilized) is often very complex, especially since many secondary complications can occur after the original injury, making SCIs very resource demanding. Learning what kind of problems can arise and how to stay on top of them is critical. Also finding a physician who is comfortable managing these problems is essential.

neuropathic pain (symptom: shooting and burning pain in the extremities)

Neuropathic pain, which is common after an SCI, can manifest as **shooting and burning pain in the extremities**. It's paradoxical and very unfair that even though you cannot use your legs or feel them, they may still cause pain. Why this occurs is not totally understood, but one of the reasons this happens is that the mental map of sensation still exists in your brain and without reliable input from the legs, the brain can go haywire. This problem can be treated with drugs such as gabapentin, Lyrica and amitriptyline. Narcotic drugs are ineffective for this type of pain and can cause dependence (5).

orthostatic hypotension (symptom: light-headed on standing)

The SCI patient may have difficulty regulating her/his own blood pressure after injury. This happens because of loss of sympathetic tone in the veins (loss of the neurons which help keep the pressure in your circulatory system). This can result in sudden drops in blood pressure when standing upright since blood collects in the veins of the legs (known as orthostatic hypotension). Compression stockings and vasopressor drugs (drugs that increase vascular tone) such as midodrine may help prevent this.

autonomic dysreflexia (AD) (symptoms: sweatiness, headache, blurry vision, redness in face)

A condition known as autonomic dysreflexia (AD) may also occur in SCI patients whose injuries occur above the T6 level, disrupting the sympathetic nervous system (again, the system which regulates your blood pressure and heart rate). When this disconnect occurs, your sympathetic nervous system sometimes over-reacts to stimuli and activates independently. **AD can result in dangerous elevation of the blood pressure**. AD can be triggered by many kinds of stimuli but is **commonly triggered by a full bowel or bladder** that sends input to the sympathetic nervous system to activate independently and actually results in dramatic increases in blood pressure that can be life-threatening. In addition to a raised blood pressure— 20mmhg or more above the patient's baseline—AD typically manifests with sweatiness, headache, blurry vision and redness of the skin above the level of the SCI. If this occurs, a patient should immediately be propped upright, have his/her clothing loosened (to allow cooling), and have his/her blood pressure carefully monitored. The offending stimulus should be removed (typically by draining the bladder with a catheter or disimpacting the bowel (evacuating stool, usually with fingers). Drugs such as nitroglycerin or a calcium channel blocker such as nifedipine may be used to lower the blood pressure (9).

pressure sores (with an SCI you won't feel them)

When you sit normally, your body tells you when you have been there for too long and you get a sensation of discomfort and change position. SCI patients lose the signal that your body tells you when it's time to move and so can stay on a patch of skin for much longer than normal. Prolonged pressure on a given spot causes the blood flow to that area of skin to break down and ultimately the skin also breaks down. Pressure sores are common in SCI patients since they have lost the ability to sense pain on bony areas, have decreased mobility and spend an increased amount of time in bed or in wheelchairs. **Pressure sores develop when there is continual pressure over a bony area** (the sitting bones, heels or hips particularly). If left unchecked pressure injuries can turn into major ulcerations and lead to life-threatening infections. **Pressure ulcers are prevented with careful monitoring, and frequent adjustments of position so that not any one area has pressure on it for more than 2 hours**. Furthermore, there are many different mattresses, cushion supports and pads which can be used to protect bony surfaces. Vigilance is key to prevent a pressure sore.

bladder and bowel care

Bladder dysfunction is very common in SCI patients. Because SCI patients may not be able to void independently and must use catheters, they are at increased risk for bladder infections and must be carefully monitored for this. However, because SCI patients lack sensation of their bladders, they do not have regular bladder infection symptoms. Thus, infections may be difficult to detect, with the patient often only experiencing nonspecific symptoms such as fever, chills, nausea, and fatigue. Other symptoms such as blood in the urine or foul-smelling urine should also be quickly considered but may not necessarily indicate infection as they can result from frequent catheterization. In patients who have had indwelling catheters for more than 5 years, there is an increased risk of bladder cancer because of constant irritation. These patients should undergo annual screening for bladder cancer with cystoscopy by a urologist (10). Bowel dysfunction is also very common in SCI patients resulting in fecal incontinence and difficulty with evacuation. Bowel care can be optimized by ensuring enough fiber is present in the diet and also through the use of stool softeners and laxatives.

breathing and respiration

With SCI, particularly those above T10, patients have weakened muscles of respiration and are at increased risk for pneumonia. This is because SCI patients whose spines have been injured high up can have a decreased ability to breathe deeply, cough and clear secretions. Patients with difficulty breathing may require chest physiotherapy, compression and percussion (tapping on the chest to mobilize and break up thick secretions) and suctioning to avoid pneumonias. Furthermore, patients should obtain yearly vaccinations for influenza and pneumococcus and should avoid smoking, which can make patients more prone to pneumonia and the pneumonia more difficult to treat.

osteoporosis

Osteoporosis is a major concern in patients who have SCI as they are no longer able to weight bear on their bones. Thus, the long bones undergo rapid deterioration with as much as 50% of bone mineral density lost within 3 years of injury. This puts SCI patients at great risk for fractures, which can occur even during simple daily tasks such as transfers (for example moving from bed to wheelchair). Patients may not even realize that they have suffered from a fracture because they will not have pain. it's also possible for fractures to trigger autonomic dysregulation (see autonomic dysreflexia (AD) above).

Most fractures are managed non-operatively unless there is a threat to the skin, and SCI patients have a great capacity for healing fractures. This is likely related to increased blood flow to the extremities resulting from lack of circulatory regulation of blood vessels but it's not entirely clear. Patients with SCI should undergo yearly DEXA scans to screen for osteoporosis and commit to adequate intake of vitamin D and calcium (see chapter 23 on these nutrients).

The Spinal Cord Injury Team

Spinal cord injury devastates all aspects of life and turns an independent person into someone who requires considerable daily assistance from both family and medical personnel. The social implications can be tremendous and to help decrease the challenges of living with an SCI, it is extremely important to have a good team assembled around you. This means you need a physician who is comfortable managing secondary problems from spinal cord injury as discussed above, and you need a physical therapist who can help you regain and maintain your skeletal muscle and keep your body in working order. Also, occupational therapists can help you adapt your house to make living easier and more comfortable. These professionals cannot cure your injury but can help keep you as healthy and as active as possible.

Early rehabilitation may be accomplished at a specialized inpatient spinal cord rehab center where a multidisciplinary team consisting of physical therapists, occupational therapists, orthotists (who make and fit braces as needed), nursing staff, social workers, pain management specialists, and psychiatric support counselors. Rehab includes learning how to use adaptive equipment such as power wheelchairs, trying to improve walking with gait training and strengthening exercises, and other aspects of self-care such as self-catheterization and rectal stimulation. Following inpatient rehabilitation, it is critical to assemble a team that can continue to support you as an outpatient. This team is generally centered around a primary care provider with experience in supporting patients with SCI.

Care for the spinal cord injury patient can be overwhelming for patients, families and physicians. Thus, it is imperative to access as much as possible online resources for support and education. Some are listed here:

- **https://msktc.org/sci/factsheets**

- **https://www.myshepherdconnection.org/sci**

- **https://actionnuggets.ca/actionable-nuggets-4th-ed-2019/**

- https://newmobility.com

Spinal Cord Stroke (Ischemia)

An acute ischemic stroke is defined as an occlusion (blockage) of blood flow resulting in death of neural (nerve) tissue. Most people are familiar with strokes of the brain (cerebrovascular infarcts); however, spinal cord strokes can also occur, though thankfully are rare, accounting for about 1% of all strokes. Because they are so rare, they are poorly understood by most. Likely the most common cause of a spinal cord stroke occurs following thoracic aortic surgery to treat an aneurysm (an enlargement of, in this case, the aortic artery in the chest). Nonetheless there are many causes of spinal cord ischemia including embolisms, arteriovenous malformations, sickle cell disease, use of drugs such as cocaine which cause vasospasm (sudden constriction of a blood vessel), aortic dissections (tearing of the aorta), and hypotension.

Like cerebrovascular strokes (those that occur in the brain), in most cases spinal cord strokes strike suddenly. The extent of symptoms depends on the area of the spine that is damaged. Pain in the extremities is the most common symptom. The anterior part of the spinal cord is typically affected and results in loss of motor function and sensation in the extremities. Loss of motor function first occurs as a flaccid paralysis (paralysis in which muscle tone is absent) which is followed by spastic paralysis (when the muscles are contracted) in the following weeks. Back pain is common.

The prognosis for **spinal cord infarctions** (tissue death) varies depending on the extent of the damage but in general is guarded (meaning doctors are not able to completely predict what tissue will recover). However, with appropriate treatment, many spinal cord stroke patients will improve and be able to walk within 1 week (11). Treatment generally consists of maintaining the blood pressure, moderate doses of steroids and possibly even draining the cerebrospinal fluid (CSF). When draining the CSF, the CSF pressure in the spinal canal is kept low (at less than 10mmhg) and this allows more blood to enter the spinal cord (12). Treatments readily used in brain strokes to break down blood clots (intravenous thrombolytics), such as tissue plasminogen activator (TPA), are currently not indicated in spinal cord strokes (13). Similarly, blood thinners are not currently used in spinal cord infarcts.

Conclusion

Spinal cord injury is perhaps one of the most feared injuries by both doctors and patients alike. This is because SCIs are poorly understood, result in terrible disability, and treatments for both the initial injury and the secondary complications are limited. Nonetheless, the field is rapidly expanding, and doctors and researchers are working tirelessly to improve outcomes. It may be that one day there is a viable treatment for spinal cord injury.

Frequently Asked Questions

- **Is sex possible after spinal cord injury?**

     Ok, it may not be a frequently asked question, but many people are too afraid to ask. One of the most challenging aspects of having a spinal cord injury may be loss or change in your sexual function, not only because of how it impacts the intimacy you have with your partner, but also because finding help to figure this out can be difficult, embarrassing and awkward. Not many doctors will come out and start giving you instruction on how you can have a fulfilling sex life after a SCI. Luckily there are many free resources online on how to maximize your sexual life after a spinal cord injury—a very comprehensive one from Mt. Sinai Rehab: https://www.sexualitysci.org/. Another resource is the book *Sexual Sustainability* by Marcalee Alexander, MD.

In brief, while there are some adjustments to be made, it is possible to have sex after spinal cord injury. The level of sexual function you can have will be different depending on the severity of your injury but, regardless, it is possible to have a healthy and fulfilling sex life after SCI. It is important to know that it is possible to have non-genital orgasms and orgasms without ejaculation. Don't try and force your body to do something you may no longer be capable of—that is a set up for disappointment. Focus instead on the areas of your body which you can derive pleasure from (for example, shoulders, nipples) and use all the senses you have available to you. Communication with your partner is also critical and helps build intimacy—leading you on a path for success. Be confident, and comfortable with who you are while also hearing what your partner needs. Most important is that you are patient with yourself and your partner. Never give up.

References

1.   Rydevik B, Brown MD, Lundborg G. Pathoanatomy and pathophysiology of nerve root compression. Spine. 1984 Feb;9(1):7–15.

2.   Fehlings MG, Vaccaro A, Wilson JR, Singh A, W. Cadotte D, Harrop JS, et al. Early versus Delayed Decompression for Traumatic Cervical Spinal Cord Injury: Results of the Surgical Timing in Acute Spinal Cord Injury Study (STASCIS). Di Giovanni S, editor. PLoS ONE. 2012 Feb 23;7(2):e32037.

3.   Gupta R, Bathen ME, Smith JS, Levi AD, Bhatia NN, Steward O. Advances in the management of spinal cord injury. J Am Acad Orthop Surg. 2010 Apr;18(4):210–22.

4.   Bouton CE, Shaikhouni A, Annetta NV, Bockbrader MA, Friedenberg DA, Nielson DM, et al. Restoring cortical control of functional movement in a human with quadriplegia. Nature. 2016 12;533(7602):247–50.

5.   Kwon BK, Banaszek D, Kirshblum S. Advances in the Rehabilitation of the Spinal Cord–Injured Patient: The Orthopaedic Surgeons' Perspective. Journal of the American Academy of Orthopaedic Surgeons. 2019 Nov;27(21):e945–53.

6.   Reinhold M, Knop C, Beisse R, Audigé L, Kandziora F, Pizanis A, et al. Operative treatment of 733 patients with acute thoracolumbar spinal injuries: comprehensive results from the second, prospective, internet-based multicenter study of the Spine

Study Group of the German Association of Trauma Surgery. European Spine Journal. 2010 Oct;19(10):1657–76.

7.   Marino RJ, Ditunno JF, Donovan WH, Maynard F. Neurologic recovery after traumatic spinal cord injury: data from the model spinal cord injury systems. Archives of Physical Medicine and Rehabilitation. 1999 Nov;80(11):1391–6.

8.   Hicks KE, Zhao Y, Fallah N, Rivers CS, Noonan VK, Plashkes T, et al. A simplified clinical prediction rule for prognosticating independent walking after spinal cord injury: a prospective study from a Canadian multicenter spinal cord injury registry. Spine J. 2017 Oct;17(10):1383–92.

9.   Cragg J, Krassioukov A. Autonomic dysreflexia. :1.

10.   Mishori R, Groah SL, Otubu O, Raffoul M, Stolarz K. Improving your care of patients with spinal cord injury/disease. J Fam Pract. 2016 May;65(5):302–9.

11.   Romi F, Naess H. Spinal Cord Infarction in Clinical Neurology: A Review of Characteristics and Long-Term Prognosis in Comparison to Cerebral Infarction. Eur Neurol. :4.

12.   Coselli JS, LeMaire SA, Köksoy C, Schmittling ZC, Curling PE. Cerebrospinal fluid drainage reduces paraplegia after thoracoabdominal aortic aneurysm repair: Results of a randomized clinical trial. Journal of Vascular Surgery. 2002 Apr;35(4):631–9.

13.   Nasr DM, Rabinstein A. Spinal Cord Infarcts: Risk Factors, Management, and Prognosis. Curr Treat Options Neurol. 2017 Aug;19(8):28.

Figures:

The Neuron

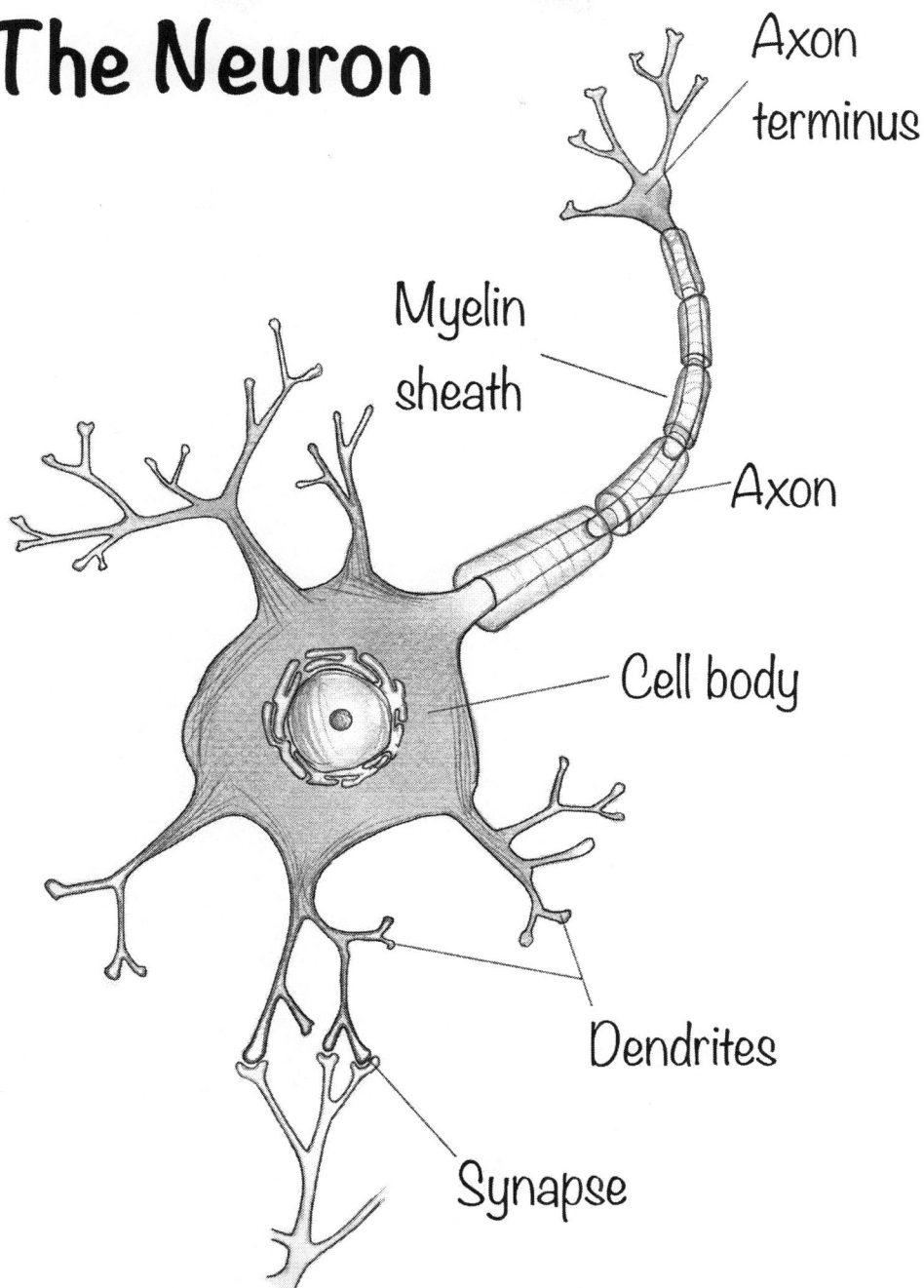

The Neuron. The neuron is the basic subunit of the nervous system and consists of several parts: the cell body is the metabolic core of the cell and has dendrite processes which communicate with other cells; the long axon is the "electrical wire" responsible for conveying a neural impulse through the body and the axon terminus; at the axon terminus this signal is transferred to another nerve or organ across a synapse.

Spinal cord injury:

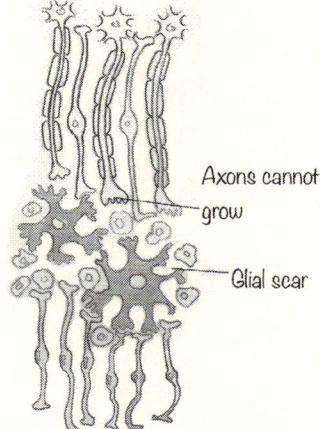

Brain Cross Section

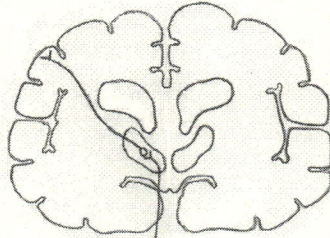

The spinal cord is composed of many neurons, but can be represented by neuron diagrams such as this one with three neurons that compose the sensory system (the circles represent cell bodies and the lines the axons)

Spinal Cord Cross Section

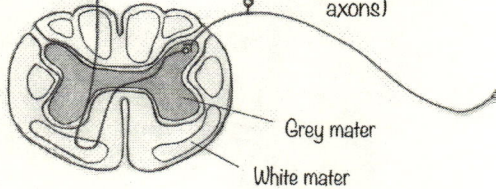

Grey mater

White mater

Normal Spinal Cord Architecture

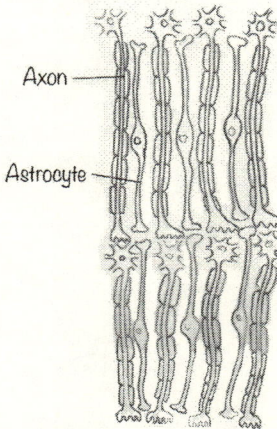

Axon

Astrocyte

Spinal Cord Injury

Axons cannot grow

Glial scar

A microscopic representation of the spinal cord showing normal axon and astrocyte arrays (left). When damage occurs (right) a scar forms that prevents axons from regenerating.

Spinal cord architecture and injury. Neurons in the spinal cord are be represented as lines in this diagram. Although in realty there are many, in this diagram only one is depicted for simplicity. A typical arrangement for sensory neurons consists of three neurons linked serially. Neurons carry signals up through the spinal cord to reach the brain. White matter consists of the signaling neuronal tracts which are highly myelinated. Gray matter consists of support cells and cell bodies, including astrocytes. One neuron depolarizes and sends a chemical signal to the next neuron causing depolarization. In this way the signal is transmitted up to the brain (top two pictures). The spinal cord consists of a highly organized neural pattern of axons and support cells (bottom left). When the spinal cord is injured, a glial scar may form preventing regeneration of the terminal axon (bottom right).

Chapter 17

Injury to the Nerves Once they Leave the Spinal Canal (Peripheral Nerve Injury and Neuron Regeneration)

Summary

Nerves are the cellular wires that connect your central nervous system (the brain and spinal cord) to the body. The nerves exit the spinal cord and join to form the "peripheral nerves" that course through the arms and legs. Unlike the spinal cord, the nerves do not have a bony spinal canal to protect them and are susceptible to injury. Typical ways nerves are injured include lacerations from sharp objects or crush injuries from fractures of the bone. Luckily, nerves have the capacity to regrow but sometimes need surgical assistance. Thus, nerve injury is much less disabling and more treatable than spinal cord injury but can still take long periods to recover.

Case

Mr. Cactus is a 40-year-old forester. One day while using a chain saw at work he sustains a serious laceration to his right wrist, severing multiple tendons as well as his median nerve (the nerve which supplies sensation to the palm). Because the chainsaw destroyed a piece of the nerve, the severed nerve cannot be easily reconnected with surgery. To help the nerve regrow surgeons use a nerve conduit (a device which can span a gap in a damaged nerve) to reconnect the nerve. His recovery takes months as he waits for the nerve to regrow, but eventually he does regain sensation in his fingers and palm (although his sensation is still slightly diminished from before the accident).

An Intro to Nerves

It's important to understand the difference between a nerve and the spinal cord. **Nerves are the "cables" which transmit information to and from the spinal cord to the body and organs**. They consist of groups of long neurons (see the previous chapter for a description of the neuron) which stretch all the way from the spinal cord to the extremities. Nerves originate from the spinal cord (begin) as nerve roots which branch and reconnect through a network called a plexus. There are four main plexuses in the body: the cervical (neck), brachial (arms), lumbar (back) and sacral (pelvis). It's a little bit confusing, but a plexus is like a freeway junction: nerve roots go into the plexus and come out redirected as peripheral nerves. The "peripheral nerve" originates from the plexus to travel out to the extremity .

The purpose of having a plexus is to introduce redundancy into the electrical system of your body. It allows organs and muscles to be supplied by more than one nerve source so if injury occurs to a nerve there is backup to some degree.

As indicated above, the basic unit of a nerve is a neuron. As a quick review, a neuron is composed of a cell body, a long axon which is the electrical wire like part, and the axon terminus. At the end of a peripheral nerve's axon terminus, there is a minute gap, known as a synapse, between the neuron and the organ or next neuron it is transmitting signals to. The synapse is where neurotransmitters (chemical messengers) are released that activate the receiving organ tissue or next neuron.

Keep in mind, **only the axons (the long part of the neuron) are part of the peripheral nerves**. Once neurons leave the spinal cord, they are just long axons (the cell bodies are in the spine. There are no cell bodies in the extremities. This is important to understand because it affects how likely a peripheral nerve can recover after injury, since all the machinery to rebuild the nerve is in the cell body close to the spine.

Peripheral nerves are highly organized structures with axons grouped into bundles of neurons or "fascicles." Fascicles are *surrounded* by connective tissue known as *peri*neurium that create discrete pockets of axons. *Within* the perineurium, another tissue called the *endo*neurium cushions and protects the individual axons. Bundles of fascicles are surrounded by a dense *protective layer* known as *epi*neurium. Damage to the myelin, or any of these protective layers can result in nerve dysfunction.

Like spinal cord injury, when a peripheral nerve is compressed, irritated or damaged, it can result in pain, numbness, and paralysis. However, overall, **nerves are much more robust structures compared to the spinal cord**, in large part because they have multiple protective layers. Individual neurons are protected by layers of myelin, tough protective shock-absorbing proteins which allow them to withstand compression, and only some cells in the spinal cord possess that. Also, as just mentioned above, nerves have a hierarchal structure with progressive bundling of fibers contained in successive protective layers of collagen. The outer most layer is the epineurium, the middle layer is the perineurium, and the innermost layer is the endoneurium. Peripheral nerves can stretch and bend because they are structured similarly to a spring, with redundant tissue that allows them to elongate. Nerves are also packed in padding or areolar tissue which further protects them from some compression. This areolar tissue is in addition to the epi-, peri- and endo-neuriums, and exists outside of the nerve casing. All this extra protection means the nerves are more durable than the spinal cord. However, nerve injury is much more common than spinal cord injury mainly because they are superficial and do not have the bony casing of the spinal cord.

Seddon's Classification for Nerve Injury			
Name	**Degree**	**Layers damaged**	**Prognosis**
Neuropraxia	**Mild:** nerve is damaged, but the overall structure is preserved	Endoneurium, perineurium and epineurium are all intact. **Myelin is disrupted.**	**Good:** Usually recovers in several days to weeks.
Axonotmesis	**Moderate:** the nerve is partially transected (cut), but portions remain intact	Epineurium and perineurium are preserved, **endoneurium is damaged as is the myelin sheath. Nerve undergoes degeneration**	**Regeneration is possible** but takes weeks to months (1mm per day). Surgery is typically unnecessary as nerve is still in continuity.
Neurotmesis	**Severe:** this is a complete nerve transection.	**All layers are disrupted.**	Independent regeneration is not possible and **requires surgery** to reconnect the ends of the nerve.

Nerve roots (the structures which exit immediately from the spine) are more vulnerable than peripheral nerves because they only possess some of the peripheral nerve's features just listed above. For example, as the nerve root leaves the spinal column the nerve root does not have a casing called epineurium, which is derived from the meninges (the spinal canal's protective membranes). This makes nerve roots more easily irritated by any compression than a peripheral nerve.

As with spinal cord injury, there are several classification systems doctors use to evaluate nerve injury. I give an example here though these classifications systems are only important for doctors to know. The simplest system, Seddon's Classification (see table above), describes both how the nerve is injured and gives prognosis.

How Nerves Heal

Neurons are long structures that heal in a strange way. Remember, nerves lack a cell body (the cell body being in or near the spinal cord) and thus do not have a metabolic core that helps regeneration. One might think that if a nerve is cut it would simply mend in the area where it is broken. This, however, is not the case because, again, nerves do not have cell bodies. Nerves undergo what is called **Wallerian degeneration**, which means **nerves are not capable of mending breaks in the axon** (the long part of the nerve). Instead, the entire axon downstream of the injury degenerates and the nerve must grow completely back from the site of injury.

Nerves are bundles of many axons (the long part of the neuron). When injured the axon bundles are disrupted and although they do have the potential to regrow, cannot mend the site of injury as described above. To heal, the cell body (located near the spine) must grow a new axon starting as a bud at the site of injury. To do this the cell body swells as it switches priority from the production of neurotransmitters to structural proteins needed to grow a new axon. In some cases, if the trauma imparted is severe enough, the entire nerve above and below the injury may die and healing will be more difficult. The nerve bud, which has many feelers like a sea anemone (think of the many axons which are trying to find their way), originates at the site of injury and searches out and elongates along the previous tract of the nerve. If the nerve lacks a tract the bud may be unable to find its original path. It may wander to a location it shouldn't or grow into a neuroma (a benign tumor).

Therefore, despite axon regeneration, functional recovery may not occur (meaning the nerve grows back but doesn't resume normal function). If functional recovery is to occur, the growing axon bud must find its way back to the original structure it controlled. To help the body heal, the far end of the cut or damaged nerve emits factors that draw the axon growth back towards it in a process known as neurotropism. However, even if the nerve ends are connected back together surgically, there is no way of guaranteeing that the correct axon buds will connect to their original partners. Imagine cutting a big telecommunications cable, if the individual wires were not color-coordinated how would you know which ones to connect back together? Thus, it is possible for mixing and matching of motor and sensory neurons. In one particularly sinister healing process, autonomic fibers (those that control automatic functions of the body), can be connected into pain and sensation fibers causing chronic pain (1).

Let's recap, as I know these concepts may be difficult to grasp. A nerve is a bundle of many neurons, which are very long cells that originate from the spinal cord and travel out to the body. Because a neuron is so long (and so much of its axon is so far from its cell body), neurons do not have the capacity to mend breaks. If injured, a neuron must regrow from the site of injury all the way to its target (the original structure it controlled, for example, a finger). This process is called Wallerian degeneration.

Wallerian degeneration starts 2-3 days after the injury and the cell body typically takes a month to ramp up production to generate a new nerve. Nerves then regrow at a rate of 1mm per day. So, if you sustain an injury near the spine, it may take a year or longer to recover function in the extremity supplied by those nerves. When the muscle becomes disconnected from its nerve supply it can no longer function properly. It's akin to cutting off the electricity to a light bulb but not as simple. Muscles shrink (atrophy) when they are disconnected, so it's also like a potted plant that wilts when you stop watering it. The term for when a muscle or any structure loses its nerve supply is "denervation." Denervated muscles remains viable for 2 years following an injury but within 4 weeks will start to atrophy, and at one year will start to scar and thicken (become fibrotic). Once fibrosis starts the muscle will not recover even if the nerve is reconnected or regrows.

Different nerves carry lots of different types of signals to and from the brain. These are carried by different neurons within the larger nerve itself. Classically, the order of recovery that occurs following an injury is: sympathetic (affecting involuntary functions such as heart rate), pain, temperature, touch, proprioception (knowing where different parts of your body are), and motor (2).

Treatment and Prognosis

Like spinal cord injury, there is no perfect formula for the treatment of a peripheral nerve injury, although the disability is typically much less and the prognosis for healing much better. As stated above, when a nerve is cut, the axon buds want to regrow along the same tract. To help this process, surgeons can surgically reconnect a nerve using a technique called nerve repair. Nerve repair was pioneered by Sydney Sunderland in the 1940s and to date only about 50% of patients regain useful function even after a surgical repair of a transected (cut) nerve. Nerve repair is only possible for peripheral nerves, which, as discussed above, originate from the plexus,

---

that network where individual nerve roots connect with other nerve roots and are redirected as peripheral nerves. Nerve repair is not done for nerve roots which originate the spine.

Today nerve injuries are repaired with small sutures that connect a disrupted nerve—called an **epineural repair**. No advantage has been shown in attempting to reconnect the more microscopic aspects of the nerve (2). If the nerve ends cannot be connected (for example, in a crush injury where a significant portion of the nerve is destroyed) **grafts and conduits** that recreate the tract of the nerve and allow a correct path for nerve growth are employed. There are many different techniques for repairing a nerve and to date none have really been found to be superior to another.

If the nerve does not heal and there is significant motor weakness, a technique called a **tendon transfer** may be performed by an extremity surgeon. In a tendon transfer, muscles which are still innervated but not critical, can be transferred to critical denervated tendons restoring some function. Tendon transfers are typically only used to restore critical functions such as grip, and wrist or finger extension.

Conclusion

Nerves do have the potential to regenerate, but the process is very long as the nerve must regrow from the site of injury to its target at a rate of 1mm per day. To facilitate healing a surgeon can reconnect a severed peripheral nerve either directly or by using a nerve conduit or graft. While this helps ensure proper healing of the nerve, the recovery time is unchanged and still can take many months. The prognosis is generally good, but some patients may still be left with some disability.

Frequently Asked Questions

- **Why can nerve root repairs not be performed in or near the spine?**

As explained above, for neuron regeneration to occur the cell body must be intact. Injury or damage to the nerve root in or near the spinal cord can result in damage to the cell body making the possibility of recovery much less likely. Furthermore, the anatomy in this area is much more complex and difficult to access, so surgery to repair a nerve root potentially puts other critical structures at risk. You could end up with a worse problem than what you started with.

References

1.   Sunderland SS. The anatomy and physiology of nerve injury. Muscle Nerve. 1990 Sep;13(9):771–84.

2.   Lee SK, Wolfe SW. Peripheral Nerve Injury and Repair. J Am Acad Orthop Surg. 2000;8(4):10.

Figures:

Neuron Regeneration:

The Neuron:

Dendrites
Nucleus
Schwann cell
Synapse
Cell body
Myelin sheath
Axon
Muscle cell

Damage/ compression from disc herniation

Wallerian degeneration

Cell nucleus swells

New axon grows

Growth cone/ Axon bud

The muscle cell undergoes atrophy and fibrosis

Axon regenerates

Muscle may not return to original size

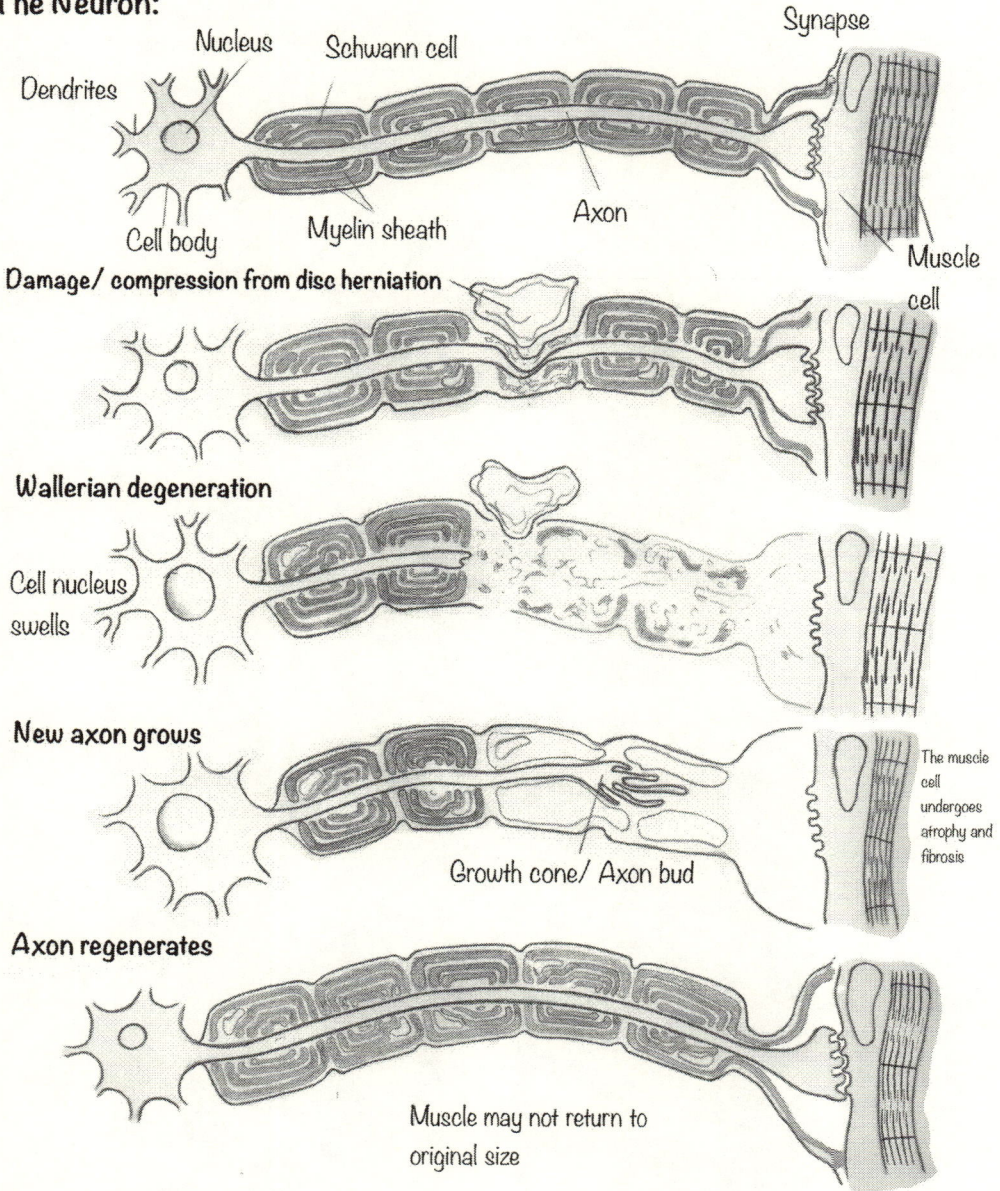

Neuron Wallerian degeneration. A normal nerve cell contains a cell body, an elongated axon covered by a myelin sheath and a synapse (top). Pressure exerted by bone spurs, or a disc can cause damage to the axon (second from top). The neuron degenerates downstream from the injury (third from top). The nerve regenerates by sprouting an axon growth bud which must find its way down the original path. If the nerve does not regenerate fast enough the muscle may atrophy (second from bottom). Myelin reconstitutes the nerve sheath (bottom).

The Brachial and Lumbar Plexuses

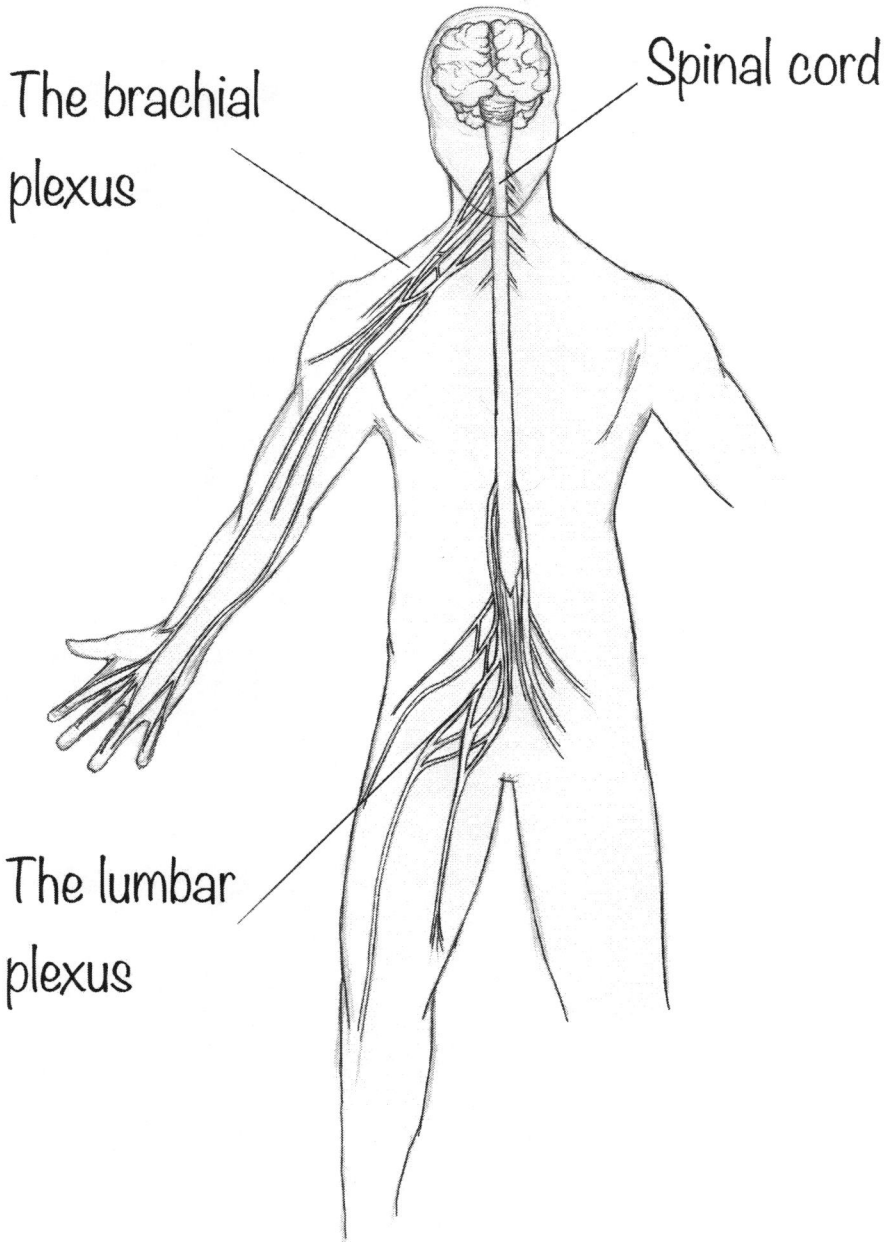

The brachial plexus

Spinal cord

The lumbar plexus

Plexuses. The lumbar and cervical plexuses that form in the upper arm coalesce from nerve roots which exit the spine and are the main neural highways that control function in the legs and arms respectively. Peripheral nerves originate from the plexuses.

The Plexus Highway

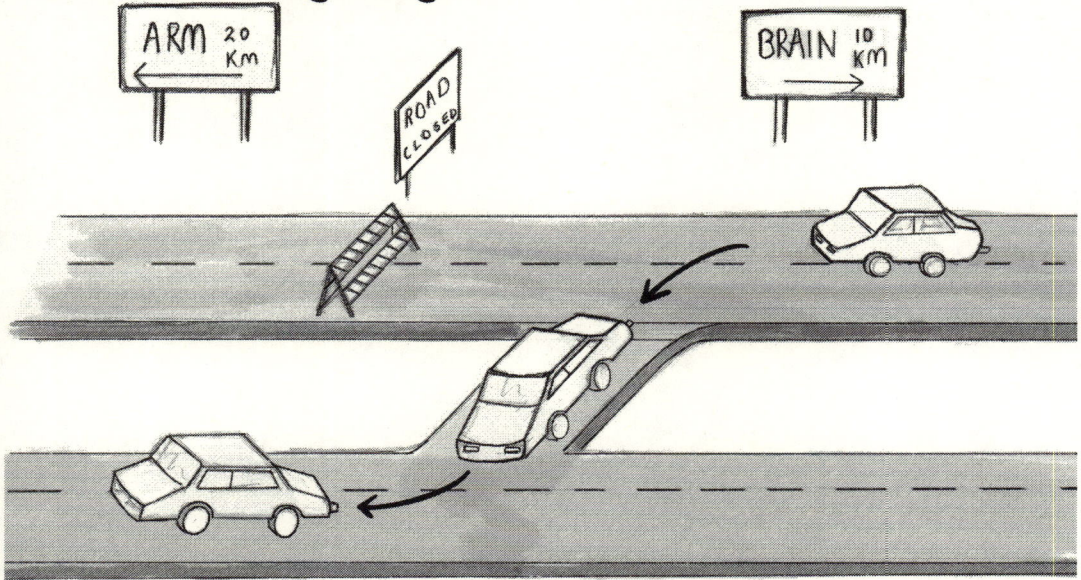

A plexus allows more than one route for a nerve to reach a destination

The Function of Plexuses. Plexuses create redundancy in the neural network allowing signals to pass through different channels if one is blocked or injured.

Chapter 18

Nerve Problems Affecting the Extremities Aka Peripheral Nerve Entrapments

Summary

This is a book about the spine and so we spend most of the time discussing nerves problems as they exist in the spine. However, nerves come off your spinal cord as nerve roots and become peripheral nerves that go to the arms and legs where they may still become pinched or irritated causing similar symptoms to spinal compression. When a peripheral nerve becomes compressed (known as entrapment) it can mimic the symptoms of spinal conditions, namely pain, numbness, and weakness. To differentiate these problems requires a detailed examination by your physician; sometimes he or she will use a test called electromyography or nerve conduction studies to help. These studies directly measure how muscles and nerves are working and can help confirm or rule out diagnoses. As a rule, spine nerve root problems will affect many different areas of your body, whereas peripheral nerve entrapments tend to be more localized.

Case

Mr. Goldenrod is an 81-year-old rancher who presents with arm pain he has been told is coming from his spine. Although he has some neck pain, most of his complaints seems to be focused in the first three fingers of the right hand and is much worse at night. In addition to the pain, he also has numbness in the same fingers. We perform a careful work up including a detailed physical exam, a cervical MRI, and a nerve conduction study. His neck MRI does show some pinched nerves and degeneration, but his nerve conduction is positive for carpal tunnel syndrome. When I examine him, I feel that most of his problems are coming from the carpal tunnel—a structure in the hand which can compress the median nerve which supplies the palm. We think it's from a lifetime of working with his hands. I explain that he has two problems. Although his neck may benefit from a procedure, surgery of the spine is much riskier than carpal tunnel surgery and I think we should try that first to see how much improvement he gets. We can do the carpal tunnel surgery and, if he is no better, pursue cervical surgery at that time. After a carpal tunnel release his symptoms are 80% improved and he does not think he needs any more treatments.

Introduction

Nerve entrapment can occur not only in the spine but also outside of the spine. When the nerve root is pinched or compressed in the spine it is called radiculopathy but when the entrapment or compression happens outside the spine it is known as **peripheral nerve entrapment.** Peripheral nerves are **the nerves which originate from the spine and travel into the extremities (arms and legs)**. Symptoms of peripheral nerve entrapment can easily mimic spinal problems. Sometimes, spinal nerve compression may even coexist with peripheral nerve compression in a condition known as double crush syndrome. This condition can be perplexing for physicians because a clear source of pain treated with decompressive surgery may not relieve symptoms if the nerve is also compressed in another remote area.

This chapter, which is divided into two sections—nerves supplying the upper extremities and nerves supplying the lower extremities—will introduce you to the various nerve problems of the extremities so that you may at least begin to understand your symptoms. The neurology of the extremities can be confusing even to those who have studied it for many years, so don't be overwhelmed.

Finally, in this chapter as you read about the various muscles of the extremities and which nerves affect them, it might be helpful to remember that when **extensor** muscles contract, they cause the body part to straighten, extend or even bend back. When **flexors** contract, that part of the body shortens, bends forward, closes.

Adductors bring that part of the body toward the center of the body. **Abductors** move the body part away from the center.

This chapter is designed as a reference that may or may not be read in its entirety. You may choose just to read about the specific nerve/syndromes you are interested in, but I also recommend reading about electromyography and nerve conduction studies, because that is a very common way for these problems to be diagnosed. Some **common terminology** I use in this chapter are the words "arm" and "Leg." **Arm = upper arm + forearm and leg = thigh + below the knee/shin/calf.**

Here is **a table of anatomic terms indicating direction** you will find helpful for this chapter:

Term	Meaning
Anterior	front (Your face is in the anterior part of your head.)
Posterior	back (Your buttocks are in the posterior part of your body.)
Lateral	To the outside of something (the shoulder is lateral to the heart)
Medial	To the inside of something (the heart is medial to the shoulder)
Proximal	closer to the body (Your elbow is proximal to your hand.)
Distal	farther from the body (Your hand is distal to your elbow.)
Superficial	closer to the surface (The skin is superficial to the bone.)
Deep	closer to the interior (The bone is deep to the skin.)
Dorsal	On the back surface (the spine is dorsal to the abdomen)
Palmar/Volar	On the front surface (the palm is palmar to the back of the hand)

Electromyography and Nerve Conduction Studies (EMG/NCS): Diagnosing Nerve Entrapments

Your nervous system is a complicated switchboard and sometimes figuring where your pain is coming from can be difficult. Nothing beats a detailed examination by an experienced physician in diagnosing problems of the nerves. However, your doctor may refer you to have an electromyogram (EMG) and nerve conduction study (NCS) to confirm a diagnosis. These tests are typically performed by a neurologist or physiatrist who has received specific training in electrophysiology.

Nerve conduction studies can be used to test the function of specific peripheral nerves, while electromyography is used to test how muscles are working. Importantly EMG/NCS may be used to rule out other serious causes of nerve dysfunction such as multiple sclerosis or myopathy (abnormal muscle weakness). In an **electromyogram** a small needle electrode is inserted into the muscle and the doctor measures muscle contractions. They can tell if there are active problems with the muscle or its nerve supply by the electrochemical signal produced by the muscle contraction. In a **nerve conduction study**, the doctor measures how fast electrical impulses travel across the nerves (nerve conduction). Nerve conduction is performed by giving you small electrical shocks that travel down the nerve and are measured with electrodes distally. Nerves that are pinched or otherwise compromised will not transmit the signal as fast which is recorded by the device. If these tests sound uncomfortable, well, to some degree they are. To use the electrical analogy, nerve conduction studies tell the doctor how well the wire (nerve) is working, and electromyography can tell if the lightbulb (muscle) is functioning.

After the test, the doctor generates a report based on the interpretation of the results. This report will usually say if any peripheral or spinal nerve entrapment is present and how severe it is. For example, a report may say you have evidence of "severe median nerve compression" or "severe carpal tunnel syndrome." EMG and NCS accuracy are totally dependent on the person who is doing the test (two doctors may get different results on the same patient). It's best to go with a doctor who is very experienced and properly trained. Also, it's important to have a physician who helps you interpret the results, as it is possible to have an EMG/NCS report that does not match your clinical examination and thus may be incorrect. Doctors who perform EMG/NCS may not even tell you what they find and leave that up to the ordering physician (they may view themselves principally as proceduralists who generate a report rather diagnosticians). The reason for this is because, the true diagnosis may be ambiguous and it's the responsibility of your main treating physician to determine how to use the report and the next treatment steps if any. The EMG/NCS report must thus be considered in the context of your clinical presentation by the ordering physician.

It's important to understand that **EMGs and NCSs are much more useful for diagnosing peripheral nerve problems than spinal problems**—in fact they can rarely diagnose spinal problems. Even if you have a serious problem in your spine, doctors will often be unable to pick it up with EMG/NCS. Conditions like lumbar or cervical stenosis rarely show up on EMG/NCS (1). Therefore, I mainly use EMG/NCS to rule out other conditions that may mimic spinal problems like carpal tunnel syndrome.

Upper Extremity Entrapment Neuropathies: Peripheral Nerve Problems That Affect the Arms, Wrists and Hands

Anatomy

The cervical nerve roots exit from the cervical spine and as they reach the shoulder, they pass between two neck muscles known as the anterior and middle scalene muscles, where they form a network called the **brachial plexus**. The brachial plexus then passes under the clavicle (collar bone) and above the first rib, crosses the chest and exits into the arm. At this location, **the brachial plexus branches into many different peripheral nerves, the five most important being the median, radial, ulnar, axillary, and musculocutaneous nerves**. Think of the course of a nerve like that of train tracks through the countryside, over hills and under tunnels. The nerves pass through muscles, and under ligaments that keep them in place but may also cause entrapment. I do my best to explain the course of each nerve below, but the three-dimensional anatomy of a nerve pathway is challenging even for surgeons. For this reason, I have also included some diagrams at the end of the chapter to help illustrate what is going on. Keep in mind that symptoms are determined by which of these nerves is irritated and where.

The nerves most affected by compression are the median, ulnar and radial nerves (in that order). While it's possible to have axillary and musculocutaneous nerve compression, they are much less common, and much harder to diagnose. The median nerve is frequently compressed because it courses under a thick ligament in the wrist called the transverse carpal ligament. More on this below.

Median Nerve Neuropathy

The median nerve is a peripheral nerve that supplies some muscles in the forearm, wrist and hand that allow you to flex or bend those body parts, for example when you want to grip an object. The median nerve also supplies sensation to most of the palm and first 4 fingers (thumb through ring finger). **The median nerve is the source of the most common peripheral nerve entrapment syndrome: carpal tunnel syndrome.**

For those interested, this paragraph gives more detail about the route of the median nerve through the arm and hand. If you are not interested, skip to the next paragraph. The median nerve originates from the brachial plexus and travels in the upper arm near the brachial artery (a major vascular supply to the arm). It then enters the forearm by going under the lacertus fibrosus (part of the biceps tendon) and between the pronator teres muscle and then travels between the flexor digitorum superficialis (FDS) and flexor digitorum profundus (FDP) muscles towards the wrist. At the wrist the median nerve crosses under the **transverse carpal ligament**, which forms the roof of the carpal tunnel. The carpal tunnel is a circular space formed by the transverse carpal ligament and the hand bones (the scaphoid and trapezium bones laterally, the pisiform and hook of hamate medially). Because this is a confined space, any thickening of tissue within the carpal tunnel can cause compression on the nerve.

There are several branches of the median nerve, supplying motor function to some forearm muscles, to the thumb, index and middle fingers and supplying sensation to the palm of the hand and several fingers. Specifically, the median nerve controls motor function to the superficial forearm muscles (pronator teres, flexor carpi radialis, and palmaris longus). The anterior interosseous nerve (AIN), the first branch of the median nerve, supplies the intermediate forearm muscles (flexor digitorum superficialis FDS, flexor digitorum profundus, flexor pollicis longus, and pronator quadratus). Near the wrist the recurrent motor branch supplies muscles of the thumb (opponens pollicis, abductor pollicis brevis, and flexor pollicis brevis and the first and second lumbricals). The palmar cutaneous branch supplies palm sensation. Finally, digital branches control sensation to the surface of the thumb, index, and middle fingers as well as the lateral half of the ring finger.

There are several constriction points where the median nerve can be compressed along its course to the hand. **High median nerve problems (compression around the elbow)** affect the finger flexor muscles of the forearm (those that let you make a grip). High median nerve issues may be caused by compression from several structures:

- **Ligament of Struthers: This is an accessory ligament present in 1% of the population that the median nerve may pass under around the elbow.**

- **Bicipital aponeurosis: This fibrous connective tissue lies between the lacertus fibrosus and the brachialis tendon (on the elbow).**

- **Between the two heads of the pronator tendon (at the elbow)**

High median nerve compression (around the elbow) may cause a deep ache in the forearm as well as weakness and numbness of the hand and forearm.

Carpal tunnel syndrome (CTS), (a low median nerve problem) results from **compression of the median nerve at the wrist** by the transverse carpal ligament. Carpal tunnel syndrome is the most common compressive neuropathy in the upper extremity, occurring in 3.72% of the population (2). CTS is a clinical diagnosis meaning there is no test with 100% accuracy, but generally is confirmed with an

EMG/NCS. People with CTS generally complain of **tingling, pain and numbness in thumb, index, long and ring fingers**. It's usually worse at night (night pain) or by bending the wrist and may be relieved by shaking the hand out. There may be weakness of the thumb in opposition (touching the base of the small finger with the thumb) and **hand clumsiness**. In severe cases there may even be wasting of the muscles (atrophy) around the thumb. Numbness may be worse when you hold your flexed wrists together (bend both wrists and put them together, hands facing down--this is known as Phalen's test). Pain may also radiate to the fingers when you tap on (Tinel's sign) or compress the wrist crease. Pain may radiate into the hand and up the forearm while numbness is generally confined to the hand

Treatment guidelines for CTS have been outlined by the American Academy of Orthopedic Surgeons (AAOS)(3). For patients with early CTS without evidence of nerve loss on EMG/NCS, a **non-surgical treatment** course such as a **steroid injection** or **splinting of the wrist** may be tried for 2-7 weeks. If treatment fails or if there is evidence of nerve /muscle loss, surgery is recommended. While surgical treatment seems superior to conservative therapy for symptom relief, there should be no rush to have the procedure done as carpal tunnel syndrome typically does not progress rapidly and may actually improve on its own (4,5).

There are **many surgical techniques** available, ranging **from open release to endoscopic release**, but **all accomplish** the same thing, which is **the release of the transverse carpal ligament,** and all have good results. Carpal tunnel release (CTR) is the most common hand surgery performed in the United States.

Open carpal tunnel release was originally performed through a large incision in the palm but has been refined such that it can now be done through a 2-3 cm incision. This is currently the gold standard treatment for CTS (4). Endoscopic CTR is a more modern alternative to the open technique and uses a small camera and an even smaller incision. This technique was developed to offer faster recovery and less operative pain. Both techniques have their benefits and risks. Open CTR is very reliable; however, it may have some scar tenderness related to the incision. Endoscopic CTR is done through a smaller incision with a potential faster recovery, but it has an increased risk of complications due to the increased difficulty of the technique.

Ulnar Nerve

The ulnar nerve is another peripheral nerve in the arm that runs around your elbow. It powers the flexor muscles of the forearm, wrist, and hand, enabling them to put force behind movements such as pinching and gripping. The ulnar nerve **also** provides **sensation to the ring and small finger.**

Like the median nerve, the ulnar nerve branches from the brachial plexus on the inside of the upper arm. It wraps around your elbow in a bony groove known as the cubital tunnel that is covered with a band known as Osborne's ligament. The cubital tunnel is a very common site of compression (this is your "funny bone") not only because the nerve is pinned against a hard surface, but also because of the motion at the elbow. The ulnar nerve then enters the forearm by passing through a muscle known as flexor carpi ulnaris (FCU). The nerve continues to run through the forearm and enters a second canal (Guyon's canal) at the wrist, which is formed by the transverse carpal ligament deep and the volar carpal ligament superficially. Guyon's canal is still another site where the ulnar nerve may be compressed, although this is much less common.

The ulnar nerve functions to provide motor strength to the forearm muscles (FCU and FDP), and hand muscles (those on the small finger side of the hand, the interossei, the 3rd and 4th lumbricals, flexor pollicis brevis, and adductor pollicis brevis). As already noted, it provides sensation to the little finger and half of the ring finger, as well as the ulnar side of the wrist proximal to the hand.

Cubital tunnel syndrome occurs from compression of the ulnar nerve at the elbow. It is the second most common upper extremity entrapment neuropathy (second to carpal tunnel) (6). Patients with cubital tunnel syndrome complain of **numbness and tingling from the elbow down to the small and ring finger** that becomes worse when the elbow is bent. Furthermore, if motor weakness is present, **your grip may become weaker,** and you may not be able to keep your small finger together with the others when you extend them. **Visible atrophy** (wasting away**) of the hand** which is usually most prominent near the thumb (1st dorsal interossei) can occur in severe cases. Cubital tunnel syndrome may easily be confused with nerve entrapment in the neck at C8/T1 as those are the nerve roots which supply the ulnar nerve and will have similar symptoms.

Like carpal tunnel syndrome, cubital tunnel syndrome is a clinical diagnosis which is typically supported by EMG/NCS. The initial **conservative management of mild cases** of cubital tunnel syndrome should consist of **a splint which pads the elbow** and prevents bending particularly at night (known as night splinting). However, in moderate to severe cases with signs of nerve loss on EMG or muscle wasting on exam, surgery should be considered to prevent ongoing nerve damage.

Cubital tunnel release is performed through a small 4 cm incision on the inside of the elbow. The surgical techniques are generally divided into two categories: in situ (on the site) decompression and decompression with transposition. **In situ decompression** means that the nerve is released without changing its position. With this approach, Osborne's ligament, the superficial fascia of the FCU muscle and the medial intermuscular septum are all opened, unroofing the cubital tunnel. In cases where the nerve is hypermobile (that is, it moves out of its groove at the elbow) a

decompression with transposition is considered. In a transposition, the nerve is surgically moved out of its groove to sit more anteriorly. Your surgeon will usually make this decision during surgery by moving the elbow in and out of flexion to see if the nerve slips out of its groove. It is hypothesized that moving the nerve out of its groove prevents recurrence of compression from ongoing traction at the elbow. Most randomized studies of compressed ulnar nerves without accompanying signs of subluxation (partial dislocation) show no difference between in situ decompression and decompression with transposition (6). Ulnar nerve transposition is a more involved operation with an associated increased complication rate and OR time, and thus is only used in cases where it is deemed necessary by your physician. Common post-op problems include loss of sensation about the incision.

Compression at Guyon's canal (at the wrist) may result in motor and/or sensory problems depending on exactly where the compression is located. Sensory loss is limited to the hand, which makes it easy to differentiate from cubital tunnel syndrome. Also motor function of the forearm muscles is preserved. This syndrome is much less common than cubital tunnel syndrome.

Radial Nerve

The radial nerve supplies some upper arm muscles and the extensor muscles of the forearm, wrist, and fingers. (The extensor muscles allow you to straighten or bend back (extend) these body parts, for example, when you put up your hand to signal someone to stop.) Injury to the radial nerve can affect your ability to use these muscles (resulting in a wrist drop) as well cause numbness in the forearm and hand.

Like both the median and ulnar nerves, the radial nerve originates from the brachial plexus. This nerve travels through the upper arm right under the triceps muscle and wraps around the humerus bone (upper arm bone). The nerve then enters the forearm through the radial tunnel, another anatomic space near the elbow where compression can occur. The nerve then splits into two major branches: the posterior interosseous nerve (PIN) and the superficial radial nerve.

The radial nerve supplies motor strength to muscles that straighten the elbow (triceps, and brachialis), **and the forearm extensor muscles that straighten the wrist and fingers** (brachioradialis, extensor carpi radialis longus, extensor digiti minimi, extensor carpi ulnaris, extensor digitorum communis, extensor carpi radialis brevis, extensor indicis, extensor pollicis brevis, extensor pollicis longus, abductor pollicis longus, and supinator). **It also provides sensation to the back of the arm, forearm, and the dorsal part of the thumb, index, long and ring fingers**.

Radial nerve injuries may be divided into "high" and "low." High injuries occur above the elbow and result in loss of sensation to the forearm and weakness of all the forearm extensor muscles that power wrist and finger extension. **Low injuries (below the elbow)** preserve forearm sensation but result in loss of sensation to the dorsum/back of the hand and only finger extension is lost. Trauma is by far the most common injury to the radial nerve; however, compressive injuries can occur.

There are **three main radial nerve compression syndromes**. In general, **physical therapy and injections are the mainstays of treatment for all three** and surgery is rarely if ever used to treat any of these:

Posterior interosseous nerve (PIN) syndrome occurs because of compression of the PIN nerve at the arcade of Frohse (a fibrous band between the two heads of the supinator muscle, located near the elbow). This results **in motor loss of thumb extension**, sometimes making it impossible for you to extend your thumb and fingers, but wrist extension and sensation will be preserved.

Radial tunnel syndrome is a controversial diagnosis, but this condition causes **pain over the lateral aspect of the forearm**, which is the thumb side of your forearm when the palm of your hand is facing forward. It is differentiated from PIN syndrome by the addition of sensory symptoms. The condition is so named because the compression occurs when the radial nerve enters the radial tunnel which is an anatomic space in the forearm composed of the extensor carpi radialis and the brachioradialis muscles laterally and the biceps and the brachialis muscles medially.

Wartenberg syndrome results from compression of the superficial radial nerve under the brachioradialis and the extensor carpi radialis longus tendons (on the lateral side of your forearm). This results in **numbness and pain over the back of the hand, thumb, index, long and ring fingers.**

Thoracic Outlet Syndrome (TOS)

Thoracic outlet syndrome (TOS) occurs when the brachial plexus itself (the network of nerves from which the peripheral nerves arise) becomes compressed in an anatomic space known as the thoracic outlet. TOS is confusing for physicians and patients alike as it can mimic both peripheral nerve entrapment and cervical spine disease. It may either be neurogenic (affecting the nerves) or vascular (affecting the blood vessels).

What and where is the thoracic outlet? The thoracic outlet is a triangular channel containing your subclavian artery/vein and the brachial plexus. The collar bone (clavicle) is the top boundary, the first rib is the bottom, and your scalene muscles are the front and back (the scalene muscles connect the cervical spine to the ribs). The nerves or blood vessels in the thoracic outlet can be compressed by both soft tissue and bone such as a cervical rib (the cervical spine usually doesn't have any ribs attached, so any cervical ribs are abnormal vestigial (useless) structures that just take up space in the thoracic outlet).

Thoracic outlet syndrome (TOS) causes variable symptoms and currently there is no gold standard way to make a diagnosis. Only after careful examination and other conditions are ruled out can your physician diagnose TOS. Overall, TOS affecting the nerves (neurogenic TOS) is much more common than TOS affecting the blood vessels (vascular TOS). **Thoracic outlet syndrome affecting the nerves presents with weakness, numbness/tingling, and pain in the upper extremity**. The pain is often vague and diffuse affecting the neck, shoulder, trapezius muscle and arm. Numbness and tingling characteristically occurs in all 5 fingers (unlike in carpal or cubital tunnel syndromes which only occurs in three). TOS can be differentiated (distinguished) from other peripheral nerve problems by a greater degree of symptoms across the arm (that is, the whole arm is numb as opposed to a discrete part).

Vascular TOS may result from compression of either the subclavian vein or the subclavian artery. Venous TOS results in obstruction of drainage in the arm causing swelling and discoloration. Arterial TOS is less common and may present with numbness and coolness of the arm.

Thoracic outlet syndrome is typically treated conservatively with physical therapy, weight loss, and injections but sometimes requires surgical decompression (1). Vascular TOS may be treated by a vascular surgeon who removes the first rib to decompress the thoracic outlet.

Is the Problem an Entrapped Peripheral Nerve or a Pinched Nerve Root in the neck:

Differentiating Upper Extremity Neuropathies from Cervical Radiculopathies

Making the diagnosis between peripheral and cervical nerve problems can be challenging as there is much functional overlap. **Cervical nerve root problems typically present with muscle weakness affecting an entire group of muscles that individually are innervated by different peripheral nerves. Also, neck pain is common.** Cervical nerve impingement will also cause pain traveling down the arm from the neck. Regardless of which nerve root is being compressed, the resulting arm pain is often similar, though the location of the pain may range from shoulder pain to forearm/hand pain (7,8). Motion of the neck may worsen the arm pain.

In peripheral nerve entrapments, the neck is unaffected and functional loss is limited to the area supplied by that nerve. Entrapment pain becomes worse with use of the arm, particularly flexion of the wrist (carpal tunnel) and elbow (cubital tunnel). There will be conduction delay on electrodiagnostic studies with entrapment of the peripheral nerves (neuropathies).

Overlap Between Nerve Root and Peripheral Nerve Symptoms	
Nerve Root	**Muscle/Peripheral Nerve**
C5	Deltoid (axillary nerve) and biceps (musculocutaneous nerve)
C6	Biceps (musculocutaneous nerve) and supinator (radial nerve)
C7	Triceps (radial nerve) and Flexor carpi radialis (median)

C8 nerve compression can easily be confused with ulnar nerve compression. However, C8 compression presents with loss of sensation in the forearm while ulnar nerve lesions do not affect sensation in the forearm (just the hand). The C8 nerve root controls most thumb function (abductor pollicis brevis, flexor pollicis brevis, and opponens pollicis—muscles whose function are controlled by the median nerve) while the ulnar nerve just controls your ability to spread your fingers (interossei muscles).

It is also possible for a nerve to be compressed both in the neck and in the periphery in a condition known as **double crush syndrome**. This is most common between carpal tunnel syndrome and compression of the C5 or C6 nerve roots. In these situations, decompression of the neck or arm alone will not produce complete relief and two surgeries may be necessary.

It's important to realize that diagnosis of these conditions requires training and experience. If you are feeling like you have a good grasp of this topic then great, but if you are feeling a little confused, rest assured you are not alone. This information is presented to help you better understand a diagnosis rather than diagnose yourself.

Lower Extremity Entrapment Neuropathies: Peripheral Nerve Problems That Affect the Legs and Feet

Anatomy

In the leg, symptoms associated with nerve damage can be traced to both lumbar spine problems and peripheral nerve problems. Once again, it's important to understand how the body is structured. Nerves to the lower extremity originate from the lumbar nerve roots starting at L2 and going to S1. These nerves form two networks on either side of the spine known as the lumbar and sacral plexuses from which nerves branch out and travel down the leg. There is overlap between the lumbar and sacral plexuses, and these definitions are just used to help name the nerve roots.

The major nerves which travel down the leg are the femoral nerve, obturator nerve, lateral femoral cutaneous nerve, the superior and inferior gluteal nerves, and the peroneal nerve and tibial nerve (the peroneal and the tibial nerves are branches of the sciatic nerve). It's possible for problems to arise from any of these nerves.

Femoral Nerve

The femoral nerve is formed in the lumbar plexus (the neural network formed by nerve roots exiting the lumbar spine), located within the psoas, the large muscle adjacent to the spine. The nerve joins up with the femoral artery and vein and enters the thigh under the inguinal ligament (a common site for hernias). This nerve then branches into an anterior branch that supplies the anterior thigh and a posterior branch which travels down the side of the leg to become the saphenous nerve in the calf.

The **femoral nerve is a mixed motor and sensory nerve. It gives motor strength to the quadriceps muscles** (rectus femoris, vastus medialis, vastus lateralis, and vastus intermedius) **and 2 of the hip flexors** (sartorius and pectineus). The saphenous nerve is a sensory nerve supplying the medial (inside) aspect of the leg.

Femoral neuropathy may cause weakness on one side of the quadriceps muscles making it difficult to straighten the knee or cause it to buckle with loading. This may make it particularly difficult to walk up and down stairs. **Numbness** can occur in the anterior thigh and medial leg (supplied by the saphenous nerve). Lumbar neuropathy can be differentiated from femoral neuropathy because L2-4 nerve root impingement will also affect hip and ankle motion while femoral neuropathy will not.

Femoral nerve injury can most commonly occur during surgery (such as undergoing an anterior hip replacement procedure, which requires being in a flexed position for longer than the nerve can sometimes tolerate or during a lateral lumbar fusion where retractors are placed inside the psoas muscle near the femoral nerve). In almost all cases non-operative management with **physical therapy** is used to treat femoral neuropathy (9).

The **saphenous nerve** that is responsible only for sensation of the medial leg may be compressed as it exits the thigh through a small fascial opening. Braces or other prolonged tight-fitting clothes at the knee may also cause compression. Saphenous neuropathy typically presents with pain and numbness on the inside of the leg.

Saphenous neuropathy will not show on nerve conduction studies. **Treatment is** again **conservative** with removal of offending compressive structures such as braces or tight-fitting clothes.

Obturator Nerve

Like the femoral nerve, the **obturator nerve** is formed in the lumbar plexus in the psoas muscle but, instead of exiting laterally, it exits medially, supplying the middle compartment of the thigh. It provides motor power to the medial adductor compartment of the thigh (adductor longus and brevis, obturator externus and a portion of adductor magnus) as well as sensation to the inside of the thigh. The adductors are the muscles on the inner thigh that bring your legs toward the center of your body (when you squeeze your thighs together, that is the adductor muscles working).

Obturator neuropathy is rare, and notoriously difficult to diagnose, but **can cause thigh and groin pain**. It is also possible to experience **weakness** in muscles **of adduction**. Like femoral neuropathy, isolated injury to this nerve that supplies the adductors is rare outside of direct trauma which can occur in pelvic surgery or total hip replacement. It may also be caused by lithotomy positioning such as used during labor. **Treatment** of obturator neuropathy is generally non-operative with **physical therapy** and **nonsteroidal anti-inflammatories**. In cases where there is no improvement surgical exploration and decompression may be considered (10).

Lateral Femoral Cutaneous Nerve (LCFN)

The **lateral femoral cutaneous nerve (LCFN)** exits the lumbar plexus lateral to the psoas muscle and courses around the internal aspect of the pelvis to exit between the pelvis and the inguinal ligament (located in the crease where the abdomen meets the thighs). **It is a pure sensory nerve to the lateral thigh meaning it does not control any muscles**. Lateral femoral cutaneous neuropathy may also be referred to by a Greek term: *Meralgia paraesthetica*. Symptoms include **numbness** and **tingling in the lateral thigh** and is typically made worse from standing when the nerve stretches from hip extension (moving your thigh backwards). The LCFN is vulnerable to compression at the inguinal ligament caused by external pressure (for example, having a belt that's too tight or heavy (like a policeman's utility belt), obesity, pregnancy, pressure from external padding during surgery, trauma, or tumors). It may also be caused by surgical procedures, such as those which require prone positioning (lying on your belly) or even in anterior iliac crest bone graft harvests where this nerve is vulnerable to damage.

Lateral femoral cutaneous neuropathy may be easily confused with L2-3 nerve root compression as both produce anterior thigh pain and numbness. However, the lateral femoral cutaneous nerve is purely sensory and will not disturb motor function, unlike lumbar radiculopathy, which will affect hip flexor strength.

LCFN neuropathy will usually **improve with conservative measures** such as **removal of the compressive structure** such as finding a better belt or not using one, and **weight loss**. **Steroid injections** may also help decrease inflammation. Surgery to treat generally consists of release or transection, but it is controversial as to whether this is helpful or not (11).

Superior and Inferior Gluteal Nerves

Both the superior and inferior gluteal nerves exit the pelvis from the sciatic notch, which is located on the ilium, one of the bones that make up the pelvis. These nerves power hip abduction— moving the hips away from the center of the body (gluteus minimus and medius) and hip extension—as when you are straightening a leg in the process of walking (gluteus maximus). Injury to one of these nerves results in an inability to keep the pelvis level during normal walking (called a Trendelenburg gait). It is rare for either to be injured without medical cause (iatrogenic cause), for example, during a total hip replacement or from a misplaced injection. Treatment is physical therapy and supportive care.

Sciatic Nerve

The **sciatic nerve** is a large nerve which exits the pelvis through a bony arch known as the greater sciatic notch. The piriformis muscle also exits the pelvis through the greater sciatic notch to attach to the top of the hip bone. The sciatic nerve typically exits below the piriformis but may also travel through or above this muscle. It then passes down the posterior thigh between the hamstring muscles. It consists of two discrete divisions (the peroneal and tibial). The peroneal division is more vulnerable to injury as it is tethered in two places (in the pelvis and at the knee). The short head of the biceps is the only hamstring muscle that is not innervated by the tibial division of the sciatic nerve. So, if this hamstring muscle is exhibiting nerve damage symptoms, then it is likely from a lesion affecting the peroneal, not the tibial division of the sciatic nerve.

The **sciatic nerve supplies all the muscles in the posterior thigh and calf** (including the hamstrings and plantar flexors of the foot and ankle). **It provides sensation in the calf and foot** but not the thigh (which is provided by the posterior femoral cutaneous nerve).

Sciatica is a term commonly thrown around by patients and doctors alike. But what does it mean? While precise definitions vary, **sciatica** can be summarized as **pain that radiates from the buttocks down the leg along the course of the sciatic nerve** (12). Compression of any part of this nerve may result in sciatica with the most common cause being irritation of the lumbar nerve roots L4-S1 in the spine.

Sciatic nerve damage results in **weakness of muscles and numbness** depending on where the lesion is located. Weakness can affect the hip, calf, and foot. The closer the damage is to the pelvis the more severe the injury will be. Trauma, such as a hip dislocation or a pelvic fracture, is the most common cause of injury. This nerve may also be compressed by the piriformis muscle in the pelvis, known as piriformis syndrome. Even carrying a large wallet in your back pocket may result in sciatica. An EMG and nerve conduction study may be useful in localizing the lesion.

piriformis syndrome: This is a cause of sciatica not related to the spine. What causes the problem is not well understood but may be related to previous gluteal trauma, or to scarring around the piriformis muscle. It may also be related to an abnormal course of the sciatic nerve around the piriformis. It commonly presents with **sciatica** and **buttock pain that is made worse with sitting**. This may be tested for by checking for pain while performing a resisted hip abduction (pushing, against pressure, to move the hip away from center) and external hip rotations (rotating the hip away from the center of your body) (two functions of the piriformis muscle). Nonetheless, piriformis syndrome is a very difficult diagnosis to make (13).   Piriformis syndrome usually responds to conservative treatment like **physical therapy** and **non-steroidal anti-inflammatories**. Injections of the piriformis muscle with **corticosteroids or Botox** may also be tried. In cases that fail to improve with these measures, surgical release may be considered but there is limited scientific evidence that it is superior to non-operative treatment.

peroneal neuropathy: The peroneal nerve branches from the sciatic nerve around the knee and wraps around the top of the fibula (the small bone on the outside of the calf), where it can be compressed. Because of this unique anatomy, peroneal neuropathy is the most common isolated neuropathy in the lower extremity. **The peroneal nerve** then travels down the leg into the foot. This nerve **provides motor power to a hamstring muscle in the thigh** (biceps femoris), **and to foot dorsiflexors**—which allow you to point your toes to your nose (the peroneal muscles, tibialis anterior, extensor hallucis longus and several other small muscles in the foot). The peroneal nerve provides sensation to the lateral leg and the first web space on the foot.

Peroneal nerve injury presents with a **foot drop** (that is, you cannot dorsiflex your ankle—you cannot lift the front part of your foot off the gas pedal). You may experience your foot slapping the floor with every step because you cannot elevate your ankle. This is very similar to what you might experience if you have compression of the L4 or L5 nerve roots in the spine. **Numbness of the top of the foot** also occurs. However, if the lumbar spine nerve roots are involved, foot plantar flexor and hip abductor muscles will likely also be affected, which are spared in peroneal neuropathy.

Peroneal neuropathy is more common than the other lower extremity neuropathies because this nerve is vulnerable as it wraps around the hard bone of the fibula (the bone on the outside of the lower leg). The nerve is close to the skin here and may be compressed from kneeling for extended periods or from knee-high braces or casts. Because the nerve is close to the skin, nerve conduction studies are particularly useful in helping to differentiate perineal neuropathy from lumbar radiculopathy.

Even partial or complete foot drops may resolve overtime, and so **initial treatment** is generally **conservative with physical therapy and discontinuing compressive clothing or braces**. Foot drop may be managed with **an ankle foot orthosis**—a brace to help keep your foot from slapping the ground when you walk. Surgery is considered in severe cases with foot drop especially if there is an internal cause to the compression of the nerve (such as a tumor or an expanding cyst pinching the nerve). If no obvious internal cause is found (such cases are called idiopathic) a trial of 3 months of non-operative treatment should be performed before surgical decompression. Decompression is accomplished by releasing any tight or compressive tissue about the nerve as it courses around the fibula (14).

tibial neuropathy: The **tibial nerve is a branch of the sciatic nerve** and travels down the thigh and in the posterior part of the calf. It then wraps around the medial ankle and travels across the bottom of the foot. **It supplies motor strength to muscles in the posterior thigh** (adductor magnus, all hamstring muscles—biceps femoris, semimembranosus, semitendinosus), **all muscles of the posterior calf** (including the gastrocnemius and the soleus) as well as all the **plantar flexors of the foot**. **Sensation to the bottom of your** foot is also provided by the tibial nerve.

Patients typically present with **weakness of plantar flexion of the ankle and toes** (the muscles you use to press the gas pedal of your car). Sensation In the posterior calf is provided by the **sural nerve** which has dual innervation from both the tibial and the peroneal nerve. Thus, **numbness** may be sporadic in tibial neuropathy. Tibial neuropathy is very rare; this nerve is only injured in specific situations such as compression from a tumor around the knee or from compression at the tarsal tunnel in the ankle (tarsal tunnel syndrome). **Treatment** for these conditions include **physical therapy, braces, and non-steroidal anti-inflammatories** (15).

Is the Problem an Entrapped Peripheral Nerve or a Pinched Nerve Root in the Low Back: Differentiating Lower Extremity Neuropathies from Lumbar Radiculopathies

Just like in the upper extremity, nerve problems of the lower extremity are often confused with spine problems. It's up to your doctor to make the diagnosis, but there are some tips which you can try on yourself. If you think your problem is coming from the spine, you should look out for symptoms of back pain and pain shooting down the leg (commonly known as sciatica). Pain caused by lumbar nerve root compression usually radiates to the buttock, back of the thigh and back of the calf (16). The pain is typically worse with extension (straightening) of the leg and flexion (bending) of the hip. Also, if you notice more than one muscle group is causing problems such as both hip and foot weakness, this is most likely a spinal and not peripheral nerve problem (17). If your pain gets worse with sitting and you have tenderness over your buttock you may have piriformis syndrome but this diagnosis should only be considered if your lumbar spine is normal (18).

Conclusion

Peripheral nerve entrapments are commonly confused with spine problems and vice versa. Electrical tests of the nerve and muscle known as nerve conduction studies (NCS) and electromyography (EMG), respectively, can help rule out certain but not all peripheral nerve entrapments, and thus may be commonly used to help make a diagnosis. While these tests can diagnose peripheral nerve problems, they are rarely useful for spinal problems. Most peripheral nerve entrapments can be treated conservatively; however, if symptoms persist surgery may be an option. It is possible to have compression of a nerve both in the spine and outside of the spine in a condition known as double crush syndrome. In such cases surgical release of both areas may be-required to experience meaningful symptom improvement.

Frequently Asked Questions

- **Is it still worth getting a carpal tunnel release if my electrodiagnostic test says, "severe carpal tunnel syndrome?" Will the nerve regenerate?**

     Studies have shown that there is no real correlation between the severity of electrodiagnostic carpal tunnel syndrome and improvement after surgery. So even with severe carpal tunnel syndrome it is possible to get improvement (19). Your nerve will regenerate to a certain degree if it and the muscle it supplies have not become fibrosed (scarred).

- **How soon should I start to experience relief of my symptoms after carpal tunnel release?**

    Typically, after 1-2 weeks.

References

1.   Kuhn JE, Lebus V GF, Bible JE. Thoracic outlet syndrome. J Am Acad Orthop Surg. 2015 Apr;23(4):222–32.

2.   Papanicolaou GD, McCabe SJ, Firrell J. The prevalence and characteristics of nerve compression symptoms in the general population. J Hand Surg. 2001 May;26(3):460–6.

3.   Keith MW, Masear V, Amadio PC, Andary M, Barth RW, Graham B, et al. Treatment of carpal tunnel syndrome. J Am Acad Orthop Surg. 2009 Jun;17(6):397–405.

4.   Verdugo RJ, Salinas RA, Castillo JL, Cea JG. Surgical versus non-surgical treatment for carpal tunnel syndrome. Cochrane Database Syst Rev. 2008 Oct 8;(4):CD001552.

5.   Padua L, Padua R, Aprile I, Pasqualetti P, Tonali P, Italian CTS Study Group. Carpal tunnel syndrome. Multiperspective follow-up of untreated carpal tunnel syndrome: a multicenter study. Neurology. 2001 Jun 12;56(11):1459–66.

6.   Staples JR, Calfee R. Cubital Tunnel Syndrome: Current Concepts. J Am Acad Orthop Surg. 2017 Oct;25(10):e215–24.

7.   Rainville J, Joyce AA, Laxer E, Pena E, Kim D, Milam RA, et al. Comparison of Symptoms From C6 and C7 Radiculopathy: SPINE. 2017 Oct;42(20):1545–51.

8.   McAnany SJ, Rhee JM, Baird EO, Shi W, Konopka J, Neustein TM, et al. Observed patterns of cervical radiculopathy: how often do they differ from a standard, "Netter diagram" distribution? Spine J. 2019 Jul;19(7):1137–42.

9.   Fox AJS, Bedi A, Wanivenhaus F, Sculco TP, Fox JS. Femoral neuropathy following total hip arthroplasty: review and management guidelines. Acta Orthop Belg. 2012 Apr;78(2):145–51.

10.   Tipton JS. Obturator neuropathy. Curr Rev Musculoskelet Med. 2008 Dec;1(3–4):234–7.

11.   Grossman MG, Ducey SA, Nadler SS, Levy AS. Meralgia paresthetica: diagnosis and treatment. J Am Acad Orthop Surg. 2001 Oct;9(5):336–44.

12.   Ropper AH, Zafonte RD. Sciatica. Longo DL, editor. N Engl J Med. 2015 Mar 26;372(13):1240–8.

13.   Cass SP. Piriformis Syndrome: A Cause of Nondiscogenic Sciatica. Curr Sports

Med Rep. 2015 Jan;14(1):41–4.

14.   Poage C, Roth C, Scott B. Peroneal Nerve Palsy: Evaluation and Management. J Am Acad Orthop Surg. 2016 Jan;24(1):1–10.

15.   Lareau CR, Sawyer GA, Wang JH, DiGiovanni CW. Plantar and Medial Heel Pain: Diagnosis and Management. J Am Acad Orthop Surg. 2014 Jun;22(6):372–80.

16.   Furman MB, Johnson SC. Induced lumbosacral radicular symptom referral patterns: A descriptive study. Spine J [Internet]. 2018 May [cited 2018 Jun 3]; Available from: http://linkinghub.elsevier.com/retrieve/pii/S1529943018302547

17.   Jeon CH, Chung NS, Lee YS, Son KH, Kim JH. Assessment of Hip Abductor Power in Patients With Foot Drop: A Simple and Useful Test to Differentiate Lumbar Radiculopathy and Peroneal Neuropathy. Spine. 2013 Feb;38(3):257–63.

18.   Hopayian K, Song F, Riera R, Sambandan S. The clinical features of the piriformis syndrome: a systematic review. Eur Spine J. 2010 Dec;19(12):2095–109.

19.   Rivlin M, Kachooei AR, Wang ML, Ilyas AM. Electrodiagnostic Grade and Carpal Tunnel Release Outcomes: A Prospective Analysis. J Hand Surg. 2018 May;43(5):425–31.

Figures:

The Median Nerve:

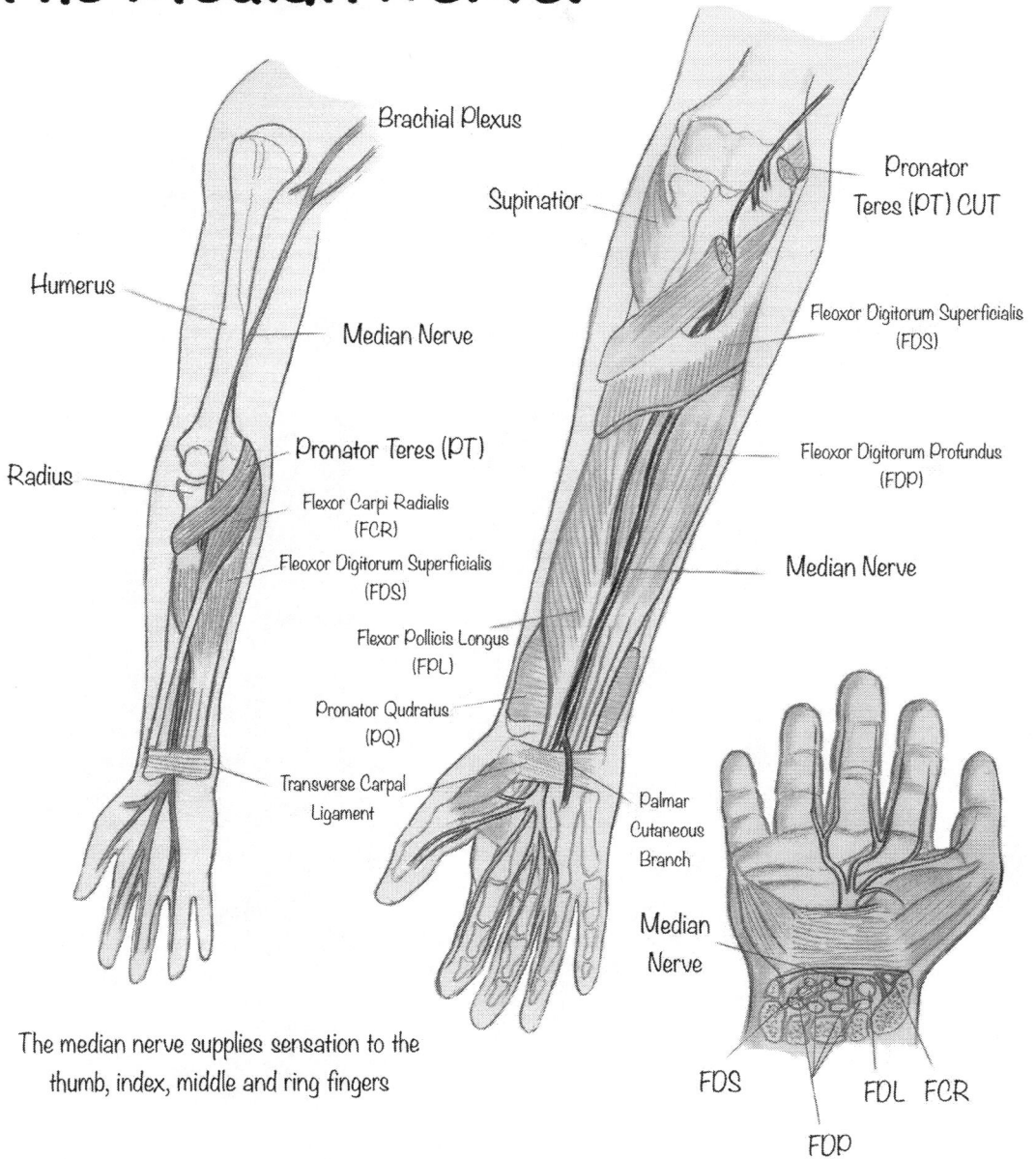

Brachial Plexus

Supinatior

Pronator Teres (PT) CUT

Humerus

Median Nerve

Fleoxor Digitorum Superficialis (FDS)

Radius

Pronator Teres (PT)

Flexor Carpi Radialis (FCR)

Fleoxor Digitorum Superficialis (FDS)

Fleoxor Digitorum Profundus (FDP)

Median Nerve

Flexor Pollicis Longus (FPL)

Pronator Qudratus (PQ)

Transverse Carpal Ligament

Palmar Cutaneous Branch

Median Nerve

The median nerve supplies sensation to the thumb, index, middle and ring fingers

FDS

FDL FCR

FDP

The median nerve. The median nerve originates from the medial and lateral cords of the brachial plexus and courses through the upper arm and forearm (left two images). The median nerve travels under the transverse carpal ligament in the carpal tunnel to supply the thumb, index, middle and ring fingers (bottom right).

The Ulnar Nerve

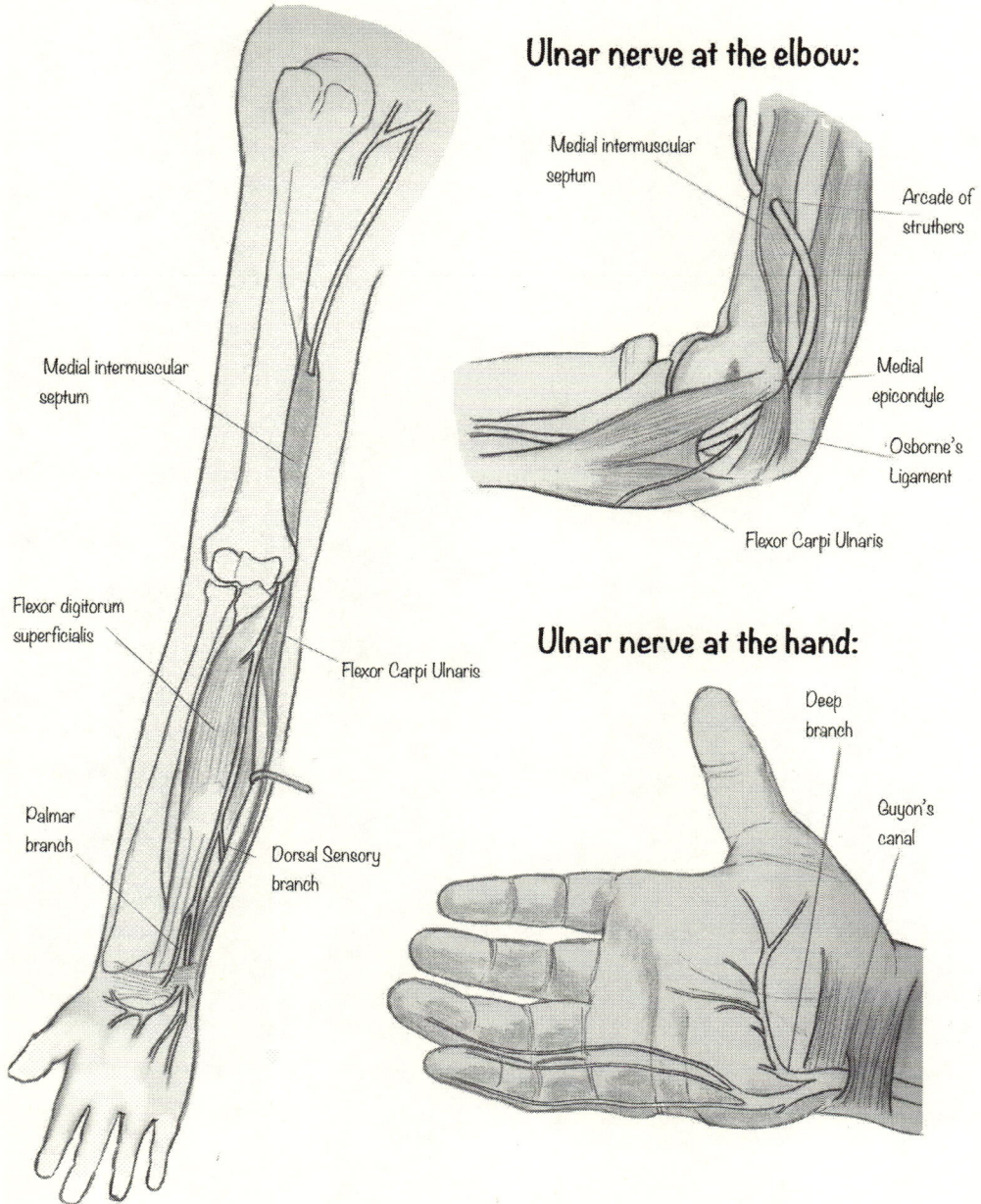

Medial intermuscular
septum

Flexor digitorum
superficialis

Flexor Carpi Ulnaris

Palmar
branch

Dorsal Sensory
branch

Ulnar nerve at the elbow:

Medial intermuscular
septum

Arcade of
struthers

Medial
epicondyle

Osborne's
Ligament

Flexor Carpi Ulnaris

Ulnar nerve at the hand:

Deep
branch

Guyon's
canal

Ulnar nerve. The ulnar nerve originates from the posterior cord of the brachial plexus and travels through the arm and forearm (left). A common site of entrapment is around the elbow under Osborne's ligament (top right). The ulnar nerve enters the hand through Guyon's canal to supply the small and ring fingers (bottom right).

The Radial Nerve

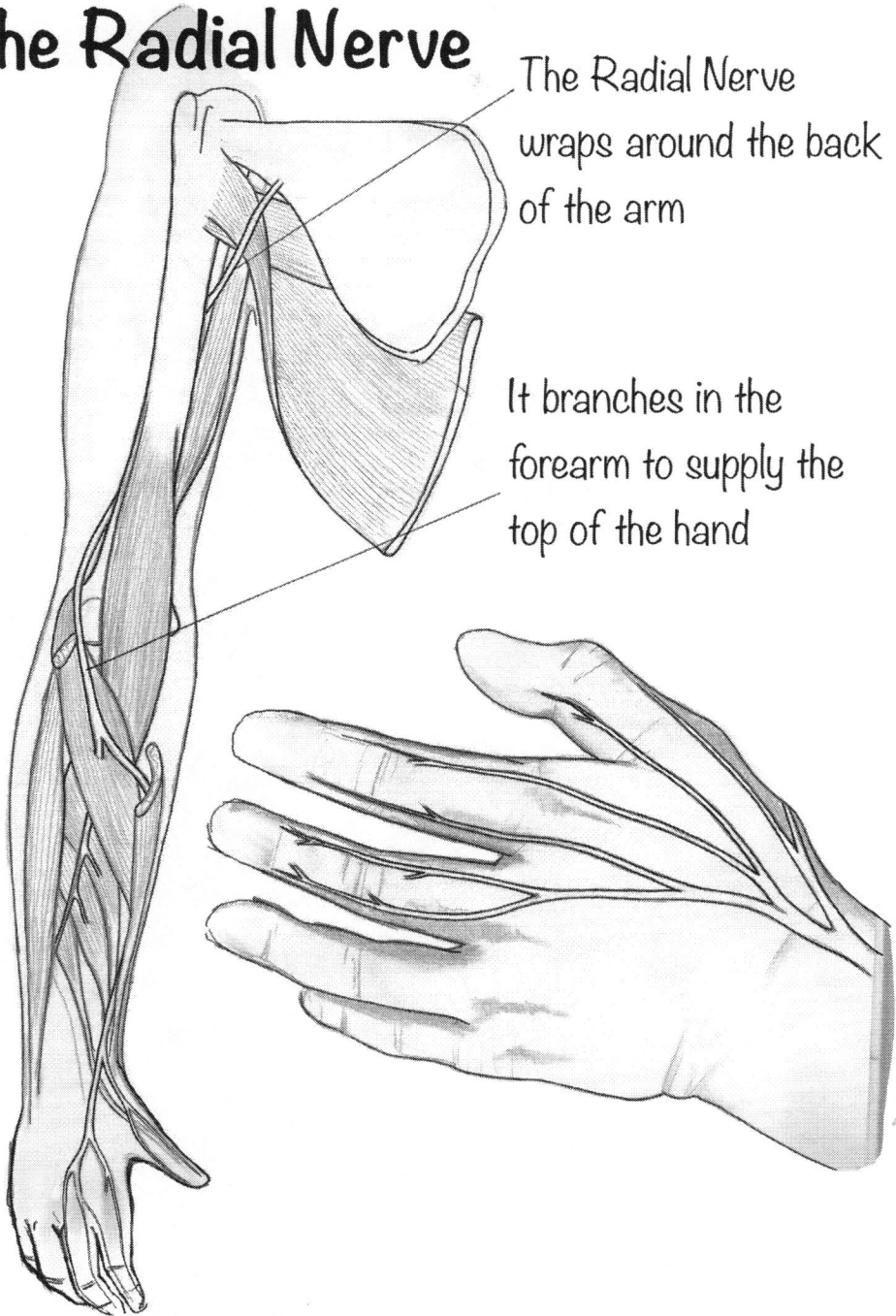

The Radial Nerve wraps around the back of the arm

It branches in the forearm to supply the top of the hand

The radial nerve. The radial nerve originates from the posterior cord of the brachial plexus and travels in the posterior compartment of the arm supplying the triceps muscle and the extensors of the forearm.

The Thoracic Outlet

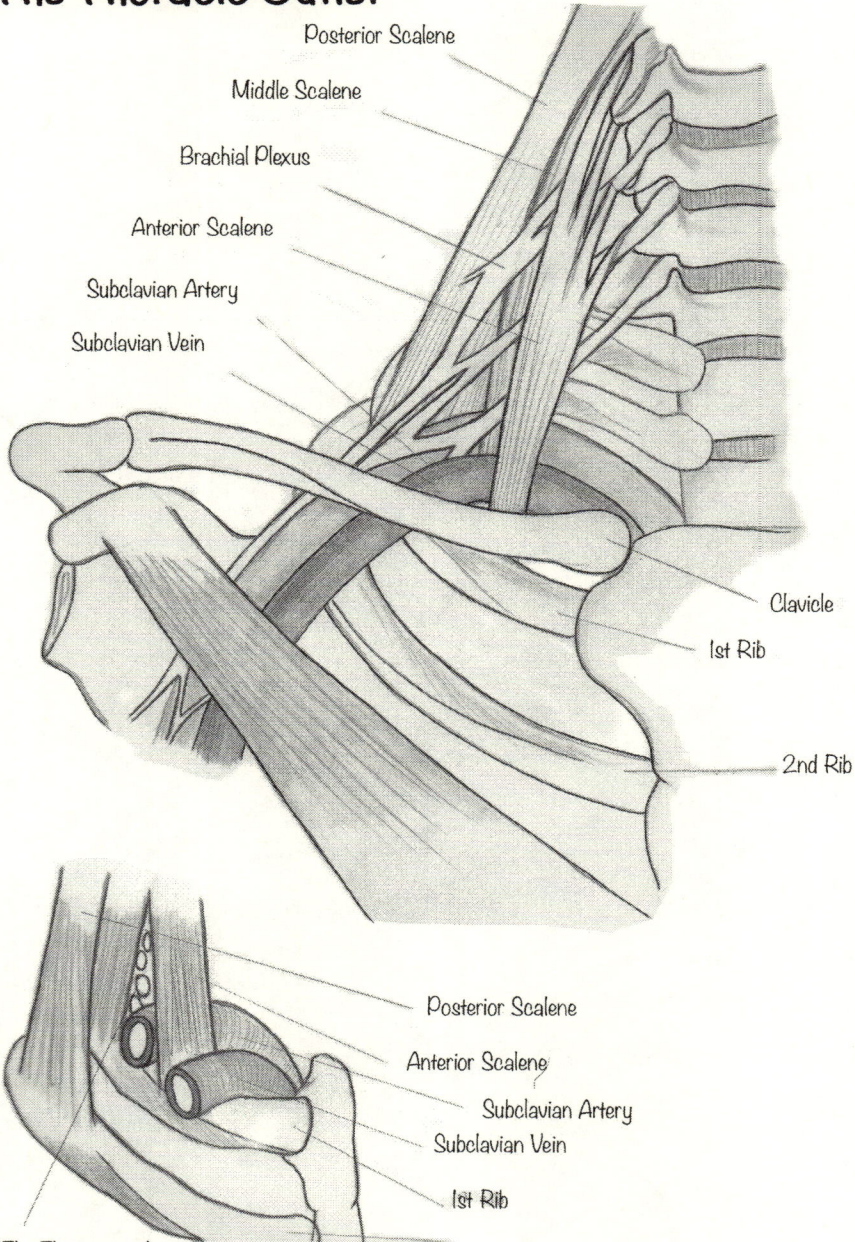

Posterior Scalene

Middle Scalene

Brachial Plexus

Anterior Scalene

Subclavian Artery

Subclavian Vein

Clavicle

1st Rib

2nd Rib

Posterior Scalene

Anterior Scalene

Subclavian Artery

Subclavian Vein

1st Rib

The Thoracic outlet
Containing the brachial plexus

Thoracic outlet. The thoracic outlet as viewed from the front (top).
The thoracic outlet is an anatomic space that is formed between
the scalene muscles, the clavicle and the first rib through which the
brachial plexus nerves travel (bottom).

Good Spine Habits and Treating Your Spine Without Surgery

"In the first 30 years of your life you make your habits. For the last 30 years of your life, your habits make you"
-Steve Jobs

Chapter 19

Medical Treatments for Back Pain

Summary

There is a broad array of so called "non-operative" treatments for spine pain. This can range from simple things such as heat and ice, to more invasive (entering through the skin) procedures like epidurals and radiofrequency ablation. Many different medications also exist to treat pain and while they can be very helpful, it's important to understand that they all have side effects. Non-steroidal anti-inflammatory drugs (NSAIDs) and oral steroids are the mainstay of treatments for spine-related pain and are useful in short courses. Other medicines such as anticonvulsants, and antidepressants may be used in conjunction with anti-inflammatories. If basic medications fail to control your pain, you may try an epidural injection or other invasive forms of pain control. Although it sounds counterintuitive, exercise and stretching play a critical role in maintaining your spine but this is a large topic and so its discussed in chapters 21 and 22.

Case

Mr. Khaki is a 46-year-old schoolteacher who one day, while playing handball, suddenly develops back pain and radiating pain down his leg (sciatica). The pain is severe enough that he must take off work and constantly take Tylenol extra strength but with little improvement. He comes in to see me and I suspect he is suffering from a lumbar disc herniation. I explain that disc herniations are very inflammatory and so powerful anti-inflammatory medications such as steroids are needed to resolve the problem. I prescribe him a Medrol Dosepak, a scheduled taper of a drug called methylprednisolone, which is an oral steroid medication that you take for about a week gradually decreasing the dose each day. Immediately after taking the medicine his pain is improved, although the medication makes him feel "anxious." We prescribe him physical therapy and in 4 weeks he is back to normal.

Introduction

When spine surgeons say "conservative care" in most cases they are referring to treating a problem without surgery. Spine surgery should be the last available option to treat a problem. In general, you should have your condition evaluated by a doctor who specializes in spine care (typically either a neurologist, physiatrist, or a spine surgeon) and a conservative approach should be attempted for at least 6-8 weeks at a minimum if there is no urgent reason to head to surgery. It is also perfectly acceptable for your primary care doctor to initiate some simple treatments currently while you wait to see a specialist. If you are being told you need back surgery for a pain or ache that is relatively acute, that is, severe and sudden in onset, you need to think twice. **Most strains and aches in the back and even nerve pain/ radiculopathies caused by disc herniations will resolve within this 6–8-week period with nothing more than supportive care.** Thus, a trial of conservative care is often necessary rather than jumping straight to surgery. Conservative or non-operative treatment is best accomplished if guided by a professional who can look out for signs that your condition is worsening.

Ice/Heat Therapy

Ice and heat are simple, relatively safe therapies which I use in my practice and on myself all the time. For the treatment of muscular pain and ligamentous strains both are anecdotally effective (individual reports of success as opposed to reports of success based on scientific studies). Ice works by decreasing inflammation in an inflamed area and thus may be more useful for acute injuries. Heat may be applied by an electric heating blanket or pad or a hot water bottle. Ice may be applied in the form of a gel ice pack or a circulating ice machine such as Game Ready®. To avoid burns or irritation when using either hot or cold, care should be taken to ensure there is no prolonged contact with exposed skin (so nothing longer than 10-30 min). I have seen many patients come in with burns from a heating pad because they fell asleep on it. In one large study heat was found to produce better short-term pain relief than an oral placebo. There is no significant evidence available to compare the effectiveness of hot versus cold therapy (1).

I recommend ice therapy for acute low back pain and neck pain. I typically recommend a flexible gel ice pack (such as a Flexikold pack®). These are useful because they contour to the shape of your neck and can easily be acquired online or from the drug store. One of these should be applied to the area of muscular pain for 10 minutes in the morning and 10 minutes in the evening. Again, make sure to avoid direct contact with heat or cold to the skin by placing a towel or pillowcase in between the source and your skin.

Prostaglandins and Pain—How Non-Steroidal Anti-Inflammatory Drug (NSAID) Therapy Works

Non-steroidal Anti-inflammatory drugs (NSAIDs) represent a large pharmaceutical class of drugs as there are almost 20 different varieties. The most well-known members of this family are aspirin, acetaminophen (Tylenol®) and ibuprofen (Advil® or Motrin®). **NSAIDs may be used sparingly to treat the symptoms of pain, inflammation, and fever**. Because they are frequently prescribed, let's try to understand how NSAIDS work, both how they stop pain and how they can cause side effects.

NSAIDs work by blocking an enzyme in your body called cyclooxygenase (COX), which is responsible for producing prostaglandins. The **COX enzyme** is present in almost all tissues of the body and has many functions. COX is responsible for converting arachidonic acid into prostaglandins, which are chemically responsible for the sensation of pain. There are two main forms of this enzyme, called COX-1 and COX-2, and they each have different functions in the body. COX-1 is a so-called "housekeeping" enzyme which has broad roles in the stomach (making a protective gastric mucus), kidneys, and vascular system. COX-2 is more exclusively involved in inflammation and, thus, plays a major role in pain.

To understand how NSAIDs treat inflammation, we should briefly discuss the chemistry of arachidonic acid—the chemical source of the pain-causing inflammatory molecules called prostaglandins. First, phospholipids (which are fatty molecules that are part of the cell membrane) are broken down into arachidonic acid by an enzyme called phospholipase A2 (this enzyme is inhibited by corticosteroids). Arachidonic acid is an essential fatty acid which is further broken down as described above by either COX-1 or COX-2. (Remember that the COX enzyme is inhibited by NSAIDs.) When you have a problem in your spine such as arthritis or a tear of a ligament, prostaglandins are activated. This is your body's way of trying to resolve the problem because prostaglandins activate the inflammatory response—the first step in the body's healing efforts.

But what exactly is **inflammation**? When prostaglandins are released, they tell your body to increase blood flow to the area (which results in swelling, warmth, and redness, which are themselves painful). This brings inflammatory cells to the area to try and repair any damage. However, prostaglandins that are released also directly irritate your nerves/spinal cord to induce the sensation of pain (2). This is to alert you—there is something wrong—and pain is your body's way of trying to tell you that. There are people who are born without the ability to sense pain, and this is very detrimental. They cannot sense when they are doing damage to the body and thus do things like keep their hands on a burning stove...not good.

The Different NSAIDs

There are several divisions or classes of NSAID drugs. They may be classified into short-acting NSAIDs (less than 6 hours) including ibuprofen, diclofenac, and indomethacin. Long acting NSAIDs (greater than 6 hours) include celecoxib, meloxicam, nabumetone and naproxen. NSAIDs may also be classified into nonselective COX inhibitors (that is, they affect both COX-1 and -2) and selective COX-2 inhibitors (select to affect only COX-2 inhibitors).

COX-2 inhibitors received a lot of attention in the 1990s because of a recall of a popular COX-2 inhibitor Vioxx® (rofecoxib) after it was found to cause heart conditions (like heart attack). Now **Celebrex®** is the only COX-2 inhibitor on the market.

Tylenol is a little different from the rest of the NSAIDS in that it does not typically reduce inflammation. Instead, it is thought to exert its effects by reducing COX/prostaglandin-signaling directly in the brain and spinal cord. As such it does not have the same side effect profile as the remainder of the NSAIDs in that it does not cause gastric (stomach) bleeding or affect blood clotting. Tylenol is metabolized (processed) in the liver, however, and high amounts can result in liver damage.

NSAIDs are useful drugs for the short-term treatment of back pain (3,4). However, there is only sparse evidence they offer significant long-term effect over placebo (5). For patients who have contraindications to NSAIDs, **acetaminophen has the lowest side effect profile (4)**.

The Negative Side of NSAIDs

NSAIDs have several adverse effects. These effects seem tied to not only the dose of the drug, but also the duration of therapy. For example, it has long been held that the longer you take NSAIDs, the greater the risk of GI perforation (tears or cuts in the digestive tract), bleeding and ulceration (6). Your doctor may prescribe a proton pump inhibitor such as omeprazole to help reduce the risk of this. While using an NSAID, any stomach pain should be taken very seriously, and close attention should be kept for signs of bleeding (such as abnormally dark stools or vomiting blood). Recently it has been refuted that NSAIDs play a significant role in GI bleeding, introducing some doubt in this long-held assumption, but care should still be taken (7)

Common Non-selective NSAIDs			
Drug name	**Oral dose**	**Maximum daily dose**	**Characteristics**
Acetaminophen (Tylenol®)	325-650mg every 4-6 hours or 1000mg every 6 hours	3000mg	Does not inhibit platelet function (Platelets help stop bleeding.) Risk for liver toxicity
Diclofenac (Cambia®)	50mg every 8 hours	150mg	Short acting
Ibuprofen (Advil®)	400mg every 4-6 hours	3200 (acute), 2400 (chronic)	Short acting
Meloxicam (Mobic®)	7.5-15mg daily	15mg	Long acting Relatively selective for COX-2 and does not inhibit platelet function
Naproxen (Aleve®)	250mg-500mg every 12 hours	1250mg (acute), 1000mg (chronic)	Long acting
Selective COX-2 Inhibitor NSAIDs			
Celecoxib (Celebrex®)	200mg daily or 100mg every 12 hours	400mg	Decreased GI (gastro-intestinal) toxicity, and platelet dysfunction Similar renal (kidney) effects to non-selective NSAIDS

Patients with a history of cardiovascular disease (coronary artery disease, angina, myocardial infarction) or even a history of risk factors for cardiovascular disease should avoid NSAIDs as they increase the risk of cardiac complications. Moreover, NSAIDs increase your blood pressure and can cause you to become hypertensive because they cause you to retain sodium and thus retain water (8). Finally, NSAIDs can cause kidney injury in about 1-5% of patients (9). Most side effects caused by NSAIDs can be prevented by limiting the dose and time you are on them.

Recently there has been evidence that chronic use of NSAIDs can contribute to the development of chronic pain—that is pain which does not go away. A study published in the journal Science Translational Medicine conducted in patients with low back pain found that inflammation was a key regulator in preventing patients pain from transitioning from acute to chronic. Although, over the short course NSAIDS help reduce pain, they also decrease inflammation which helps stop the pain. This is thus another reason to only use NSAIDs for short periods of time (10).

NSAIDs in Spinal Fusion

Unfortunately, because of their anti-inflammatory properties, **NSAID use should be minimized after spinal fusion surgery because they increase the risk of non-union (failure of the fusion to heal) (11)**. Specifically selective COX-2 NSAIDs have been shown to impair healing in fractures (we extrapolated the same to be true of fusions because both heal by a similar mechanism), while this was not shown for non-selective COX inhibitors (11). Short-term courses of NSAIDs around the time of surgery seem to be safe; however, long-term use should be avoided until the fracture or spinal fusion is healed (12,13).

Topical NSAIDs

NSAIDs may be **applied topically** which is advantageous as it delivers a high concentration of the medication to the area where it is needed, while limiting the systemic absorption in the rest of the body and thus **limiting side effects**. For example, gastric bleeding is low with the use of topical NSAIDs as are other adverse effects. The most commonly used topical NSAID is Diclofenac patches (Flector patch®) and Diclofenac Gel (Voltaren®) which can be used for either acute or chronic pain with good results (14).

Topical NSAIDs

Drug name	Dose	Maximum daily dose	Characteristics
Diclofenac Gel (Voltaren Gel)	1-2% (apply 2-4 grams)	16 grams of 1% or 8 grams of 2%	May cause rash
Diclofenac Patch (Flector Patch)	1 patch	2 patches a day	May cause rash

Topical Anesthetics

Topical anesthetics are perhaps most well known for their use in dental procedures as a numbing agent. These drugs **block the transmission of electrical signals along nerves and can block the superficial sensation of pain**. The most used topical anesthetic is **lidocaine** and comes in the form of a patch. A single patch may be applied to an area of pain for 24 hours. These patches are typically used to treat neuropathic (nerve problem) pain, such as numbness and tingling. There is no major clinical trial evidence that this type of therapy offers long term benefit, but it is relatively safe and thus may be useful for some patients (14).

Topical Anesthetics			
Drug name	Dose	Maximum daily dose	Characteristics
Lidocaine (Lidoderm Patch®)	5% lidocaine patch containing 700mg	1 patch every 24 hours	Rash, itching, nausea
Lidocaine Cream (Aspercreme®)	5% lidocaine	3 applications per day	Redness, swelling
Capsaicin Cream	0.075% capsaicin	4 times daily	Local irritation and burning

Capsaicin Cream

Capsaicin is a chemical produced naturally in chili peppers and is what is responsible for producing the burning sensation when you eat them. It may be used topically in the form of a cream. Capsaicin causes analgesia (relieves pain) by depleting a substance called substance-P that, when released by tissue, triggers pain. **It has been shown to reduce neuropathic pain in randomized trials (15)**. Of note, it may cause a local burning sensation which some can find quite disturbing, although this tends to improve with continued use.

Antidepressants

There are **several antidepressant medicines** which **are** also **effective at treating neuropathic pain**. Since these medications not only treat mood disorders, but also may be used independently to treat pain, the name "antidepressant" is a bit of a misnomer. There are two main classes of antidepressants which are used: **tricyclic antidepressants** and **serotonin norepinephrine reuptake inhibitors (SNRIs)**. These drugs act at the synaptic cleft (area where two neurons meet) to block the reuptake (reabsorption) of serotonin and norepinephrine, two neurotransmitters in the body. These drugs must be used for several weeks before a noticeable effect occurs and thus must be taken as prescribed and not in a "once off" as needed fashion.

Antidepressant medications can have several side effects. **Tricyclic antidepressants** have **anticholinergic properties** (blocking a neurotransmitter of the autonomic nervous system that is responsible for secretions), which can result in blurred vision, dry mouth, constipation, and urinary retention. Tricyclic antidepressants also have **antihistamine properties** which can result in sedation (sleepiness), confusion, delirium, and weight gain. Finally, they block a portion of the sympathetic nervous system known as alpha 1 receptor which can result in orthostatic hypotension (low blood pressure on rising from sitting or lying down). Tricyclic antidepressants may also have **cardiac side effects** and cause arrhythmias (irregular heartbeats) and congestive heart failure. Thus, these medicines are contraindicated in patients who have severe cardiac disease, or a prolonged QT interval (this is a finding on EKG). They may also lower your seizure threshold and thus should not be used in patients with a history of seizures. Finally, tricyclic antidepressants, unlike SNRIs, may be **fatal in overdose**. These side effects may be more pronounced in the older individual. Some of these side effects may be reduced by introducing the medication in a very small dose and slowly increasing it over several weeks to an effective dose.

Common Tricyclic Pain Medications			
Drug name	Oral dose	Maximum daily dose	Characteristics
Amitriptyline (Elavil®)	10-25mg initial dose which is increased in increments of 10-25 mg each week up to 150 mg	150mg	Anticholinergic, antihistamine, and anti-alpha-1 properties.
Nortriptyline (Pamelor®)	10-25mg daily at bedtime, may increase as tolerated every 3 days	150mg	Anticholinergic, antihistamine, and anti-alpha-1 properties.
Common SNRI Pain Medications			
Drug name	Oral dose	Maximum daily dose	Characteristics
Duloxetine (Cymbalta®)	30-60mg initial dose daily, may increase up to 120mg	120mg	Headache, dry mouth, drowsiness, fatigue, nausea, sexual dysfunction in men

Despite the side effects, **tricyclic antidepressants** have been shown in randomized, controlled trials to be **effective in the treatment of chronic low back pain** compared to placebo (16). There is also evidence that it is **useful in the treatment of neuropathic pain (17).**

Duloxetine is the most used **serotonin norepinephrine reuptake inhibitor (SNRI) to treat chronic musculoskeletal pain**. Unlike the tricyclic antidepressants, duloxetine is FDA-approved for the treatment of chronic low back pain, osteoarthritis, and neuropathic pain.

Side effects with duloxetine may be less severe than those with tricyclic antidepressants but may still result in constipation, fatigue, insomnia, and dizziness. It should be avoided in those with kidney or liver impairment. Duloxetine is, however, very well tolerated—in one study only 1 in 25 patients discontinued treatment due to side effects (18). In male patients, impotence has been reported while taking this medication.

Serotonin norepinephrine reuptake inhibitors should not be combined with other antidepressants as this may result in a serious condition known as **serotonin syndrome** which is characterized by tachycardia (a fast heart rate), hyperthermia (become hot), and tremors. Also, important to know about antidepressants is that once you start them you cannot just stop taking them without experiencing side effects. Notably, even tapering off the medicine rapidly can result in increasing anxiety, dizziness, dysphoria (a feeling of unease), and headache. You should wean yourself from this medicine over a 2–4-week period under the supervision of your doctor.

Muscle Relaxants

Muscle relaxants do pretty much what the name implies. They **relax skeletal muscle, reduce painful spasms, and provide pain relief**. Individual muscle relaxants are similar in their effectiveness and all have been shown to be useful in the treatment of non-specific low back pain (19). These medicines are all generally sedating and thus should mainly be used before bed.

 Cyclobenzaprine (Flexeril®) in particular is sedating and should mainly be used before bed. Muscle relaxants should not be used by anyone who needs to operate machinery or be alert. They may also worsen glaucoma or urinary retention because of their anticholinergic (drying) properties. Elderly patients have increased risk of side effects with these drugs, and they should not be used by patients with a history of dementia or delirium. While there is some potential for dependency with these drugs, it is generally low (20).

Benzodiazepines are also classified as muscle relaxants but are sedating drugs and in general should not be used in the treatment of back pain. They have a high potential for abuse (21). They work by increasing gamma-aminobutyric acid (GABA-A, a neurotransmitter) signaling activity in neurons and are commonly used to treat spasticity (abnormal muscle stiffness, sometimes spasms) in patients who suffer from stroke or cerebral palsy.

Baclofen is a gamma-aminobutyric acid-B (GABA-B) agonist (activator) and is commonly used to treat spasticity and muscle spasm. Baclofen is safe for long term use and does not seem to be habit forming or cause the body to develop tolerance to the drug. However, baclofen should not be stopped abruptly because you may experience withdrawal symptoms. Baclofen may be used during the day.

Tizanidine is a drug which stimulates the sympathetic nervous system (specifically an alpha-2 adrenergic agonist). It is another muscle relaxant that has been shown to be effective in the treatment of spasticity, especially that resulting from a spinal cord injury (22). It may also be used in the treatment of low back pain.

Common Muscle Relaxers			
Drug name	Oral dose	Maximum daily dose	Characteristics
Cyclobenzaprine (Flexeril®)	5-10mg daily	40mg	Sedation, anticholinergic properties, including urinary retention
Methocarbamol (Robaxin®)	1.5g every 8 hours for 2 days, followed by 750mg every 8 hours	4.5g	Sedation, anticholinergic properties, including urinary retention
Tizanidine (Zanaflex®)	2-4mg every 6-12 hours	16mg	Sedation, anticholinergic properties, including urinary retention
Baclofen	5mg-10mg 3 times daily	30mg	Confusion, headache, hypotonia (loss of muscle tone), nausea, vomiting.

Anticonvulsants (Antiseizure Medications)

Gabapentin is an antiseizure medicine which has pain-relieving properties particularly effective at targeting nerve pain. Like the neurotransmitter γ-aminobutyric acid (GABA), Gabapentin decreases the nerve's "excitability." It works by binding to the $\alpha2-\delta$ subunit of voltage-gated calcium channels on nerve membranes, which inhibits neurotransmitter release. These channels can accumulate on nerves which have chronic damage. Because these drugs are used to decrease neural activity, they are helpful in managing seizures. Gabapentin is traditionally used for conditions such as diabetic neuropathy and neuropathic pain from spinal cord injury; however, evidence exists that it may help in lumbar spinal stenosis (23). Gabapentin has been shown in large randomized, controlled trials to be effective for the treatment of neuropathic type pain (24). However, in a large double-blinded, randomized, controlled trial, pregabalin—a drug very similar to gabapentin— did not significantly reduce sciatica pain. Gabapentin is rarely used in isolation in the treatment of spinal pain, but it may be helpful as an adjunct to other analgesics. Gabapentin may also be used to help control your pain after having spine surgery (25).

Gabapentin and pregabalin (Lyrica®) are very similar drugs and are essentially

Common Anticonvulsant Medicines			
Drug name	**Oral dose**	**Maximum daily dose**	**Characteristics**
Gabapentin (Neurontin®)	Starting dose: 100mg TID (three times a day)	3600mg	Sedation Respiratory depression Dizziness Blurred vision Edema (swelling) Must slowly taper off drug when stopping to reduce withdrawal
Pregabalin (Lyrica ®)	25-150 mg once daily	600mg	Sedation Respiratory depression Dizziness Blurred vision Edema (swelling) Weight gain Must slowly taper off drug when stopping to reduce withdrawal

used interchangeably. Pregabalin is absorbed faster and thus may begin to work faster than gabapentin; however, there is no evidence showing its overall superiority compared to gabapentin. Lyrica ® is purported to have less side effects than gabapentin but there is no good evidence that this is true (26). The cost of Lyrica® is much higher as it is not available in generic form (27).

The common side effects from gabapentin and pregabalin include dizziness, somnolence (drowsiness), gait disturbance (27).

A final word about gabapentin: it should not be stopped abruptly. If gabapentin is stopped suddenly, you may experience **gabapentin withdrawal syndrome** with symptoms that mimic those of alcohol withdrawal syndrome: sweating, irritability, anxiety, headache. While rare, this syndrome typically occurs in patients who have been taking high doses of gabapentin (greater than 800mg daily) for long periods of time. This is extremely rare with short term use at low doses (less than 800mg daily). Please discuss with your doctor before discontinuing this medicine and make a plan for ending with a slowly tapered dose (28).

Opioids

Opioids should be avoided in the treatment of low back pain. There is a very high risk of abuse and dependence with these medicines (29). It's such an important topic, please see chapter 20 on narcotic medicines.

Steroids

Glucocorticoids (commonly called steroids) are a synthetic form of the natural hormone cortisol. These are totally different from the anabolic steroids you hear about professional athletes using. **Cortisol** is naturally released when the adrenal glands are stimulated by corticotropin (ACTH) which is secreted from the pituitary gland in your brain. Stress, your circadian rhythm, and hypoglycemia (low sugar) can all cause your body to release cortisol. **Cortisol is a stress hormone**, so called because it helps your body deal with stressful situations by allowing the production of glucose and by interrupting non-essential metabolic pathways such as inflammation and tissue repair. The hypothalamic-pituitary-adrenal (HPA) axis works as a feedback loop such that cortisol, once released, causes a suppression of ACTH and a subsequent decrease in the further release of cortisol.

Steroids are exceptionally powerful anti-inflammatories, making them useful in treating many painful conditions. Like NSAIDs, they inhibit the synthesis of proinflammatory substances in the body, including arachidonic acid, IL-1, TNF-α and prostaglandin E2. Steroids may also stabilize cell membranes and thus may be useful in epidural injections (discussed below). In general steroids are much more potent than NSAIDs because they inhibit phospholipase A2, the enzyme that initiates the cascade of chemical reactions that result in inflammation whereas, as discussed earlier, NSAIDs inhibit the COX enzyme, further down the line in that inflammation-producing process.

Because steroids are such potent anti-inflammatories, they also are potent **immunosuppressive** drugs and can increase your risk of infection. Steroids have **other adverse effects** on the **musculoskeletal system** including osteoporosis, osteonecrosis (bone death due to lack of blood supply), muscle atrophy (wasting away), weakness, as well as poor tissue healing. Steroids effect the **gastrointestinal system** and may cause or worsen peptic ulcers or pancreatitis. Thus, if your doctor prescribes a steroid, she or he may also prescribe a medication that decreases stomach acid such as ranitidine or omeprazole.

Steroids may also cause several **metabolic disturbances** such as increasing your blood glucose (sugar) level, retaining salt— causing you to retain water and your blood pressure to go up—as well as high cholesterol, and low potassium. Steroids may also cause **mental disturbances** such as mania, psychosis or delirium and can cause damage to your eyes, resulting in cataracts.

Finally, because your body produces its own steroids, systemic (not topical) administration of steroids can interfere and inhibit your own natural synthesis of steroid hormones. In this way you become dependent on the medicine.

Common Oral Steroids

Drug name	Oral dose	Potency relative to hydrocortisone (cortisol)	Duration	Characteristics
Methylprednisolone (Medrol Dosepak)	6-day course (21 tablets at 4mg strength) starting at 24 mg and tapering down to 4mg.	5X	12-36 hours	There are varied side effects, please see above.
Prednisone	6-day course (21 tablets at 4mg strength) starting at 30 mg and tapering down to 5mg.	4X	12-36 hours	There are varied side effects, please see above.
Hydrocortisone (Cortef*)	20-200 mg a day divided per your physician	1X	12-36 hours	There are varied side effects, please see above.

Common Injectable Steroids

Drug name	IV dose	Potency relative to hydrocortisone (cortisol)	Duration	Characteristics
Dexamethasone (Decadron®)	4-10mg	30X	36-72 hours	Dexamethasone is a corticosteroid commonly used in a hospital. You will generally not be required to manage it on your own.

So why would anyone ever consider using steroids with all these ill effects? The good news is that **most side effects only occur when either taking a very high dose of steroids or taking them for a long period of time**. While short term (less than 30 days) use may be rarely associated with an increased risk of sepsis (infection), venous thromboembolism (blood clots) and fracture, short courses of the drugs typically do not cause problems (30). Steroids come in different preparations that determine their overall potency and duration of action. The most common route of administration is oral; however, they may be given intravenously (in a vein) as well as intraarticular (in a joint) or epidural (around the spinal canal). **To avoid the side effects discussed above steroids are commonly administered in a tapered fashion.** A popular dosing regimen is the Medrol Dosepak which contains 21 tablets, 4mg each. On day 1 you take 6 tablets, totaling 24 mg, on day 2 you take 5 tablets, totaling 20mg, on day 3, 4 tablets, (16 mg), day 4, 3 tablets (12mg), day 5, 2 tablets (8mg) and day 6, 1 tablet (4mg).

To reduce the risk of side effects of steroids on the musculoskeletal system, **while on steroids it is important to exercise and take vitamin D and calcium**.

Cannabinoids/ CBD

With the onset of the opioid pandemic, the need for alternative treatments for pain is evident. Cannabis has arisen as a potential form of pain treatment, particularly some of the specific chemical compounds found in cannabis known as cannabinoids. The active ingredients in cannabis are tetrahydrocannabinol (THC) and cannabidiol (CBD) both of which activate the cannabinoid receptors in the body—how they affect pain control is not currently well understood but they may have anti-inflammatory properties. Although the cannabis plant is legalized for medical use in some areas, because of its psychoactive properties it is not in mainstream use in the treatment of pain.

The psychological effects of cannabis are caused by the THC chemical component. CBD, which does not cause intoxication but still helps with pain, has turned out to be more relevant for mainstream application. CBD comes in many different preparations and can be ingested orally or applied topically. It is generally available over the counter. CBD and cannabis seem to help with pain and serve as a useful alternative to narcotics, but most studies to date on CBD or cannabis are quasi-experimental and not rigorous enough to be able to make formal recommendations (31). Side effects may include decreased coordination, decreased lung function, dry mouth and sedation (32).

Other Supplements

There are many supplements out there with purported benefits for treating achy joints. Two common forms which I get asked about routinely are curcumin and glucosamine/chondroitin.

Curcumin is a yellow pigment compound found in the plant spice Turmeric which is common in eastern dishes such as curry. There is a dizzying array of purported medical benefits to ingesting curcumin, but it is relevant as a treatment for back and neck pain because of its anti-inflammatory properties. Curcumin ingestion of around 1000mg a day can decrease pain from knee osteoarthritis and may be beneficial for spine osteoarthritis although this has not been strictly tested (33). Importantly, curcumin is a relatively safe compound to ingest, but should be avoided in those with kidney stones or gallstones as these may become worse. It should also likely be avoided in pregnant individuals.

Glucosamine and Chondroitin are compounds found in cartilage, the smooth tissue which covers joints and allows for easy movement. The theory is that by ingesting these compounds, the cartilage can be nourished and preserved thus alleviating or preventing arthritis. Although some studies have shown a cartilage preserving effect of glucosamine and chondroitin (34,35) it has not been shown in randomized controlled placebo studies to relieve pain (36). It is currently unclear whether they offer any clinical benefit, but they are well tolerated with no discernable side effects.

Lumbar Epidural Steroid Injections

Injections are commonly used in the spine to both treat pain (therapeutic) and diagnose sources of pain (diagnostic). Because the spine is so complicated and has many moving parts that can cause pain, surgeons sometimes use injections to help pinpoint where your pain is coming from. Local anesthetic (numbing medicine) is injected into a potential site of pain and if the pain is relieved, gives some proof that that is indeed the source of the pain.

In some cases of lumbar spine disease, lumbar epidural steroid injections may be used to manage low back pain and lower extremity pain. These injections are typically done under X-ray (fluoroscopic guidance) or CT guidance by a physiatrist, pain specialist or spine surgeon. A long needle is used to deliver a small amount of contrast agent (dye which is visible under X-ray to help confirm you are in the correct location), a steroid, as well as local anesthetic to the spinal canal or nerve root. Steroids, as discussed above, are potent anti-inflammatory drugs that, if delivered to the site of a disc herniation where there is ongoing active inflammation, may result in significant relief of pain. While they do nothing for the compressive effects of herniations and stenosis, they can totally stop the inflammatory process which is responsible for pain, thus often "curing" the problem. **Local anesthetics** are numbing medications which can directly relieve pain from inflamed or compressed nerve roots and are commonly also administered in epidurals. In contrast to steroids, which influence the inflammatory process, local anesthetics simply stop the transmission of pain signals. Local anesthetics only last for about 6-12 hours depending on the type used and thus are also useful for diagnostic purposes. If the pain is relieved from the injection, it gives your doctor more confidence that that area is the source of your pain.

Epidural steroid injections should not be performed on patients with any active infection (especially on the skin), uncontrolled diabetes, spinal malignancy, or those who have trouble with profuse bleeding (coagulopathy) or are on blood thinners (anticoagulants) (37). If you are on a blood thinning agent, make sure to tell your doctor before the procedure.

Epidural procedures are performed in a special suite or in the operating room— so generally not in the doctor's office. There are several different approaches to performing epidural injections, depending on where your surgeon decides to introduce the needle, a decision which is usually based on your anatomy and the location of your pain. These approaches are intralaminar (in between the lamina), transforaminal (through the foramen), or caudally (through the sacrococcygeal ligament). There is no consensus on how often epidural steroids injections should be performed, but they are generally done in a series of 3, at 3-7 weeks apart. If the first epidural is not effective, you should discuss the pros and cons of repeating it with your doctor.

Epidural steroids injections may be associated with **adverse events**. In a study of 207 patients the overall complication rate of epidural steroid injections was 10%. In this study the most common complication was headache (3%) and tended to be temporary, possibly related to a small leak of the cerebrospinal fluid caused by the needle. Increase in back pain was reported in 2.4% of patients. Other adverse events included facial flushing, increased leg pain, rash, fainting, dizziness, temporary leg weakness, increase in blood glucose levels, hypertension, and nausea (38). Rarer complications include infection, damage to nerves and blood vessels and even paralysis or paraplegia (37). Finally epidural steroid injections should be avoided if surgery is planned within 3 months as they have been linked to increased rates of post-operative infection, particularly in spinal fusions (39,40).

Epidural steroid injections are useful for short term symptomatic relief of leg pain and can possibly be used to delay surgery (41). They are particularly useful when there is an active inflammatory process associated with the problem such as, for example, with a disc herniation or nerve root irritation. An epidural steroid injection has absolutely no effect on structural bony compression or abnormal anatomy and, while many patients get relief from pain following an injection, numbness and weakness from nerve root impingement will persist (37,42). Let me repeat, they will not whisk away disc herniations or evaporate stenosis. Furthermore, in a large randomized, double-blind clinical trial of 160 patients with leg pain who received either saline placebo or steroid/local anesthetic combination, the steroid injection improved leg pain at 2 weeks; however, back pain and leg pain were lower at 3-6 months and 6 months, respectively, in the saline group. This indicates that epidural steroids may have a rebound phenomenon, that is, when they wear off, your pain is actually worse (43). On the other hand, in smaller a study of 55 surgical candidates undergoing epidural steroid injections, 29 decided not to have surgery at 1 year following an injection series. In this study steroid injections were more effective than local anesthetic alone in preventing surgery (44).

In addition to being therapeutic, epidural steroid injections can also serve a diagnostic purpose and help surgeons identify troublesome spinal levels. If your pain is either reproduced by the injection or relieved when the doctor infuses numbing medicine, this can be very helpful in predicting the success of surgery (45,46). If your pain is relieved (greater than 50% reduction) it helps confirm the level of origin of your pain as well as the possibility that it can be corrected. In chronic cases, structural damage to the nerve may be permanent and may not respond as well to epidural injections (47).

So, what's the bottom line. I think epidural steroids are particularly useful for acute disc herniations where most of the pain may be coming from inflammation, and the underlying problem has an excellent chance at healing on its own. I think epidurals are also useful if I cannot figure out exactly where the pain is coming from based on imaging and physical exam. Where I think epidurals are less useful are cases where there are significant neurological symptoms such as numbness or weakness or in cases where there is disease that will ultimately require surgery. Nonetheless, I think in most cases it's worth giving epidurals a shot before you consider surgery as they are quick, safe and help a lot of people. Here it is critical to work with a good surgeon to help decide what the is the correct path for you.

Other Areas of Pain Management

There are many other ways pain can be managed. In the next section we discuss some treatments which pain specialists, physiatrist or physical therapists typically administer. Some spine surgeons may use these treatments, but most will not offer these services.

transcutaneous electrical nerve stimulation (TENS)

The principle of transcutaneous electrical nerve stimulation is based on **the gate control theory of pain** (see chapter 2 What Causes Pain in the Spine). The gate control theory of pain states that small fiber pain nerves which enter the spinal cord (specifically at the substantia gelatinosa, an anatomic area in the dorsal horn of the spinal cord) can be modulated by descending neurons from the brain to block pain transmission. **In plain English: your brain can suppress pain signals**. TENS units take advantage of this loophole in your pain system to try and suppress pain signals with a distracting electrical signal that mimics one that comes from your brain.

TENS units are composed of a small battery generator (the size of a Walkman), electrical leads, and electrodes that are placed on the body. The generator can deliver different stimulation and pulse frequencies. The electrodes are placed by your physician or physical therapist. **TENS may be used to treat acute musculoskeletal pain, and pain from spine vertebral insufficiency fractures** (weakened bone fractures). It is in general not effective for neuropathic (nerve-related) pain. Patients who are pregnant or have implanted devices such as pacemakers or spinal cord stimulators, or patients with significant sensory impairment should not use TENS machines. TENS units should also not be placed on the neck in a way that they may induce syncope (fainting). Otherwise, TENS is a safe modality of pain treatment with few side effects.

spinal cord stimulators

Spinal cord stimulators work by applying an electrical current directly onto the spinal cord from an implanted electrode. This is similar in concept to a TENS unit except spinal cord stimulators are a much more invasive form of pain control. The idea behind the spinal cord stimulator is that stimulation of certain nerve fibers can block the transmission of pain in pain- sensing fibers (again think gate control theory of pain), but the true mechanism is unknown.

Spinal cord stimulators have two main components, an electrode lead, and a battery pack (also called the generator). The electrode is implanted into the spinal canal and the battery pack is generally placed under the skin and has a life span of 4-8 years. Patients must undergo a successful trial period where a temporary external stimulator is implanted without formally implanting the final implant. If this trial stimulator offers no relief from pain, a formal stimulator is not implanted. Following implantation, the stimulator's programming may be adjusted to fine tune its effects. Spinal cord stimulation does not treat the source of the pain, but instead influences how your brain interprets pain signals.

Spinal cord stimulators may improve your pain, if you are an appropriate candidate;

however, they will not improve your function. As with any invasive spinal procedure, there are also associated complications. The stimulator may fail to relieve your pain, or even result in significant injury to your nerves, spinal cord damage and even death. Spinal cord stimulators are most used to treat complex regional pain syndrome and in cases of failed back surgery where it may be dangerous to perform revision surgery. I typically recommend their use for patients who will clearly not benefit from surgery and so spinal cord stimulators are somewhat of an end-of-the-line treatment for me.

radiofrequency ablation (RFA)

Radiofrequency ablation (RFA) blocks the transmission of pain to the brain by using an electrical current to create a heat lesion on a targeted pain-transmitting nerve. In essence, RFA fries the nerves that are transmitting pain. RFA relies on the theory that destroying the nerves that transmit pain results in the brain perceiving and therefore conveying a feeling of less pain. The injury or condition is not changed, but the pain you were feeling from it is blocked. Like spinal cord stimulation and TENS, RFA does not treat the actual pathology, and instead is a palliative technique employed only to reduce pain. RFA can be used to treat back and neck pain. RFA can only be used on sensory nerves (using it on motor nerves would cause paralysis) and so only certain areas may be treated. Common areas of ablation are the medial branch of the dorsal nerve root, which supplies the facet joints in the lumbar spine, the lumbar dorsal root ganglion which can be involved in chronic pain, the cervical medial branch of the dorsal nerve which supplies the cervical facets. Blocking these nerves causes anesthesia (numbing) of painful arthritic facet joints without any effect on motor function.

It is important to note that prior to undergoing an RFA procedure, the diagnosis of facet pain must be confirmed with a series of medial branch block injections. A medial branch block consists of an injection of local anesthetic targeting the affected facet and nerve to be burned. Because there is a high false positive rate (one block giving relief but not accurately diagnosing the problem) it is only considered a true positive result when greater than 50-80% of patient reported relief occurs after each of two different medial branch blocks. This result confirms that RFA may be therapeutically beneficial and only following this may the formal RFA procedure be performed.

The actual RFA procedure is **performed percutaneously** (that is, through the skin, not requiring a formal incision, and usually under light sedation). A small RFA probe is targeted under fluoroscopic X-ray guidance. The position of the needle is confirmed to be in a safe position by electrical stimulation to ensure no motor nerves are being contacted. The area is then numbed with local anesthetic and the RFA current is run through the probe burning the nerves carrying the pain signal from the facet joint. After the procedure the patient may experience increased pain and dysesthesias (abnormal sensations) for 3-4 weeks, following which the relief may take effect. These symptoms typically can be treated conservatively with anti-inflammatories.

In appropriately selected patients, the RFA procedure, when properly performed, has been shown to produce results superior to placebo injections (48).

spinal pumps

I include spinal pumps in this section because it is a treatment offered by pain specialists, but really these should be used only very rarely and are not part of mainstream non-operative treatment of spine pain. Like spinal cord stimulators, **spinal intrathecal (inside the spinal canal) pumps are implanted within the spinal canal to deliver powerful narcotics such as morphine directly to the spinal cord**. Spine pumps typically consist of a small catheter which is implanted into the spinal canal and attached to a pump and a reservoir located under the skin of the abdomen which may be refilled. Before implantation the patient should undergo a trial where opioids are delivered to the spinal canal to see if the drug relieves pain. Moreover, patients undergoing spinal pump implantation must have a designated support person available 24/7 to aid the patient in case the pump runs out of medication because of risk of withdrawal. Spinal pumps are generally reserved to control pain from cancer which has failed surgical or radiation treatment or to treat rare forms of chronic pain caused by overwhelming pathological processes that do not respond to surgical treatment. Purported benefits are that the overall dose of narcotics used are quite small compared to oral narcotic agents (see chapter 20 on narcotics) but more effective because they are delivered directly to the source of pain transmission. I think they are mainly useful as palliative type treatments where nothing can be done to treat the problem that is causing pain. It's important to note that pain pumps must be periodically refilled with narcotic medication which involves a medical professional injecting the medicine into a reservoir in the device through the skin.

Conclusion

No one wants to be in pain and patients are usually desperate for relief. Before jumping to surgery, you should consider some non-operative treatment modalities such as basic anti-inflammatories or even an epidural steroid injection—both are very effective at relieving pain. Depending on your pain type, there are various medications which can help alleviate your suffering. It's important to note that even though these medications are considered "conservative" care, they can have side effects. Also, if they are not giving you the help you need, remember that taking medications for prolonged periods can also cause problems. Give them a shot under the supervision of a physician, but if they fail to give you relief it may be time to consider other forms of therapy.

Frequently Asked Questions

- ### What is the best TENS unit?

  There are many different TENS units and so it is difficult to choose one that is good. The industry standard TENS unit is made by EMPI and runs for around $300.

- ### Who can help me adjust my TENS unit?

  Your physical therapist typically will have more experience with adjusting TENS units than your surgeon.

References

1.   French SD, Cameron M, Walker BF, Reggars JW, Esterman AJ. A Cochrane Review of Superficial Heat or Cold for Low Back Pain: Spine. 2006 Apr;31(9):998–1006.

2.   Ricciotti E, FitzGerald GA. Prostaglandins and Inflammation. Arterioscler Thromb Vasc Biol. 2011 May;31(5):986–1000.

3.   White AP, Arnold PM, Norvell DC, Ecker E, Fehlings MG. Pharmacologic Management of Chronic Low Back Pain: Synthesis of the Evidence. Spine. 2011 Oct;36:S131–43.

4.   Roelofs PD, Deyo RA, Koes BW, Scholten RJ, van Tulder MW. Non-steroidal anti-inflammatory drugs for low back pain. Cochrane Back and Neck Group, editor. Cochrane Database Syst Rev [Internet]. 2008 Jan 23 [cited 2020 Apr 24]; Available from: http://doi.wiley.com/10.1002/14651858.CD000396.pub3

5.   Rasmussen-Barr E, Held U, Grooten WJA, Roelofs PDDM, Koes BW, van Tulder MW, et al. Nonsteroidal Anti-inflammatory Drugs for Sciatica: An Updated Cochrane Review. SPINE. 2017 Apr;42(8):586–94.

6.   Richy F. Time dependent risk of gastrointestinal complications induced by non-steroidal anti-inflammatory drug use: a consensus statement using a meta-analytic approach. Ann Rheum Dis. 2004 Jul 1;63(7):759–66.

7.   Fleischman AN, Li WT, Luzzi AJ, Nest DSV, Torjman MC, Schwenk ES, et al. Risk of Gastrointestinal Bleeding with Extended Use of Nonsteroidal Anti-inflammatory Drug Analgesia After Joint Arthroplasty. J Arthroplasty [Internet]. 2021 Feb 10 [cited 2021 Feb 25];0(0). Available from: https://www.arthroplastyjournal.org/article/S0883-5403(21)00141-8/abstract

8.   Warner TD, Mitchell JA. COX-2 selectivity alone does not define the cardiovas-

cular risks associated with non-steroidal anti-inflammatory drugs. The Lancet. 2008 Jan;371(9608):270–3.

9.   Whelton A. Nephrotoxicity of nonsteroidal anti-inflammatory drugs: physiologic foundations and clinical implications. Am J Med. 1999 May 31;106(5B):13S-24S.

10.   Parisien M, Lima LV, Dagostino C, El-Hachem N, Drury GL, Grant AV, et al. Acute inflammatory response via neutrophil activation protects against the development of chronic pain. Sci Transl Med. 2022 May 11;14(644):eabj9954.

11.   Li Q, Zhang Z, Cai Z. High-Dose Ketorolac Affects Adult Spinal Fusion: A Meta-Analysis of the Effect of Perioperative Nonsteroidal Anti-Inflammatory Drugs on Spinal Fusion. Spine. 2011 Apr;36(7):E461–8.

12.   Sivaganesan A, Chotai S, White-Dzuro G, McGirt MJ, Devin CJ. The effect of NSAIDs on spinal fusion: a cross-disciplinary review of biochemical, animal, and human studies. Eur Spine J. 2017 Nov;26(11):2719–28.

13.   Pradhan BB, Tatsumi RL, Gallina J, Kuhns CA, Wang JC, Dawson EG. Ketorolac and Spinal Fusion: Does the Perioperative Use of Ketorolac Really Inhibit Spinal Fusion? Spine. 2008 Sep;33(19):2079–82.

14.   Derry S, Wiffen PJ, Kalso EA, Bell RF, Aldington D, Phillips T, et al. Topical analgesics for acute and chronic pain in adults - an overview of Cochrane Reviews. Cochrane Pain, Palliative and Supportive Care Group, editor. Cochrane Database Syst Rev [Internet]. 2017 May 12 [cited 2020 May 31]; Available from: http://doi.wiley.com/10.1002/14651858.CD008609.pub2

15.   Effect of treatment with capsaicin on daily activities of patients with painful diabetic neuropathy. Capsaicin Study Group. Diabetes Care. 1992 Feb;15(2):159–65.

16.   Urquhart DM, Wluka AE, van Tulder M, Heritier S, Forbes A, Fong C, et al. Efficacy of Low-Dose Amitriptyline for Chronic Low Back Pain. JAMA Intern Med. 2018 Nov;178(11):1474–81.

17.   Moore RA, Derry S, Aldington D, Cole P, Wiffen PJ. Amitriptyline for neuropathic pain in adults. Cochrane Pain, Palliative and Supportive Care Group, editor. Cochrane Database Syst Rev [Internet]. 2015 Jul 6 [cited 2020 Jun 7]; Available from: http://doi.wiley.com/10.1002/14651858.CD008242.pub3

18.   Citrome L. Vortioxetine for major depressive disorder: An indirect comparison with duloxetine, escitalopram, levomilnacipran, sertraline, venlafaxine, and vilazodone, using number needed to treat, number needed to harm, and likelihood to be helped or harmed. J Affect Disord. 2016 May 15;196:225–33.

19.   van Tulder MW, Touray T, Furlan AD, Solway S, Bouter LM. Muscle relaxants for non-specific low-back pain. Cochrane Back and Neck Group, editor. Cochrane Database Syst Rev [Internet]. 2003 Apr 22 [cited 2020 Apr 25]; Available from: http://doi.wiley.com/10.1002/14651858.CD004252

20.   Preston KL, Guarino JJ, Kirk WT, Griffiths RR. Evaluation of the abuse potential of methocarbamol. J Pharmacol Exp Ther. 1989 Mar;248(3):1146–57.

21.   Friedman BW, Irizarry E, Solorzano C, Khankel N, Zapata J, Zias E, et al. Diaz-epam Is No Better Than Placebo When Added to Naproxen for Acute Low Back Pain. Ann Emerg Med. 2017 Aug;70(2):169-176.e1.

22.   Simpson DM, Gracies JM, Yablon SA, Barbano R, Brashear A, the BoNT/TZD Study Team. Botulinum neurotoxin versus tizanidine in upper limb spasticity: a place-bo-controlled study. J Neurol Neurosurg Psychiatry. 2008 Dec 9;80(4):380–5.

23.   Yaksi A, Özgönenel L, Özgönenel B. The Efficiency of Gabapentin Therapy in Patients With Lumbar Spinal Stenosis: Spine. 2007 Apr;32(9):939–42.

24.   Finnerup NB, Sindrup SH, Jensen TS. The evidence for pharmacological treat-ment of neuropathic pain: Pain. 2010 Sep;150(3):573–81.

25.   Kurd MF, Kreitz T, Schroeder G, Vaccaro AR. The Role of Multimodal Analgesia in Spine Surgery: J Am Acad Orthop Surg. 2017 Apr;25(4):260–8.

26.   Robertson K, Marshman LAG, Plummer D. Pregabalin and gabapentin for the treatment of sciatica. J Clin Neurosci. 2016 Apr;26:1–7.

27.   Goodman CW, Brett AS. A Clinical Overview of Off-label Use of Gabapentinoid Drugs. JAMA Intern Med. 2019 May 1;179(5):695.

28.   Norton JW. Gabapentin withdrawal syndrome. Clin Neuropharmacol. 2001 Aug;24(4):245–6.

29.   Frieden TR, Houry D. Reducing the Risks of Relief — The CDC Opioid-Prescrib-ing Guideline. N Engl J Med. 2016 Apr 21;374(16):1501–4.

30.   Waljee AK, Rogers MAM, Lin P, Singal AG, Stein JD, Marks RM, et al. Short term use of oral corticosteroids and related harms among adults in the United States: popu-lation based cohort study. BMJ. 2017 Apr 12;j1415.

31.   First L, Douglas W, Habibi B, Singh JR, Sein MT. Cannabis Use and Low-Back Pain: A Systematic Review. Cannabis Cannabinoid Res. 2020;5(4):283–9.

32.   Vivace BJ, Sanders AN, Glassman SD, Carreon LY, Laratta JL, Gum JL. Cannabi-noids and orthopedic surgery: a systematic review of therapeutic studies. J Orthop Surg. 2021 Jan 14;16(1):57.

33.   Mathieu S, Soubrier M, Peirs C, Monfoulet LE, Boirie Y, Tournadre A. A Me-ta-Analysis of the Impact of Nutritional Supplementation on Osteoarthritis Symptoms. Nutrients. 2022 Apr 12;14(8):1607.

34.   Hochberg MC. Structure-modifying effects of chondroitin sulfate in knee osteo-arthritis: an updated meta-analysis of randomized placebo-controlled trials of 2-year duration. Osteoarthritis Cartilage. 2010 Jun;18:S28–31.

35.   Lee YH, Woo JH, Choi SJ, Ji JD, Song GG. Effect of glucosamine or chondroi-tin sulfate on the osteoarthritis progression: a meta-analysis. Rheumatol Int. 2010 Jan;30(3):357–63.

36.   Clegg DO, O'Dell JR, Weisman MH, Moreland LW, Molitor JA, Shi H. Glucos-amine, Chondroitin Sulfate, and the Two in Combination for Painful Knee Osteoarthri-

tis. N Engl J Med. 2006;14.

37.   Young IA, Hyman GS, Packia-Raj LN, Cole AJ. The Use of Lumbar Epidural/ Transforaminal Steroids for Managing Spinal Disease: J Am Acad Orthop Surg. 2007 Apr;15(4):228–38.

38.   Botwin KP, Gruber RD, Bouchlas CG, Torres-Ramos FM, Freeman TL, Slaten WK. Complications of fluoroscopically guided transforaminal lumbar epidural injections. Arch Phys Med Rehabil. 2000 Aug;81(8):1045–50.

39.   Yang S, Werner BC, Cancienne JM, Hassanzadeh H, Shimer AL, Shen FH, et al. Preoperative epidural injections are associated with increased risk of infection after single-level lumbar decompression. Spine J. 2016 Feb;16(2):191–6.

40.   Kreitz TM, Mangan J, Schroeder GD, Kepler CK, Kurd MF, Radcliff KE, et al. Do Preoperative Epidural Steroid Injections Increase the Risk of Infection After Lumbar Spine Surgery? 2020;6.

41.   Wilson-MacDonald J, Burt G, Griffin D, Glynn C. Epidural steroid injection for nerve root compression: A RANDOMISED, CONTROLLED TRIAL. J Bone Joint Surg Br. 2005 Mar;87-B(3):352–5.

42.   Gerling MC, Bortz C, Pierce KE, Lurie JD, Zhao W, Passias PG. Epidural Steroid Injections for Management of Degenerative Spondylolisthesis. 2020;102(15):8.

43.   Karppinen J, Malmivaara A, Kurunlahti M, Kyllönen E, Pienimäki T, Nieminen P, et al. Periradicular Infiltration for Sciatica: A Randomized Controlled Trial. Spine. 2001 May;26(9):1059–67.

44.   Riew KD, Yin Y, Gilula L, Bridwell KH, Lenke LG, Lauryssen C, et al. The Effect of Nerve-Root Injections on the Need for Operative Treatment of Lumbar Radicular Pain: A Prospective, Randomized, Controlled, Double-Blind Study*. J Bone Jt Surg-Am Vol. 2000 Nov;82(11):1589–93.

45.   Stanley D, McLaren MI, Euinton HA, Getty CJ. A prospective study of nerve root infiltration in the diagnosis of sciatica. A comparison with radiculography, computed tomography, and operative findings. Spine. 1990 Jun;15(6):540–3.

46.   Dooley JF, McBroom RJ, Taguchi T, Macnab I. Nerve root infiltration in the diagnosis of radicular pain. Spine. 1988 Jan;13(1):79–83.

47.   Derby R, Kine G, Saal JA, Reynolds J, Goldthwaite N, White AH, et al. Response to steroid and duration of radicular pain as predictors of surgical outcome. Spine. 1992 Jun;17(6 Suppl):S176-183.

48.   Bogduk N, Dreyfuss P, Govind J. A Narrative Review of Lumbar Medial Branch Neurotomy for the Treatment of Back Pain. Pain Med. 2009 Sep;10(6):1035–45.

Figures:

Anatomic representation of nerves exiting lumbar spine

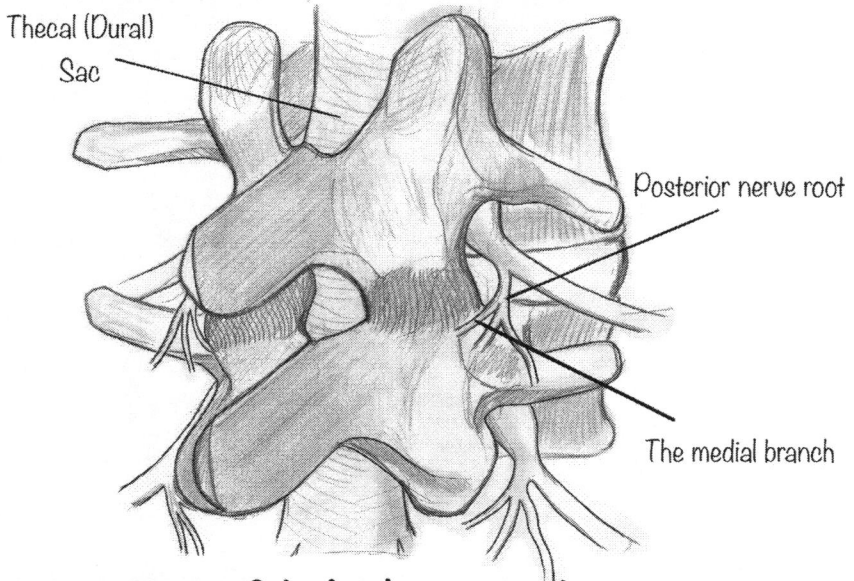

Thecal (Dural) Sac

Posterior nerve root

The medial branch

Fluoroscopic image of the lumbar spine during an interventional procedure

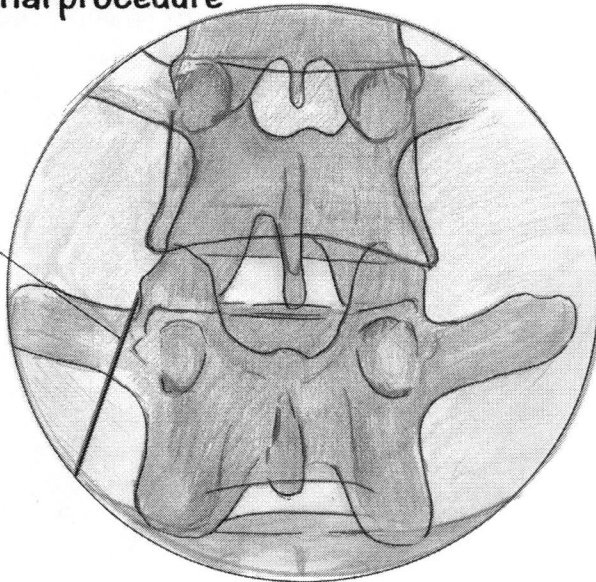

Needle inserted under x-ray guidance for injection of the medial branch

Medial branch. Nerve roots exit from the neural foramina (opening) between vertebrae and branch anteriorly and posteriorly. The posterior branch branches yet again into a medial, intermediate, and lateral branch. The medial branch supplies the facet joint and can be a source of pain transmission (top). The medial branch can be blocked with injections and radiofrequency ablation procedures reducing pain. Here we have a fluoroscopic image depicting a medial branch block with a needle injecting medicine near the facet (bottom).

Lumbar Epidural Steroid Injections (ESI)

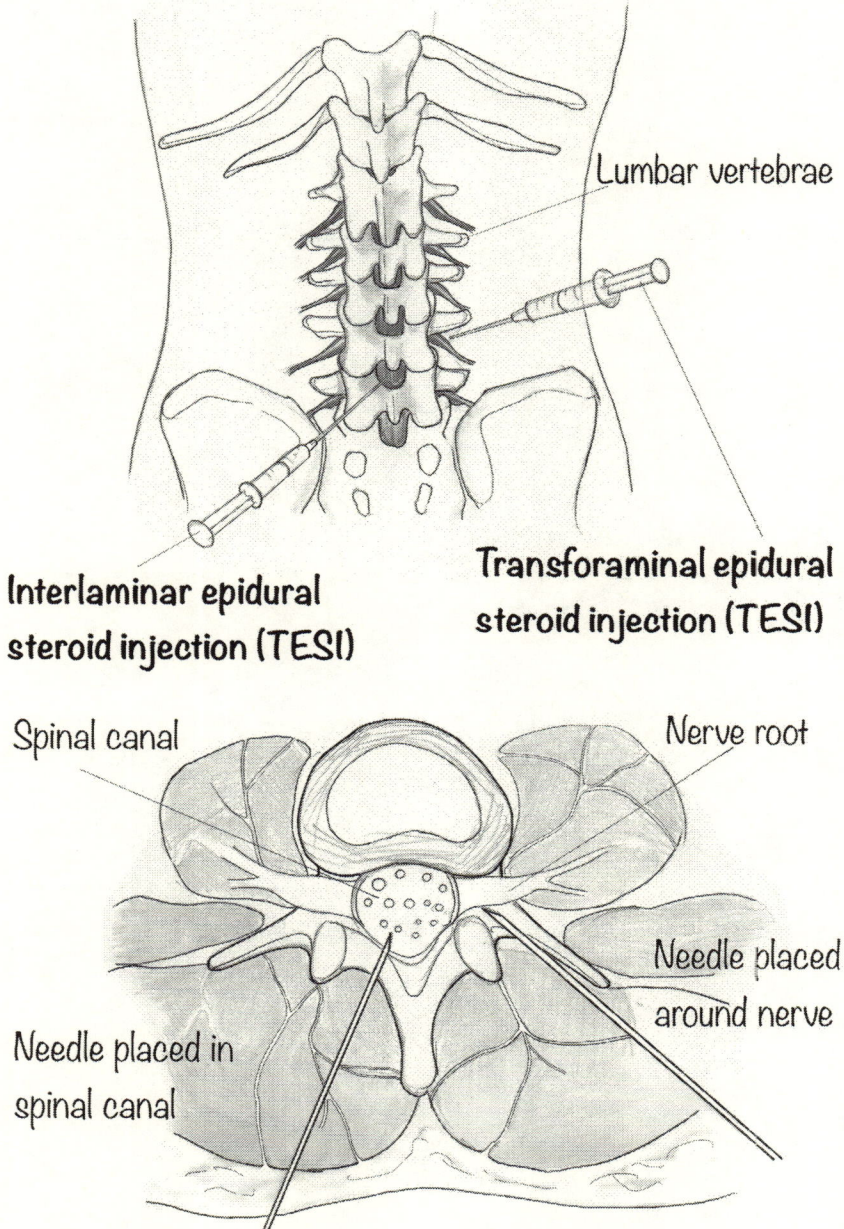

Lumbar vertebrae

Interlaminar epidural steroid injection (TESI)

Transforaminal epidural steroid injection (TESI)

Spinal canal

Nerve root

Needle placed around nerve

Needle placed in spinal canal

Lumbar epidural steroid injections (LESI). A LESI may be performed through the lamina (interlaminar) or through the foramen (transforaminal) of the spine (top of image). The injections are viewed in cross section (bottom).

Chapter 20

Narcotic Pain Medicine

Summary

Opioid medications (narcotics) are used across the medical field to help control pain and ease suffering. They work by creating not only analgesia (pain relief) but a disconnect between your brain and the pain sensation you are experiencing. Our knowledge of how this powerful class of drugs works has grown over the past decade. We now have more insight into how they cause tolerance, dependence and ultimately sensitization to pain. Opioids should mainly be used in the acute treatment of pain such as from a broken bone, or from surgery. They work poorly if given for periods of greater than 4 weeks and ultimately can result in increased pain levels. They have many side effects including constipation and nausea and can cause profound respiratory depression.

Case

 Ms. Chiffon is a 63-year-old office worker who has been suffering from back pain and leg pain for about a decade. She has degenerative disc disease and lumbar stenosis that is severe, causing bad sciatica in her legs. Her pain comes

in episodes and fluctuates. To help control her pain her primary care provider gives her a prescription for hydrocodone. This seems to help for a period but eventually no longer suppresses her pain. She returns to the doctor for something stronger and is given Percocet (a drug containing the narcotic oxycodone with about 10 times the strength of hydrocodone). This too loses its effect over several months and she finds herself increasing the dose such that she takes 10mg every 2-4 hours. Her primary care provider, at wits' end, decides to change to an even stronger opioid known as methadone to try and ease her suffering. Ultimately this too fails and she decides she must see a spine surgeon. I recommend fusion and decompression surgery but advise her that there is no way to complete the surgery with the level of narcotics she is currently on. Her pain will be unmanageable after the surgery and no narcotics will work to ease her surgical pain as she has developed a tolerance and her body will no longer respond to those drugs. We work with her primary care provider to decrease the level of narcotics she is on over several months. What is strange is that even off the medicines her pain does not increase, in fact it seems more tolerable. Ultimately, we get her off her narcotics, she has surgery and now is doing fine.

Introduction

The term narcotic comes from the Greek *narko* which means to "make numb." The term was originally associated with any drug with sleep-inducing properties, but since has been associated with drugs derived from the opium poppy, the most familiar being morphine. Morphine is named aptly after the Greek god of dreams *Morpheus* and is an opiate compound—as in derived from opium. The term opioid refers to both endogenous (naturally occurring in the body) and exogenous (derived outside the body) chemicals. The history of opioid drugs is long and complicated, but they have been in medicinal use essentially since the dawn of time. They are such an important medicine in spine care, both for how they can be helpful and harmful, that I dedicate an entire chapter to their use.

Endogenous Opioids—How do They Work?

Every person is programmed with an endogenous (your body's own) opioid system that drives reward behavior through chemical signaling in the brain and body. Reward behavior simply means that the behavior makes you feel good temporarily or, put another way, that you experience euphoria, for example, eating a piece of cake or bag of potato chips makes you feel so good you want to do it again (and get the reward of feeling good again). The system consists of naturally occurring opioid neurotransmitter (chemical messenger) proteins which act on opioid neurotransmitter receptors (molecular sites that sit on a cell membrane, accepting a specific chemical transmitter and relaying the signal into the cell). Opioid neurotransmitters include three main groups of proteins: the endorphins, dynorphins and enkephalins. Opioid neurotransmitters bind to three main neuroreceptors on the cells of neurons: mu (μ), kappa (κ), delta (δ), as well as others. The mu (μ) and delta (δ) receptors affect reward and addiction. Mutation in any of these receptor types may explain various sensitivities to opioid compounds as well as drug addiction.

Each of these protein transmitter/receptor families share a common protein structure upon which different chemical side chains are attached. The **endorphins** are produced mainly in the central nervous system (brain and spine) and are the protein family most responsible for pain control in the human body. However, it is important to keep in mind **the opioid-signaling pathways have diverse effects outside of pain control, including effects on the motor system and gastrointestinal tract**. For example, the mu receptor is responsible not only for supraspinal (affecting the perception of pain) and spinal (directly affecting pain transmission) analgesia, but affects respiration, food intake, gastric motility (moving food through the digestive tract), cognitive function, learning, memory, and immune function. The mu receptor also drives the psychological effects of opioids such as euphoria, tranquility and reward-driven behavior (eating more ice cream).

Opioid pain medicines act mainly on the mu receptor to inhibit the transmission of pain traveling from the periphery through the spinal cord to the brain. They do this by making the neuron cells that transmit pain less excitable, so it takes a greater pain stimulus to trigger the sensation of pain than it would if the neurons were not inhibited by the opioid medicine. These medicines also activate descending pathways from the brain that close the pain gate in the spinal cord, thereby suppressing the transmission of pain up to the brain (see earlier chapters, especially chapter 2, for an explanation of the gate control theory of pain). Furthermore, they have effects on the brain and emotional state, making pain more bearable. Essentially, they make you not care so much about pain. Also important is that opioids trigger the sensation of euphoria (the reward system) and just plain make you feel good (temporarily).

Side Effects

There are many side effects possible with opioid therapy because they not only affect pain neurons but many other cell types in the body.

Opioids decrease your ability to fight infections by suppressing the immune system.

Opioids decrease the drive to breathe. This obviously can be lethal and commonly how overdose occurs. If this occurs then the effects of opioids should be reversed with an antagonist (a substance that blocks opioids from binding to the mu receptor) most commonly Naloxone.

Opioids have a profound effect on the gastrointestinal tract causing a decrease in gastric motility – the ability of your stomach and intestines to move food through. This occurs even at very small doses and can result in profound constipation. In addition, they may precipitate gall stones and gall bladder pain because they also result in a reduction of the gall bladder's ability to empty.

Opioids may cause an inability to urinate because they can cause an increase in urinary sphincter tone, making it difficult for the sphincter to relax and allow the passage of urine.

Opioids can result in a release of histamine in the skin and thus cause significant itching.

Opioids also have effects on your cardiovascular system causing your heart rate to slow.

Opioid-induced Hyperalgesia

Hyperalgesia refers to the process of becoming more sensitive to pain. This can occur paradoxically with opioid administration, that is, instead of getting pain relief with opioids, the patient becomes more sensitive to pain. The physiology of this process is not entirely clear but has to do with an alteration in the biology of the endogenous (the body's own) opioid system. Opioid- induced hyperalgesia typically occurs after a period of chronic (ongoing) opioid exposure (1). It is unclear at what stage or for how long you can take opioids before this occurs, but this increased sensitivity to pain throughout your body has been reported in less than a month (2).

In opioid-induced hyperalgesia (abnormally heightened sensitivity to pain), pain is generally diffuse and ill-defined. That is why I <u>only</u> recommend opioid use for the treatment of acute pain, such as the pain after surgery. I do not believe opioids should be used for chronic pain (pain which lasts more than 4 weeks) as opioids end up causing more problems than they solve. I have had patients who were taking tremendous doses of opioids, helped these patients come off them entirely after years of use and seen them have the same or LESS pain than they were experiencing with the heavy, daily use of narcotics. The one exception to this rule in my practice is the use of opioids for palliative pain control, that is, for pain control in cases where no other treatments are feasible.

Addiction/Physical Dependence and Abuse

Opioids activate the reward system in your brain, meaning that when you take them you experience a pleasurable or a rewarding experience (euphoria). The reward system exists to drive beneficial behaviors such as eating high calorie foods (to prevent starvation). Opioids however hijack this natural system to artificially create a reinforcing sensation in your body which only drives you to take more opioids. **Addiction** is defined as both a physiological and behavioral compulsion to take a drug continuously for its psychological effect and to avoid the symptoms of withdrawal. Both the μ (mu) and δ (delta) receptors as well as dopamine (another neurotransmitter) receptor mediate reward and subsequent addiction.

When opioids are administered for a short time for an acute (severe but short-lasting) condition, the opioids decrease your sensation of pain. They do this by deactivating a G-coupled cellular messaging system named cyclic adenosine monophosphate (cAMP), thereby reducing the overall level of cAMP in your body. cAMP affects genetic expression enhancing pain transmission in the cell and, since a short use of opioids decreases cAMP production, at first taking opioids results in you feeling less pain.

However, administering opioids for chronic pain over a longer period of time results in upregulation (an increase) and activation of cAMP (3), **producing not less pain but more pain**—in essence, something changes in the cellular machinery that responds to opioids with use over time. This molecular change is what drives addiction and increased pain sensitivity.

Those who are dependent on opioids may experience an adverse **withdrawal syndrome** when they stop taking opioids, characterized by cravings, irritability, anxiety, insomnia, abdominal pain and nausea, and pain sensitivity. These symptoms are due to the increased activity around the brain known as the locus coeruleus, which is responsible for the response to stress (these neurons are typically suppressed with opioids). The addicted patient's effort to avoid these symptoms results in a physical dependence on the drug. To avoid withdrawal symptoms the dosage may be decreased by 10-20% every 2 days until you are completely off, safely.

Addiction can lead to abuse of opioid drugs which, unfortunately, is a very common problem in the United States, affecting over 3 million people (4). **All opioids carry a risk for abuse.** At higher risk are those who have either a personal or familial history of drug abuse, are a younger age (under 40 years), experience mental disorders, or are experiencing more severe pain. Because of the high risk of addiction and dependence, many physicians defer prescribing opioids to a doctor who is familiar not only with appropriate dosing and medical effects but also the legal aspects—all opioids are now controlled substances which are closely monitored by government agencies. Many states require the prescribing physician make sure that the patient is not obtaining the drug from multiple sources by checking a prescription drug monitoring program (PDMP) prior to dispensing any opioids. Patients should only receive opioid medications from **one prescriber**. Furthermore, opioids are typically not dispensed in longer than 1-week courses.

Tolerance

Over time, opioids predictably lose their effects and higher doses are required. This is mainly because your body can eliminate the drug from your system faster and faster the more opioids you take. Moreover, continued use of opioid drugs causes your body to adapt to the high levels of opioid drugs by both decreasing the number of receptors for them on neurons and making the receptors less effective (they become desensitized) causing the cellular response to reverse. To get the same effect you now need to take double, triple or even quadruple the amount of drug. Again, we are not sure exactly when this happens, and the timing is a little different for everyone, but rest assured, it will eventually happen to you if you keep taking them.

Types of Opioids

There are several classifications of opioid drugs. They may be classified based on the degree to which they affect the potency of opioid receptors, either by stimulating (agonists) or inhibiting (antagonists) the opioid receptors.

agonists

Agonists are drugs that artificially stimulate the receptor to do what it does naturally—in the case of opioid receptors, to give pain relief by making you feel euphoric. Antagonists bind to the receptor but do not stimulate it—see the section below to understand their medical benefit.

- **Partial Agonists: buprenorphine**

- **Agonists: morphine, codeine, methadone, fentanyl, hydromorphone, oxycodone, tramadol**

- **Agonist-Antagonists: butorphanol, nalbuphine, pentazocine, dezocine**

- **Antagonists: naloxone, naltrexone**

IV (intravenous) opioids

Morphine is a naturally occurring plant chemical derived from the seed capsules of the poppy flower. It may be administered orally, rectally or parenterally (via injection) and it acts fast and typically lasts for 2-3 hours. It is used mainly for moderate to severe acute pain. It can cause severe respiratory depression, itching, nausea and constipation among other symptoms.

Dilaudid (hydromorphone) is a derivative of morphine which is 6-8 times as potent and thus mainly used as an IV medicine in the hospital setting to treat severe pain.

oral opioids

Tramadol is a synthetic opioid with a half-life of 6 hours. This medicine is contraindicated in patients who are taking antidepressants such as monoamine oxidase (MAO) inhibitors because it also has effects on the monoamine system by inhibiting reuptake (reabsorption) of serotonin and norepinephrine, neurotransmitters which affect your mood. Unlike its sister opioids, tramadol has a low potential for dependence and produces minimal respiratory depression and it is about 1/10 of the strength of morphine. I prescribe this medication for many of my outpatient surgeries (surgeries with same day discharge from the hospital).

Hydrocodone is a synthetic opioid that is typically orally administered in combination with another pain medication like acetaminophen. It has a high potential for addiction.

Oxycodone is a derivative of morphine with a longer half-life in the body (roughly 3-6 hours). Unlike tramadol, both oxycodone and hydrocodone have a high potential for addiction and dependency.

Opioid Agonists		
Drug Name	**Half Life**	**Morphine Equivalency (Strength Relative to Morphine)**
Tramadol	6-9 hours	0.1X
Morphine	2-3 hours	1X
Hydrocodone	3-6 hours	1X
Oxycodone (Roxicodone®)	3-6 hours	1.5X
Hydromorphone (Dilaudid)	2-3 hours	7X
Fentanyl	3-4 hours	100X

antagonists

An antagonist is a substance which binds to a receptor but instead of activating it, it deactivates it or does nothing. Antagonists also block the true agonist from activating the receptor and thus **can be used to** *reverse* **the effect of opioids. Naloxone** is an opioid antagonist, meaning that it binds to the opioid receptor but does not cause any of the known effects of opioids. It can be used to reverse the ill effects of opioids by blocking their binding to receptors that influence respiratory depression, sedation, analgesia and slow gastric transit. They are commonly used to reverse an overdose of opioids in patients who are at risk for respiratory depression.

Opioids and the Spine Surgical Patient

Not only do opioids have a profound impact on health if used for prolonged courses, they can also impact the results of surgery. Many spine patients use opioids to try to avoid surgery and, in some cases, continued non-operative treatment is associated with an increased risk of long-term opioid therapy. Up to 42% of lumbar stenosis patients report opioid use, 21% of whom continued for up to 24 months (5). In a large prospective study, patients who used opioids prior to their surgical treatment had significantly worse baseline pain and quality of life, and thus are more likely to need surgery (6). However, studies have shown that even short term opioid use leads to worse clinical outcomes following a routine spine surgery, a lumbar microdiscectomy (7).

Conclusion

Opioids are very powerful drugs that give us the potential to do surgery with less pain. They are, however, a double-edged sword and can cause many problems such as dependence, and a host of side effects. Ultimately, they sensitize you to pain if taken for too long and increase your tolerance to their effects, making them ineffective long term.

Frequently Asked Questions

- **I have chronic low back pain, should I take Opioids?**

     Most likely no. Opioids are excellent for short term pain control. They should not be used for the treatment of chronic low back pain.

- **Opioids have been about the only thing to help me with my pain, it's how I continue to function, how do you expect me to stop them?**

     Unfortunately, I get this question all the time. Prior to the epidemic of opioid over- prescription, these drugs used to be given out like candy. This mainly benefited the drug companies which are now paying for it in major lawsuits (8). The problem with long term opioid use is the addictive nature of the drugs—you become dependent on them and they change the way you perceive pain for the worse. Are the opioids relieving your pain or merely preventing withdrawal symptoms? On top of this, they have many negative side effects and do not actually treat the problem which is causing you pain. Furthermore, the prescription of opioids is now governed by a host of laws where a physician could possibly have his/her license revoked for inappropriate or over administration (9). There are cases where opioids are appropriate as there may not be a good treatment option but this is a careful decision usually made in coordination with a pain management doctor.

References

1.   Higgins C, Smith BH, Matthews K. Evidence of opioid-induced hyperalgesia in clinical populations after chronic opioid exposure: a systematic review and meta-analysis. Br J Anaesth. 2019 Jun;122(6):e114–26.

2.   Yi P, Pryzbylkowski P. Opioid Induced Hyperalgesia. Pain Med. 2015 Oct;16(suppl 1):S32–6.

3.   Camí J, Farré M. Drug addiction. N Engl J Med. 2003 Sep 4;349(10):975–86.

4.   Results from the 2015 National Survey on Drug Use and Health: Detailed Tables, SAMHSA, CBHSQ [Internet]. [cited 2020 Jun 16]. Available from: https://www.samhsa.gov/data/sites/default/files/NSDUH-DetTabs-2015/NSDUH-DetTabs-2015/NSDUH-DetTabs-2015.htm

5.   Krebs EE, Lurie JD, Fanciullo G, Tosteson TD, Blood EA, Carey TS, et al. Predictors of Long-Term Opioid Use Among Patients With Painful Lumbar Spine Conditions. J Pain. 2010 Jan;11(1):44–52.

6.   Radcliff K, Freedman M, Hilibrand A, Isaac R, Lurie JD, Zhao W, et al. Does Opioid Pain Medication Use Affect the Outcome of Patients With Lumbar Disc Herniation?: Spine. 2013 Jun;38(14):E849–60.

7.   Virk S, Sandhu M, Qureshi S, Albert T, Sandhu H. How does preoperative opioid use impact postoperative health-related quality of life scores for patients undergoing lumbar microdiscectomy? Spine J. 2020 May;S1529943020302850.

8.   Hoffman J. $26 Billion Settlement Offer in Opioid Lawsuits Gains Wide Support. The New York Times [Internet]. 2020 Nov 5 [cited 2022 Jan 6]; Available from: https://www.nytimes.com/2020/11/05/health/opioids-settlement-distributors.html

9.   Webster LR, Grabois M. Current Regulations Related to Opioid Prescribing. PM R. 2015 Nov;7(11 Suppl):S236–47.

Chapter 21

Alternative Therapy: Ergonomics, Exercise, Physical Therapy, Acupuncture, Chiropractor and Others

Summary

The body is a machine, and it is important that it receives regular maintenance to keep working optimally. This includes avoiding repetitive motions or strenuous positions common in most lines of work, including in the office setting. The field of ergonomics can help to prevent such injuries, offering better, less strenuous ways to work. Regular exercise, focusing on some form of core strength to help maintain the structure of your spine, as well as cardiovascular exercise to keep your body fit, is critical. Physical therapists can help guide you in exercise and train you in a home program that can be helpful in keeping back pain at bay. Other alternative treatments such as going to a chiropractor or using acupuncture can be very helpful in certain scenarios. The treatments in this chapter are so called "alternative therapy" because they are not considered part of mainstream medicine. Talk with your physician before pursuing treatments in this chapter. If you want to try an alternative treatment, it should be done under physician supervision and stopped immediately if it's not helpful.

Case

Mr. Thistle is a 54-year-old computer programmer who suffers from chronic low back pain and obesity. He sits at his desk most of the day staring at a computer and typing rapidly. He has visited me in my clinic looking for a solution to his problem, but I tell him there is nothing surgery can do to help. He wants a quick fix in the form of surgery, but I tell him surgery will only hurt him. There are treatments to cure his problems, but they will take work. He needs to get more exercise, lose weight, and practice better habits at work. In other words, he needs to change his lifestyle and discontinue his unhealthy habits, which are the source of his problems. His back pain is starting to interfere with his home life as he can no longer play with his children—for them he knows he needs to make a change. He is determined not to be beaten by his back pain and under the instruction of a physical therapist starts to exercise. He starts slow, carefully building flexibility, strength, and cardiovascular endurance. He builds a regular core strength routine into his day and takes brisk walks 4 times a week. Suddenly his back pain is getting better. At work, he no longer sits for prolonged periods, making sure to stand, stretch and walk every 30-40 minutes. He changes to a desk chair with good lumbar support and starts to diet, losing 20 pounds. After several months of this behavior his back pain is gone, and it seems crazy that he was even contemplating spine surgery.

Introduction

This chapter is devoted to the discussion of alternative therapies that can be a good addition to the traditional mainstream medical care of your spine that is, medications and surgery). Used with careful supervision they have provided many with significant relief and in specific cases perhaps even helped to avoid surgery. Importantly, some of the methods noted in this chapter have very low risk (compared to surgery) so regardless of whether they work, they can be worth a try before considering spinal surgery. However, before pursuing the treatments in this chapter, it is critical to have a physician perform a full clinical exam and diagnostic workup (observe, ask questions, and order tests as needed). This is to ensure you do not ignore serious problems which are best treated with medicine or surgery or risk worsening the condition with ineffective treatments. Nothing in this chapter will fix a serious problem in the spine, so get checked out first and make sure you do not have a serious problem before trying one of these alternative therapies. Finally, keep in mind most of the advice in this chapter is driven by common sense.

Basic Mental Health

It may sound silly, but your overall mental health plays an important role in how you interpret pain. Have you ever noticed you are aware of your body aches more after a stressful day at work while on the weekend at the beach you have relatively no pain? Stress, anxiety, and insomnia all play a critical role in how your mind interprets pain. Are you getting at least 7-8 hours of sleep a night? Do you find yourself fixated on your pain while you are at work or are in stressful situations? If you have trouble with sleep, back pain and spine pain can become even more difficult to deal with. This is because your mind exerts control on the interpretation and processing of pain. Per the gate control theory of pain (see chapter 2), your brain has the power to enhance or shut down pain perception.

You must remember that your mind has a finite amount of power. If it is drained by anxiety, stress, and insomnia, it loses the ability to regulate pain. I devote an entire chapter to the discussion of psychology and how you can harness the power of your mind to fortify your body (see chapter 28 on the impact of psychology on spine surgery).

Weight Loss

Losing weight merits an entire chapter of its own, chapter 24. Suffice to say, losing weight can be excellent for relieving back pain.

Ergonomics

Despite your best intentions, **back pain or spinal problems may arise** without any significant event such as a fall or collision but, rather, **just from daily use**. Perhaps you notice your neck hurts after a long day at the office or from holding a phone against your head. Musculoskeletal problems of the spine can arise from overuse or incorrect use of certain muscles and from repetitive motions. Ergonomics refers to the science, engineering and design of household objects and furniture to reduce stress and strain on the human body. **The overarching goal of ergonomics is to prevent your spine from being in an abnormal posture for extended periods.**

However, it is also important to exercise common sense regarding ergonomics and therapy. If something hurts your spine, it's probably not good to keep doing it even if advertisements and friends swear by it. Just because something is advertised to reduce strain on the body doesn't mean it accomplishes that. And sitting for hours even in the best chair is bad for your back and body as a whole. **Be aware of your body**.

office ergonomics

Office work includes a lot of opportunity to strain your low back and neck because of all the repetitive motions and stationary positions that it involves. Applying the principles of ergonomics to the office setting can reduce injury. For example, it is critical to have any desk top monitor set at a comfortable eye level height to prevent neck strain. Obviously holding a phone against your head with your neck craned to hold the phone in place is not good for anyone who suffers from neck pain. A hands-free headset can help reduce this strain. A supportive adjustable chair with a lumbar support can help prevent your low back from resting in a poor posture for hours and reduce back pain symptoms (1). You really should not be sitting in a chair in one position for greater than 30-40 minutes. For many people, even with an ergonomic chair, if they have poor posture, they will still be placing undue stress on the spine and its discs. Sit with your back tall, and a slight arch in the lumbar spine. Use a footrest. And let your head float on your neck instead of jutting it out in front of your chest as you intently view your computer. Ideally your knees should be even with or slightly lower than your hips.

sleep ergonomics

Your mattress also plays a critical role in preventing your spine from collapsing into an abnormal posture and staying like that overnight. For this reason, firm mattresses are preferable to softer ones that allow your back to sag and collapse. Having the right pillow is also important to prevent neck pain. Just like you should maintain a neutral neck position at a desk, you should also do so while sleeping. This means having your neck supported in a position where it is in line with your body. This usually requires at least two pillows, especially if you sleep on your side (to fill the space between your bed and your head that your shoulder creates). Everyone has different pillow preferences, but I recommend soft latex filled pillows. They are spongy and do not collapse as much as down pillows offering more consistent support. I also recommend sleeping on your back with a pillow under the knees or on your side with your neck supported.

driving ergonomics

Your car, where you may spend a considerable amount of time, also plays a role in supporting your spine. Firstly, you should examine your driving style. Do you often aggressively pump the gas and then suddenly brake? This is likely putting significant strain on your spine from frequent accelerations and decelerations and so you should consider shifting to a smoother driving style. Although switching cars is not always practical, when looking for a new car, you should carefully examine the seat. Is it comfortable? Does it support your entire spine? Does it have lumbar support to help maintain your low back curvature? (Yes, some car seats have built in lumbar support). Is there a neck and head rest to prevent your head from snapping back in the event of a rear-end collision? Does the car have deforming bumpers which can absorb some of the shock of an impact, thereby protecting you in the event of a collision?

Physical Therapy

Physical therapy (PT) may be an excellent choice to treat your neck or low back pain, depending on your spine problem. It is typically prescribed by physicians and guided by physical therapists who are trained in musculoskeletal disease. Working closely with physicians, physical therapists can help guide exercise that promotes strengthening and flexibility. The fundamental tenet behind PT is that **movement** is good for your body and guiding you in exercise are physical therapists' most important function. They may also be trained in other "**modalities**" such as icing, massage, traction, transcutaneous electrical stimulation, deep tissue release, ultrasound, and matrix rhythm therapy, which can be comforting treatments of disc herniations and low back pain. However, all these modalities are less important than the actual exercise—yet often they are easier for a physical therapist to provide than getting you to exercise. If your PT is not emphasizing exercise, you should switch therapists.

PT can really improve pain but if selected for the wrong reasons or the wrong disease it can easily worsen spinal conditions. Thus, it is important to work with a physician to determine what is the safest course of action. Most courses of physical therapy should be attempted for six weeks with sessions twice or three times a week. The therapist should also prescribe a home exercise program for you to perform daily on your own. If significant improvement is not noted in six weeks, it is best to re-consult your physician on the next best course of action.

Exercise

It may seem counterintuitive, but **the skeleton and muscles require motion to prevent degeneration**. Your bones need to be loaded to stay strong. Your joints need to move to stay supple. The facet joints of the spine, just like the knee or hip, are synovial joints meaning they contain a lubricating fluid which facilitates gliding motion but also feeds nutrients to the cartilage surface. Without motion, the joint fluid cannot circulate, and the cartilage becomes diseased and brittle, resulting in arthritis. Muscles and bones similarly require pressure and tension to maintain their strength.

Motion helps strengthen your spine, but, also, the many joints and discs in the spine require motion to obtain nutrition and lubrication. In fact, exercise is one of the only non-operative modalities shown to improve back pain and function and should be an integral part of healthy life (2,3). In general bed rest is terrible for low back pain and a sedentary lifestyle has been shown to be a risk factor for increased low back pain (4). **Moderate exercise is critical to maintaining a good back and neck**.

There are other benefits to exercise. Cardiovascular workouts are protective against diabetes, cardiovascular disease, obesity, cancer and even brain atrophy (gradual wasting away) (5)! As little as 15 minutes of daily exercise has been associated with a 3-year increase in life expectancy (6)! The recommendations from the American Heart Association for lowering cholesterol and blood pressure are 40 minutes of aerobic exercise 3-4 times a week (6).

three components of effective back exercises

So, what type of exercise should you do for your back? I have many patients say, "I have too much pain to exercise." While it's true that some exercises can worsen your problem there are so many different types of exercises available, it's easy to find alternative types that work for you. No matter what type of exercise works for you there are 3 main components: **flexibility, strength-building,** and **cardiovascular conditioning**. Flexibility allows your ligaments and muscles to move without breaking and allows optimal nutrition to the joints. Your core muscles act as a suspension system for your spine. Strength in the core spinal muscles unload the bones and ligaments by providing the power to keep your spine upright (think of a suspension bridge where your spine is the road, and the muscles are the cables which hold the road off the water—you don't want the cables to sag). Cardiovascular conditioning ensures good blood flow and oxygenation of the tissues. Let's discuss some of the specific areas which I believe are critical for maintaining your spine.

flexibility

You may not realize it, but when one area of your body is stiff, other suppler areas of the body compensate. For example, patients who have stiff shoulders elevate their arms by using more shoulder blade (scapula) motion and through bending the spine. Patients who have stiff hips, bend more through the spine when they try to pick something off the ground. The spine is a chain, and when certain areas become stiff it forces more motion out of the other segments. In your lower extremity, for example, hip, knee, and ankle stiffness can all impact your spine (with the parts closer to the spine, such as the hips, playing a more important role). Similarly, in the upper extremity, shoulder stiffness can put more demand on the spine. When the hips cannot move well, your spine must move more to make up for this. Thus stiffness in other areas of the body can result in low back problems (7). To ensure that undue stress is not placed on the spine, it is paramount to maintain flexibility not only in the spine, but, also, in the lower and upper extremities.

In the era of the "desk job" and the sedentary lifestyle, stiffness can creep up on you without you even realizing it. Then you go to pick up something off the ground, take out the trash or unload the laundry and you pull something that is stiff. Better to prevent things like this from happening by staying ahead of the game—**keep your flexibility a priority with a regular daily stretching program**:

- **Cat and camel stretches: This is a simple stretch to begin your exercise program with. Perform this by getting on all fours. First, extend the spine (with firm abdominals, exhale, and push chest toward floor, look up slightly arching your back). Then flex the spine (inhale, lift lower rib cage and round back, relaxing neck) and follow by gentle rotation clockwise and counterclockwise and some lateral bending (think of wagging your tail from side to side).**

- **Back extension: lie flat on your stomach and push up with your arms arching your back.**

- **Hamstring stretches: this can be done several ways. One way is to place your hands on a wall with one leg in front of the other and lean into the wall. Hold for 10 seconds and switch to the other side. Another way is to sit on the ground with one leg outstretched and the other foot touching the knee. Lean forward and try to hold your toes.**

- **Iliotibial and paraspinal stretch: lay on the ground and cross your knee over your body such that it touches the ground on the other side. Breathe and hold for 10 seconds. Repeat on the other side.**

- **Gluteal and external rotator stretch: lie on the ground and bend one knee up off the ground. Place the other foot on that knee and pull your knee towards your chest. Repeat on the other side.**

- **Quadriceps stretch: Lying on your side, pull the ankle that is up behind such that your knee and thigh are stretched. Repeat on the other side.**

- **Upper extremity and torso stretch: sitting up, bend one elbow behind your head and, using your other hand, pull on the elbow. Allow the shoulder to stretch and the lumbar and thoracic spine to bend laterally. Repeat on the other side.**

Try to have a stretching routine that lasts for at least 5 minutes. Do each stretch 5-10 times daily. Take two deep breaths for each stretch to maximize the amount of oxygen getting to the tissues during the stretch. Obviously, there are many different stretching programs out there and this is just an example. Find one you like and try to practice it daily.

core strength

Your "core" is a complex system of muscles that consists of the major muscles that support your trunk and pelvis (the torso). Conceptually, the core is a "box" of 29 paired muscles with the abdominals and paraspinals forming the front and back of that "box" and the diaphragm and pelvic floor forming the roof and floor (8). These 29 muscles include the abdominal muscles (rectus abdominus, internal and external obliques, transversus abdominus), the posterior spinal musculature (the erector spinae, multifidus, quadratus lumborum), the muscles of the pelvis (pelvic floor, gluteus maximus), and the diaphragm. A select group of these muscles attach to the thoracolumbar fascia which acts as a natural "back belt" surrounding your abdomen.

Your core is what maintains your posture and supports your spine and pelvis. The complicated strut system helps keep the spine in balance and finely tune your posture. The muscles literally share the load with the bones and act to suspend the skeleton—they provide "active support." The core also helps to support movement of the upper and lower extremities. A spine devoid of muscles is incapable of supporting normal physiologic loads and the motion of your torso (9). In a person with a weak core, the spine bones support a greater proportion of your body weight than nature intended, causing the vertebrae, discs, and ligaments of the spine, which provide "passive support" of the torso, to undergo more rapid degeneration. Remember that the bones and ligaments do not move on their own, if the muscles weaken, they are forced to bear more weight. Moreover, if your core is not maintained, imbalance between the front and back muscles will develop, leading to strain on the weaker set (usually the back paraspinal muscles). Low back pain has been associated with weak core muscles (8).

A general spine maintenance program should include range of motion and flexibility exercises such as described above, coupled with simple core-strengthening exercises. The strengthening and flexibility programs should be progressive, meaning you first work to regain normal strength and motion of the core before trying anything too aggressive. It does not mean suddenly starting with 100 pushups and sit-ups.

Simple strengthening exercises may begin with **abdominal hollowing** and **abdominal bracing**, which are contrasting strategies to activate the abdominal musculature, particularly the transversus abdominus. Abdominal hollowing is simply drawing in the abdomen towards the lumbar spine while maintaining your posture and continuing to breathe normally. Abdominal bracing is when you contract your abdominal muscles in a static neutral position while normal breathing is maintained (10). Do 10 reps of each. After bracing, you should focus on your balance. **Balance** will help fine tune the multiple small stabilizer muscles in the back that are not readily exercised with gross movement. A simple balance exercise is to stand on one leg (if your balance is poor stand near the sink or something else you can hold on to if you feel unsteady) and abduct (bring out) the other leg out to the side and in. Do this for 20 reps on each side and close your eyes for a real challenge. **Following a guided progression of abdominal bracing, more advanced exercises may be started such as the following:**

- **Curl up/hip bridge: starting from lying supine on the floor, place your hands under the small of your back and bend your knees. Raise your torso off the ground in one unit, keeping your shoulders on the ground and hold off the ground.**

- **Side plank: lie on your side with your arm out in a straight line from the shoulder at 90 degrees and your elbow on the floor. The hips should be held off the floor. Hold for 30 seconds to a minute.**

- **Quadruped position with alternate arm /leg raises (bird dog): position yourself on all fours and sequentially elevate your arm and the opposite leg so that they are straight. Then repeat on the other side.**

- **Prone plank: Get into the push-up position with your elbows on the ground bent at 90° and toes on the ground with your knees off the ground. Hold for 30 seconds to a minute.**

- **Locust pose/superman: lie on your stomach with your arms in front of you and off the ground. Elevate one leg off the ground keeping your neck and back straight while also elevating the opposite arm. Hold the leg off the ground for 10 seconds and repeat on the other side. You can also elevate both arms and legs at the same time (a true superman position).**

A basic core strength program may be created from these exercises and others as guided by a physical therapist or trainer. As you progress, other more advanced exercises may be attempted. However, caution should be exhibited with certain exercises. Traditional sit-ups and exercises which require extreme flexion/ extension and heavy resistance against the spine should be avoided. Spinal exercises should be avoided in the first hour after waking because of increased disk pressure at this time (8).

Many other popular exercise programs strengthen the core including yoga, Pilates, and tai chi. I generally recommend these types of exercises for those who already have healthy backs and are trying to keep it that way. Some of the motions of yoga and Pilates can easily be overdone and should not be attempted by certain spine patients. Please check with your doctor before attempting this type of exercise.

cardiovascular conditioning

Walking: Walking is the essential spine exercise. It can exercise your core, build your cardiovascular system, and move the joints of the spine. Importantly, walking places very low strain and stress on the spine. It is great for getting exercise when you have a spine problem or are recovering from spine surgery. A typical walking schedule is as easy as picking a route that you like that typically takes 30 minutes to complete and to walk it at a brisk pace, once or twice daily.

Aqua therapy: The problem with many aerobic exercises (such as running, walking) is that patients with arthritis will not tolerate them very well. The joints are already painful and getting exercise can be difficult. For patients with arthritis, aqua therapy offers an alternative approach to get exercise, lose weight and build cardiovascular reserve. This is because your body is buoyant in water and thus the weight on your joints is reduced, much like being in a lower gravity. Nonetheless, the viscosity of water provides enough resistance for the muscles to provide exercise. The most basic form of aqua therapy is getting into a pool, the water between waist and chest level (enough that a good portion of the torso is covered, but not so high you are lapping water), and walking back and forth in the lap lane swinging your arms gently against the water for 30 minutes. Many pools may offer water aerobics classes which may be a useful way to get exercise. Obviously, common sense must be exercised and working yourself to extreme fatigue in water can be dangerous. Unfortunately, aqua therapy does require access to a pool or body of water.

Running: Running is an excellent form of cardiovascular exercise. While overuse injuries (particularly knee injuries such as patellofemoral syndrome, as well as iliotibial band syndrome and plantar fasciitis) may be caused by running, the spine is rarely injured from running (11). Contrary to popular belief, long distance runners are not at increased risk for osteoarthritis and running may actually protect against it (12). As you age your body undergoes a natural decrease in aerobic capacity which running may help prevent (13). However, if you have just had spine surgery, running is much too jarring and should be avoided.

Other Alternative Therapies

My disclaimer for the therapies introduced in this section of the chapter is that while they can be helpful, they cost money and have no real proven effect on curing spinal problems. If they help you and you enjoy them, I think it's fine to use them, so long as there is no major spinal problem that you are ignoring. If you give them a shot and the effect is only temporary, you may want to reconsider continued use since each visit will cost you money.

acupuncture

Acupuncture is a part of ancient Chinese medicine to treat pain. Small needles are placed in the skin according to set patterns. Interpreted through the lens of modern science, the sensation of the needles can distract your nervous system and mind from your pain. In this way, it is like spinal cord stimulation which activates the dorsal columns (an area of the spinal cord) to close the gate for pain transmission in the spinal cord. Acupuncture may be used to treat chronic low back pain or neck pain from whiplash (14,15). Acupuncture treatments, while useful in treating pain, tend to be short-lived and can become costly. Make sure your acupuncturist is properly trained and uses disposable needles.

chiropractic medicine

Chiropractic manipulation is an alternative medicine that is based on the idea that spinal disorders arise from malalignment of the spine and that manipulations can "realign the spine." Although many patients do find relief from chiropractic treatments, the benefits are generally short-lived and require many sessions, which can become costly.

Bishop et al conducted a prospective study on the use of chiropractic medicine to treat those with acute low back pain without red flags (signs of a serious condition) and showed improvement in outcome measures and concluded that it could be a feasible component of primary care (16). The one caveat to this is that I almost never recommend neck manipulation without a careful screening for any neck problems. Serious accidents resulting in stroke, paralysis and death have occurred when neck manipulation was performed unwittingly on patients with serious cervical spine problems (17).

low level (cold) laser therapy

Many alternative medical practitioners offer low level laser therapy, also known as cold laser therapy, as part of non-operative treatment to treat pain. The cold laser's beam is generally directed at areas of pain and can be used on a variety of sites. The theory is that photons delivered through the skin at levels low enough to not be harmful will induce biologic activity and healing. There are many claims that lasers increase blood flow and stimulate natural opioid release, but, ultimately, the effects are not well-understood or proven. Many studies on the use of cold laser therapy fail to give adequate technical details or fail to adhere to strict treatment protocols (18). While this treatment may be relatively safe and may offer some relief, it is critical you see a medical doctor and have a working diagnosis of your problem before you pursue treatments such as this.

Conclusion

The paramount message of this chapter is that exercise is important not only for your overall health, but also for that of your spine. Physical therapists are specially trained to help you stretch and maintain strength. They get you to exercise and this can relieve many musculoskeletal pains. You should develop your own independent exercise program focusing on flexibility, strength, and cardiovascular conditioning. There are other treatments that exist to help with back pain such as chiropractic manipulation and acupuncture. These should be used only after serious causes of spine pain are ruled out.

Frequently Asked Questions

- **Why can't you just do the surgery to cure my problem?**

    While some problems require surgery to fix, we must remember that surgery won't help everyone. Furthermore, surgery carries some risk. Some problems stem from a poor lifestyle and thus the cure is to change the lifestyle. This undoubtedly is hard and takes work, but it can be empowering to take control of your health.

References

1.   Iii BCA, Robertson MM, DeRango K, Bazzani L, Moore A, Rooney T, et al. Effect of Office Ergonomics Intervention on Reducing Musculoskeletal Symptoms. :6.

2.   Linton SJ, van Tulder MW. Preventive Interventions for Back and Neck Pain Problems: What is the Evidence? Spine. 2001 Apr;26(7):778–87.

3.   Taimela S, Diederich C, Hubsch M, Heinricy M. The Role of Physical Exercise and Inactivity in Pain Recurrence and Absenteeism From Work After Active Outpatient Rehabilitation for Recurrent or Chronic Low Back Pain: A Follow-Up Study. Spine. 2000 Jul;25(14):1809–16.

4.   Lemes ÍR, Pinto RZ, Turi Lynch BC, Codogno JS, Oliveira CB, Ross LM, et al. The Association Between Leisure-time Physical Activity, Sedentary Behavior, and Low Back Pain: A Cross-sectional Analysis in Primary Care Settings. Spine. 2021 May 1;46(9):596–602.

5.   2013 AHA/ACC Guideline on Lifestyle Management to Reduce Cardiovascular Risk. :24.

6.   Wen CP, Wai JPM, Tsai MK, Yang YC, Cheng TYD, Lee MC, et al. Minimum amount of physical activity for reduced mortality and extended life expectancy: a prospective cohort study. The Lancet. 2011 Oct;378(9798):1244–53.

7.   Vad VB, Bhat AL, Basrai D, Gebeh A, Aspergren DD, Andrews JR. Low back pain in professional golfers: the role of associated hip and low back range-of-motion deficits. Am J Sports Med. 2004 Mar;32(2):494–7.

8.   Akuthota V, Ferreiro A, Moore T, Fredericson M. Core Stability Exercise Principles: Curr Sports Med Rep. 2008 Jan;7(1):39–44.

9.   Panjabi M, Abumi K, Duranceau J, Oxland T. Spinal stability and intersegmental muscle forces. A biomechanical model. Spine. 1989 Feb;14(2):194–200.

10.   Grenier SG, McGill SM. Quantification of Lumbar Stability by Using 2 Different Abdominal Activation Strategies. Arch Phys Med Rehabil. 2007 Jan;88(1):54–62.

11.   Taunton JE. A retrospective case-control analysis of 2002 running injuries. Br J Sports Med. 2002 Apr 1;36(2):95–101.

12.   Vigdorchik JM, Nepple JJ, Eftekhary N, Leunig M, Clohisy JC. What Is the Association of Elite Sporting Activities With the Development of Hip Osteoarthritis? Am J Sports Med. 2017 Mar;45(4):961–4.

13.   Spiker AM, Johnson KB, Cosgarea AJ, Ficke JR. A Primer on Running for the Orthopaedic Surgeon. J Am Acad Orthop Surg. 2020 Jun 15;28(12):481–90.

14.   Lam M, Galvin R, Curry P. Effectiveness of Acupuncture for Nonspecific Chronic Low Back Pain: A Systematic Review and Meta-analysis. Spine. 2013 Nov;38(24):2124–38.

15.   Cameron ID, Wang E, Sindhusake D. A Randomized Trial Comparing Acupuncture and Simulated Acupuncture for Subacute and Chronic Whiplash: Spine. 2011 Dec;36(26):E1659–65.

16.   Bishop PB, Quon JA, Yee BW, Arthur BE, Fedder PG, Forbes JC, et al. 143. Chiropractors treating patients with acute lower back pain in a spine treatment pathway model: a five-year prospective cohort study. Spine J. 2019 Sep;19(9):S69.

17.   Oppenheim JS, Spitzer DE, Segal DH. Nonvascular complications following spinal manipulation. Spine J. 2005 Nov;5(6):660–6.

18.   Clijsen R, Brunner A, Barbero M, Clarys P, Taeymans J. Effects of low-level laser therapy on pain in patients with musculoskeletal disorders: a systematic review and meta-analysis. Eur J Phys Rehabil Med. 2017 Aug;53(4):603–10.

Figures:

The Core Muscles

Front (Anterior):

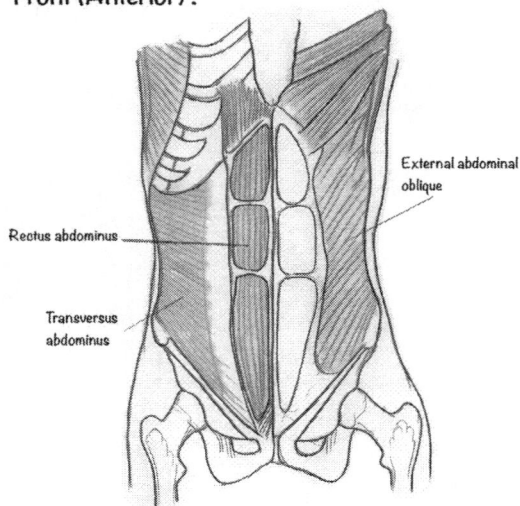

External abdominal oblique

Rectus abdominus

Transversus abdominus

Back (Posterior):

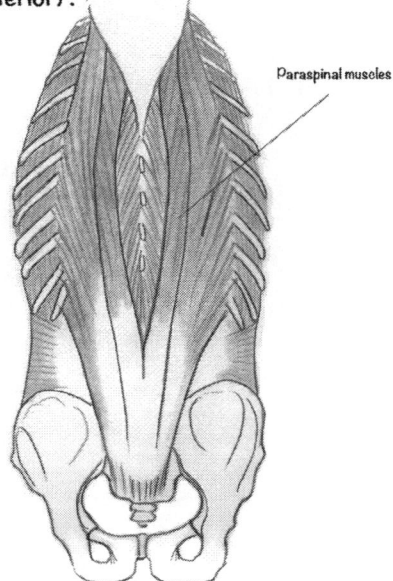

Paraspinal muscles

Core muscles. The core muscles as viewed from the front consist of the rectus abdominus, the internal (beneath the external, not shown) and external obliques and the transversus abdominus (located beneath the obliques, not shown) (top). The core muscles as viewed from behind consist of the paraspinals (bottom).

Core Exercises

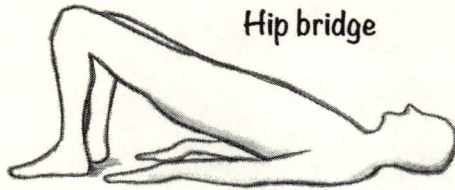

Hip bridge

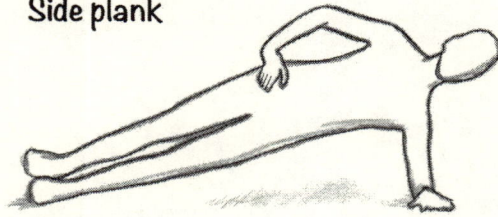

Side plank

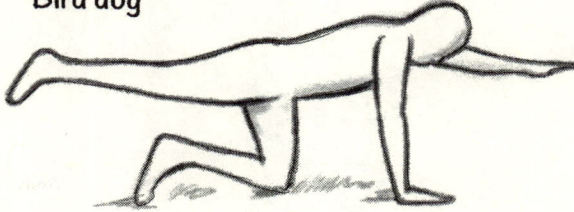

Bird dog

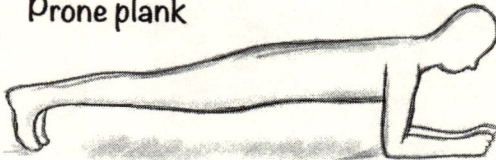

Prone plank

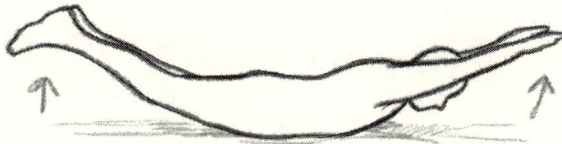

Superman

Core exercises. Please see core strength section for more detailed instructions.

Core Stretches

Camel stretch

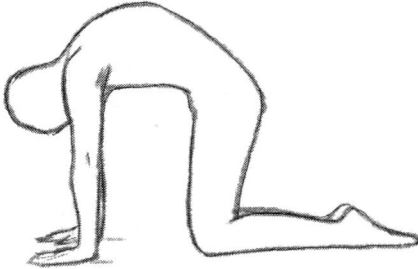

Paraspinal IT band

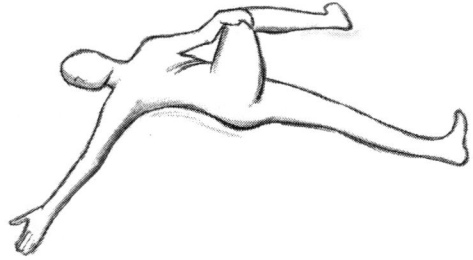

Cat stretch

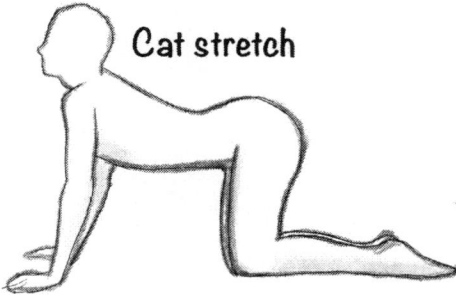

Gluteal stretch

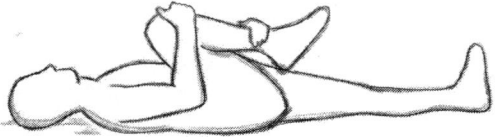

Back extension

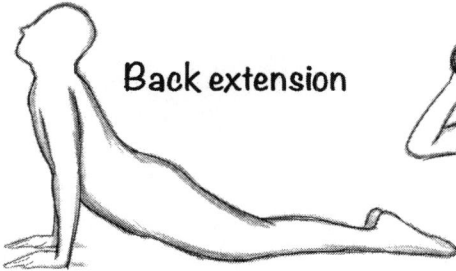

Quadriceps

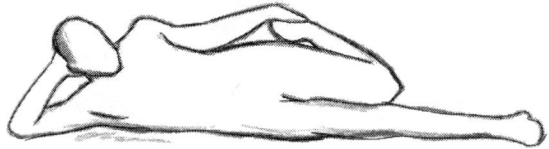

Hamstring

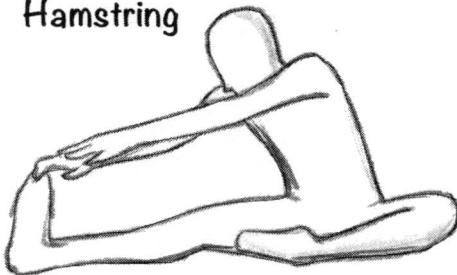

Torso

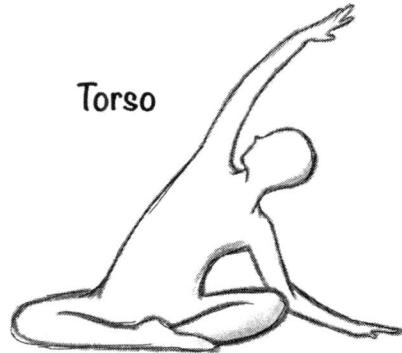

Core Stretches. Please see section on flexibility for detailed instructions.

Chapter 22

Sports and the Spine—Dos And Don'ts

Summary

Sports are an incredible part of the American life, and many people will continue to participate in sports despite injury. Most sports are harmless and healthy to participate in for your spine. However, the high energy/speed sports such as ice hockey, football, rugby, diving, and skiing are the most notorious for causing spine injury. In addition, other non-contact swing sports with a large rotational component (that is, twisting your torso) such as golf and tennis are also capable of causing spine problems. You can avoid catastrophic injury by avoiding high impact or contact sports entirely. If you can't do this, avoid injury by doing sports only when you are awake, alert and focused—many injuries occur when the muscles are fatigued and you are not paying attention. It is certainly possible to return to sports after injury or surgery, but recovery must be slow and gradual.

Case

Golf is one of the most physically demanding sports on your spine. I can think of no case better to exemplify this than that of Tiger Woods, the prodigy golf-

ing star. **Wood's back problems seem to have started around 2014 when he announced that he would miss the Masters Tournament that year because of a spine surgery for a lumbar disc herniation. Later that year he had to withdraw from a tournament after he took an awkward shot irritating his back, causing worsening low back pain. Woods required a second revision microdiscectomy surgery in 2015, and then again, a month later, forcing him to withdraw from competition. This string of surgeries kept Woods out of competition for the ensuing years, while he worked to rehabilitate his back. Unfortunately, he never felt strong enough to play again and underwent an anterior lumbar interbody fusion (ALIF) to try and salvage his spine. This surgery ultimately allowed him to make a fantastic comeback to win the Masters Championship Tournament in 2019 (1). He exemplifies, both how a lumbar spine issue can derail your sports aspirations, but also what incredible power the body has to heal and return to fitness at the highest levels.**

Introduction

One of the most common questions I get in the spine clinic is "What can I do and what can I not do?" The orthopedic surgeon lives to keep his patients active and living the lifestyle that they want, whether that is walking a block or getting back to competitive sport. While we long to stay active, sports are also a common source of back problems and injury. As we get older we all need to find creative ways to stay active and enjoy life. Sometimes this means finding new hobbies or finding ways to exercise that have less impact on our bodies. Spine injuries and disorders can cause major setbacks. I have seen this countless times in middle-aged patients who wonder where the glory days went. This psychological state of mind alone causes significant duress regardless of the injury. It's important to remember that with most spine disorders, recovery is possible and you can get back in the game.

In this chapter we examine the impact of sport on the spine and how to get back in the game after surgery. For more information about the surgeries themselves see chapters discussing those procedures. As a reminder, I use the term "Level" to refer both to individual vertebra (for example, L4) as well as a disc spaces (for example, L4-5).

Sports and Spine Injury

The spine is strong, but still consists of a chain link of bones strung together with ligaments. If it is twisted, pulled or bent in a forceful way, injuries are possible. Most of the time these injuries are minor and amount to pulled muscles that quickly recover. However, though rare, major injuries to the spine resulting in paralysis or the need for surgery are possible in contact and high-speed sports. Roughly 9% of all spinal cord injuries in the United States are sustained from sports (2). Certain sports have a very high risk of spinal cord injury and spine fractures, including diving, football, hockey, horseback riding, rugby, and skiing. In the 1960s, American football players used to tackle with the crown of their heads, a practice known as spear tackling, which resulted in multiple, major catastrophic injuries. Spear tackling was banned in 1976 (2). Whether you are a pro athlete or a weekend warrior, major injury to the spine can occur if you are participating in a high-risk sport. Of course, not all sports-related spine injuries are major, and there is a spectrum of even mild injuries, ranging from sprains to minor fractures of the spine.

Certain spinal conditions may increase the risk of major injury and should be considered before sport participation. Cervical stenosis or congenital (occurring at birth) cervical stenosis is a condition where the spinal canal in the neck is narrow leaving less room for the spinal cord and increases the chance of a neurologic deficit following a spinal injury. It is also possible to have a congenitally narrow lumbar spine which can result in back injury at a much younger age.

Some Conditions with an Increased Risk of Spinal Injury
Congenital stenosis (either lumbar or cervical)
Spinal cord compression
Spinal instability of any variety
Transient spinal cord injury or paralysis
Klippel-Feil syndrome (born with fused cervical vertebrae)

Major Contact Sports

Major contact sports such as American football, ice hockey and rugby are responsible for a large amount of serious spine injuries every year. In football, 4.8% of patients who participated in the National Football League pre-draft combine between 2003 and 2011 reported a cervical (neck) spine problem (2). Both neck and low back disc herniations (see chapter 7) are common in these sports.

Alpine Sports

Alpine sports such as skiing and snowboarding are another common source of spinal injury, especially spine fractures in the mid to low back and in the neck. This is mainly due to high speed/ high impact falls and jump failures (3). While the overall rate of major spinal injury is relatively rare compared to other musculoskeletal injuries, spinal cord injury was reported to occur at a rate of 2.2% of alpine spinal injury patients (spinal injuries account for 2.2% of all alpine injuries). To be safe on the slopes, stay aware— you should not be listening to music while skiing—and you should avoid skiing in overcrowded areas where collision is most likely. When it comes to spine injury, snowboarding, because it has fixed boot bindings, is even more dangerous than skiing, and represents the most dangerous sport after football and ice hockey. As expected, spinal injury is more common in snowboarding compared to skiing—9 out of every 1000 snowboarders will incur a spinal injury per day on the slopes.

Golfing and the Spine

Golf is a popular sport in the United States and can be enjoyed regardless of age. Golf may seem like a benign, non-contact sport; however, golf imparts significant force and demand on the spine. During the golf swing, the spine experiences a tremendous amount of torsion, compression and shear. Loads approximately 8 times your body weight are transmitted through the spine during the swing which is similar to what a D1 lineman experiences when hitting a blocking sled; such loads are more than sufficient to rupture intervertebral discs (4). Considering about 33% of golfers are older than 50 years of age with pre-existing degenerative conditions, this force has the potential to worsen spinal problems. The demands of golfing predisposes golfers to muscle strain, intervertebral disc herniation, compression fractures and facet (spinal joint) damage.

Your golfing technique may have an impact on whether you will develop spinal injury. There are two main swings in golf: the modern and the classic. The two are distinct based on the amount of separation between the degree of motion at the hips and the degree of motion at the shoulders, known as the X-factor. In the classic golf swing, the hips are allowed to turn with the shoulders, resulting in a decreased X-factor. Thus, in the classic swing the spine is held erect during follow-through, resulting in the spine moving in an "upright I" position.

In the modern golf swing the hips are held stationary and this is coupled with large shoulder rotation, which dramatically increases power of the swing while, unfortunately, also increasing torsional strain on the spine. The modern swing also focuses on a hyperextension "reverse-C" position of the spine during follow-through (the end of the swing), which increases compression forces across the back. The goal of the modern swing is to wind up the spine as much as possible and release it like a spring. In contrast, the classic swing allows for much more hip motion and thus decreases the wind-up load on the spine. The X-factor is decreased and the finish has less arc. As a result, the classic swing causes much less spinal injury.

Although pros can have issues with their spines from overuse, amateurs have more inconsistencies in their swings which require more trunk muscle activation to compensate for unintended motions and have an increased risk of injury. With golf, there is a cumulative effect on the spine—the more high power swings taken, the greater the risk of injury over time (4).

Several preventive measures have been proposed to help golfers reduce injury. The abdominal muscles should be regularly strengthened. The multifidus muscle, lying on either side of your spinal column, is critical for spine stabilization and also should be regularly exercised. The bird dog exercise is good for this (assume quadruped position and lift one arm and, simultaneously, lift the leg on your opposite side; hold.) When playing golf, the ball may be moved closer to the golfer to generate a more upright swing. The hip-shoulder angle is reduced by allowing the hips to move with the swing—in a more classical fashion. Despite our best efforts, golf may pose a risk to your back.

Exercise and Spine Injury

Exercise is part of a healthy lifestyle and critical for muscle, joint and bone health. However certain exercises are more demanding of the spine than others and may result in increased injury. As described above, the contact sports such as American football, rugby, ice hockey, and boxing, as well as those where high-speed injury are possible (skiing, diving are two) are responsible for the majority of acute spine injuries. Nonetheless, non-contact sports also place large loads on the spine. Swing sports such as tennis and golf require a significant amount of rotation and may place you at risk for back injury. Golf requires that a tremendous amount of rotational force be generated by the spine and low back injuries are very common (5). Other non-contact sports that place a significant amount of repetitive load across the spine, such as rowing, may increase risk of back injury.

There are some fitness programs which have come across the spine radar recently for causing serious injuries. CrossFit® which combines regular calisthenics with Olympic style lifting is one of those programs that seems to be popular at the time of this writing. CrossFit®, where high impact lifting and jumping exercises are employed, are also notorious for causing spinal injury (6). The likely problem with CrossFit® is that amateurs are now trying to get their bodies to perform activities for which they lack the conditioning. If you have a back problem, this is probably not the exercise program for you.

Injury Prevention

It seems like common sense but there is really nothing you can do to avoid injury if you are participating in a high impact activity. If you take a hit, it is chance whether you suffer an injury or not. Having said that, maintaining good core strength and flexibility are critical for avoiding spine overuse and injury (see chapter on alternative spine treatment). Strength allows your muscles to have increased control over the motion of the bones, and flexibility will allow your spine to absorb greater shocks with less risk of breaking. Strength is particularly important for the core abdominal and back muscles which brace and protect the spine (7). Most injuries will occur when you are not paying attention, or your muscles are already tired and stiff. Kinesio tape, a type of elastic tape that can be placed superficially on the body over areas of motion such as the back has not been shown definitively to prevent or treat injury. However, it may be used as an adjunct to other strength and flexibility therapies discussed in detail in the alternative therapies chapter (chapter 21) (7).

Which exercises are good for avoiding spine injuries? As stated in the previous chapter, walking is the best spine exercise because of the low demand it places on the spine. Biking is also an excellent sport to consider for spine injury patients, particularly recumbent biking. In the recumbent bike, there is minimal load exerted through the spine and good alignment may be maintained. The elliptical trainer is also a great low-impact activity which was designed specifically to allow athletes to recover from injury while maintaining fitness. While it's not impossible, I have yet to come across anyone who gets a herniated a disc doing one of these activities. Remember certain sports have an increased rate of spinal injury and back pain: skiing, football/rugby and rowing—so avoiding these may be a good idea if your back hurts. Approximately 600,000 to 1 million football related injuries occur in the United States per year and about 10-25% involve the back and neck (7).

For those who cannot resist high speed/high impact activities, the rate of spinal injury in sports can be decreased by avoiding things such as alcohol and by avoiding participating in sports when you are very tired and more likely to make mistakes. These choices lead to poor decision making, decreased coordination and thus increased risk of injury. Properly fitting protective equipment such a spine vests are available for high impact activities; however, the effectiveness of such devices is unknown. In football, cowboy collars—a cushioning device placed around the neck—may be used to prevent hyperextension injuries.

Returning to Sport Following Spinal Surgery or Spine Injury

There are no golden rules for return to play following spine surgery or spinal injury and in most cases common sense must be exercised. Nonetheless, most patients undergo spinal surgery so that they can continue to participate in the activities they enjoy. For patients in their golden years, being able to continue to participate in low-impact activities such as swimming, golfing, tennis and hiking are major components in the decision to undergo surgery.

In general, following a spine surgery or spine injury, before returning to sport you should be totally pain-free, without significant neurologic deficit (abnormal function) and with full strength and near normal range of motion (8). Returning to collision sports is generally never recommended following spinal surgery.

FOLLOWING SURGERY: Indications to NOT Return to Contact Sport OR To Return with Caution
Neurologic deficit (nerve damage to part of the body)
Occipital-Cervical Arthrodesis (fusion of the neck to the skull)
Poor range of motion (may occur following extensive spinal fusion)
Major sagittal imbalance of the spine (such as flat back or hunch back)
Spinal instability
Spinal fusion—more than 3 levels in low back or more than 2 levels in neck

Many fractures of the spine are benign and are not contraindications (reasons to avoid) to returning to sport. Such fractures include spinous process fractures and fractures of the transverse process. Major fractures to the vertebral body should be cleared by a spine surgeon before return to sport is considered.

Returning to sport following major reconstructive spine surgery may be impossible, but return to sport after minor spine surgery is common. Most of us are not pro-athletes, but we can use data based on their recoveries to consider our own recovery potential. Lumbar (low back) disc herniation is one of the most common injuries in the athlete and a lumbar microdiscectomy (removing the part of the disc causing pain) is a very common treatment used to get people back in the game. Following a lumbar microdiscectomy approximately 81% of patients return to sport at the same level as prior to their injury (9). It's best to gradually re-enter sports after this surgery, starting with strength training and activation of core musculature. Keep in mind that the strength of the disc only reaches 65% by 6 weeks after a microdiscectomy (10). In studies that examine tissue under a microscope, the disc is typically near fully repaired by 12 weeks and thus return to sport around this time is feasible, but return should be gradual.

Return to sport following lumbar fusion is more complicated and may be delayed, depending on surgeon preference. In general, guided strength training may be resumed as early as 3 weeks after surgery safely (11). Rates as high as 100% have been reported for return to golf, swimming and biking by 3 to 9 months (12). It is typically faster to return to biking after a lumbar fusion compared to either golf or swimming. Sports may increase the rate of adjacent level disease, meaning the discs above and below the fusion wear down faster. While lumbar fusion can significantly decrease the amount of pain experienced during recreational activity, performance may be reduced because of muscle loss and stiffness. For example, in golf, driving distance is typically reduced and handicap increased following lumbar surgery (12). You may have to adjust your golf swing to a more classic style to decrease the amount of rotation you are putting through your spine.

Following surgical treatment of cervical disc herniations with anterior cervical discectomy and fusion (ACDF) performed at a single or double level, the majority of competitive athletes (80%) return to play and were more likely to return to play than those who underwent non-operative care (14,15). Return to sport following a single level fusion is more common than return to sport following larger spinal fusions. Following single level cervical surgery (ACDF, foraminotomy or laminectomy) 81% of patients are generally able to return to recreational sport. Roughly 70% return to golf, 31% for tennis, 81% return to swimming following single level cervical surgery (16).

Spine surgery is designed to remove pain that can impede motion, strength and quality of life. It's important to keep in mind that these numbers are not diminishments (it's not that prior to surgery 100% of spine patients can participate in sports and only 80% return after treatment). Most patients with spinal injuries/problems have pain and/or functional limitations and so are NOT actively engaged in sports or recreational activities. Thus, these statistics are very encouraging, because they show how spine surgery may help those who have lost the ability to do what they love get back in the game.

Recommended Time to Return to Golf Following Spine Surgery (13)	
Surgery	Return time
Lumbar laminectomy /decompression	4-8 weeks
Cervical fusion	3 months
Lumbar fusion	6 months

Conclusion

Sports are very important to some people and staying in the game as we age is also important. It's much better to focus on injury prevention, than trying to solve problems with surgery after the fact. This means taking good care of your core muscles, stretching regularly, and avoiding high impact activities where you roll the dice with your spine. If you do suffer an injury, there is a good chance spine surgery can help get you back; however, it's important to remember that surgery is not a panacea and comes with many risks.

Frequently Asked Questions

- **When can I go back to swimming after spine surgery?**

    Typically, by 6 weeks. You need to make sure with your surgeon that your wound is totally healed. Getting even a partially healed incision wet or submerged can risk major infection (pool water is generally not very clean).

References

1.   vCard D. A Timeline of Tiger Woods' Spine Surgeries - MINSTX.COM [Internet]. Minimally Invasive Neurosurgery of Texas. 2020 [cited 2021 Aug 18]. Available from: https://minimallyinvasiveneurosurgerytexas.com/tiger-woods-spine-surgery-timeline/

2.   Schroeder GD, Vaccaro AR. Cervical Spine Injuries in the Athlete: J Am Acad Orthop Surg. 2016 Sep;24(9):e122–33.

3.   Bigdon SF, Gewiess J, Hoppe S, Exadaktylos AK, Benneker LM, Fairhurst PG, et al. Spinal injury in alpine winter sports: a review. Scand J Trauma Resusc Emerg Med. 2019 Jul 19;27(1):69.

4.   Gluck GS, Bendo JA, Spivak JM. The lumbar spine and low back pain in golf: a literature review of swing biomechanics and injury prevention. Spine J. 2008 Sep;8(5):778–88.

5.   Cole MH, Grimshaw PN. The Biomechanics of the Modern Golf Swing: Implications for Lower Back Injuries. Sports Med Auckl NZ. 2016 Mar;46(3):339–51.

6.   Hopkins BS, Cloney MB, Kesavabhotla K, Yamaguchi J, Smith ZA, Koski TR, et al. Impact of CrossFit-Related Spinal Injuries. Clin J Sport Med Off J Can Acad Sport Med. 2019 Nov;29(6):482–5.

7.   Hryvniak D, Frost CD. Spine Injury Prevention. Clin Sports Med. 2021 Jul;40(3):429–44.

8.   Huang P, Anissipour A, McGee W, Lemak L. Return-to-Play Recommendations After Cervical, Thoracic, and Lumbar Spine Injuries: A Comprehensive Review. Sports Health. 2016 Feb;8(1):19–25.

9.   Reiman MP, Sylvain J, Loudon JK, Goode A. Return to sport after open and microdiscectomy surgery versus conservative treatment for lumbar disc herniation: a systematic review with meta-analysis. Br J Sports Med. 2016 Feb;50(4):221–30.

10.   Ahlgren BD, Lui W, Herkowitz HN, Panjabi MM, Guiboux JP. Effect of anular repair on the healing strength of the intervertebral disc: a sheep model. Spine. 2000 Sep 1;25(17):2165–70.

11.   Kernc D, Strojnik V, Vengust R. Early initiation of a strength training based rehabilitation after lumbar spine fusion improves core muscle strength: a randomized

controlled trial. J Orthop Surg. 2018 Jun 19;13(1):151.

12.   Jain NS, Lin CC, Halim A, Knight B, Byrne CT, Alluri R, et al. Return to Recreational Sport Following Lumbar Fusion. Clin Spine Surg. 2020 May;33(4):E174–7.

13.   Abla AA, Maroon JC, Lochhead R, Sonntag VKH, Maroon A, Field M. Return to golf after spine surgery. J Neurosurg Spine. 2011 Jan;14(1):23–30.

14.   Hsu WK. Outcomes following nonoperative and operative treatment for cervical disc herniations in National Football League athletes. Spine. 2011 May 1;36(10):800–5.

15.   Watkins RG, Chang D, Watkins RG. Return to Play After Anterior Cervical Discectomy and Fusion in Professional Athletes. Orthop J Sports Med. 2018 Jun;6(6):2325967118779672.

16.   Richards A, Pines A, Rubel NC, Mauler D, Farnsworth J, Zhang N, et al. Return to Golf, Tennis, and Swimming After Elective Cervical Spine Surgery. Cureus. 2020 Aug 24;12(8):e9993.

Figures

Spine Mechanics in Golf

Modern swing:

Most rotation comes from shoulders and torso

Hips are stationary

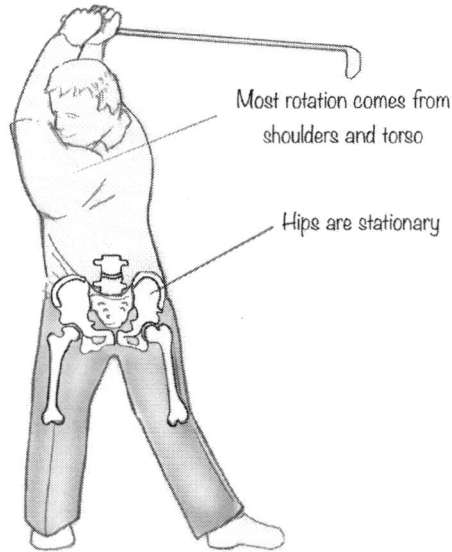

Classic swing:

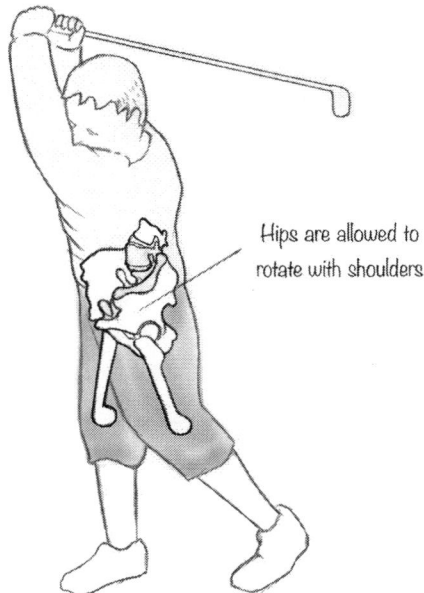

Hips are allowed to rotate with shoulders

The Spine in Golf. A cartoon depicting the difference between a modern swing (top) and the classic swing (bottom). The modern swing keeps the hips and knees planted and rotation comes through the lumbar spine. The classic swing allows for more rotation through the hips and knees taking some pressure off the lumbar spine

Chapter 23

Calcium, Parathyroid Hormone, Vitamin D and the Spine

Summary

Bones are alive and change constantly as we grow and age. Many patients are interested in how to help keep their bones healthy but browsing the supplement aisle in the grocery store can be overwhelming. It is not critical to understand all areas of bone metabolism (how bones grow or degrade), but basic knowledge of how calcium, parathyroid hormone and Vitamin D work can help you navigate the complicated world of supplements and bone health. Calcium is regulated very tightly in your blood stream because it is critical for cellular function. Bones serve as the body's primary reservoir of calcium and thus will be degraded when your calcium is low. The parathyroid glands help to regulate your calcium levels by releasing parathyroid hormone when calcium is low in the blood. Parathyroid hormone (PTH) works by telling your bones to break down and release calcium back into your body. Vitamin D works in concert with parathyroid hormone to increase your calcium absorption from the intestines and suppress release of parathyroid hormone. Thus, dietary intake of both calcium and vitamin D are essential. Calcium can be obtained from the diet, but Vitamin D should be supplemented especially if you are at risk for low levels.

Case

Ms. Magenta is a very active retired 70-year-old artist. She goes to Pilates 4 times a week and has a trainer who works with her for strength and flexibility. Her mother suffered from osteoporosis, having multiple spinal compression fractures, and she is very worried she will have the same problems. She has had a DXA bone density scan which showed she has osteoporosis and does not want it to progress. She doesn't want to take pharmaceutical osteoporosis treatments as she has heard horror stories about the side effects but wants to try natural remedies. She reads online about Vitamin D and calcium but is unsure how much she should take and whether there are other supplements like chondroitin she should be taking. She also has a family history of coronary artery disease and has read that taking extra calcium can increase her risk of a heart attack. Confused she goes to her primary care provider who checks her Vitamin D level which come back at 22ng/dl (low). She is counseled that she may need pharmacologic treatment, but certainly with her low vitamin D levels supplementation is indicated. Furthermore, she is recommended to have regular biannual DXA scans to trend any worsening of her osteoporosis and to keep up her physical activity.

Introduction

The bones are living organs just like the heart or lungs. They have their own biology and are affected by disorders of metabolism that can have a profound impact on their health. The spine is obviously composed of many bones which depend on three different compounds for optimal health: calcium, Vitamin D, and parathyroid hormone. Bone metabolism is a complicated subject, but I include it in this book because I do believe it is very important for overall spine health. If you are interested in mineral supplementation and how some anabolic osteoporosis drugs work, then I suggest reading deeper into this chapter. If you are not interested in it, just read the summary, and move on to the next chapter.

Calcium in the Body

Calcium is an element (Ca) that is very important in the human body, not just for bones, but for many cellular functions. The majority (99%) of human calcium is stored in the bone as part of the crystal hydroxyapatite ($Ca_{10}PO_46OH2$). Hydroxyapatite is what gives bones their compressive strength (allowing you to run and jump on them without them shattering). The remaining 1% of calcium is tightly regulated in the blood stream at a level between 8.5-10.5 mg/dl. Maintaining calcium in this range is essential as Ca ensures proper nerve function, muscle contraction, blood coagulation, cell division and many other things critical for life. In a typical adult diet 1000mg are ingested per day, 200mg of which is absorbed from the intestines and another 200mg which is excreted in the urine. The remaining 800 mg simply pass through the bowel. There is a daily turnover in the bone of about 500-600mg of calcium meaning this amount is released and reincorporated into the bone. Depending on how much parathyroid hormone you have in your blood stream will determine whether calcium remains in the blood or is absorbed into the bones. **The recommended daily intake of calcium is around 1000-1200mg per day and should not exceed 2500mg/day (1).**

Calcium may be obtained through either calcium rich foods (dietary calcium) or through processed tablets, or so-called calcium supplements. In general dietary calcium such as that found in dairy and vegetables are absorbed better than that from calcium supplement tablets (2). There is a lot of conflicting evidence about calcium supplementation out there. The problem with calcium supplements is that in addition to increasing your calcium they may also cause side effects. For example, calcium supplements may cause gastrointestinal symptoms such as constipation and bloating or urinary problems like kidney stones. There is worry that calcium supplementation can increase the risk of cardiovascular disease but currently this is not totally clear. It is uncertain whether routine supplementation with calcium is necessary and thus **dietary calcium is the recommended form of intake** (2). Taking calcium over a certain level will not result in more calcium being stored in the bones or even a significant reduction in fractures. Those who have low dietary intake of calcium or some malabsorptive problem should certainly consider calcium supplementation (3). This is particularly important for post-menopausal women, women who are breast feeding, those with osteoporosis or osteopenia, and vegans. For everyone else, dietary calcium is probably sufficient. You can get calcium in your diet from the following sources:

Sources of calcium (in order of calcium content)	
Dairy	• Yogurt (200-400mg per 6 oz serving) • Cheese (200-400mg per 1 oz serving) • milk (200-400mg per 8 oz serving)
Fish	• Salmon • sardines (200-300mg per serving)
Fruits and vegetables	• Cruciferous vegetables such as raw kale, bok choy, broccoli, (50-100mg per 4 oz or 100 g serving) • Nondairy milk (oat or soy) (300mg per 8oz serving) • Beans (80mg per 4 oz or 100g serving) • Almonds (70mg per 1 oz serving (23 nuts)) • Orange (60mg per orange, 4-5 oz)

Certain compounds in food can increase or decrease the absorption of calcium. For example, casein and lactose (found in milk) and non-digestible sugars such as inulin found in plants) are thought to increase calcium absorption (3). The absorption of calcium seems to be similar between milk and dark leafy vegetables but may be lower for compounds containing oxalate such as spinach, rhubarb and beans (4).

There are two main forms of calcium supplementation on the market: calcium citrate and calcium carbonate. While calcium carbonate is the cheapest form of supplementation it must be taken with a meal and calcium citrate seems to have better bioavailability (it can be more efficiently put to use in the body) (1). Other forms of calcium supplementation such as "bone meal" containing hydroxyapatite derived from animal bones are not recommended because they have been found to contain high amounts of heavy metals. Furthermore, there is insufficient evidence that hydroxyapatite has any benefit on the skeleton (1).

Parathyroid hormone

You have 4 small parathyroid glands near your thyroid gland in the neck. They appeared in evolutionary history at the time when animals moved from the calcium-rich sea to land, where there was low calcium in the environment. The parathyroid glands secrete a hormone known as parathyroid hormone (PTH). The chief function of PTH is to act as a "thermostat" to regulate your blood calcium in a very narrow range. As noted above, calcium is critical for most cellular function and disturbances in the levels in your blood can result in problems. The parathyroid glands ensure your calcium is kept in the exact range by controlling how much calcium is absorbed from the intestines and how much is released from bones.

When your blood calcium levels become low, the cells of the parathyroid gland sense the change and release parathyroid hormone. Parathyroid hormone stimulates the kidney to resorb (pull back into the body) calcium and excrete more phosphate. PTH also stimulates the conversion of the inactive 25-OH Vitamin D to the active form 1,25-OH Vitamin D which helps to increase intestinal absorption of calcium. Finally, PTH acts on the bone to cause release of calcium and phosphate PTH binds to receptors on osteoblast bone cells which then release a molecule known as RANKL which stimulates bone-eating cells (osteoclasts) to break down bone and release calcium.

High blood calcium and Vitamin D levels suppress PTH release, just as low blood calcium and Vitamin D levels stimulate release of PTH. In conditions where your PTH is abnormally high your bones will rapidly lose calcium, and this can be a cause of osteomalacia (or poor mineralization of the bones) that can lead to weak brittle bones.

Parathyroid Hormone-related Peptide (PTHrP)

Although not one of the main components of bone metabolism, I think it's important to mention PTHrP, because it can be used as a powerful drug to treat osteoporosis (see section on osteoporosis treatment). However, it is certainly a more esoteric area of bone metabolism and thus it's not a problem if you choose to skip this section.

PTH and PTHrP are related protein hormones that both stimulate the same receptor (the PTH1R receptor). However, unlike PTH, PTHrP is produced by many different organs in the body and seems to have a more diverse set of actions on the body than PTH. For example, PTHrP is critical for skeletal development in the embryo and limb development and plays a role in breastfeeding and smooth muscle relaxation. Importantly PTHrP is associated with some cancers and the development of hypercalcemia (too much calcium in the blood) as PTHrP causes the release of calcium from bones and bone breakdown. Interestingly, PTHrP has slightly different effects on the PTH receptor than PTH and can be used as a treatment for osteoporosis if given intermittently.

Magnesium

The element magnesium (Mg) is directly linked with maintenance of calcium in the blood stream. A low magnesium level can affect the bones because it can stimulate the parathyroid gland to produce PTH, which in turn draws down the calcium in the bones. However, extremely low magnesium (hypomagnesemia) can result in low blood calcium (hypocalcemia) due to lowering the PTH levels. Why this occurs is not entirely clear.

Found in the majority of food groups magnesium is generally only going to be low because of poor absorption, GI (gastrointestinal) loss of function, the use of drugs such as proton pump inhibitors (PPIs like omeprazole), alcoholism, and renal (kidney) loss of function with the use of diuretics. Symptoms can include cramping, fatigue, and seizures.

High magnesium (hypermagnesemia) may be caused by ingestion of laxatives (magnesium sulfate or magnesium citrate) or IV (intravenous) supplementation. A high magnesium level may also cause low blood calcium because it inhibits PTH release. A high magnesium level may cause nausea, vomiting, heart problems and neurological symptoms such as confusion.

In addition to magnesium's relationship to the parathyroid glands, it is critical for many enzymatic processes involved in metabolism. Most of the magnesium in the body is found in the cells, with only a small amount in the blood stream.

In general, if your magnesium levels are normal and you are not symptomatic, you do not need routine supplementation. The elderly and alcoholics may benefit from magnesium supplementation under the guidance of physician which can be taken orally or intravenously (5).

Vitamin D

Vitamin D is a fat-soluble vitamin (meaning it will not dissolve in water). Vitamin D plays a major role in many metabolic functions in the body and has a major role in the prevention of chronic illnesses such as cancer, cardiovascular disease, depression, and infection. Vitamin D is also crucial for bone metabolism and bone health and muscle strength. Vitamin D deficiency is very common in both adults and children with an estimated 50% of men and women in the United States suffering from either Vitamin D insufficiency or deficiency (3).

Sources of Vitamin D	
Vitamin D2 (ergocalciferol)	**Natural:** Shiitake mushrooms
	Packaged: Prescription 50,000 IU capsule, over-the-counter multivitamin 400IU
Vitamin D3 (cholecalciferol)	**Natural:** Cod liver oil, Mackerel (canned), Salmon, Sardines, Tuna (canned), Exposure to sunlight
	Packaged: Over-the-counter supplements--400, 800, 1000, 2000 and 5000 IU.

I find the biology of vitamin-D processing in the body interesting, but it can be summarized in one sentence: you need either sunlight or dietary intake of vitamin D to get enough. If you would like to know how it works in the body, continue reading or you can skip to the next section.

The precursor to Vitamin D (25-OH-D) is either ingested or is produced in the skin when a chemical 7-dehydrocholesterol (7DHC) present in the skin is exposed to sunlight and converted to 25-OH-D. A diet high in fishy oils is a good way to get vitamin D but this is really the only food that contains vitamin D naturally (see above). Thus, most vitamin D is obtained from exposure to sunlight. Typically, somewhere from 15-30 minutes of exposure to sunlight twice a week is necessary depending on your latitude. Clothing and sunscreen both prevent vitamin D production. In certain areas even sunlight will not produce enough vitamin D. Almost no vitamin D is produced from the skin at latitudes above the 35° north parallel (just north of Santa Barbara in California) from October through April (6).

There are two main forms of vitamin D: Vitamin D2 (ergocalciferol) which is plant-derived and Vitamin D3 (cholecalciferol) which is animal-derived. Both are referred to as "Vitamin D" and are inert in and of themselves but ultimately can be converted to active vitamin D in the kidney. Exposure to UV light at a certain wavelength converts 7-DHC to cholecalciferol which is then converted to 25-OH-D by the liver. This is the main form of vitamin D that is measured in the lab. 25-OH-D is then converted to its active form 1,25-OH-D in the kidney by the enzyme 1-a-hydroxylase.

As stated above, this process is influenced by low blood calcium levels as well as high PTH levels. Vitamin D acts on the intestines to increase absorption of calcium and phosphorous. Without Vitamin D, your intestines become very inefficient in calcium absorption. Vitamin D levels are inversely related to PTH levels where low Vitamin D levels can increase your PTH levels and vice versa. As your vitamin D levels drop you develop what's called secondary hyperparathyroidism, meaning your PTH levels will increase because of the low vitamin D. Increased PTH acts as a check to increase your vitamin D and calcium levels. In a hyper parathyroid state, your body cannot maintain adequate bone mineral density because calcium is always being drawn out of the bones by PTH.

Sunlight does not produce toxic levels of Vitamin D even with continued exposure and the Vitamin D precursor (7-DHC) degrades into two metabolites (lumisterol and tachysterol) with excessive exposure to sunlight. Thus, you cannot develop hyper vitamin D from sunlight (although you may develop a sunburn). Patients with a significant amount of pigmentation in the skin have less conversion of 7-DHC to 25-OH-D. Vitamin D toxicity is rare with oral intake but has been associated with taking 50,000 IU daily.

Vitamin D levels less than 20ng/ml are considered deficient. A level from 21-29 ng/ml is considered insufficient due to the response of the intestines to levels greater than 30ng/ml which results in a 65% increase in absorption of calcium. Vitamin D becomes toxic at blood levels higher than 150ng/ml. Vitamin D levels are directly correlated with bone mineral density meaning the higher your levels the better your bone mineral density will be (7). Vitamin D deficiency is most caused by low exposure to sunlight or poor dietary intake but may also be associated with renal disease and malabsorption (inability to absorb through the intestines). Vitamin D is important for many organ systems and deficiency is associated with increased risk of colon cancer, prostate cancer, and breast cancer. Taking oral vitamin D is associated with reduced fracture risk (8).

VITAMIN D Levels	
Deficiency	less than 20 ng/ml
Insufficiency	21-29 ng/ml
Preferred range	30-60 ng/ml
Toxicity	higher than 150 ng/ml

Adults should consume at minimum 1000 IU of vitamin D per day. While both Vitamin D2 and D3 are effective at treating deficiency, Vitamin D2 (ergocalciferol) is inferior to Vitamin D3 (cholecalciferol) in maintaining blood vitamin D levels (about 30% as effective). Vitamin D3 seems to last longer in the blood (9). Your doctor may prescribe high dose vitamin D2 (50,000 IU weekly) or higher levels of vitamin D3 to get your vitamin D levels up. Treatment of vitamin D deficiency should be guided by your physician.

Conclusion

The bones are living organs with a specific biology that is quite complex. The three primary chemicals that determine overall bone health are calcium, parathyroid hormone, and vitamin D. Our understanding of the small details of how bone metabolism works is constantly improving, but it's clear that disturbances in bone metabolism can lead to problems in the spine.

Frequently Asked Questions

- **Is there any difference between using Vitamin D2 (Ergocalciferol) vs Vitamin D3 (Cholecalciferol) supplements?**

    Vitamin D3 (cholecalciferol) has been shown to be superior in elevating Vitamin D levels in the blood but both are effective (9,10). I use both in my practice as some pharmacies only have one form or another but I prefer D3. For all intents and purposes D2 works fine; you may have to take more of it.

References

1.   Straub DA. Calcium Supplementation in Clinical Practice: A Review of Forms, Doses, and Indications. Nutr Clin Pract. 2007 Jun;22(3):286–96.

2.   Bauer DC. Clinical practice. Calcium supplements and fracture prevention. N Engl J Med. 2013 Oct 17;369(16):1537–43.

3.   Cashman KD. Calcium intake, calcium bioavailability and bone health. Br J Nutr. 2002 May;87(S2):S169–77.

4.   Office of Dietary Supplements - Calcium [Internet]. [cited 2022 Jan 30]. Available from: https://ods.od.nih.gov/factsheets/Calcium-HealthProfessional/

5.   Wang R, Chen C, Liu W, Zhou T, Xun P, He K, et al. The effect of magnesium supplementation on muscle fitness: a meta-analysis and systematic review. Magnes Res. 2017 Nov 1;30(4):120–32.

6.   Webb LX. Analysis of Surgeon-Controlled Variables in the Treatment of Limb-Threatening Type-III Open Tibial Diaphyseal Fractures. J Bone Jt Surg Am. 2007 May 1;89(5):923.

7.   Holick MF. Vitamin D Deficiency. N Engl J Med. 2007;16.

8.   Bischoff-Ferrari HA, Willett WC, Wong JB, Giovannucci E, Dietrich T, Dawson-Hughes B. Fracture Prevention With Vitamin D Supplementation: A Meta-analysis of Randomized Con-

trolled Trials. JAMA. 2005 May 11;293(18):2257.

9.   Shieh A, Chun RF, Ma C, Witzel S, Meyer B, Rafison B, et al. Effects of High-Dose Vita-min D2 Versus D3 on Total and Free 25-Hydroxyvitamin D and Markers of Calcium Balance. J Clin Endocrinol Metab. 2016 Aug;101(8):3070–8.

10.   Martineau AR, Thummel KE, Wang Z, Jolliffe DA, Boucher BJ, Griffin SJ, et al. Differen-tial Effects of Oral Boluses of Vitamin D2 vs Vitamin D3 on Vitamin D Metabolism: A Random-ized Controlled Trial. J Clin Endocrinol Metab. 2019 Dec 1;104(12):5831–9.

Figures:

Vitamin D Sources:

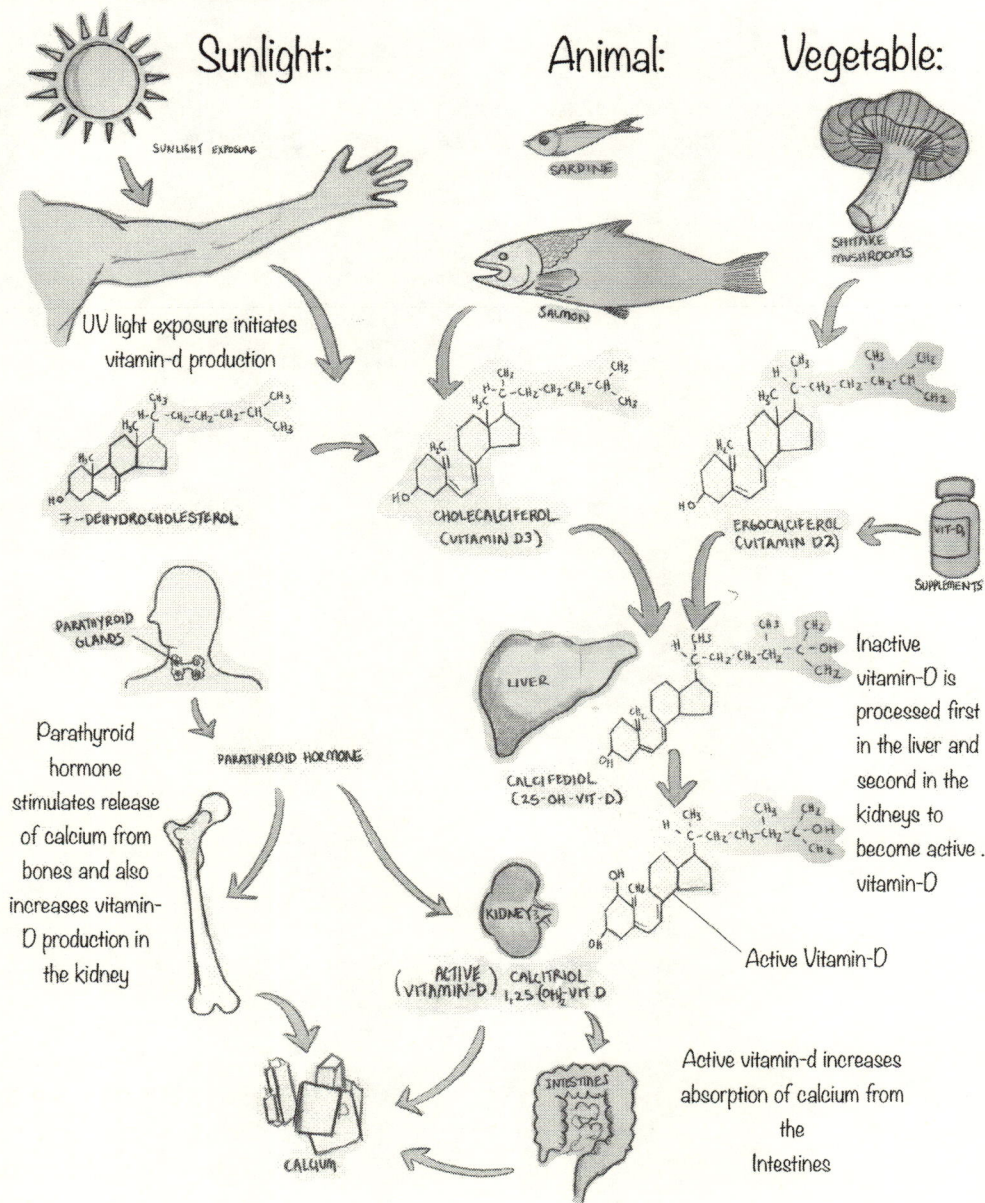

Sunlight:

SUNLIGHT EXPOSURE

UV light exposure initiates vitamin-d production

7-DEHYDROCHOLESTEROL

PARATHYROID GLANDS

Parathyroid hormone stimulates release of calcium from bones and also increases vitamin-D production in the kidney

PARATHYROID HORMONE

Animal:

SARDINE

SALMON

CHOLECALCIFEROL (VITAMIN D3)

LIVER

CALCIFEDIOL (25-OH-VIT-D)

KIDNEYS

(ACTIVE VITAMIN-D) CALCITRIOL 1,25 (OH)₂ VIT D

INTESTINES

CALCIUM

Vegetable:

SHITAKE MUSHROOMS

ERGOCALCIFEROL (VITAMIN D2)

VIT-D SUPPLEMENTS

Inactive vitamin-D is processed first in the liver and second in the kidneys to become active vitamin-D

Active Vitamin-D

Active vitamin-d increases absorption of calcium from the Intestines

Calcium and Vitamin D. Bone metabolism is complicated but is driven by Vitamin D and parathyroid hormone. Inactive Vitamin D (cholecalciferol or ergocalciferol) can either be obtained from sunlight, supplementation or from certain foods (dairy, mushrooms, or fish). Inactive Vitamin D is activated sequentially in the liver and then the kidney. Active Vitamin D stimulates the intestines to absorb calcium for deposition into bones. The master regulator of calcium metabolism is parathyroid hormone (PTH) which is released in response to low calcium in the blood. PTH stimulates the breakdown of bone to release calcium into the bloodstream. PTH also stimulates the conversion of inactive Vitamin D to active Vitamin D resulting in increased calcium uptake from the intestines.

Chapter 24

Obesity, Diabetes, Smoking: Lifestyle Factors That Affect Spine Degeneration and Spine Surgery

Summary

Obesity and smoking have a major negative impact on your health. Luckily, both obesity and smoking can be treated with changes in your habits. Obesity makes your spine carry more weight and ultimately do more work. This causes it to wear down faster and have problems at an earlier age. Furthermore, obesity can lead to diabetes which can also cause accelerated disc degeneration. Smoking also destroys intervertebral discs and can lead to complications following spine surgery. Smoking increases your risk of a spinal fusion failing, wound complications and general medical complications such as heart attack or embolism. Obesity, diabetes, and smoking not only cause changes in your body that make the need for spine surgery more likely, they also increase the risks of something going wrong when you do have spine surgery. Obesity and diabetes can both be combatted with a low calorie/high nutrient diet. There are many methods that can be used to quit smoking, perhaps the best of which is to quit cold turkey.

Case 1

Mr. Peru is a 63-year-old mechanic. He had a problem with his L4-5 intervertebral disc where he developed stenosis and spondylolisthesis. He had it treated
with a lumbar fusion decompression by a capable surgeon across town and did
well for a time. However, he is a heavy smoker and obese. His wound becomes
infected and ultimately contaminates the hardware, which requires several
washouts. When he gets out of the hospital, he still has back pain and over the
next year it just gets worse to the point where he is in more pain than ever. This
pain causes him to smoke and eat more to decrease his anxiety. He comes to see
me for a second opinion, and we do a comprehensive work up. His BMI (body
mass index) is high (45.3) and yet he is malnourished with low levels of Vitamin
D and protein. A CT scan reveals that the bone graft of the fusion has failed
to heal. We try to correct course, replacing his vitamin D and try to get him to
lose weight. I implore him to try and quit smoking and lose some of the weight.
I explain that even if I went in again, under the current circumstances it would
not only be risky but the same problems could repeat themselves. He doesn't
know if he can quit and he is also addicted to his American diet. He states, how
can I lose weight if I can't exercise? How can I stop smoking if I am in pain?
I try to convince him that he can accomplish these things, but ultimately, he
decides to go on disability.

Case 2

Mr. Gold is a retired 78-year-old retired plumber who presents with back and
leg pain from a degenerative spondylolisthesis at L4-5 causing severe stenosis.
He is morbidly obese with a BMI around 41 and he is a smoker but worked all
his life. Now that he is trying to enjoy his retirement after a long career, his
back is preventing him from enjoying the activities he loves. Similar to Mr.
Peru, he has addictions to cigarettes and food and is a diabetic, but there is
something different about his attitude. When I explain how his diet and smoking are negatively impacting his health, specifically his spine, I see a light go on
and he says "no one ever explained that to me." He has been self-reliant his entire life building a career and a tight knit family. For them, he decides to make
changes to his lifestyle. He institutes a low calorie but highly nutritious diet
focused on non-processed plant-based foods. He stops smoking cold turkey.
He starts physical therapy and exercises more, bringing his BMI down to 35
over several months. Ultimately, he has a successful lumbar fusion, which eliminates his back and leg pain. A year out, he is a new man. His health has greatly
improved and he feels lucky he was able to get through a successful surgery
unscathed.

Introduction

Your spine is a complicated machine that, like any other machine, if run poorly will wear out faster. There are certain conditions and habits that we know have a direct negative impact on the spine. These include being overweight, diabetes, and smoking. Not surprisingly, these lifestyle factors also negatively affect healing from spine surgery and increase your risk of complications. Smoking and poor eating are called modifiable risk factors for surgery because patients can make a change in lifestyle that improves their chances of a good outcome. This contrasts with non-modifiable risk factors such as your age which cannot be changed. In western medicine we are obsessed with fancy surgery and pills to treat disease, but some of the most powerful interventions are those which focus on changing habits.

Obesity

We all know what obesity looks like, but in medicine we have a definition for it. Obesity is defined as having a body mass index (BMI) greater than or 30 kg/m2. Body mass index is measured by calculating your weight (in kilograms) divided by your height (in meters) squared. Basically, you are obese if, for your height, you are carrying over a certain amount of weight.

BMI = body weight in kg/ (height in m)2

Table 1: Body Mass Index (BMI) Classification	
Classification	**BMI (kg/m^2)**
Underweight	less than 18.5
Normal	18.5-24.9
Overweight	25-29.9
Obese Class 1	30-34.9
Obese Class 2	35-39.9
Obese Class 3	greater than or 40

Body mass index is not a perfect measure of obesity. For example, non-obese, very fit and muscular individuals may have an elevated BMI because muscle is denser than fat. Thus, another simple way to assess obesity is your waist to height ratio (WHtR). Ideally your waist measurement (performed with a measuring tape around the abdomen at the level of the navel totally relaxed) should be less than half of your height. Waist to height ratio has been shown to be more predictive of having diabetes and cardiovascular disease than BMI (1).

WHtR = waist measurement (cm) divided by height measurement (cm): if it's less than 0.5 you are not obese.

I like WHtR because the message is simple: keep your waist to less than half of your height.

Obesity is an epidemic in the United States, affecting 37% of the population (2), and is associated with many health issues, including an increased risk for diabetes, high cholesterol, hypertension, coronary heart disease, heart failure, stroke, venous thrombosis, multiple types of cancer, chronic kidney disease, respiratory disease, and infection.

Obesity has also been associated with specific negative effects on the spine. For example, in large population-based studies a high body mass index has been associated with low back pain and early disc degeneration (3,4). Patients who are obese and also have spine problems or pain in their low backs report more significant symptoms and decreased function compared to non-obese patients (5). This makes intuitive sense. The more weight you carry on your body, the more your bones and ligament must carry as well. Your bones don't suddenly get stronger and your ligaments more robust when you become overweight. They still must do the same work as they did when you were skinnier.

It is always more difficult to perform surgery on someone overweight. Positioning is more difficult, incisions need to be larger to get where you need to go, at times larger or custom instruments are required to perform the operation, and, overall, procedures take more time. Obesity has also been linked to post-operative complications following surgery, particularly in the lumbar (low back) spine. For example, in a large prospective study, patients who had a BMI greater than 30 did worse with non-operative measures than those with a normal BMI. Moreover, while obese patients had similar outcomes to non-obese patients after undergoing lumbar surgery for degenerative spondylolisthesis, obese patients had a higher infection and reoperation rate compared to non-obese patients (6). While obese patients may still benefit from spinal surgery if indicated, they have a higher risk of infection, longer length of stay in the hospital and greater likelihood of medical complications and hospital readmission (7,8).

In many cases the reduced mobility caused by spinal pain is cited by patients as a reason for weight gain. However, while some studies have reported patients are able to achieve weight loss once their spines are fixed with spinal surgery, the research is conflicted (9–11). This is because weight loss is achieved by not only increased activity but also changes in diet (12). I have seen many people who have become trapped in their bodies—unable to move because of pain, but no way to easily fix it because they are too obese to have surgery safely. You do not want to become trapped in this situation.

how to achieve weight loss

The food industry is very interested in keeping you snacking, which is why they invest heavily in developing foods that are more and more addictive. Suffice to say, the food industry is interested in keeping you fat. They also commonly brand or label foods as "healthy" or "athletic" that are no different from candy off the shelf.

In addition to this, there are many name-branded and fad diets in existence that collectively represent a multi-billion-dollar industry (13). With the significant media blitz that results from these forces, it is difficult to determine what information, if any, is correct. How can you select healthy foods or effective diets when there is so much false information out there. Some diets suggest a low carbohydrate diet while others suggest a high protein diet.

So let's boil it down to the most basic concept: **calories from either fat or sugar (carbohydrates) get converted to fat in the body—which is how you get fat**. Despite conflicting suggestions, this one simple principle guides almost all diets. To lose weight you must limit dietary intake of the macronutrients fat and sugar. In other words, for a diet to be successful you need to limit your overall caloric intake. If you decrease your caloric intake and increase caloric expenditure through exercise you will lose weight. Studies have shown that there is little difference between the success rate of different fad diets—however, the diets with the lowest intake of carbohydrates and fat tend to be the most successful. This makes intuitive sense, as these are the macronutrients with the highest number of calories.

To understand how low fat/carbohydrate diets work we need to discuss a little about metabolism—how your body changes food into stored energy for later use. When you consume sugar (carbohydrates) it is broken down and absorbed into the blood stream. This stimulates the release of a hormone known as insulin from the pancreas, which tells your body to absorb sugar from the blood stream into cells—especially fat cells. Fat cells absorb the sugar and then convert it directly into a fat molecule. "A minute on the lips, forever on the hips" is an appropriate way to describe sugar metabolism. Sugar does not pass go and does not collect 100 dollars; in the presence of insulin sugar gets incarcerated directly into fat in fat cells. When you are obese and carry excess fat, something changes in your body's ability to utilize insulin. The fat cells do not multiply but rather become so swollen with fat they are unable to convert sugar into fat and fat starts spilling into the blood stream (14). Obese people have higher circulating levels of fat which is thought to interrupt insulin-signaling further (15). More on this later.

When you restrict your carbohydrate intake, your body is forced to use the fat in storage. Not all carbohydrates are created equal, and some have much more impact on your blood glucose (the sugar in your blood stream). The measure of how much a food raises your blood sugar is called the Glycemic Index (GI). Another measure, called the Glycemic Load (GL), combines how fast a given food can raise your blood sugar with how much sugar is in a single serving of that food. In other words, GL allows you determine the actual impact a serving of a certain type of food has on your blood sugar, a very useful piece of information. Foods which have a high GI and GL include refined cereals and grains, sugary soft drinks, candy. If you are curious about the GI and GL of a food a convenient website is: http://www.glycemicindex.com/.

The puzzle is finding the right combination of diet for you which is both sustainable and healthy. Many of us are looking for a "holy grail" which simply does not exist. The ideal diet is one that you can easily follow and stick to (13). It makes no sense to eliminate carbohydrates only to gorge on high fat meals. The best diet is one you tailor to your own life and follow ardently.

As stated above, the most effective dieting style is one which limits both fat and carbohydrate intake and increases intake of fiber and nutrient-rich foods such as fruit and vegetables (13). This diet was proposed by many famous doctors including Dr. Dean Ornish. Dr. Joel Fuhrman, another nutrition guru, has fully outlined how to lose weight using this diet in his book Eat to Live which I highly recommend reading. (The success stories appearing throughout the book will motivate you!) The concept is simple: to eat as much natural produce as possible and strictly limit foods which are calorically dense with low nutrients. This is similar to a macrobiotic diet which is popular in Japan/Asia where animal products and processed foods only account for a very small portion of the diet. The most important study to popularize this diet has been the China Study which showed dramatically lower rates of both cancer and cardiovascular disease in groups which primarily consume plant matter (16). Dr. Fuhrman boils this down to a simple equation: Health = Nutrition/calories, which means you should eat the most nutritious foods with the least number of calories to achieve optimal health. This means avoiding two primary groups of foods: fat and carbohydrates. This means avoiding foods which are common in the standard American diet such as sugars, trans-fats, high calorie density snacks and drinks, refined grains all of which are high in calories, low in nutrients and not filling. These foods are typically processed (meaning they have been converted from their original form, for example, turning wheat into flour into bread or pasta) which removes much of the nutritious content, leaving only empty calories. He further simplifies this method of dieting with another equation: refined foods+ fat = MAKES YOU FAT. Refined and processed carbohydrates drive insulin surges which encourages the body to convert sugar into fat rapidly. Fat, on the other hand, needs no help, it goes directly on to your waist without any ifs ands or buts. Again, "A minute on the lips, forever on the hips."

The thing which I find appealing about this diet is that there is no reliance on calorie counting or the need to keep track of how much food you eat. This diet is instead about consuming as much as you want of nutrient-rich foods, while eliminating foods which have no nutritional content but have tons of calories. Thus, you replace your diet high in fat and refined sugars with plant material. Plants are an excellent source of nutrients but have a very low caloric density due to their high fiber content. This means they fill you up without raising blood sugar and driving fat production. A common myth about plants is that they do not contain protein—this is simply false. All plants contain the essential amino acids (the scientific name for protein). You do not need to eat meat to get enough protein. Consider the horse: an animal which is very high in muscle yet typically has a 100% vegetarian diet. How did the horse become so muscular if it only eats plants? The answer is that plants contain plenty of protein. The plants that humans can eat to get the protein they need include nuts, seeds, beans and spirulina.

 I recommend this diet to many of my patients, some who find it overly strict. But if followed correctly it is certainly effective. And even partial adherence to this program can bring some results. Below is a simplified summary of the process:

Foods which one can eat an unlimited amount of: raw and cooked vegetables, beans and fruits.

- **Dark green leafy vegetables (arugula, spinach, chard, kale, etc.) offer the highest ratio of nutrition/calories, followed closely by other green vegetables (broccoli, romaine, Brussel sprouts, green beans and so on). Finally, there are other non-green vegetables (onions, mushrooms, carrots, tomatoes, to name a few).**

  - 1lb daily raw; no limit

  - 1lb daily cooked; no limit

  - Salad is the main component of this diet, eat it before every meal to fill up and decrease cravings for carbohydrates and fat.

- **Fresh fruit also offer a high ratio of nutrients to calories but are not as good as green leafy vegetables.**

  - Unlimited but minimum 4 daily

- **Beans, sprouts, tofu, legumes**

  - 1 cup daily

Foods which should be limited to one serving daily: starchy vegetables (pota-

toes, rice, squash, grains), nuts, dried fruit

- **Potatoes, squash, corn, rice, whole grains: limit to 1 cup/day**

- **Nuts should be limited to 1oz/day**

Foods which should be avoided completely: animal and dairy products (meat, cheese, creams which are high in fat), sugars (candy/soda/juice), alcohol, processed foods high in carbohydrates (pasta, bread, cake, cookies and basically anything that comes in a package), fruit juice, and oils.

- **These foods are empty calories and dramatically increase weight.**

There are some fats which are essential to the body (the so called essential fatty acids, including omega-3, or polyunsaturated fatty acids). These acids are considered essential to add to your diet because they cannot be produced by the body's own metabolism. Dr. Fuhrman recommends Omega-3 supplementation. These can either be consumed in foods such as flax and soy or taken in over-the-counter supplementation (fish oil sources of omega-3 supplementation should be avoided because of the potential for ingesting mercury or other contaminants). A single tablespoon of flax seeds mixed in a smoothie is all that is required. At all costs you should avoid trans-fats, saturated fats and partially hydrogenated fats. Vitamin B12 and Vitamin D should also be supplemented as a diet low in animal products is also low in these vital nutrients. Vitamin D is important for immune system and bone health. Vitamin B12 (also known as cobalamin) is typically obtained from meat and dairy and is important for DNA and RNA synthesis. B12 is critical for red blood cell health and formation well as for normal neurologic function (19).

Ultimately dieting should be about common sense. Food writer Michael Pollan has some common-sense rules to follow for healthy eating (20).

- **Don't eat anything that your great grandmother wouldn't recognize as food (that is, a CLIF BAR, or another highly-processed edible. I say this with a heavy heart as I am very fond of CLIF bars).**

- **Don't eat anything with more than 5 ingredients or with ingredients you cannot pronounce.**

- **Shop only in the perishable section of the grocery store.**

- **Never eat until you are completely full.**

- **Try not to eat between meals.**

- **Don't buy food where you buy gasoline (my own caveat to this is the produce section of Costco).**

Diabetes

A person with diabetes is unable to adequately metabolize (process) sugar, which results in high levels of blood glucose (hyperglycemia). As discussed above, the hormone responsible for regulating blood glucose levels is insulin. Diabetes is caused by the body's inability to produce insulin (type 1 diabetes) or the body's resistance to insulin acting in a normal way, causing too much glucose (sugar) in the blood (type 2 diabetes).

When you eat some form of carbohydrate (such as bread or candy) the body releases insulin, which allows the absorption of carbohydrates into cells. In a diabetic state you either lack insulin entirely (type 1) or are resistant to its effects and thus sugar remains in the blood stream at very high levels (type 2). Type 2 diabetes is by far the most common form of diabetes in adults and is highly linked with being obese (21). As mentioned earlier, this is thought to be related to high levels of fat in the blood which can block insulin effectiveness (15).

High blood glucose has a number of negative effects on the body. High sugar levels cause glycosylation (attachment of sugar) to enzymes and proteins responsible for your health, which causes them to malfunction or degrade more rapidly. This can affect anything in your body from your kidneys, heart, immune system, your eyes to your musculoskeletal system. Diabetes may also have a profoundly negative effect on the nervous system, causing the destruction of your nerves in a process called "diabetic neuropathy." This can result in problems with sensation, peripheral pain (usually in the hands and feet), decreased motor strength and joint destruction. There is evidence that diabetes is also linked to degeneration of the intervertebral discs and thus causes spine problems to occur sooner than they otherwise would (22,23).

Diabetes is typically **diagnosed as a fasting blood glucose level of 126 mg/dL** or a random blood glucose level greater than 200 mg/dL. As stated above, glucose attaches to enzymes and proteins in the blood at high concentrations. One of the simplest ways of diagnosing and monitoring diabetes is by looking at the percentage of hemoglobin A1C, which is a form of glycosylated hemoglobin (HbA1C). This is a useful measure that tells the clinician what your sugar levels have been over the past 3 months, as the hemoglobin protein has a lifespan of 3 months in the blood stream. A HbA1C level of **greater than 6.5% is diagnostic for diabetes**. HbA1C levels greater than 7.5% are associated with increased risk of morbidity and mortality in surgery (24).

Diabetes also has a negative impact on the results of spine surgery. In spine surgery diabetes has been associated with longer hospitals stays, as well as increased non-home discharges (nursing facilities), increased medical complications, increased readmissions, poor outcomes and death (25–27). Furthermore, because diabetes has such a profound effect on nerves it may impair your ability to recover from neurologic problems caused by spinal pathology (28).

Smoking/Nicotine Products

Smoking is directly responsible for approximately 500,000 deaths in the United States per year (29). Smoking impacts many aspects of your health, including an increased risk of cardiovascular disease (including heart attacks and stroke), cancer, infection, diabetes, osteoporosis and many other chronic conditions. Moreover, smoking has a specific impact on your spine. While there are many ingredients in tobacco smoke that are harmful, the number one culprit is nicotine.

Smoking is a known cause of spinal disc degeneration and back/neck problems. In studies comparing twins (one who smoked, and one who didn't) 18% greater disc degeneration was noted in the twin who smoked (30). Patients who smoke are also more likely to report back pain (31). Smokers typically report that their spinal symptoms are more severe than those who do not smoke (32). Smokers are hospitalized at a higher rate for spinal conditions than non-smokers (33).

Smoking also increases the risk in spinal surgery. In a large study examining the effects of smoking on spinal fusion, smoking almost doubled the rate of failure of the fusion to solidify (heal) (34). In one study, a history of smoking resulted in longer ICU stays for spine trauma patients (35). Smoking—similar to diabetes—can result in poor neurological improvement following decompression surgery for pinched spinal cord or nerves (36). In general, smoking increases the risk of pulmonary and cardiovascular complications in all surgeries (37).

Types of Named Diets			
Diet Type	Name	Details	Pitfalls
Low Carbohydrate	Atkins	Carbohydrates should be limited to 60-130 grams per day and foods with a high glycemic index should be limited as well. These diets have been shown to be at least as effective as low-fat diets (17).	Low carbohydrate dieters may be directed to overconsume another macronutrient diet such as fat.
Low Fat	Ornish	Fat should be limited to less than 30% of the total caloric intake. Low-fat diets may cause certain vitamin and nutrient deficiencies.	Low fat dieters may be driven to consume more carbohydrates and sugar.
Portion-Controlled Diet	Jenny Craig, Weight Watchers.	Similar to low calorie diets, these programs provide prepackaged meals which contain a set number of calories and can be used to replace meals.	These diets require tremendous will power to both keep track of calories and portions. Many will find them only successful for short periods of time. They are also very expensive.
High Protein Diet	Paleolithic ("Paleo") Diet	The idea behind this diet is to replace fat and carbohydrates with protein (primarily from animal meat) and fiber, which is thought to be more filling and more consistent with what our caveman ancestors may have eaten.	Does not consider negative effects of a diet high in animal meat.
Intermittent Fasting		There are many different types of intermittent fasting, but the idea is to not eat for a period of time at regular intervals.	Many will find this type of diet difficult to follow as it creates significant hunger pangs!
Vegetarian	Fuhrman diet	Only vegetable matter is consumed and animal products are partially or completely abstained (Vegan). This diet has been demonstrated to improve cardiovascular health and lower blood glucose,	A total vegetarian diet may lack certain vitamins and require supplementation with omega-3 fatty acids, Vitamin B12, Zinc, Vitamin D and Calcium

If you are planning to undergo spinal surgery and you smoke, try to stop. Obviously, this is a very difficult task. However, when faced with the increased morbidity and mortality associated with surgery if you continue smoking, it is well worth quitting.

Ideally you should stop smoking at least 8 weeks prior to any spine surgery (38). There are several methods which can be used to make this process as easy as possible:

- **Behavioral therapy such as counseling, and quit lines (1-800-quit-Now)**

- **Pharmacologic therapy—drugs such as Bupropion have been shown in randomized controlled trials to be effective in helping smokers quit (39,40).**

- **At the end of June 2021, pharmaceutical manufacturer Pfizer announced they are stopping the global production of Chantix (varenicline). The halt of this smoking cessation pill is due to a discovery of higher levels of nitrosamines — possible carcinogens — in Chantix than what's considered acceptable.**

- **Nicotine supplementation should be avoided because, as stated above, many of the negative effects of smoking come from nicotine. So there really is no difference from a spine standpoint to using nicotine patches compared to smoking cigarettes.**

- **Research has shown that eating broccoli (one stalk per day) helps reduce the carcinogenic properties of smoking and helps return your body to normal health while you are quitting. Broccoli, kale and turmeric have also been shown to decrease inflammation and reduce the potential for developing cancer or cancer spread related to smoking (41–43).**

Your doctor can help you further navigate this difficult task, but rest assured there are few medical interventions more helpful to your health than quitting smoking.

Conclusion

Obesity, diabetes and smoking all work to destroy your spine. They don't stop there, though, they make surgery to fix your spine riskier and recovery more complicated. Together they represent three major anti-spine health factors. What's amazing, is that they are all to some degree controllable by lifestyle—even diabetes. Hopefully, understanding how they negatively impact your spine will help you or any loved ones who might be struggling with these issues to make some changes that can pay huge dividends for your spine, both its general health and its ability to recover from spine surgery should you need it.

Frequently Asked Questions

- **What if I cannot go completely to a plant-based diet?**

I once ate a large proportion of meat in my diet. I told myself, "meat is healthy" despite what I heard. I thought "My parents fed me meat and tons of dairy so it must be good for you." Now, having been faced with an insurmountable amount of evidence which shows the negative health impact of meat and sugar I have come to terms with not eating any of it, and really do not miss it. Nonetheless, occasionally I go out with friends or to restaurants where almost all food items are meat. In these situations, I do occasionally eat meat or consume sugar, with the understanding that I'm only eating a small amount and only once in a while. That having been said I typically refuse to serve my children refined sugar. I think of refined sugar as similar in addictive properties to cigarettes or even opiates. I would never offer my kids cigarettes or opiates, so why would I offer them sugar?

References

1.   Browning LM, Hsieh SD, Ashwell M. A systematic review of waist-to-height ratio as a screening tool for the prediction of cardiovascular disease and diabetes: 0·5 could be a suitable global boundary value. Nutr Res Rev. 2010 Dec;23(2):247–69.

2.   Flegal KM, Kruszon-Moran D, Carroll MD, Fryar CD, Ogden CL. Trends in Obesity Among Adults in the United States, 2005 to 2014. JAMA. 2016 Jun 7;315(21):2284.

3.   Heuch I, Hagen K, Heuch I, Nygaard Ø, Zwart JA. The Impact of Body Mass Index on the Prevalence of Low Back Pain: The HUNT Study. Spine. 2010 Apr;35(7):764–8.

4.   Urquhart DM, Kurniadi I, Triangto K, Wang Y, Wluka AE, O?Sullivan R, et al. Obesity Is Associated With Reduced Disc Height in the Lumbar Spine but Not at the Lumbosacral Junction: Spine. 2014 Jul;39(16):E962–6.

5.   Fanuele JC, Abdu WA, Hanscom B, Weinstein JN. Association Between Obesity and Functional Status in Patients With Spine Disease: Spine. 2002 Feb;27(3):306–12.

6.   Rihn JA, Radcliff K, Hilibrand AS, Anderson DT, Zhao W, Lurie J, et al. Does Obesity Affect Outcomes of Treatment for Lumbar Stenosis and Degenerative Spondylolisthesis? Analysis of the Spine Patient Outcomes Research Trial (SPORT): Spine. 2012 Nov;37(23):1933–46.

7.   Djurasovic M, Bratcher KR, Glassman SD, Dimar JR, Carreon LY. The Effect of Obesity on Clinical Outcomes After Lumbar Fusion: Spine. 2008 Jul;33(16):1789–92.

8.   Puvanesarajah V, Werner BC, Cancienne JM, Jain A, Pehlivan H, Shimer AL, et al. Morbid Obesity and Lumbar Fusion in Patients Older Than 65 Years: Complications, Readmissions, Costs, and Length of Stay. SPINE. 2017 Jan;42(2):122–7.

9.   Akins PT, Inacio MCS, Bernbeck JA, Harris J, Chen YX, Prentice HA, et al. Do Obese and Extremely Obese Patients Lose Weight After Lumbar Spine Fusions? Analysis of a Cohort of 7303 Patients from the Kaiser National Spine Registry: SPINE. 2018 Jan;43(1):22–7.

10.   Garcia RM, Messerschmitt PJ, Furey CG, Bohlman HH, Cassinelli EH. Weight Loss in

Overweight and Obese Patients Following Successful Lumbar Decompression: J Bone Jt Surg-Am Vol. 2008 Apr;90(4):742–7.

11.   Knutsson B, Michaëlsson K, Sandén B. Obese Patients Report Modest Weight Loss After Surgery for Lumbar Spinal Stenosis: A Study From the Swedish Spine Register. Spine. 2014 Sep;39(20):1725–30.

12.   Wu T, Gao X, Chen M, van Dam RM. Long-term effectiveness of diet-plus-exercise interventions vs. diet-only interventions for weight loss: a meta-analysis. Obes Rev Off J Int Assoc Study Obes. 2009 May;10(3):313–23.

13.   Johnston BC, Kanters S, Bandayrel K, Wu P, Naji F, Siemieniuk RA, et al. Comparison of weight loss among named diet programs in overweight and obese adults: a meta-analysis. JAMA. 2014 Sep 3;312(9):923–33.

14.   Spalding KL, Arner E, Westermark PO, Bernard S, Buchholz BA, Bergmann O, et al. Dynamics of fat cell turnover in humans. Nature. 2008 Jun 5;453(7196):783–7.

15.   Grieger M, Stone G. How No to Die. Macmillan; 2016.

16.   Campbell TC, Parpia B, Chen J. Diet, lifestyle, and the etiology of coronary artery disease: the Cornell China study. Am J Cardiol. 1998 Nov 26;82(10B):18T-21T.

17.   Nordmann AJ, Nordmann A, Briel M, Keller U, Yancy WS, Brehm BJ, et al. Effects of low-carbohydrate vs low-fat diets on weight loss and cardiovascular risk factors: a meta-analysis of randomized controlled trials. Arch Intern Med. 2006 Feb 13;166(3):285–93.

18.   Mullin GE. Search for the Optimal Diet. Nutr Clin Pract. 2010 Dec;25(6):581–4.

19.   Shipton MJ, Thachil J. Vitamin B12 deficiency - A 21st century perspective. Clin Med Lond Engl. 2015 Apr;15(2):145–50.

20.   DeNoon DJ. 7 Rules for Eating [Internet]. WebMD. [cited 2022 Jan 22]. Available from: https://www.webmd.com/food-recipes/news/20090323/7-rules-for-eating

21.   Ginter E, Simko V. Type 2 diabetes mellitus, pandemic in 21st century. Adv Exp Med Biol. 2012;771:42–50.

22.   Alpantaki K, Kampouroglou A, Koutserimpas C, Effraimidis G, Hadjipavlou A. Diabetes mellitus as a risk factor for intervertebral disc degeneration: a critical review. Eur Spine J. 2019 Sep;28(9):2129–44.

23.   Kakadiya G, Gandbhir V, Soni Y, Gohil K, Shakya A. Diabetes Mellitus-A Risk Factor for the Development of Lumbar Disc Degeneration: A Retrospective Study of an Indian Population. Glob Spine J. 2020 Sep 23;2192568220948035.

24.   Halkos ME, Puskas JD, Lattouf OM, Kilgo P, Kerendi F, Song HK, et al. Elevated preoperative hemoglobin A1c level is predictive of adverse events after coronary artery bypass surgery. J Thorac Cardiovasc Surg. 2008 Sep;136(3):631–40.

25.   Qin C, Kim JYS, Hsu WK. Impact of Insulin Dependence on Lumbar Surgery Outcomes: An NSQIP Analysis of 51,277 Patients. SPINE. 2016 Jun;41(11):E687–93.

26.   Guzman JZ, Iatridis JC, Skovrlj B, Cutler HS, Hecht AC, Qureshi SA, et al. Outcomes and Complications of Diabetes Mellitus on Patients Undergoing Degenerative Lumbar Spine Surgery: Spine. 2014 Sep;39(19):1596–604.

27.   Guzman JZ, Skovrlj B, Shin J, Hecht AC, Qureshi SA, Iatridis JC, et al. The Impact of

Diabetes Mellitus on Patients Undergoing Degenerative Cervical Spine Surgery: Spine. 2014 Sep;39(20):1656–65.

28.   Kusin DJ, Ahn UM, Ahn NU. The Influence of Diabetes on Surgical Outcomes in Cervical Myelopathy: SPINE. 2016 Sep;41(18):1436–40.

29.   World Health Organizaton. WHO-NMH-PND-17.4-eng.pdf [Internet]. [cited 2020 Jul 7]. Available from: https://apps.who.int/iris/bitstream/handle/10665/258503/WHO-NMH-PND-17.4-eng.pdf;jsessionid=E2CDDAC41F525F56363083E4D93EF863?sequence=1

30.   Battié MC, Videman T, Gill K, Moneta GB, Nyman R, Kaprio J, et al. 1991 Volvo Award in clinical sciences. Smoking and lumbar intervertebral disc degeneration: an MRI study of identical twins. Spine. 1991 Sep;16(9):1015–21.

31.   Scott SC, Goldberg MS, Mayo NE, Stock SR, Poîtras B. The association between cigarette smoking and back pain in adults. Spine. 1999 Jun 1;24(11):1090–8.

32.   Vogt MT, Hanscom B, Lauerman WC, Kang JD. Influence of Smoking on the Health Status of Spinal Patients: The National Spine Network Database. Spine. 2002 Feb;27(3):313–9.

33.   Kaila-Kangas L, Leino-Arjas P, Riihimäki H, Luukkonen R, Kirjonen J. Smoking and Overweight as Predictors of Hospitalization for Back Disorders: Spine. 2003 Aug;28(16):1860–8.

34.   Glassman SD, Anagnost SC, Parker A, Burke D, Johnson JR, Dimar JR. The effect of cigarette smoking and smoking cessation on spinal fusion. Spine. 2000;25(20):2608–15.

35.   Du JY, Weinberg DS, Moore TA, Vallier HA. Smoking Is Associated With Longer Intensive Care Unit Stays in Spine Trauma Patients. J Orthop Trauma. 2020 Jul;34(7):e250–5.

36.   Kusin DJ, Ahn UM, Ahn NU. The Effect of Smoking on Spinal Cord Healing Following Surgical Treatment of Cervical Myelopathy: Spine. 2015 Sep;40(18):1391–6.

37.   Schmid M, Sood A, Campbell L, Kapoor V, Dalela D, Klett DE, et al. Impact of smoking on perioperative outcomes after major surgery. Am J Surg. 2015 Aug;210(2):221-229.e6.

38.   Jung KH, Kim SM, Choi MG, Lee JH, Noh JH, Sohn TS, et al. Preoperative smoking cessation can reduce postoperative complications in gastric cancer surgery. Gastric Cancer. 2015 Oct;18(4):683–90.

39.   tonstad. Effect of Maintenance Therapy With Varenicline on Smoking Cessation: A Randomized Controlled Trial. :8.

40.   Tonstad S. Bupropion SR for smoking cessation in smokers with cardiovascular disease: a multicentre, randomised study. Eur Heart J. 2003 May;24(10):946–55.

41.   Riso P, Martini D, Møller P, Loft S, Bonacina G, Moro M, et al. DNA damage and repair activity after broccoli intake in young healthy smokers. Mutagenesis. 2010 Nov;25(6):595–602.

42.   Riso P, Vendrame S, Del Bo' C, Martini D, Martinetti A, Seregni E, et al. Effect of 10-day broccoli consumption on inflammatory status of young healthy smokers. Int J Food Sci Nutr. 2014 Feb;65(1):106–11.

43.   Gupta GP, Massagué J. Cancer metastasis: building a framework. Cell. 2006 Nov 17;127(4):679–95.

Figures:

Insulin Metabolism

High fat / high sugar diet:

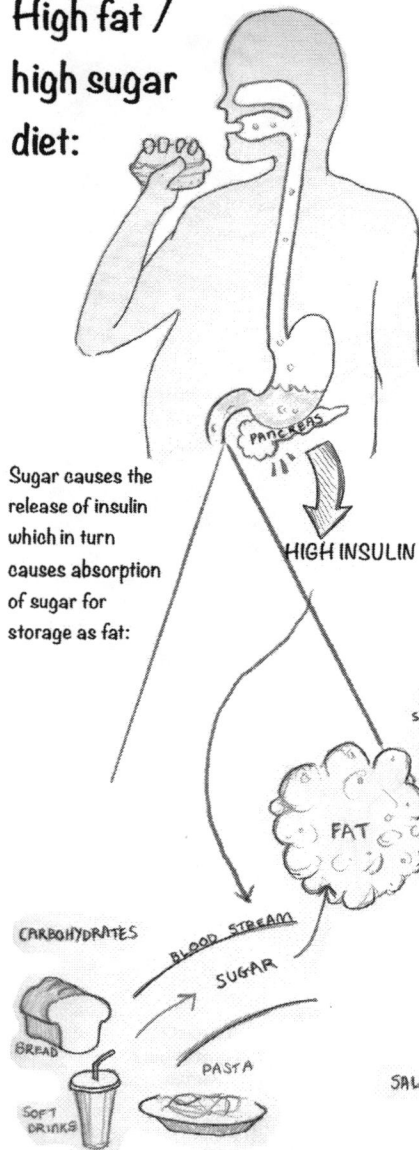

Low fat / low sugar diet:

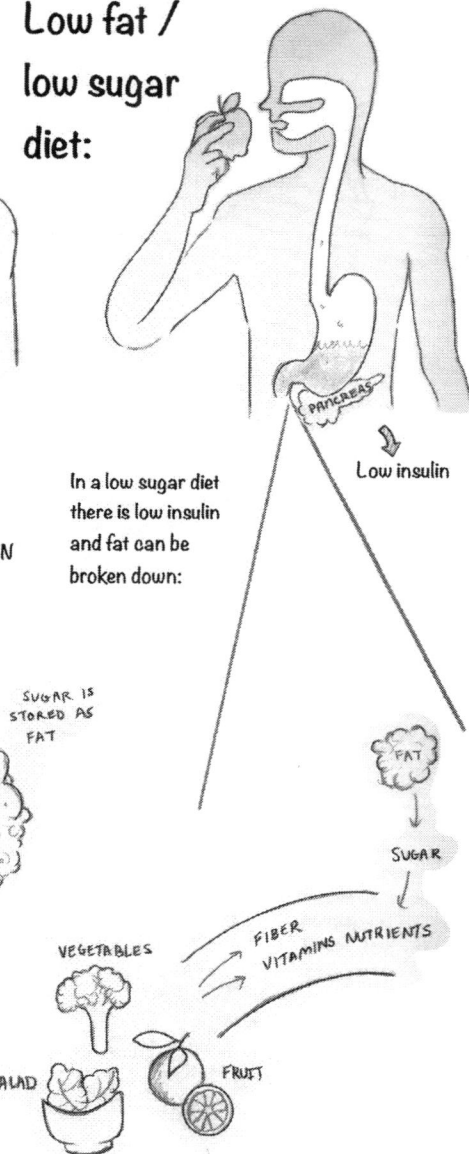

Sugar causes the release of insulin which in turn causes absorption of sugar for storage as fat:

HIGH INSULIN

In a low sugar diet there is low insulin and fat can be broken down:

Low insulin

SUGAR IS STORED AS FAT

FAT

FAT

SUGAR

CARBOHYDRATES

BLOOD STREAM

SUGAR

PASTA

BREAD

SOFT DRINKS

VEGETABLES

FIBER VITAMINS NUTRIENTS

SALAD

FRUIT

Insulin metabolism. Food rich in carbohydrates such as bread, soda, and pasta stimulate dramatic secretion of insulin from the pancreas which converts the carbohydrate sugar directly into fat. Such foods are very low in nutrients (left). Vegetables and fruits do not stimulate the release of insulin at high rates and are also full of nutrients. In a low insulin setting when carbohydrates are not being taken in, fat can be burned to use as energy (right).

Chapter 25

Care of the Aging Spine: Keeping Your Back Working For You in Your Golden Years Instead of the Other Way Around

Summary

As we age, our cells become less functional, and bodily tissues lose the ability to replenish and regenerate. The spine is not excluded from this process and undergoes predictable degeneration as we age. For some, spinal degeneration turns into serious pain and disability that can end in the need for surgery. For others, this is not the case, and they continue to have active lifestyles despite degeneration in the back and neck. What separates these groups? What can we do to make sure our backs work for us as opposed to having to work for our backs (going to the doctors, getting treatments and surgery)? While the answers to these questions remain somewhat unknown, there are many non-surgical interventions to not only extend the life span of our spines, but also of our lives. These include practices such as following a healthy low-calorie diet, not smoking, treating osteoporosis, and practicing a balanced exercise regimen.

Case

Mr. Silver is a healthy 70-year-old male. He retired from a career as a teacher at the age of 65 and has been very busy in retirement. He pays close attention to his health and makes sure he does at least 40-50 minutes of vigorous exercise 4-5 times a week. This can consist of a brisk hike, bicycle riding or even swimming and he enjoys switching between these activities. He used to be an avid runner but finds hiking, biking, and swimming to be more tolerable to his bones and joints these days. He participates in yoga and to outside viewers his posture, gait and flexibility reflect that of a young man, although he will tell you he feels stiff at times. He has never smoked, and only occasionally drinks wine. In addition to these basic tenets of lifestyle, he is very active with his grandkids and enjoys a full circle of friends with whom he regularly socializes. Although he can drive himself to the doctors, he is never short of volunteers who want to come with him for support. He has no pain, has not had a fracture from weakened bones, and takes no medicines.

Introduction

Getting older is inevitable. The turn of the century Italian philosopher Giacomo Leopardi had this to say about aging: "Old age is the supreme evil, because it deprives us of all pleasures, leaving us only the appetite for them, and it brings with it all sufferings. Nevertheless, we fear death, and we desire old age." We all want to continue living, but the price for continued life is getting older, including an aging skeleton. Unfortunately aches and pains are going to be in everyone's future, but as a physician I have noticed that there seems to be a trick to aging gracefully. Looking at colleagues and patients, I have seen those who "cruise" into old age, and those who "bruise" into old age. In other words, some have no issues in old age, and others have endless problems. While genetics likely play a crucial role in aging, we cannot control our genes (yet). However, we do have the power to change environmental factors and lifestyle choices that accelerate aging. In medicine we talk about a patient's genotype and phenotype. The genotype simply refers to the type of genes a person has (for example, a person has a gene for brown hair), while the phenotype refers to the actual expression of those genes (that is, a person has brown hair). Our environment plays a role in determining the phenotype as expressed with this equation (1):

Phenotype = Genotype + (diet and lifestyle).

The phenotype we all want is one that allows us to live a long, healthy life. We must assume we are stuck with our genotype, but this equation begs the question: what are the things we can do to age gracefully?

What Is Aging and Why Does It Happen?

Aging is simply the process of becoming older. Superficially, as we age, we appear to have more wrinkles and blemishes in the skin, and perhaps grayer hair. We don't have the same strength, endurance and even body shape as we did when we were younger. But on a molecular and cellular level in the body, what is driving these changes?

Cells are the building blocks that form all our tissues. As we age, our cells age too. Stem cells, which are cells that are capable of becoming a range of different tissues (bone, muscle, blood etc.) lose the capacity to undergo differentiation—the ability to change from one cell type to another (2). This is problematic because stem cells are responsible for replenishing damaged tissue, for example, damaged cartilage in joints. So, the body cannot regenerate as effectively.

Unlike the cells in young bodies, cells in the older person's body also lose some of their metabolic capacity and start to accumulate waste proteins, resulting in malfunction. This is thought to occur because of several different reasons: 1. DNA damage arising from exposure to free radicals (free radicals are high energy molecules in the body capable of destroying or damaging other molecules); 2. Shortening of telomeres (telomeres are structures on the end of your DNA that protect it from degradation); 3. Advanced glycosylation end products (AGEs) (destructive molecules created from sugar) abnormally bond with other normal proteins and fat molecules and, over time, these altered molecules accumulate; 4. Our cells may be intrinsically programed genetically to age and stop working (1).

Thus, the body loses its ability to replace old or damaged cells and those older cells start to malfunction. This disrupts the complex biological processes in the body.

Cellular aging processes affect the musculoskeletal system, and we know that three things happen: 1. bones lose density, becoming weaker and more brittle (aka osteoporosis and osteopenia); 2. muscle mass and density decreases (aka sarcopenia); and 3. the smooth cartilage which covers our joints wears down. In the spine all three of these processes occur in addition to degeneration of the intervertebral discs—the structures which are responsible for linking our vertebrae together.

What Happens to the Spine as We Age?

The spine, which is composed of vertebral bones, as well as the facet joints and intervertebral discs that connect them, degrade as we age (3). In addition to this, the muscles surrounding the spine tend to atrophy (waste away), shrink, and become less functional –a condition called sarcopenia.

The facet joints, which are small, paired joints that link adjacent vertebrae together tend to become arthritic as we get older. What this means is that the smooth cartilage surface of the joints become worn down and bone starts to rub on bone. This abnormal contact can result in the development of bone spurs (osteophytes) that try to stabilize the joint. This results in increased stiffness of the spine and potentially even pinched nerves.

The intervertebral discs undergo characteristic changes as we age. The discs have two main components: a tough outer ring called the annulus fibrosis and an inner jelly like material called the nucleus pulposus. The discs are normally very elastic and springy which helps them to better absorb shocks between the vertebrae. Another unique feature of the discs is that they are not exposed to a very good blood supply and tend to get nutrients and oxygen from the bone. Special cells called notochordal cells that help maintain this structure start to disappear as we age. When these cells start to disappear, chemicals that break down the structure of discs increase in concentration. The discs become dried out and brittle making them more susceptible to injury. In addition, they start to collapse because they can no longer support the weight of the body. As the intervertebral discs are worn away, the vertebral bodies may come into contact with one another and start to form reactive bone spurs as well.

The vertebrae (the cylindrical bones that make up the spinal column) can become weakened from osteoporosis and may start to collapse and lose some of their height and shape (please see chapter 12 on osteoporosis for more information). Changes in the vertebral shape and height as well as the disintegration of the discs lead to an overall more slouched (kyphotic) posture and even a decrease in your overall height.

Your hips, knees, pelvis, neck, and abdominal muscles will try to fight this change in posture, but they too become atrophied and will no longer have the same strength. Because you are more slouched forward your hips and pelvis will try to compensate to keep you upright by flexing. You may bend your knees to try and maintain your posture. A good deal of back pain will originate from aged muscles and joints straining to correct a kyphotic back posture.

So, is it all doom and gloom? Hardly. You will be happy to know that most degenerative changes have no impact on our quality of life. The prevalence of degenerative disc disease is greater than 90% in those over 60 years of age, but the vast majority have no symptoms at all. So, let's explore the tricks to keeping your spine working for you even as you age.

What Can We Do to Delay Aging?

There is no holy grail. The science behind aging is still in its infancy, but there are many promising theories on how we can prevent or delay aging. First, we discuss some strategies to delay cellular aging followed by good practices to keep your back young.

strategies to prevent or delay cellular aging

Cellular aging seems to be related to the generation of free radical and AGE molecules in the body, so it would make sense that decreasing these in your body would slow the aging process.

Advanced glycosylated end products (AGEs) are nasty molecules that form when sugar combines with protein or fat and accumulate in many different tissues as we age. AGE accumulation causes damage and malfunction of cells, leading to the changes we see with aging. Decreasing the number of AGEs in the body may thus slow aging. AGEs can either be produced in the body (when sugar combines with proteins or fats) or is ingested. High levels of sugar in the blood stream, as is present in diabetics or those who eat a high amount of processed sugar can increase the concentration of AGEs in the body. AGEs are also present in processed foods, foods which have been cooked with dry heat at high temperature (grilling, broiling, frying, etc.) and in cigarette smoke (4). Thus, maintaining a healthy diet low in sugar, processed, fried, or grilled substances, and avoiding cigarette smoke is critical to reducing your AGE burden. It is also possible that exercise decreases AGEs (1).

Decreasing free radical oxidation in the body is also theorized to slow the aging process. Once again, free radicals are high energy molecules that can cause damage to DNA as well as other critical enzymes in the body. While there is currently no evidence that antioxidant supplementation increases life span, a diet rich in antioxidants (think of colorful foods) may help balance the amount of free radicals in the body and delay aging (1). Smoking and alcohol intake also increase free radicals in the body, so limiting or not consuming these products can increase longevity.

Calorie restriction (limiting the number of calories you eat every day) has been shown to increase longevity in laboratory animals and potentially could have a similar effect in humans. It's not clear exactly why this increases lifespan but may have to do with reducing the metabolic rate of the body and thus the reduced generation of free radicals and AGEs. Caloric restriction means decreasing the number of calories you eat without causing malnutrition. This can be done by reducing your overall daily or weekly food consumption by 15-20% (5,6).

strategies for protecting the aging spine

Osteoporosis, or loss of bone mineral density, occurs to everyone to some degree. Prevention is critical for maintaining the structural integrity of your spine and can be accomplished by avoiding smoking, alcohol, insufficient exercise, and poor nutrition. Osteoporosis can lead to fractures of the weakened vertebral bone that are known as insufficiency compression fractures, meaning the bone fractures under a stress that does not harm healthy bone. Insufficiency compression fractures have direct impact on your overall mortality (7). Preventing and treating compression fractures is important for extending life. Please see chapter 12 on osteoporosis for more information.

preventing degenerative disc disease

Like osteoporosis, almost all people (more than 90%) will show some form of disc degeneration by the age of 60. This seems to be increased in people who participate in high impact or high load sports such as football, hockey, gymnastics to name a few. Interestingly runners do not seem to be affected by degenerative disc disease. Most of degenerative disc disease is predicted by genetics, but there are some external factors which can accelerate deterioration. These include a sedentary lifestyle with prolonged sitting, trauma, smoking, alcohol, as well as excessive strain caused by labor intensive jobs such as construction or those jobs that require heavy lifting.

weight loss and obesity

Your entire torso is supported by the L5-S1 disc, which is about the diameter of a soda can. If your torso is larger, more pressure is exerted on this disc. Obesity is directly related to increased degenerative disc disease, because the discs must shoulder a heavier weight and break down faster. Reducing and maintaining your right weight is a critical component of extending the life of your spine.

exercise

The overall benefits of exercise have been shown to outweigh the consequences from increased wear on the body (8). As we age, our sedentary behavior increases, meaning we sit around more. This increases the risk of unhealthy sugar metabolism, and death (9). The key is to find exercise that does not increase pain or come with a significant risk of injury, both of which become more common as we age. Swimming, walking, and hiking are all excellent recreational activities with a low risk of injury. Aqua therapy, otherwise known as water aerobics, can also be an excellent way for seniors to get exercise. Water unloads painful arthritic joints and can help recondition muscles for traditional land-based exercise. Cross training (that is, doing different types of exercises) can also help prevent overuse of muscle and ligamentous groups. Exercise is important for preventing both sarcopenia and osteoporosis and should involve a combination of cardiovascular and strength training (10).

At least 150 minutes of moderate intensity (for example, brisk walking, aqua therapy, hiking) or 75 minutes or vigorous intensity cardiovascular work such as running or biking broken up into 3-5 sessions, should be performed per week. Strength training should be done 2-3 times per week and involve at least 12 reps of 10 exercises that target major muscle groups (biceps, chest, abdominals, back, shoulders, quads, hamstrings and calves) (9). Flexibility exercises should be performed at least 10 min daily—this helps prevent stiffness and further damage and deterioration to joints (please see chapter 21 on alternative therapy for instructions on core strength and flexibility exercise). Yoga is a relatively safe and effective way to do this and can decrease your back and neck pain—although its best if you have supervision if you are not comfortable with the postures.

Yoga postures that help to reduce spinal pain (11)	
Adho Mukha Svanasana	Downward dog
Adho Mukho Virasana	Child's pose
Ardha Uttanasana	Forward bend with flat back
Supta Pavanamuktasana	Lying knee pose
Utthita Parsvakonasana	Extended side angle
Utthita Trikonasana	Triangle pose

posture and lifestyle modifications

Being conscious of your posture is critical as you age. As discussed, the spine tends to bend forward as you get older, so always maintaining an erect posture while walking and sitting will help keep your spinal muscles active. Also, while sitting you should try to not allow your spine to sag or your low back to curve forward. Think about sitting on your hips and keeping your back upright. Sitting should be limited to 40 minutes at a time to prevent any excess pressure on the discs (sitting in one position tends to place abnormal forces on the disc).

If your job or life involves heavy labor or lifting it can put strain on your back and discs over the years. Regularly lifting greater than 50 lbs. over waist with poor mechanics is a recipe for disaster. Use common sense and pay attention to your body. If you are having pain with lifting it either means you have a problem with your back, or you are lifting incorrectly. While it may not be possible to leave a job or lifestyle to decrease the load on your spine, it is possible to modify how you work and lift.

Always lift with your back straight, using your legs to elevate an object and not by bending your spine. Keep your gaze up to help avoid bending the back. If you start to hurt, take a break, or try modifying the task. Understand that accidents are more likely to happen when you are tired and distracted.

balance

Falls are a common cause of orthopedic injuries in the elderly because even low impact trauma can cause serious fractures due to weak bones. Falls also become more likely because there is a decrease in your ability to balance as you age related to a decline in strength and flexibility (12). Losing your balance not only increases your risk for fractures, but also increases the risk of mortality, possibly because hip and spine fractures can cause a serious decline in health. Working on your balance daily should be a priority. A balance exercise program can consist of standing on one leg and abducting your other leg out to the side, followed by hip extension (moving your leg behind you) and hip flexion (pretending to kick a soccer ball in front of you), using a nearby chair to hold onto in case you lose your balance. Do 10 sets on each side. Activities like Tai Chi and strength training can help increase your balance.

It's not just about you!

Having a rich network of family and friends is very beneficial to your spine and overall health. Those with supportive people around them live longer. The reason for this is obvious to me as a physician. You have people to take you to your doctors' appointments! It seems ridiculous but accessing medical care as you age becomes more difficult for many reasons. You may lose the ability to drive, and your overall physical mobility is decreased. You may not be able to hear what the doctor says or have trouble remembering exactly what he said. Having a caring friend and family member may be the difference between getting an elective spine surgery, and being bed bound in a nursing home. In addition to this practical benefit, multiple studies have shown that those who have a rich network of family and friends live longer happier lives (13).

Conclusion

Though there is no silver bullet or magic pill to keep our spines healthy as we age, there are many choices we make daily that can keep our spines healthy. Furthermore, the same habits that promote a healthy spine promote a healthy body and mind. Caring for your spine requires avoiding a harmful diet (high calorie and high sugar), smoking, and obesity. If your job involves heavy labor always be mindful about how you are using your bones and muscles to avoid undue pain and stress. You should also regularly exercise, focusing on cardiovascular, strength and flexibility. Make sure you have a rich social network and can access expert spine and medical care.

Frequently Asked Questions

- **Even if I need spine surgery, if I'm old, it will be too dangerous right? How old is too old for spine surgery?**

    This is a common question and thus I devote an entire chapter to discussing spine surgery in the elderly (chapter 34). The short answer is that most people who have spine surgery are greater than age 65 (so spine surgery is not just for young people), and your ability to tolerate surgery depends more on your overall health.

References

1.   da Costa JP, Vitorino R, Silva GM, Vogel C, Duarte AC, Rocha-Santos T. A synopsis on aging—Theories, mechanisms and future prospects. Ageing Research Reviews. 2016 Aug;29:90–112.

2.   Roberts S, Colombier P, Sowman A, Mennan C, Rölfing JHD, Guicheux J, et al. Ageing in the musculoskeletal system: Cellular function and dysfunction throughout life. Acta Orthopaedica. 2016 Dec 16;87(sup363):15–25.

3.   Prescher A. Anatomy and pathology of the aging spine. European Journal of Radiology. 1998 Jul;27(3):181–95.

4.   Singh R, Barden A, Mori T, Beilin L. Advanced glycation end-products: a review. Diabetologia. 2001 Feb 5;44(2):129–46.

5.   Most J, Redman LM. Impact of calorie restriction on energy metabolism in humans. Experimental Gerontology. 2020 May;133:110875.

6.   Calorie Restriction and Fasting Diets: What Do We Know? [Internet]. National Institute on Aging. [cited 2022 Jul 30]. Available from: https://www.nia.nih.gov/news/calorie-restriction-and-fasting-diets-what-do-we-know

7.   Kado DM, Browner WS, Palermo L, Nevitt MC, Genant HK, Cummings SR. Vertebral fractures and mortality in older women: a prospective study. Study of Osteoporotic Fractures Research Group. Arch Intern Med. 1999 Jun 14;159(11):1215–20.

8.   Kamalapathy PN, Hassanzadeh H. Spinal Care in the Aging Athlete. Clinics in Sports Medicine. 2021 Jul;40(3):571–84.

9.   Lee PG, Jackson EA, Richardson CR. Exercise Prescriptions in Older Adults. 2017;95(7):8.

10.   Tournadre A, Vial G, Capel F, Soubrier M, Boirie Y. Sarcopenia. Joint Bone Spine. 2019 May;86(3):309–14.

11.   Crow E, Jeannot E, Trewhela A. Effectiveness of Iyengar yoga in treating spinal

(back and neck) pain: A systematic review. Int J Yoga. 2015;8(1):3.

12.   Araujo CG, de Souza E Silva CG, Laukkanen JA, Fiatarone Singh M, Kunutsor S, Myers J, et al. Successful 10-second one-legged stance performance predicts survival in middle-aged and older individuals. Br J Sports Med. 2022 Jun 21;bjsports-2021-105360.

13.   Vila J. Social Support and Longevity: Meta-Analysis-Based Evidence and Psychobiological Mechanisms. Front Psychol. 2021 Sep 13;12:717164.

Figures:

The Aging Spine

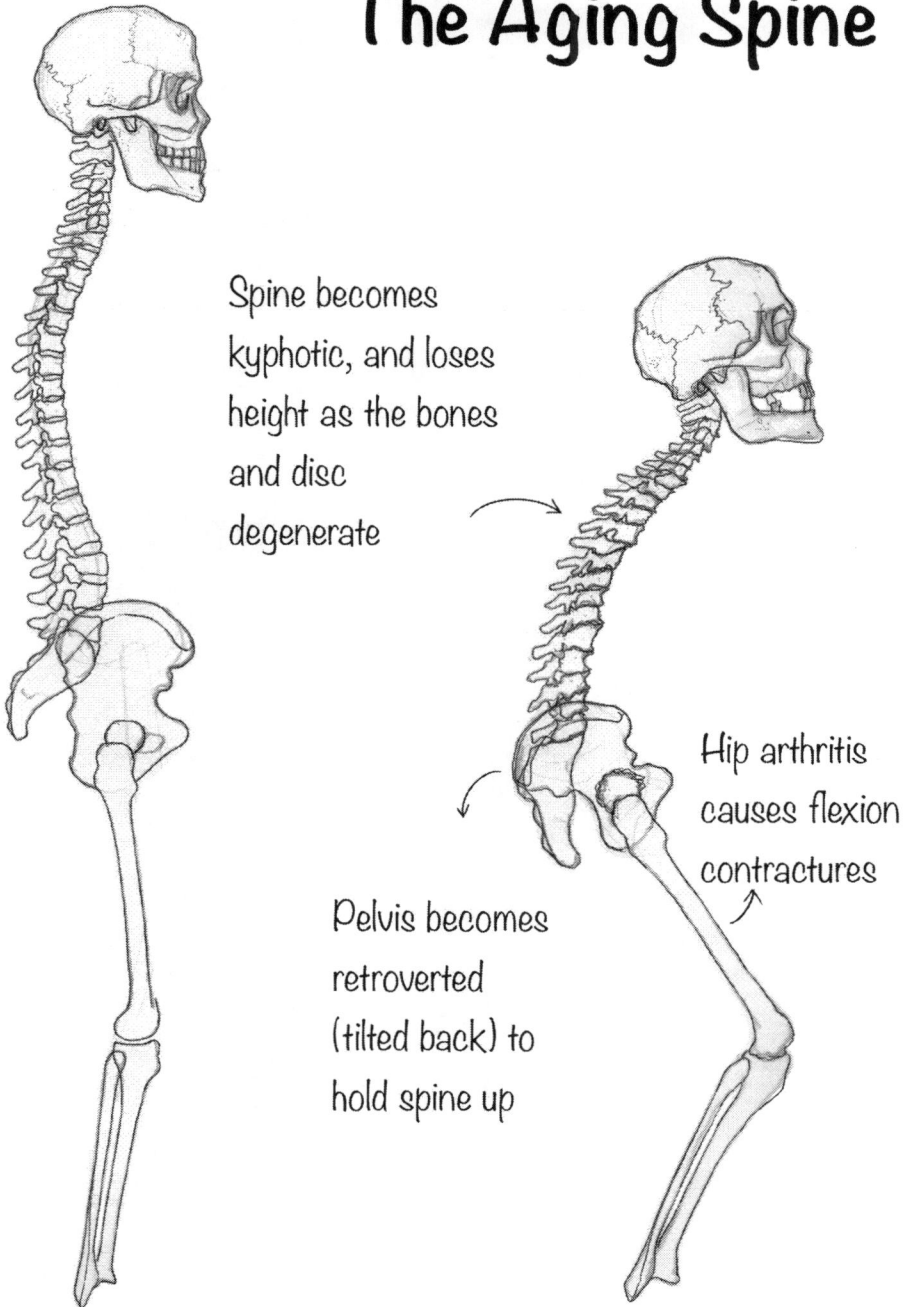

Spine becomes
kyphotic, and loses
height as the bones
and disc
degenerate

Hip arthritis
causes flexion
contractures

Pelvis becomes
retroverted
(tilted back) to
hold spine up

The Aging Spine. As you age the lumbar spine becomes more kyphotic meaning you start to bend forward. To stay upright you compensate through several mechanisms. You flex your hips and tilt your pelvis back. You crane your neck back to keep your head up. You bend at the knees to pull your back into alignment. These changes alter the biomechanics of the body and increase pain.

Disc Aging

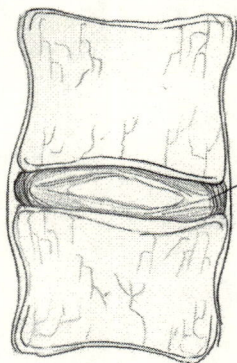

Healthy,
hydrated disc

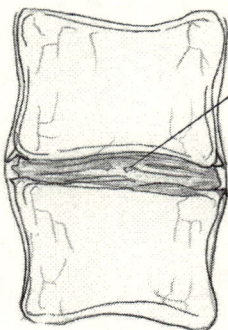

Disc starts to
fissure, crack and
dry out losing height

Small bone spurs
start to form

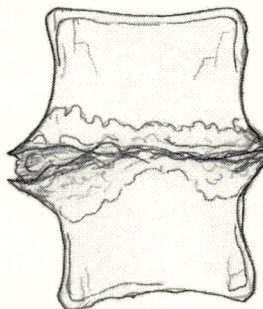

Disc totally
degenerates resulting
in bone on bone
contact

Disc Aging. Discs age in a predictable fashion. First, they lose their hydration becoming dry. This causes the disc to lose its flexibility and it cracks easily becoming more susceptible to injury. Overtime the disc wears down, allowing the bones to come into contact.

Yoga Poses:

Downward dog

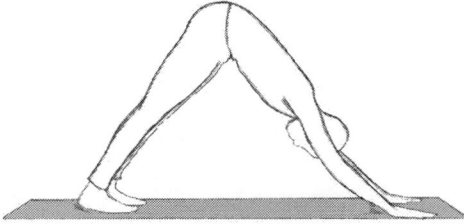

Child's pose

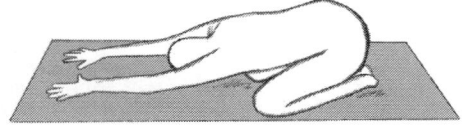

Forward bend

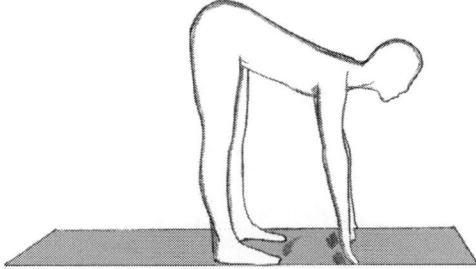

Lying knee pose

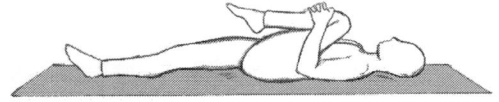

Extended side angle

Triangle pose

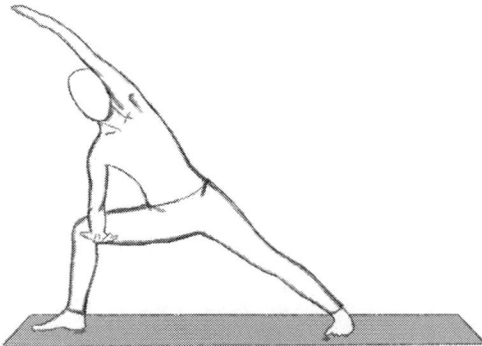

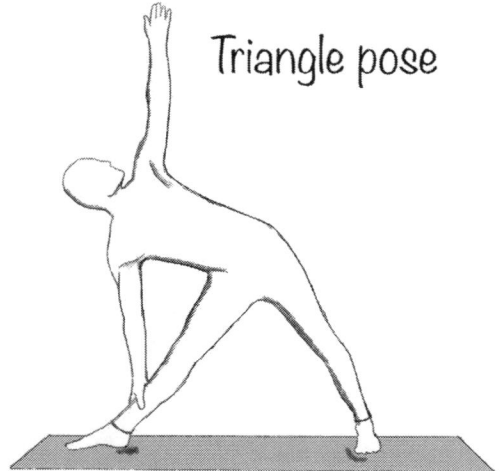

Yoga poses. Yoga can be an excellent way to maintain flexibility and strength. It is best done with an instructor at first.

Balance Exercises

Hip Abduction

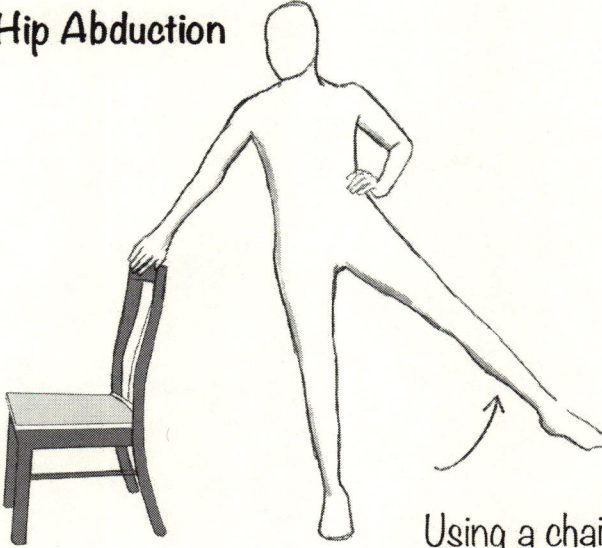

Using a chair to balance practice raising your leg in flexion, extension and abduction

Hip Flexion

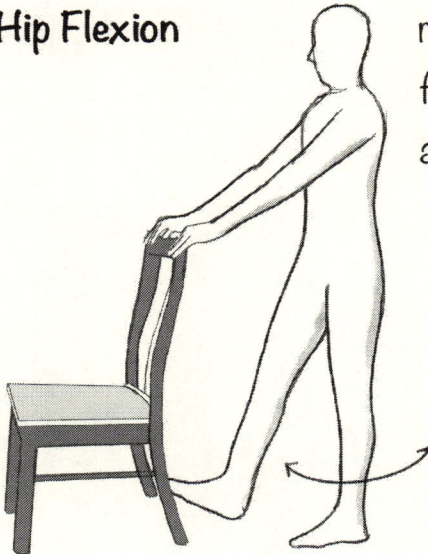

Balance exercises. Holding onto a chair abduct your leg on one side for 10 reps (top). Then do the other side. Then turn to face the chair and move one leg forward and back 10 times each. Once you get the hang of it and can maintain your balance try doing these exercises without holding on to the chair.

SECTION 4

What You Need to Know About the Different Types of Spine Surgery

"I fear the day when technology will surpass our human interaction. The world will have a generation of idiots." -Albert Einstein

Chapter 26

Finding the Right Spine Surgeon and Hospital

Summary

Many patients with spine problems like to start off with a doctor who does not perform surgery such as a physiatrist or neurologist. This may be a good option because you can hopefully get a diagnosis and undergo some conservative treatment. If you find you are getting worse, or not improving with non-operative care, then you should be referred to see a spine surgeon. Spine surgeons are either orthopedic surgeons or neurosurgeons. Ideally, you should see someone who has also completed a fellowship specifically in spine surgery in addition to his/her primary residency. Look for someone who is either "board eligible" or "board certified." Additionally, you should find a doctor with a good reputation either by talking to friends or your primary care provider. You may be tempted to only to go a tertiary center (offering more specialized care) because of its size and number of specialists; however, superior care is often provided by small local hospitals. However, tertiary care centers may be more equipped for very complicated spine cases where there may be high blood loss or the need for multiple medical specialists.

Try to go somewhere close to home if possible. When you see the spine surgeon, make sure you have your story down and be as organized as possible. Do not wait until the consultation begins to think about what to say about your problem and medical history. Think about the symptoms which bother you the most and avoid the "shopping list" method where you try to convey every ache and pain in detail. Some symptoms occur together, such as numbness and weakness and should be described that way. Write it all down so you are ready for the interview.

Case

Mr. Slate is a 57-year-old businessman who is suffering from a C5-6-disc herniation that is causing severe neck and arm pain and weakness. He receives an MRI by his primary care doctor who then recommends he see a spine surgeon. He gets his first opinion from a surgeon who recommends a C5-6 fusion. He doesn't get a good impression from this doctor and makes appointments to see 2 other surgeons. One is at a big academic center and after a quick appointment recommends a two-level cervical fusion because he thinks that the C4-5 level does not look great either. Mr. Slate then makes an appointment with a local doctor who instead recommends a C5-6-disc arthroplasty (artificial disc replacement). Mr. Slate is really unsure which opinion he should go with but ultimately decides to go with the surgeon who recommended the C5-6-disc replacement as he had a good rapport with him. This doctor took a little more time explaining the diagnosis and the various options including reviewing the possibility of a cervical fusion. Ultimately the surgery goes well but Mr. Slate is shocked to realize that there could be so many differing opinions on how to treat his problem all coming from doctors in the same field.

Introduction

For many patients, visiting the spine surgeon is a serious event in their lives marked by feeling anxious at the thought of potential spinal surgery and fretting over whether they can trust the person who is recommending it. But keep in mind that visiting the spine surgeon is visiting someone who can help guide you, shed light on the problem and ultimately help you. Nonetheless, there should be some preparation on your part, not only to optimize the working relationship with the surgeon, but to help you know you are with a good doctor. In this chapter we discuss spine surgeons and how you can find the right one and make sure the consultation goes well.

I Have a Spine Problem—Do I Need to See a Surgeon First?

Obviously, that is a difficult question to answer without seeing a surgeon (you won't know you need surgery until a surgeon recommends it). There are many types of medical physicians who deal in spine problems that are not surgeons and can offer guidance and medical treatments for pain. Physiatrists are doctors specializing in rehabilitation, often do injections to treat pain, and specialize in examination of the musculoskeletal system. Some specialize only in pain management of spinal conditions and have a good knowledge of spinal problems. Neurologists are doctors specializing in the medical treatment of brain and nerve problems, such as strokes, degenerative neurological diseases such as multiple sclerosis, and spinal problems. Neurologists are excellent diagnosticians and can help pinpoint your problem and suggest whether you need to see a surgeon. Rheumatologists specialize in joint problems such as rheumatoid arthritis and inflammation and pain and may also have knowledge of spinal disorders. Finally pain medicine specialists and so-called "interventionalists" may also be helpful, particularly at offering non-operative treatments for pain. Interventionalists consists of doctors (for example, anesthesiologists, neurologists, radiologists) who perform procedures such as injections to treat pain. Any of these doctors may be a good first stop before seeing the surgeon.

I find that some people are afraid of seeing a surgeon and would rather see a "non-operative" doctor (see below). Luckily most spinal conditions do not require surgery; however, the pickle comes in sorting out which do and which don't. There is no one more qualified to do this than the spine surgeon. Most spine surgeons I know only like to operate on conditions that they know they can help improve and thus are very conservative in selecting surgical cases. If you know you need a surgeon (particularly after seeing a non-op doc), don't hesitate to see a spine surgeon for fear of too quick a recommendation to operate; he/she will not suggest surgery lightly.

Fear of the Surgeon

There is a natural phenomenon in medicine for patients to "fear the surgeon." This is a cognitive bias based on the fear of surgery where patients will knowingly avoid going to see a surgeon and instead will repeatedly seek treatment from a practitioner who does not have surgical qualifications. This cognitive bias has created a host of "interventional" procedures and "specialists" who offer treatments that in essence are surgical procedures but have a more pleasing sound to them. I do not necessarily think this is a bad thing. Some problems will not benefit from surgery and simple procedures may be useful. Furthermore, many interventionalists are exceptionally well trained and know when a patient should be referred to a surgeon. The problem arises when treatments are offered and accepted with little hope of solving serious problems in the spine, or from practitioners with poor training. Moreover, as stated above "interventions" or "minimally invasive procedures" often have the same risk of traditional surgery. Deciding on which treatment to accept is often difficult and confusing for the patient. I would recommend if you are concerned, to see a surgeon with the proper training (see below) to see if minimally invasive procedures are appropriate. Surgery is a sacred practice, and it takes years of dedicated training to call yourself "surgeon."

Preparing to See the Spine Surgeon

Remember that going to see the doctor is a stressful event. You may have to wait and then maybe dress in a gown to be examined. Bring something that can keep you busy while you wait, such as a magazine, book or even a game/tv show on your cell phone. You can also use the time you wait to be seen by the doctor to go over what you think it's important to tell him or her. Make sure to write it down to consolidate your thoughts. Bringing a trusted friend or loved one with you to the consultation can be an excellent idea. They can offer to be a second set of eyes and ears which is particularly helpful in a situation where you are stressed and may not be listening your best. I have even seen companions come to the visit to take notes for the patient.

It is important to remember your spine surgeon wants to help you and guide you in making correct decisions. Some surgeons have different philosophies on how to accomplish this. For example, most spine surgeons will think that declining to operate on a spinal problem that will not benefit from surgery is helping the patient to avoid unnecessary surgery. This is my perspective—there is no point in attempting surgery with a low success rate. For spine surgery to be successful there needs to be a clear surgical target—one that is backed up by a combination of exam findings, radiological findings, and symptoms. If only one or two of these indicators for surgery are present, it may not be enough to justify surgery.

On the other hand, some surgeons will simply look at the MRI and determine that there is no surgical remedy—they tell you this—and that is the end of the consultation. You may leave the spine office a little perturbed that he/she didn't spend more time with you, but remember, ultimately this can be a service to you. Most become doctors because they want to help, and it is hard to tell patients you cannot help them. I always remind myself and my patients that the alternative—offering surgery when it is not beneficial—is much worse. Once a surgeon has made the decision not to operate they may present this in a way that is interpreted as callous and patients will feel as if "this guy is not helping me!" While bedside manner is critical in surgery, even more critical is not operating when it is not indicated.

the importance of organization

You may have been living with your symptoms for months—you know exactly what they are and could recite them easily, right? In most cases the answer is probably no. Most people have different ideas of what going to the doctor is like. Some people feel rushed in the medical office and feel as if they do not get to "tell their story." In most cases spine surgeons are busy people who want to get to the facts to determine what kind of treatment you need. Spine surgeons are still human, get tired and have difficulty focusing on long-winded stories just as anyone else would. You are not likely to get much benefit from a spine surgeon if you spend an hour talking about problems you are having without ever getting to the point of what is really bothering you. Therefore, focusing your story as much as you can before you see the surgeon is important, even writing it down, so that you know what points you most want to get across. Try to be as focused as possible and highlight the major symptom that is bothering you. If you can do this in less than 2 minutes even better. For example, if you have mild pain in your neck and arms, but your main complaint is severe right lower extremity pain, you should lead with that main complaint. If you have neurologic symptoms such as weakness in your extremities, numbness, difficulty with balance or gait, bowel and bladder incontinence, these should also be brought up.

Basic Information to Bring to Your Visit with a Spine Surgeon
What is your main symptom? What is causing you to seek treatment? Where exactly is the problem?
Include some details about this symptom: when did it start, what seems to trigger it or make it worse? What treatments have you tried?
Are you experiencing any of the following? Weakness/paralysis, numbness or tingling, bowel and bladder difficulty, loss of balance, falls, clumsiness?
What is your medical history? Have you had previous spinal surgeries? If yes, write them down in the following way: "procedure X, performed by Dr. X on date XXXX"

In general, the more chronological you are about your problem the better. Give a 1–2-minute summary of your problem. Start when things really became bad and what may have caused it and how you got to where you are now. Let him/her know what you have tried and if it worked or not. In a busy surgical practice time is limited, and so the more organized you are, the more likely you are to communicate effectively with your surgeon and ultimately make his or her job easier. Write down a synopsis. Do not expect the surgeon to read your mind or intuit what is wrong with you without information. I can't emphasize how critical this is and how few people take the time to do this. Think of when you go grocery shopping without a list. You inevitably forget things that you needed, buy unnecessary things you didn't need and take a lot more time in the store. When you have a list, you get exactly what you need and are very efficient with your time.

medical records

If you have had previous surgery it is important to bring your records, especially the operative notes if you can get them, as you may not know the specific technical details. These can be obtained from your hospital's medical record department. Any test results, X-rays or scans you have had performed should also be brought with you to your visit. It's not enough to bring the radiology reports (a note from a radiologist giving the interpretation of the scans). If you have had a scan done, all hospitals should be able to provide you with a copy of that study, usually in the form of a CD. You usually must go to the radiology department to get this. Spine surgeons all read their own studies and images and will want to see the hard copies. Some patients with multiple medical problems and past surgeries find it helpful to keep track of things with a single document that lists all their medical problems, medications, allergies, and surgeries so it can be presented to doctors at medical appointments, thereby avoiding having to list things out each time they make a visit to the medical office. I cannot emphasize enough how helpful this is, especially if you have a complicated medical history.

questions

Write down your questions BEFORE you see the surgeon, you will forget them in the heat of the moment and they may go unanswered. The more prepared you are, the better your consultation with the surgeon will go.

Some useful questions include the following:

- **What do you think is the cause of my symptoms? Is it likely coming from my spine?**

- **What treatments are available to help? Could surgery help me?**

Checklist for Visiting the Surgeon
Write down a synopsis of what your symptoms are.
Make sure you have access to all old spine surgery operative reports.
Bring X-ray/MRI/CT studies of your spine with you or have them sent ahead on CDs.
Write down in an organized list all your medical problems, past surgeries, medications, allergies. It's best to do this in a word processing document that you can edit over time.
Write down 2-3 questions you are interested in asking.

Selecting a Spine Surgeon

There are many factors which go into choosing a spine surgeon. In general, you will want your surgery performed by a specialist who has completed a training program in either neurosurgery or orthopedic surgery (see section below). While there may be slight differences in conditions treated between orthopedic surgeons and neurosurgeons (orthopedic surgeons tend to focus on spinal deformity and neurosurgeons tend to focus on tumors and the brain), there are no major differences in the capability of these two groups of doctors in terms of the spine. If you have an aneurysm in your spinal cord, you are probably better off seeing a neurosurgeon; however, if you have scoliosis you are better served by an orthopedist. Most general spinal cases can be done by either group.

There is a wide swath of interventionalists. These are physicians trained to perform so called "minimally invasive procedures" and they have varied training in spinal care yet offer many spinal procedures. These include procedures such as epidural steroid injections, and radiofrequency ablation—procedures performed only with needles. In general, it is reasonable to see these providers for non-operative care, but more invasive procedures are best left to surgeons—those who have trained to do surgery (1). If you are having a procedure done by an interventionalist, you should make sure orthopedists or neurosurgeons are available as a back-up in case things go wrong at the hospital.

If you are looking for care of your child for scoliosis or some other pediatric condition keep in mind that there are two different types of surgeons who operate on children and they are classified by the kind of training they have received: the spine fellowship trained surgeon and the pediatric fellowship trained surgeon. Both may perform surgery for scoliosis. The spine fellowship trains the surgeon in all aspects of the spine, whereas pediatric orthopedic surgeons only devote a portion of their training to spinal conditions and only those specific to children; their training is focused on the unique challenges of dealing with a child's still growing and ever-changing musculoskeletal system. Thus, pediatric orthopedic surgeons are comfortable treating children with many overlapping orthopedic problems such as kids with cerebral palsy or spinal muscular atrophy. Because of the complexity of spine surgery and the uniqueness of each case, you and your doctor will have to decide which of these surgeons can best deal with your child's spinal condition as both are equally qualified.

When you meet your spine surgeon ask yourself if this is someone you will work well with? Do you feel comfortable with him/her? Surgery of the spine can be a long and complicated path and making sure you trust and feel comfortable with your surgeon is critical. Does the surgeon explain the rationale for surgery and explore whether you have exhausted non-operative care? You may not just be dealing with this person for a once-off procedure. Even simple problems in spine surgery may become complicated. Your problem may require more than one procedure or may require a revision in several years. Would you want to work with this person for that long? My personal philosophy is that the patients I operate on are part of an extended family. I would look after them (if able) for as long as I humanly could.

Beyond checking out the kind of training a surgeon has had, word of mouth is perhaps the best way to find a good surgeon. Talking to your friends who have had a good experience with a surgeon is likely your best shot at finding someone who is reputable. Your primary care provider will have experience referring patients to different surgeons and will be a good resource. You can also look at online reviews, but these do not often tell the full story of a surgeon's skill. There are numerous online hacking schemes which target physicians and hold them ransom by posting false negative reviews. Furthermore, it is common to receive complaints on office wait times and other factors which obviously do not reflect surgical skill.

Your surgeon is part of a team that will be delivering your care. This includes both the office staff as well as the hospital staff. There are many factors in the hospital which can determine the result of your surgery that your surgeon has very little control over. For example, the cleanliness of the facility can impact infection rates. Nursing staff may be good or bad. Finally, you may be limited by your type of insurance which only allows you to have care at certain hospitals.

Some surgeons work as teams. Spine surgery can be long, exhausting, and stressful. In big spine cases it can be helpful to share the load with another spine surgeon to ensure the case moves along at a good pace. In spine surgery this is common for anterior lumbar access surgery (surgery performed through the abdomen) where your spine surgeon will team up with a vascular surgeon. This can be good for patient outcomes, but there have been instances of surprise bills from out-of-network physicians. In 2021 Federal legislation was passed to prevent unexpectedly huge bills (2).

spine surgery training

There are two ways to become a spine surgeon, either you go into orthopedic surgery or neurosurgery.

Your orthopedic surgeon will have undergone years of training. Typically, 4 years of pre-med, 4 years of medical school, followed by 5 years in an orthopedic surgery residency, followed by 1-2 years in a specialty spine surgery fellowship. Training programs should be accredited by the ACGME or American College of Graduate Medical Education. Non-accredited fellowships exist, as well as mentorship models which also augment a surgeon's training. Immediately following residency training there is a written orthopedic board exam to be taken. Upon successful completion of this your spine surgeon-to-be is deemed "board-eligible." Following this there is another two years during which time she or he practices her or his skills and then, finally, after passing an oral exam your spine surgeon becomes fully board certified by the American Board of Orthopedic Surgery (ABOS). Board certification lasts for a period of 10 years, after which the surgeon must recertify.

If your surgeon is a neurosurgeon, they typically complete 6-7 years of neurosurgical training. Some neurosurgeons will then complete an additional fellowship in spine surgery. Some neurosurgeons spend a year in their residency doing an "enfolded spine fellowship"; while these are typically not ACGME accredited, they may still provide excellent training. Neurosurgeons take their written boards prior to graduation and then complete an oral exam after graduation, thus becoming certified by the American Board of Neurological Surgery (ABNS). In short, coming into practice many surgeons will have already performed/ assisted in thousands of surgeries and are vetted by a thorough evaluation process.

I am an orthopedic surgeon. I think orthopedics allows you to have a complete view of the human skeleton and understand other musculoskeletal problems that may mimic spine problems. That having been said, spine neurosurgeons are also exceptionally talented. At a bare minimum your spine surgeon should have completed a fellowship in spine surgery (outside of residency) of at least 1 year and either be board-eligible or board-certified.

Selecting a Hospital

In general, you want to use a hospital that is geographically close to you so that if any problems occur after your surgery you can easily access your care team. Choosing a hospital that is geared for spinal surgery is also important. Do they have the appropriate equipment and specially trained orthopedic or neurosurgical nursing staff?

Academic centers often are prestigious and famous for the research they produce but may not necessarily provide care that is better than smaller private hospitals. In fact, according to Consumer Reports, they rarely provide care that is superior (3). While they may produce the research that fuels the advancement of surgery, care may be fragmented, and provided mostly by residents or a frequently changing staff. While this is not necessarily a bad thing—most residents are compassionate and dedicated and may improve the quality of your care—there will be some inefficiencies as a result of the educational system. Furthermore, academic centers are typically responsible for dealing with a high load of indigent care which means there is a higher burden of infections in the hospital. Nevertheless, academic centers are fully loaded with all the medical specialists and most modern equipment. Most high complexity spine cases are sent to academic centers (that is, spinal tumor reconstructions, or large deformity corrections).

One thing to be aware of is that larger academic hospitals may do a high volume of cases but this is generally spread across many surgeons. What that means is that if a hospital does 1000 spinal cases a year spread across 10 surgeons, each surgeon does roughly 100 cases. In smaller hospitals the volume may be lower but one or two surgeons generally shoulder the entire load and develop really excellent skills as a result. This means that in the smaller hospital only 500 cases may be done a year but one highly skilled surgeon does all of them and has much greater experience. Spine surgeons can become even more specialized focusing on one area of spinal pathology. For example, spine oncology (care of spine cancer) and spinal deformity are two areas where a spine surgeon may focus his/her entire time.

Many people may be concerned with having surgery at a rural hospital. But in fact, some of the best care provided in the United States is provided at rural hospitals. Such hospitals tend to be small and close-knit with a very caring staff that is dedicated to the community.

Getting Second Opinions

You are always encouraged to get second opinions.

However, in spine surgery, you will find that no two spine surgeons will think the same. There are so many ways to accomplish the overall goals of spine surgery and any surgeon will typically offer you the procedure he/she feels will mostly likely result in a great outcome in his/her hands. As discussed in this book, there are many different techniques and approaches to surgically correct a spinal condition and in most cases the outcomes are the same. The problem arises when your two surgical opinions are conflicting. How can you decide which is better for you? If the second surgeon suggests non-operative treatment you may be forced to live with that outcome by your insurance company, which may refuse to pay for the operation. What if three different doctors offer three different opinions? Which one will you choose?

I would try to limit getting second opinions to 2 doctors if possible. Then choose the doctor whose approach sounds reasonable and who you think you will work well with. If your case is a complicated one, even if you see only one surgeon, often he/she will typically get second opinions and discuss the case with trusted colleagues in pre-operative case conferences. This can be a very convenient way to get a second opinion as it costs you no time or resources and does not end in conflicting recommendations and your care will still be provided by the surgeon you know and trust.

In this modern age with limitless internet access to information, researching surgery is easy, but comprehending the results is difficult. Some doctors prowl social media groups offering faulty advice to the unaware. That is ultimately why you seek an expert opinion that you can trust to help you make the decision, or at least guide you where you want to go. I always find the informed patient much easier to treat, but you must be careful not to try and "doctor" yourself. There are many nuances to spinal surgery that are only understood after years of training and practice. While I always try to point out problem areas on imaging to my patients, comprehending a spinal MRI scan takes years of training. I would not recommend trying to interpret your own scans and diagnostics unless you are trained to do so. There is even more we don't know about the spine. Find someone who you trust, and cares about you.

Conclusion

Finding the right spine surgeon is a combination of finding someone who has completed the right training, and who matches well with your personality. Do some basic research on your spinal condition, find a doctor who is well regarded in the community and work with him/her to decide if surgery is right for you.

Academic centers are excellent for taking care of very complex spinal conditions, but for garden variety cases you may receive superior care at a local hospital.

Frequently Asked Questions

- **Is it worth flying to a destination area for surgery? Such as flying to Germany for a highly specialized surgery like a total disc replacement.**

  The answer is yes and no. Certain procedures like lumbar total disc replacement may only be available to you at specific medical centers and you may not be able to get one locally. So, if you are convinced this is the procedure you need and find a doctor who agrees, traveling far may be the only way to get the procedure done. However, I have seen people who travel far away to get surgery only to have it fail and have no easy access to their treating surgeon.

References

1.   Condon A. 6 reasons neuro, spine surgeons should be the only specialists to perform spinal fusion [Internet]. [cited 2022 Jan 25]. Available from: https://www.beckersspine.com/spine/item/53424-6-reasons-neuro-spine-surgeons-should-be-the-only-specialists-to-perform-spinal-fusion.html?origin=SpineE&utm_source=SpineE&utm_medium=email&utm_content=newsletter&oly_enc_id=6333H-0701901H2K

2.   Sanger-Katz M. A New Ban on Surprise Medical Bills Starts Today. The New York Times [Internet]. 2021 Dec 30 [cited 2022 Jan 25]; Available from: https://www.nytimes.com/2021/12/30/upshot/medical-bill-ban-biden.html

3.   Six Tips For Choosing The Right Hospital for Surgery - Consumer Reports [Internet]. [cited 2021 May 14]. Available from: https://www.consumerreports.org/cro/news/2014/08/six-tips-for-choosing-the-right-hospital-for-surgery/index.htm

Chapter 27

Preparing Yourself for Surgery

Summary

Once you have decided to have surgery, there is a lot of preparation that goes on behind the scenes. You will have to sign an informed consent stating you understand and agree to the procedure you are going to have. Because surgery will stress your heart and lungs, medical clearance is a process that reviews your health with a fine-tuned comb to ensure you are fit medically to tolerate the stress of the procedure. While this process is not foolproof, it should evaluate your cardiac risk and other risk factors for complications. You may need to undergo testing such as blood draws, echocardiograms, and chest X-rays. Prior to surgery you may have to stop certain medications such as blood thinners and anti-inflammatories. Each medication you take should be cleared by your doctor and generally all supplements should be stopped at least 2 weeks prior to surgery. Finally, you should have a basic idea of what the day of surgery will look like, where you are going to go, what to bring with you, and how you should prepare your home for when you return there after surgery.

Case

Mr. Blue is 72 years old and has been told he needs a lumbar fusion to treat his severe lumbar spinal stenosis. He has a long medical history, including hypertension currently under control with 3 anti-hypertensive agents, a heart attack which was treated with several stents, high cholesterol, urinary retention, and a "mini-stroke." He is also taking two blood thinners, aspirin, and Plavix. He lives alone in a small apartment with stairs and without any nearby family. Let's discuss two sample scenarios:

Scenario A: Mr. Blue misses his pre-operative clearance appointment because he slept in and doesn't hear back from the medical office, nor does he call to check in. He shows up to the hospital on the day of his surgery at 7 a.m. but has trouble finding the registration area. By the time he gets there its 8 a.m. and the nurses tell him they have been trying to reach him (he doesn't have a cell phone, only a land line). They take his blood pressure and it's 180/110. His surgeon comes to meet him looking concerned. He cannot find the pre-operative clearance reports. He asks Mr. Blue if he has taken his aspirin and Plavix recently to which Mr. Blue replies, "I didn't know I needed to stop those." The surgeon explains it is too dangerous to proceed with the procedure and that Mr. Blue needs to go to his pre-operative clearance appointment and see his cardiologist. Mr. Blue receives a call from the surgery scheduler who states that the next available pre op appointment is 2 months from now and that the next surgery slot is 3 months from now. Mr. Blue is upset; he is in severe pain from his back and wonders who dropped the ball.

Scenario B: Mr. Blue shows up to his pre-operative clearance appointment. There, a medical doctor takes detailed notes on all his medical conditions. His blood pressure, at 160/90, is slightly elevated and the doctor instructs Mr. Blue on how to take his anti-hypertensive medications around the time of surgery. The doctor also reviews his cardiac history and blood thinners. Based on what he sees, he recommends an echocardiogram and a visit to the cardiologist. The cardiologist notes that Mr. Blue's echo looks good and that he can discontinue his Plavix and aspirin for surgery 7 days before the procedure. Mr. Blue isn't sure where to go on the day of the procedure and asks the office staff who give him detailed instructions well in advance. On the day of surgery, he shows up 2 hours early and knows exactly where to go. His blood pressure is well controlled, and his surgeon reviews the informed consent with him. Mr. Blue has done his own research on the procedure and asks the surgeon a few last-minute questions. He then has successful surgery without complication.

Introduction

One of the most common questions I get from patients is, "What can I do to increase my chances of having a good outcome?" If you are healthy, going in for surgery can be a relatively simple task with a few minor steps to help you prepare. However, if you have many medical problems, getting ready for surgery can be overwhelming. Elective surgery should be as safe as possible, and thus most surgeons will insist on a rigorous pre-operative clearance process to make sure you are medically optimized before your procedure. Jumping through medical hurdles is a frustrating but necessary part of elective surgery. I tell all my patients they are part of the medical team and must do their part. Educating yourself on the process is a big help to your doctors and can change elective surgery from a bad experience to a good one.

Before Admission to the Hospital

decision-making/informed consent

Ultimately if your surgery is elective, it is your decision to undergo the procedure. Choices are made every day that could end in something good (winning the lottery) or something bad (a car wreck). Surgery is no different. Thus, you should be as informed as possible to make the right decision. This usually involves understanding the proposed risks and benefits of the procedure. Your surgeon will often go through an informed consent with you prior to surgery to discuss these risks. Make sure your goals, and the surgeon's goals are the same. Often people have unrealistic expectations of what surgery can do for them because they have not been thoroughly educated on the proposed procedure or are just desperate to get out of pain. While surgery can be very beneficial, it always carries risk (even in simple cases).

Informed consent is a legal document and agreement that you sign to give your permission for the surgery to take place, and to state that you understand what is going to happen to your body. In the informed consent, the procedure is typically spelled out in language that a lay person can understand. The type of surgery, the laterality (right or left side), and who will be performing the surgery are stated clearly. This consent should be explained to you by your surgeon until you are comfortable with it. In my practice this is done in a pre-operative visit but may be done in the waiting area prior to the procedure by other surgeons. The patient and I typically go over the risks and benefits as I understand them and there is time to ask questions. People react differently to informed consent. Some become terrified by what could go wrong, others feel empowered knowing exactly what they are signing up for. It's a fine balance between understanding the risks and being overwhelmed with worry over complications that rarely occur. Engage with your surgeon and ask your questions which will inform you of realistic risks before signing on the dotted line. For some patients it's easiest to accept the risk without going through all the nitty gritty of possible complications that may dramatically increase anxiety. Importantly, informed consent does not give anyone permission to do "a bad job." Excellence is still expected for every case. It can be useful to bring a family member or trusted friend with you during the informed consent to act as another set of eyes and ears as you may be anxious and not hear what the surgeon says.

Some good questions:

- **What are the chances of a complication occurring? How likely are complications to affect my outcome?**

- **What are the chances that this procedure will relieve my symptoms?**

- **How much pain am I likely to have in the post-operative period?**

your home care team

Prior to surgery, make sure you designate someone to be at home with you who can help you through this tough time once you are discharged from the hospital. The period after surgery can be difficult. Your surgeon, the medical office staff, and hospital staff are all here to support you, but someone like your significant other or a family member, or a close friend who can be with you at your home will make a big difference. Make sure that the hospital knows who this person is, and that his/her phone number is handy so that we can update them about your progress as you go through your procedure. It is important also to have an advanced directive, a document which allows your designee to make medical decisions for you should you become incapacitated.

pre-operative clearance

The first step to getting ready for surgery is obtaining pre-operative medical clearance. This may be done by your surgeon, primary care provider, or an independent third-party doctor. While your surgeon is an expert on your spine, he or she may not be comfortable managing all your other medical problems and will usually recommend someone to do the clearance. As your primary care provider is typically intimately knowledgeable about your personal health, that person may be a good option. The purpose of medical clearance is twofold: to carefully outline the risks of surgery based on the procedure and your overall health, and to get you as medically ready as you can be so you will be in the best possible shape for surgery. The process is designed to try and control as many factors as possible; however, it is critical to understand that even the smartest doctors cannot predict all serious post-op adverse events. As such the term "clearance" is a misnomer, as the purpose does not entirely clear you of risk. We try instead to understand if the procedure is going to lead to premature death, delirium, loss of function or independence. It can be useful but not totally necessary if a hospital staff physician performs your clearance so that someone is on hand who understands your unique problems.

In addition to obtaining primary clearance, you may also be required to obtain clearances from other specialists. If you see a specialist who manages a complex medical problem for you such as a cardiologist, rheumatologist, or a pulmonologist, you should obtain a clearance letter from them prior to surgery. If you are undergoing major dental work, it's critical you get dental clearance and to have any procedures done before your surgery. Dental problems are a common source of spine infections.

Anesthesia clearance: Some people with complicated medical backgrounds should speak with their anesthesiologist prior to surgery, particularly if you answer yes to any of the following questions (1):

- **Has anyone in your family (blood relatives) had a serious problem following an anesthetic?**

- **If you have been put to sleep for an operation were there any anesthetic problems/complications?**

- **Do you have any problems with pain, stiffness or arthritis in your neck or jaw?**

- **Do you have a history of difficult intubation?**

- **Do you have a history of malignant hyperthermia (severe fever reaction to certain drugs used for anesthesia)?**

- **Are you on home oxygen (O2)?**

- **Do you have severe pulmonary hypertension (pressure is too high in the artery going from the heart to the lungs)?**

Cardiology clearance: If your surgery is elective you may need to have a cardiology consult prior to surgery if any of the following describe you:

- **you have a major cardiac problem such as unstable coronary artery disease (you have active chest pain), decompensated congestive heart failure (you have swelling in your legs with difficulty breathing), a significant arrhythmia (abnormal heart rate) or severe valvular disease for any procedure with general anesthesia.**

- **you have chest pain, a history of a heart attack (myocardial infarction), congestive heart failure that is controlled, diabetes mellitus, or renal fail-**

Table to help you determine if you would benefit from cardiology clearance prior to surgery		
CARDIOLOGY CLEARANCE	Intermediate Risk Procedure • 1-5% risk of cardiac event (majority of spinal procedures)	High Risk Procedure • More than 5% risk of cardiac event (high blood loss or prolonged time such as more-than-3-level fusions)
Intermediate Risk Clinical Profile • Congestive Heart Failure (CHF) • Past Heart Attack (MI) • Kidney Failure (Creatinine > 2) • Diabetes • Chest Pain	CARDIOLOGY CLEARANCE REQUIRED: if poor functional status (cannot walk 4 blocks, cannot climb 2 flights of stairs, CHF).	CARDIOLOGY CLEARANCE REQUIRED
High Risk Clinical Profile • Decompensated CHF (heart can't maintain adequate circulation) • Unstable Coronary Artery Disease • Kidney Failure (Creatinine >2) • Diabetes • Chest Pain	CARDIOLOGY CLEARANCE REQUIRED	CARDIOLOGY CLEARANCE REQUIRED

ure (creatinine greater than 2) and are planning to undergo an intermediate risk surgery such as a 1-2 level lumbar fusion.

•   you are planning to undergo a major risk procedure with prolonged operative time, or a procedure with high estimated blood loss (which most more-than-3-level lumbar fusions are) (2).

Your exercise capacity is a strong predictor of your cardiac risk. The American Heart Association and the American College of Cardiology (AHA/ACC) recommends against cardiac tests for patients with a good exercise capacity as measured by metabolic equivalents (METS). Metabolic equivalents are a measure of your cardiovascular capacity (one MET =metabolic rate of consuming 3.5ml O2/kg/min). For example, for most people it takes about 1.5 METS to sit at a computer. Patients able to perform activities that require at least 4 METS, or more are low risk for cardiac complications during surgery. Activities which require less than or about 4 METS include walking up a steep hill or climbing two flights of stairs or walking 4 blocks in 15 minutes (3,4). If you do not have the capacity to complete 4 METS, you are at INCREASED risk of cardiac complications and will require further clearances from your cardiologist and possibly an echocardiogram. Of course, this system may be confused if your disability and your trouble moving stems from your spinal disease rather than your heart but remember it's just a guide.

Your doctor may order other tests such as a chest X-ray if you have known cardiopulmonary disease or if you are older than 50 years old. Electrocardiograms (EKG) are also recommended for patents with known cardiac disease. You may need to have a stress test to confirm your heart can handle the stress of surgery.

Dental clearance: Bad teeth are an infection risk when metal implants are put into the body. For example, an infected tooth can easily spread bacteria to the site of your surgery through your blood stream which may result in a catastrophic complication. For this reason, your surgeon may recommend you get clearance from your dentist to make sure your teeth are in good condition and that you do not have any active infections.

Understanding risk stratification: Risk stratification is an assessment process to help surgeons decide how risky it is to perform a specific surgery on a given patient. It currently is not possible to calculate risk with 100% accuracy. However, there are a variety of online tools/ scoring systems which can help calculate life expectancy (ePrognosis.org, is commonly used), and risk from surgery.

As you age, you become more vulnerable to illness and may have worse outcomes following surgery. Determining your frailty level is part of the risk stratification process of surgery. There are many instruments used to measure frailty; here is one with a simple mnemonic:

FRAIL Score: A score of 3-5 is frail, a score of 1-2 is prefrail and a score of 0 is robust. You can calculate your own score (5).

- **Fatigue: have you felt fatigued? Most or all the time over the past month? (Yes = 1, No = 0)**

- **Resistance: Do you have difficulty climbing a flight of stairs? (Yes = 1, No = 0)**

- **Ambulation: Do you have difficulty walking one block? (Yes = 1, No = 0)**

- **Illnesses: Do you have any of these illnesses: Hypertension, diabetes, cancer (other than minor skin cancer), chronic lung disease, heart attack, congestive heart failure, angina, asthma, arthritis, stroke, kidney disease? (5 or more= 1, less than 5 = 0)**

- **Loss of weight: Have you lost more than 5% of your weight in the past year? (Yes = 1, No = 0)**

Cardiac risk may be assessed with several tools. The Revised Cardiac Risk Index is a simple and easy to use scoring system to stratify your risk of a major cardiac event around surgery (6,7).

REVISED CARDIAC RISK INDEX (RCRI)	
RCRI CRITERIA	**Present?**
High risk surgery: vascular (blood vessels), and open intraperitoneal (gut) or intrathoracic (within the chest) surgery	Yes/No
History of ischemic heart disease (coronary artery disease) such as myocardial infarction (heart attack), positive exercise test, current chest pain, use of nitrate therapy, electrocardiogram with pathological Q waves)	Yes/No
History of heart failure	Yes/No
History of cerebrovascular disease (conditions that affect blood flow and blood vessels in the brain)	Yes/No
Diabetes that requires treatment with insulin	Yes/No
Pre-operative Serum Creatinine >2.0 mg/dl	Yes/No
Scoring	**Estimated Risk of a Major Perioperative Cardiac Event (cardiac death, non-fatal MI, non-fatal cardiac arrest)**
No risk factor	0.4%
One risk factor: Low risk	1.0%
Two risk factors: Moderate risk	2.4%
Three risk factors: High Risk	5.4%

laboratory testing

You may be required to undergo a few blood tests usually within 1 month of surgery. This can include tests such as:

- **Complete blood count: this is to check your baseline hemoglobin (a protein found in red blood cells), and your platelets (cells involved in blood clotting)**

- **Comprehensive metabolic panel: checks your kidney (creatinine), liver and endocrine function.**

- **Coagulation panel: measures how well your blood clots. You should alert your surgeon and medical doctors if you have a history of blood clots, or uncontrollable bleeding.**

- **Hemoglobin A1C: will be checked if you have known diabetes.**

- **Urinalysis: to detect pre-operative urinary tract infection (UTI)**

- **Pregnancy testing: should be done in all reproductive-age women.**

bone metabolism/ osteoporosis

If you are having hardware implanted in your spine, your doctor may want to assess your bone quality prior to the procedure. This is because osteoporosis (low bone mineral density) increases the risk of complications with orthopedic implants. This assessment typically consists of the following tests:

•   **Dual Energy X-ray Absorptiometry (DEXA)—a low radiation X-ray scan which looks at how dense your bone is in the hip and the spine.**

•   **Metabolic Bone labs evaluating levels in your blood of chemicals such as Calcium, Parathyroid hormone, Thyroid-stimulating hormone, Vitamin-D.**

medication review

Prior to surgery you should go through your medications both with your surgeon and your prescribing doctors to ensure you know which ones to stop and which to continue during the peri-operative period. The best way to do this is to bring in all your pill bottles holding the medications you currently take so that none are forgotten. Peri-operative refers to around the time of surgery.

Some medications that your surgeon will recommend stopping prior to surgery may surprise you. For example, you must stop your anti-inflammatory medications prior to surgery (aspirin, naproxen, and ibuprofen) and most supplements that may cause bleeding.

Aspirin and spine surgery: Withholding aspirin has been associated with a platelet rebound effect that that can increase risk of cardiac events like a heart attack. However, this risk must be weighed against the risk of bleeding during spine surgery as aspirin is a blood thinner. Patients who have had cardiac stents or bypass surgery may be maintained on aspirin at the discretion of their surgeons as the cardiac risk is high. If you have had a bare metal or drug-eluting cardiac stent placed within the last year you will likely be maintained on a low dose (81 mg) of aspirin. While the risk of major bleeding is increased on low dose aspirin, this risk is small for intermediate risk procedures such as percutaneous spinal procedures, decompressions, and single level fusions. Importantly, if continuing aspirin, other NSAIDS should be discontinued.

YOUR DAILY MEDICATIONS—CAN YOU TAKE THEM PERI-OPERATIVELY?

Medication Class	Examples	Discontinuation	Why
ACE Inhibitors and Angiotensin II Receptor Blockers (ARBS)	ACE: Lisinopril, Captopril, Benazepril ARBs: Losartan (Cozar®), Candesartan (Atacand®)	STOP morning of surgery (exceptions may be if used to treat heart failure or poorly controlled hypertension), restart within 48 hours after surgery.	May cause difficulty to manage low blood pressure.
Alpha-2 Agonists	Clonidine	Continue but not initiate.	There is no added benefit to adding clonidine to your peri-operative medications.
Anticoagulants	Please see section on anticoagulation.		
Benign Prostatic Hypertrophy Drugs (Alpha-1-Antagonists)	Tamsulosin (Flomax®), Doxazosin (Cardura®)	Continue in peri-operative period.	May help prevent urinary retention.
Beta Blockers	Propranolol, Atenolol	Continue in peri-operative period.	Patients may go into "beta blocker withdrawal" if discontinued in the peri-operative period leading to arrhythmias and high blood pressure.
Beta-2 Agonists	Albuterol (Volmax®), Salmeterol (serevent diskus®)	Continue in peri-operative period.	May reduce incidence of severe pulmonary reactions during surgery.
Calcium Channel Blockers	Diltiazem, Nimodipine, Amlodipine	Continue in peri-operative period.	Safe to continue.

YOUR DAILY MEDICATIONS—CAN YOU TAKE THEM PERI-OPERATIVELY? Continued

Medication Class	Examples	Discontinuation	Why
Diuretics	Hydrochlorothiazide (HCTZ), Furosemide (Lasix®).	Discontinue if taking for hypertension on morning of surgery. May restart 2-3 days after surgery once electrolytes are stable. May continue if using for heart failure.	May cause hypokalemia (low potassium) and hypovolemia (low volume of blood circulating).
Estrogen Therapy (Hormone Replacement Therapy)	17-beta-estradiol (Alora®, Climara®)	Discontinue at least 2 weeks prior to surgery. This may result in hot flashes and other menopausal symptoms.	Causes increased risk of venous thromboembolism (blood clot in a deep vein) and pulmonary embolism (a sudden blockage in the lungs).
Leukotriene Inhibitor	Montelukast (Singulair®)	Continue morning of surgery.	Reduces risk of an asthmatic attack.
Nonsteroidal Anti-Inflammatory Drugs (NSAIDs)	Ibuprofen (Advil®), Aleve, Mobic, Diclofenac	Discontinue at least 3 days prior to surgery, preferably 7 days.	Increases risk of bleeding and platelet dysfunction.
Oral Contraceptives		Consult your medical doctor if you are at increased risk for blood clots. It may be safe to continue if appropriate steps are taken.	Increases risk of thromboembolic disease and blood clots.

YOUR DAILY MEDICATIONS—CAN YOU TAKE THEM PERI-OPERATIVELY? Continued

Medication Class	Examples	Discontinuation	Why
Oral Diabetic Medications	Metformin (Glucophage®)	Continue until the morning of surgery and skip dose the morning or surgery. May restart once tolerating an oral diet.	Increased risk of sudden reduction in blood flow to the kidney (renal hypoperfusion) and lactic acidosis (inability of liver or kidney to clear acid from the body).
Oral Diabetic Agents (Sulfonylureas)	Glyburide (Glynase®), Glipizide (Glucotrol®), Chlorpropamide (Diabinese®)	Discontinue on the morning of surgery, may restart post-op.	Can cause hypoglycemia (low blood sugar).
Osteoporosis Medications: Antiresorptives	Alendronate (Fosamax®)	Do not take on the morning of surgery but can continue day after surgery.	Taking these medicines on an empty stomach may cause stomach upset.
Proton Pump Inhibitors/H2 Blockers	PPI: Omeprazole (Protonix®) H2 Blocker: Famotidine (Pepcid®)	Continue in peri-operative period.	Reduces risk of aspiration and stress on GI system during surgery.
Selective Serotonin Reuptake Inhibitors (SSRI)	Fluoxetine (Prozac®), Paroxetine (Paxil), Sertraline (Zoloft®)	Continue through peri-operative period. If high risk of bleeding (posterior cervical surgery), may discontinue with taper several weeks prior to surgery in consultation with psychiatrist.	Increases bleeding risk and platelet aggregation.
Statins	Simvastatin (Zocar®)	Continue in peri-operative period.	May decrease mortality and cardiovascular complication.

YOUR DAILY MEDICATIONS—CAN YOU TAKE THEM PERI-OPERATIVELY? Continued

Medication Class	Examples	Discontinuation	Why
Steroids (Glucocorticoids, Inhaled or Oral)	Prednisone	Typically, will continue in peri-operative period but please alert your physician you are on this medicine as it could impact your healing.	Stopping suddenly may precipitate a steroid crisis in your body, and make coping with the biologic stress of surgery more difficult.
Tricyclic Antidepressants	Amitriptyline (Elavil®), Nortriptyline (Pamelor®), Desipramine (Norpramin®)	Continue in peri-operative period especially if depression is severe.	May cause cardiac arrhythmias in peri-operative period (prolong cardiac QT).

supplement review

In addition to reviewing your medications, you should also review any supplements you take with your doctor. Although frequently considered natural and safe, supplements can result in complications in the post-operative period and can increase mortality and morbidity. As a rule, all supplements should be discontinued 10 days prior to surgery. The following is a list of standard supplements that can cause problems with surgery and when you should stop them. This is list is not exhaustive, and if you take supplements not listed here, please review them with your physician.

This list is not exhaustive. Review all supplements with your surgeon.

nutrition

Nutrition is critical for your healing post-operatively. If you are underweight, your surgeon may require blood tests checking albumin, prealbumin, and transferrin levels to evaluate your nutrition status. Regardless of whether you are overweight or not, you may also be required to see a nutritionist prior to surgery. A high fiber diet will help ensure you bowel movements maintain regularity, especially if you are prone to becoming constipated. Foods high in fiber are fruits, vegetables, and leafy greens. It is a common myth that you need to have high levels of sugar to heal wounds. Another sugar myth is that your "body needs the calories." While your body does need calories to heal, it does not need to be overloaded with sugar from soft drinks, candy, ice cream and other desserts, especially if you are diabetic.

DISCONTINUE THESE SUPPLEMENTS BEFORE SURGERY		
Supplement	**Discontinuation**	**Risk**
Curcumin	Discontinue 3 weeks prior to surgery	Increases bleeding risk
Echinacea	Discontinue 7 days prior to surgery	Associated with increased sedation and withdrawal
Ephedra	Discontinue 7 days prior to surgery	Associated with blood pressure problems and may cause seizures
Garlic	Discontinue 7 days prior to surgery	Increases bleeding risk
Ginger	Discontinue 7 days prior to surgery	Increases bleeding risk
Ginkgo	Discontinue 7 days prior to surgery	Increases bleeding risk
Ginseng	Discontinue 7 days prior to surgery	Increases bleeding risk
Grape seed	Discontinue 7 days prior to surgery	Increases bleeding risk
Omega-3 Fish Oil	Discontinue 3 weeks prior to surgery	Increases bleeding risk
Turmeric	Discontinue 3 weeks prior to surgery	Increases bleeding risk
Valerian	Taper 3 weeks before surgery	Associated with increased sedation and withdrawal

alcohol

Alcohol should be stopped 4 weeks prior to surgery. If you have alcohol dependence you may undergo withdrawal, which can be managed with the help of your medical doctor. Undergoing withdrawal after a major spine surgery is risky and should be avoided.

smoking

You should stop smoking at a minimum of 4 weeks but preferably 6 weeks prior to your surgery. Each week you are smoke-free prior to surgery decreases your risk of complication by roughly 20%! Why would you not bet on those odds (8)? Please see chapter 24 on the effects of smoking on spine surgery for more information.

preparing your home

You should get your living area ready for your return before you come in for surgery. The first step is to remove obstacles and things such as loose rugs and cords— anything on the floor that you may trip over. You may want to borrow or purchase a soft recliner to sit in as this can be a comfortable way to sleep after spine surgery. Make sure you have enough easy-to-prepare nutritious food at home. Cold smoothies are excellent following anterior cervical surgery where swallowing may be difficult. If you sleep upstairs, you may want to temporarily relocate to a downstairs bedroom.

things to buy prior to your surgery

Adaptive equipment: Following surgery you will typically need to avoid bending, lifting, and twisting motions and that can make activities of daily living more difficult. There are certain devices such as a sock-aid and long-handled sponges or graspers which may help you stay independent while observing your post-op precautions (some of these items may be provided by your hospital occupational therapist).

Durable Medical Equipment (DME): Certain pieces of durable medical equipment (DME) may make your post op recovery at home much more pleasant:

- **Elevated toilet seat or bedside commode: makes it easy to get on and off the toilet.**

- **Grab bars: may be installed in the bathroom/shower to help prevent slips.**

- **Shower chair: it may be difficult or dangerous to shower standing up. Purchase a chair that can be safely placed into the shower or bath so you can bathe sitting down.**

Other useful supplies: Here are a few more things that are useful to have on hand after surgery.

- **Laxatives/stool softeners: both spine surgery, and your post-operative pain medication may cause you to become constipated. It is a good idea to have some stool softeners on hand at home; these do not require a prescription. Some examples are:**

  - Bisacodyl (Dulcolax): 5-15 mg daily

  - Polyethylene glycol (Miralax): 17g powder daily

- Senna (Ex-lax): 17.2mg tablet BID (twice a day)

- **Pre-operative cleansers: Body hygiene and cleanliness are critical for decreasing the risk of a post-operative infection. I typically provide my patients with 4% chlorhexidine gluconate soap (Hibiclens). You should wash your entire body with this at least once a day for 7 days prior to surgery. In addition to Hibiclens, I also recommend patients wash their surgical areas (for example, low back if lumbar surgery) and under the arms with 5% benzoyl peroxide soap (generic over-the-counter acne soap is fine) for 3 days prior to surgery (9).**

- **Slip on shoes and slippers (for the house): As you may know, following your surgery you are typically restricted from bending, lifting, or twisting (BLTs). Reaching down to tie your shoes is one of the simplest ways to break these restrictions. Slip on shoes as well as some no-slip slippers for the house will make sure you have good traction with the ground, increase your comfort and, most importantly, ensure you do not jeopardize your surgery.**

the night before surgery

On the night before surgery, take your medications as instructed. Small sips of water are ok, but nothing to eat or drink after midnight. This is to make sure your stomach is mostly empty prior to undergoing anesthesia. If you have a full stomach, you risk having an aspiration (where the stomach contents enter the lungs) which can result in a severe pneumonia.

You are usually asked to be at the hospital at least 2 hours prior to your procedure. If the procedure is to start (leave the pre-op area for the OR) at 8, you should typically get to the pre- op area by 6 unless instructed otherwise. It's easy to get confused or lost trying to make your way to the hospital's pre-operative area, so make sure you know what the game plan is the night before surgery. Call the hospital if you are not sure where to park, who should come with you, and where to go.

what to bring with you to the hospital

Try to bring comfortable loose-fitting clothing with you such as pajamas so you don't have to wear the hospital gown during your physical therapy (PT). Glasses, hearing aids, CPAP machine and dentures should all be brought to the hospital. You will not need money, valuables, jewelry (all jewelry should be removed prior to your surgery), or home medications, except for eye drops and inhalers.

In the Hospital

On the morning of surgery, already knowing where to go and how to get there is important to reduce your anxiety and avoid delays. Ask in advance where you should be to check in. Larger hospitals often have multiple check-in locations. When you get to check-in you will be registered by a clerk and given an identification bracelet. Then you will be transferred to the "pre-op holding area" where you will change into a gown and be able to relax while everyone gets you ready for your procedure. It's a good idea to leave valuables at home or with a loved one and plan on not wearing any jewelry to the hospital. Nurses will start IVs and draw labs if necessary.

your care team

It's important to remember that besides your surgeon, your care team will consist of many other health care professionals who are dedicated to making sure your hospital stay is as safe and as comfortable as possible. This team will consist of:

Anesthesiologist: In most cases you will meet with your anesthetist prior to your procedure in the holding area. Here you will discuss the options available for anesthesia and, in coordination with your surgeon, will decide on which is best for you. I provide a summary below, but also dedicate an entire chapter to anesthesia and spine surgery (chapter 33).

- **general anesthesia: General anesthesia consists of intubation (the use of a breathing tube) and total sedation and is the most common form of anesthesia in spine surgery. A sophisticated breathing machine called a ventilator ensures you are breathing properly during the procedure, and a cocktail of medications keeps you totally unconscious and pain-free. Patients often ask "Is it possible to wake up during an operation?". The answer to this is it is possible, but it is almost unheard of. To ensure you are totally out during your surgery, your level of "awareness" may be monitored with the bispectral index (BIS), a technique which monitors brain waves to determine level of consciousness.**

- **MAC sedation: Monitored anesthesia care or MAC is a light sedation that may be used for minimally invasive spine procedures such as a spinal biopsy or kyphoplasty. Under a MAC you are sedated and given supplemental O2 but not intubated.**

- **local anesthesia: Your surgeon may inject numbing medication prior to and after making your incision. This helps numb the area and provides so called "preemptive" anesthesia, so your pain control starts before any incisions are made. In addition to local anesthesia, you may receive other**

medications such as steroids, anti-inflammatories, and gabapentin to help blunt post-operative pain. Local anesthesia is rarely used alone in spine surgery.

- **other preoperative medications: As part of the infection control protocol, you will typically receive antibiotics 1 hour prior to incision which is usually cefazolin (Ancef®). This medication does have some cross-reactivity with penicillin, so you should let the medical staff know about any penicillin allergies. Even If you have a history of intolerance to penicillin (such as diarrhea, nausea, vomiting, abdominal pain, chills, headache) or a minor reaction (itching, isolated rash, or an unknown reaction in the remote past greater than 10 years ago) cefazolin is very safe (10,11). However, if you have a history of reacting to penicillin with anaphylaxis (difficulty breathing, hives, chest tightness, swelling, fever and other symptoms), an alternative antibiotic such as vancomycin may be used.**

Case managers: Case managers help plan your discharge whether that is to home or to a rehab/skilled nursing facility.

Medical doctors/hospitalists: These doctors—usually internists—help look after any specific medical issues you have not related to your spine such as high blood pressure or diabetes and help make sure you are on the appropriate home medications. If any medical problems arise during the hospitalization, they may be consulted to help.

Nurses: You will typically be assigned a nurse for each hospital shift who will help you control your pain, give you your medications, help you use the restroom and assist you in your discharge planning. Nurses will keep the doctors informed of your progress and will be your point person should you need anything. In addition to nurses, you will likely be assigned a Certified Nurse Assistant (CNA) who will also help with many tasks in your care.

Physical therapists (PTs): PTs will help you get out of bed and get moving. PT starts in earnest the day after surgery but can occur as early as the evening after surgery. Therapists will make sure you are safe to mobilize and instruct you on how you should move when you get home and there is less support. If you have been prescribed a brace, they may help adjust it. Importantly, for spine surgery they will instruct you on proper spinal precautions, especially which movements to avoid. In the hospital you will typically get PT anywhere from 1 to 3 times a day where you will work on a process known as PT clearance. You will be cleared by PT once you prove you are safe for discharge from the hospital by walking a certain distance independently as well as climbing stairs.

Orthotists: Orthotists help you make sure you get the correct brace, and that it fits properly.

Occupational therapists (OTs): OTs are different from PTs. OTs will help you with rehab of your upper extremities and give you instruction on how to do tasks of daily living. They will help with any medical equipment you may need and instruct you on how to prepare your home for discharge.

in the pre-operative holding area

In the pre-operative area, you will typically be met by countless personnel. A pre-op nurse will look through your paperwork, make sure your consents are signed and make sure any last-minute testing gets done. The pre-op nurses will also ask you questions based on checklists to ensure you have a safe surgery and will start any intravenous (IV) lines. They confirm your identity and will ask you basic questions about your understanding of the procedure to ensure there are no serious mix-ups.

You will typically be seen by your anesthesiologist or certified registered nurse anesthetist who will do a quick exam and discuss the plan for pain control and anesthesia as noted above.

Your surgeon will come by and perform several important tasks. He will confirm your identity, review your history (and any changes), and may do a quick exam. He will then place a mark (typically his initials) on the site of your planned surgery. Go over with him what the surgery will be and what will happen, including having him mark with permanent marker the exact levels on your back that he will be treating. This sounds trivial but confirming the levels and location for surgery can help prevent a serious wrong-level procedure. If one side is hurting more than the other (more right arm pain than left arm pain, for example) you should let your surgeon know again. This process in the pre-operative area helps prevent "wrong person, wrong site, wrong procedure" surgeries which occur in the United States every year.

In spine surgery, it is considered wrong site surgery when the primary operative procedure is performed on an unintended level. Your surgeon will perform multiple checks both before and during the procedure to make sure he or she is in the right place—there are many segments which look similar in the spine, making wrong level surgery a matter of an error in millimeters. Despite many checks performed in surgery, wrong level surgery is reported by as many as 50% of spine surgeons some time in their careers. Your surgeon will typically confirm the correct level using X-ray after the incision and surgical exposure has been completed. Surgical incisions and exposures of the wrong level are common, easily corrected, and is not considered wrong site surgery (12). It is important to be as involved in this process as possible.

Confirm with the surgeon what the levels are and what the procedure is. Look over your consent and make sure everything matches what you had discussed previously.

When you are ready, you will be rolled back to the operative suite. There the anesthesiologist will put you under general anesthesia, and while you are unconscious the nursing staff will prepare you for surgery. A foley catheter (bladder catheter) may be inserted as well as any additional IV lines. You may require an arterial line which monitors your blood pressure carefully. Neuromonitoring electrode leads may be inserted on your extremities and scalp and finally you may be placed in a head rest that positions your head during surgery such that there is no pressure on your face.

A series of steps are taken at this point to ensure the surgical area is sterile. This includes a scrub nurse washing the surgical area with scrub soaps including alcohol, chlorhexidine, and iodine depending on the surgeon's preference. Once this is done sterile drapes are applied so that the chances of contamination are very low. New measures such as the application of an iodine-impregnated clear plastic drape known as Ioban® is used to cover the surgical site so that no bacteria can inadvertently enter the wound from the patient's skin. All of this may take up to an hour or more, and so even through your procedure may be scheduled for a certain time it may not actually start until 30-60 minutes after you roll into the room.

The period during the procedure can be a stressful time for family as they watch the clock on the wall. It's important for everyone to remain calm and know that the surgeons and nurses will alert family when the procedure is complete. Becoming anxious and calling into the OR frequently for updates may ease the anxiety of those waiting but may also distract the crew from doing what they really need to do— caring for you or your family member.

After your operation you will be transferred to the post anesthesia care unit (PACU) where nurses will observe you until you are awake and stable. After certain spine surgeries, you may be transferred directly to the intensive care unit (ICU) as part of standard care. After you have recovered in the PACU you will be transferred to the general med/surg floor.

a note on penicillin allergies

Contamination of the wound during surgery is a chief concern for medical professionals and patients. In addition to scrubbing the skin with antiseptics and using sterile drapes to keep the surgical field clean, one of the most important steps to prevent infection is administering antibiotics prior to incision. Cefazolin (Ancef®), a cephalosporin antibiotic which is chemically derived from penicillin, is the most common, safest, and most effective antibiotic used for this purpose. However, about

17% of patients self-report an allergy to penicillin, which can prevent the use of cefazolin.

The term "allergy" can mean many different things to patients, but to physicians this means you have developed an activation of the immune response. When the immune response is activated, it can result in itching, rash, or in severe cases anaphylaxis (a serious immune response where you develop potentially life-threatening swelling of the throat, hives, chest tightness, and fever). A history of diarrhea, vomiting, headache, fatigue, or nausea does not constitute a true allergic reaction but rather a medication intolerance. If you can, it is important to try and tell your doctors which category you fall into, so you do not unnecessarily receive a prophylactic antibiotic that is more expensive, less effective and less safe than cefazolin. Although the cross-reactivity (incidence of people who are allergic to penicillin who will also be allergic to cefazolin) is small (less than 10%) your doctor may withhold Ancef® if you have a history of penicillin allergy noted in your medical chart (10).

after the procedure

Your procedure is now complete, and the recovery process begins. While you are in the hospital your surgeon, or an associate will typically come and see you on rounds. He will typically do a quick exam to ensure your nervous system is functioning properly and ask you a set of basic safety questions. Nurses will be available to help you with basic needs like getting out of bed and going to the bathroom.

Post-op symptoms that you may experience and should pay attention to:

- **Dizziness or lightheadedness: These may result from your post-op pain medications, blood loss or both. They should be reported immediately to your nurse or doctor.**

- **Headache: If you experience a headache after spinal surgery, it should be reported to your nurse and doctor. Headaches are common for a variety of reasons, but certain headaches may be a sign of a post-op CSF (cerebrospinal fluid) leak.**

- **Nausea: Nausea is very common after surgery. It typically results from anesthesia and pain medications and your anesthetist will typically take measures to help prevent this from occurring. Rarely it is a sign of something more serious such as an ileus (where your bowels temporarily shut down) or a myocardial infarction (heart attack). To prevent vomiting, you may be treated with antiemetics such as ondansetron (Zofran®), promethazine (Phenergan®) or a scopolamine patch. In the hospital may be the** only time in your life that you are frequently asked if you are passing gas, which is used to determine if your bowels are working correctly.

- **New numbness or weakness: These symptoms should always be reported to your nurse or doctor. Some numbness may be common after your surgery; however, it should still be reported. New weakness is rarely expected and thus should be reported immediately.**

- **Pain: Pain is expected after surgery. If you have a pain block in place (a numbing agent used to control pain), you may have increased pain on the second day after surgery when it wears off. Gradually over the course of the week your pain will subside. It's helpful if you communicate your pain using a numeric scale: 0 (no pain) to 10 (worst pain imaginable). You may get patient-controlled analgesia (PCA) where you push a button to deliver pain medication through your IV (although these devices are used less commonly since the onset of the opioid epidemic). There are also other modes of pain control including oral narcotics, muscle relaxants, and ice. If you experience a sudden increase in your pain, it is important to communicate this to your doctors. It may be normal; however, he /she may want to adjust your medications. Rarely it may indicate something more sinister, which will require more tests and images.**

- **Urinary retention: after the procedure it can be common to have some difficulty with urination—especially if you already have preexisting difficulty with urination. The combination of anesthesia and narcotics do an excellent job of shutting down your autonomic nervous system and prevent you from voiding freely. Your nurse may bladder scan you and you may be prescribed medicines to help you urinate. In some cases, you may need a foley (bladder) catheter inserted or a straight catheter which is only inserted as needed.**

drains

Drains help prevent fluid from accumulating at the surgical wound while your body naturally adjusts to the surgical disruption of blood vessels. Drains are commonly used in spine surgery, but the exact use varies from surgeon to surgeon. Drains usually come out through the skin and are attached to a small receptacle that is emptied periodically by nurses. It can feel weird to have a little tube coming out of you, but, unfortunately, this can be part of the spine surgery experience. Your drain will be removed when your surgeon feels it's appropriate, usually when output decreases to a certain threshold.

hospital exercises

As mentioned above, physical therapy is an important component of your healing. The PT will work with you on safe transfers, walking and negotiating stairs. He or she will instruct you on the use of a walker or cane. In addition to working with your PT, it's important to practice a small subset of exercises on your own to prevent blood clots and deconditioning:

- **ankle pumps: Move your ankles up and down vertically 10 times every 30 min while awake**

- **quad sets: lie on your back and contract your quad muscle to drive the back of your knee down into the bed. Do 10 reps every 30 min while awake.**

- **heel slides: slide your heels up to your buttock on the bed. Do 10 reps every 30 min while awake.**

transfer training

Once you have your spine surgery, getting out of bed the normal way will put an excessive amount of strain across your back. Thus, the PTs will help you learn a safe way to get out of bed called
ing.

- **Lying on your back, hug yourself, bend your knees up and roll your hips and shoulders as a unit (keeping your spine straight), you are now lying on your side.**

- **Place your top hand (the one closest to the ceiling) on the bed in front of your chest and your bottom hand (the one closest to the bed) underneath your shoulder. Use your hands to push your body vertical again keeping your hips in line with your shoulders (no twisting).**

- **To get back into bed just reverse the process but remember to scoot back into bed as much as possible before lowering your body to its side. Once your back is straight you can lift your legs onto the bed.**

length of hospital stays

Your length of stay will vary depending on the type of surgery you have had. Here is a rough breakdown of typical lengths of stays depending on the type of surgery:

- **Outpatient-1 night inpatient: single level cervical or lumbar decompression, kyphoplasty**

- **1 night: 1-2 level anterior cervical discectomy and fusion (ACDF) or disc arthroplasty, kyphoplasty, cervical laminoplasty**

- **1-2 nights: greater than 1 level lumbar or cervical laminectomy**

- **2-5 nights: lumbar fusion, posterior cervical fusion**

- **Greater than 5 nights: major spinal deformity correction, spinal tumor or infection, and greater than 3-level lumbar fusions.**

discharge criteria

Before you can go home there are certain criteria that you must meet to ensure it is safe to do so:

- **You must "clear PT," usually by completing climbing stairs and walking a certain distance.**

- **Your pain must be reasonably well-controlled on oral pain medications.**

- **Your drain outputs must be at a certain level to allow for safe removal of drains.**

- **You should be able to void independently and have a bowel movement if possible.**

If you are not able to reach these milestones you may need to go to a rehabilitation or skilled nursing facility so you can have ongoing PT and access to medical expertise as you convalesce. A typical stay at one of these facilities can range from 1 to 6 weeks before you are fully ready to go home.

At Home Following your Surgery

post-op restrictions

I have my patients maintain spinal precautions for a certain amount of time following their procedure. For a decompression this is typically 6 weeks while the tissues heal and 3-6 months for a spinal fusion. I encourage walking both as a form of cardiovascular exercise and as a form of physical therapy for strengthening. I typically do not put a limit on the amount I allow my patients to walk after surgery, but it is important to listen to your body and to exercise common sense. It's important to remember that your spine is different now and needs to heal, thus you should not stoop, bend, or twist. Don't reach or grab for anything suddenly.

home exercises

Continue to work on your ankle pumps, quad sets, and nerve glides once you get home. While awake it should be done hourly.

outpatient physical therapy

A common question I get before surgery is, "Will I need physical therapy?" The answer depends on the type of surgery you are having. For example, if you have had a micro decompression PT may start as early as 3 weeks with the addition of exercise bike and elliptical trainer to your walking program. However, if you have had a fusion surgery performed, you may need to let your surgery heal for several months before starting PT. Talk with your surgeon.

home medications

Your surgeon and medical doctor will let you know which medicines to resume and when. You may be given the following prescriptions to take home with you:

- **Narcotic pain medication such as Percocet or tramadol. Your pain should continue to decrease over the next 2-6 weeks. If you have a sudden**

increase in pain, you should let your surgeon know. Use these medicines sparingly as they cause constipation and can be habit forming.

• **Anticoagulation medication (blood clot prevention)—typically either aspirin or low molecular weight heparin (LOVENOX).**

• **Anti-constipation medications should be used if you are taking narcotics.**

• **Anti-nausea medications such as ondansetron (Zofran).**

• **Steroid dose pack—sometimes a steroid dose pack can be used for pain and nausea control post-op at your surgeon's direction.**

You should NOT take NSAIDS without consulting with your surgeon. This includes Advil, Motrin, Mobic, and Celebrex.

incision care

There are usually so many questions about closure and dressings I dedicate an entire later chapter (Chapter 49) to the topic but here is a summary. All surgeons are different, but I typically have my patients leave their dressings in place for 7 days following surgery. I give the wound 7 days in the protected environment of the dressing, which has been shown to decrease wound infections because the dressing applied in the operating room is the most sterile (13).

In most cases absorbable sutures are used during spine surgery; however, if you do not have absorbable sutures, you may need them removed in 2-4 weeks following your procedure. Absorbable sutures mean you do not have to have your stitches removed as they will dissolve over 6-8 weeks. Your surgeon may also use a special glue (a cyanoacrylate—such as Dermabond). This leaves a protective coating over your wound that falls off over several weeks. Do not pick at it! It's like an artificial scab and prevents bad bacteria from crawling into your wound.

You may take a shower 7 days after surgery as the skin is typically sealed at this point. Some dressings are waterproof and so may be exposed to moisture earlier. Do not submerge your incision (in a tub, pool, bath, river, ocean) until you have clearance from your surgeon.

When you should call your surgeon or his office

If you ever have a question, you should not hesitate to call your surgeon or the office. While doing your best to respect boundaries, it's better to overcommunicate than to under communicate. Group your questions so that you do not make repeated phone calls to the office that will overload the staff. Your surgeon should always know about:

- **Calf pain or tenderness: This may indicate a DVT (a blood clot in your leg).**

- **Wound drainage: If your dressing becomes saturated or there is persistent drainage from your wound you should alert your doctor.**

- **Fever: Low grade temps are very common after surgery. Temps higher than 101.5° F (38° C) should be called in immediately.**

- **New weakness or numbness.**

- **Signs of infection about the incision: redness, swelling, warmth around the incision.**

- **Shortness of breath, difficulty breathing or chest pain: You should not only call your surgeon, but you should also probably go to the emergency department or call 911.**

Conclusion

In this chapter we covered everything you need to know to get you ready for surgery. You should now have a good knowledge of what is going to happen prior to your procedure but remember each facility is different and will have its own protocols. Make sure you discuss with your surgeon and the care team what the specific protocols are at your hospital. The more you know, the easier it will be for the doctors and nurses to take care of you.

Frequently Asked Questions

- **What time should I be at the hospital?**

    This is probably the most common question I get, and the answer will depend on the anticipated start time of your procedure. Typically, you should be at the hospital at least 1-2 hours before your procedure to allow nursing staff to prepare you for surgery. It's important to keep in mind that surgery schedules are very fluid. Emergencies can come in that disrupt elective schedules or certain surgeries can take longer than anticipated. You may be asked to come into the hospital much earlier or much later. You may even have to wait in the hospital. It's good to bring reading material or things you can use to distract yourself and decrease your anxiety while you wait.

References

1.   Hilditch WG, Asbury AJ, Jack E, McGrane S. Validation of a pre-anaesthetic screening questionnaire. Anaesthesia. 2003 Sep;58(9):874–7.

2.   Park KW. Preoperative cardiology consultation. Anesthesiology. 2003 Mar;98(3):754–62.

3.   Reilly DF, McNeely MJ, Doerner D, Greenberg DL, Staiger TO, Geist MJ, et al. Self-reported exercise tolerance and the risk of serious perioperative complications. Arch Intern Med. 1999 Oct 11;159(18):2185–92.

4.   Mangano DT, Goldman L. Preoperative assessment of patients with known or suspected coronary disease. N Engl J Med. 1995 Dec 28;333(26):1750–6.

5.   Gleason LJ, Benton EA, Alvarez-Nebreda ML, Weaver MJ, Harris MB, Javedan H. FRAIL Questionnaire Screening Tool and Short-Term Outcomes in Geriatric Fracture Patients. J Am Med Dir Assoc. 2017 Dec 1;18(12):1082–6.

6.   Lee TH, Marcantonio ER, Mangione CM, Thomas EJ, Polanczyk CA, Cook EF, et al. Derivation and prospective validation of a simple index for prediction of cardiac risk of major noncardiac surgery. Circulation. 1999 Sep 7;100(10):1043–9.

7.   Devereaux PJ, Goldman L, Cook DJ, Gilbert K, Leslie K, Guyatt GH. Perioperative cardiac events in patients undergoing noncardiac surgery: a review of the magnitude of the problem, the pathophysiology of the events and methods to estimate and communicate risk. CMAJ Can Med Assoc J J Assoc Medicale Can. 2005 Sep 13;173(6):627–34.

8.   Mills E, Eyawo O, Lockhart I, Kelly S, Wu P, Ebbert JO. Smoking cessation reduces postoperative complications: a systematic review and meta-analysis. Am J Med. 2011 Feb;124(2):144-154.e8.

9.   Kolakowski L, Lai JK, Duvall G, Hasan SA, Henn RF, Gilotra MN. Benzoyl Peroxide Effectively Decreases Pre-Operative Propionibacterium acnes Shoulder Burden: A Randomized Trial. J Shoulder Elbow Surg. 2018 Apr;27(4):e131–2.

10.   Goh GS, Shohat N, Austin MS. A Simple Algorithmic Approach Allows the Safe Use of Cephalosporin in "Penicillin-Allergic" Patients without the Need for Allergy Testing. J Bone Jt Surg. 2021 Dec 15;103(24):2261–9.

11.   Goodman EJ, Morgan MJ, Johnson PA, Nichols BA, Denk N, Gold BB. Cephalosporins Can Be Given to Penicillin-allergic Patients Who Do Not Exhibit an Anaphylac-

tic Response. :4.

12.   Palumbo MA, Bianco AJ, Esmende S, Daniels AH. Wrong-site Spine Surgery. J Am Acad Orthop Surg. 2013 May;21(5):312–20.

13.   Bains RS, Kardile M, Mitsunaga LK, Bains S, Singh N, Idler C. Postoperative Spine Dressing Changes Are Unnecessary. Spine Deform. 2017 Nov;5(6):396–400.

Figures:

The Log Roll

Start by lying on your back and bend the knees up

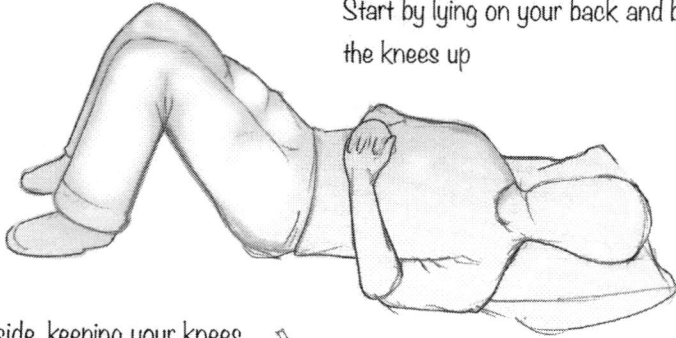

Roll to your side, keeping your knees bent and hugging yourself

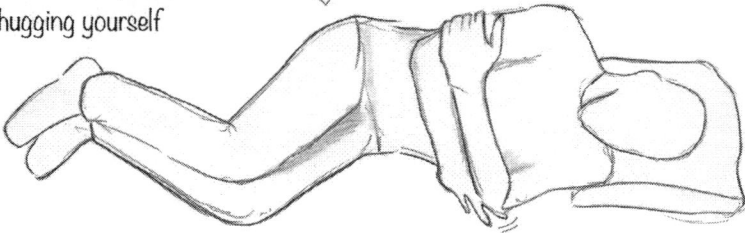

Use the arm closest to the bed to push yourself up, swinging your legs over the edge of the bed

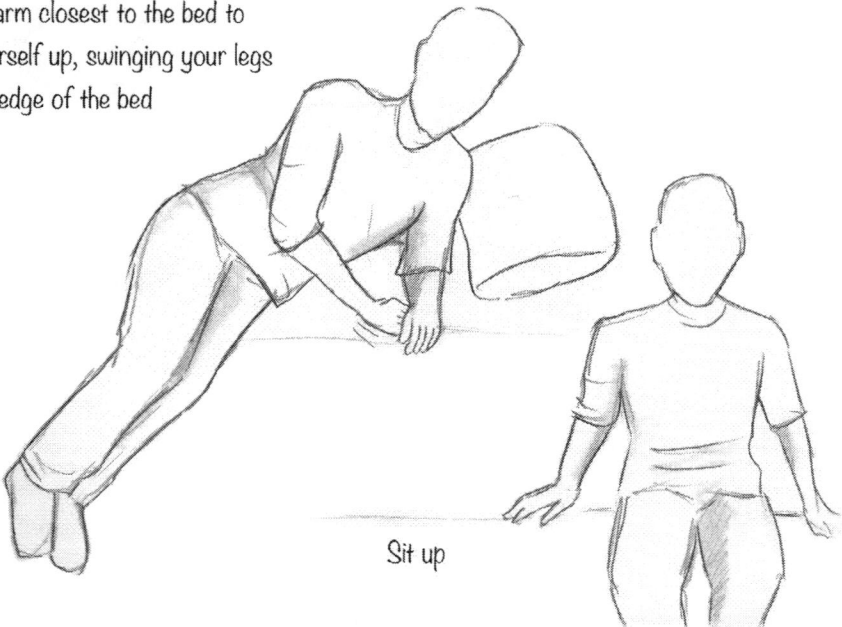

Sit up

Log roll. The log roll maneuver is a safe way to get out of the bed without putting stress on the spine. First hug yourself, bend your knees up and roll onto your side (second from top). Use the down arm to brace yourself and the up arm to push yourself erect allowing your legs to swing down (bottom).

Chapter 28

How Your Thoughts and Feelings Affect Pain and Outcomes in Spine Surgery

Summary

Pain is a sensation that your body uses to signal something to you, typically either that there is a problem, or that you are healing. Your mind interprets the pain depending on your mental state. If you are depressed, anxious or stressed your will have a lowered pain threshold (feel pain more easily). This can lead to worse problems with your back and worse outcomes from surgery. Negative thoughts and beliefs can also cause you to misinterpret pain, thinking it is something worse than it is, or that the pain from healing after surgery is bad. There are specific programs which can help you increase your mental resilience and improve your pain tolerance, including cognitive behavioral therapy, stress reduction and mindfulness. If you are going in for surgery this also takes mental preparation. You should be actively involved in your own psychological preparation for surgery. For some this means understanding as much about the problem, procedure, and convalescence as you can, others choose an "ignorance is bliss" attitude. Whichever approach you use, the amount of anxiety or distress you carry about your surgery will affect the outcome.

Case 1

Ms. Wheat is a 50-year-old homemaker who suffers from anxiety, depression, and PTSD. She suffers from neck and arm pain and is very worried something is seriously wrong. She goes online and looks for causes of neck pain and now is worried she has cancer of the neck. Her anxiety peaks and she cannot sleep because of her fear that she has cancer, and her pain gets worse. She gets an MRI scan of her neck which shows a disc herniation, but no cancer. Her primary care physician recommends she see a spine surgeon. This creates a whole new set of anxieties for Ms. Wheat who is now focused on the thought of spine surgery. She really cannot imagine having surgery on her neck and just the thought sends her into panic. By the time she sees me her pain has gotten worse, and she is haggard from anxiety. I recommend she try some conservative options but tell her that, due to the severity of the stenosis caused by the herniated disc, I think she may eventually require an operation. She tries PT and some other things but ultimately gets no better. She has surgery in the form of a cervical fusion and does well. Her pain is gone, but now she is constantly worried about her hardware. She thinks that something must not be healing right in her neck. All her X-rays and CT scans show normal healing, yet she cannot let go of the thought that something is seriously wrong.

Commentary: In this case you can see that Ms. Wheat suffers from intrusive thoughts and is prone to rumination. In no way does this constant worrying benefit; instead, it saps her energy and resilience. Although she tolerated surgery well and one problem improved, she created a new one almost immediately that she is now fixated on. Let's see how mindset can improve outcome in the next case.

Case 2

Ms. Crimson is a 68-year-old retired teacher. In her retirement she has taken up golfing. She enjoys the sport for many years but one day takes a swing too aggressively and pulls out her back and experiences searing leg pain. As a daily yoga practitioner, she aggressively tries to work out the kink in her back for several weeks, but her problem gets no better. Faced with this reality she decides to take a new approach and seek the opinion of a doctor. Her primary care doctor orders an MRI which shows a large disc herniation and decides to refer her to me for a surgical opinion. During the consultation I lay out the options but suggest surgery as the best course forward. She is not daunted by the thought of surgery but wants to know as much as she can to understand her condition. I provide her with some reliable reading material to better make an informed decision. She returns about a week later, having discussed things with her family and elects to proceed. She's active and doesn't want to waste

**time with treatments which may only offer temporary relief. She asks appro-
priate questions about how the surgery will go. While she understands there is
some risk, she also feels confident she is getting the treatment that is right for
her. The surgery goes well, and she is discharged from the hospital on the same
day. After surgery she is engaged in following restrictions and her rehab therapy. In 6 weeks, she is back on the golf course and is pleased she has navigated a
potentially life-changing problem without much fuss.**

Introduction

Have you ever heard someone say, "I have high pain tolerance?" I have found that
most people who say this have a low pain tolerance. But why would they say that? It's
all part of the intricate psychology of pain, and people believing they have high pain
tolerance provides a way for them to cope with pain, despite possibly having low pain
tolerance. In this chapter we explore how your mental state and attitude impacts pain
from spinal problems and recovery from surgery.

State of Mind

As explained in the chapter on pain, there are many complex factors which
contribute to your mind's interpretation of pain. The biochemical model of tissue
damage that is sensed and interpreted as pain in your brain is over simplified and
does not explain why some experience worse pain than others with similar injuries.
Your mind is the missing link between whether your pain is just a nuisance or
crippling. How does this work? Each neurological signal your body produces is
evaluated by your mind which, in turn, determines if the signal deserves immediate
attention or can be ignored safely. For example, consider the difference between the
pain from a good workout and that caused by cutting your hand on glass. Both result
from similar neural signals but are processed totally differently in the brain. Your
workout pain is interpreted as something "good" because you did it to try and be
healthy, while the cut is interpreted as "bad" because you didn't mean to do it and it's
damaging. Such is also the case with pain arising from your spine and from surgery.
Your expectations, beliefs and coping ability have an incredible power to color your
experience of pain, making it either more or less intense (1).

Psychosocial factors (the combination of what you think and the influence of your
social environment) are exceptionally important in your interpretation of pain.
Stress may increase your body's activation of the autonomic nervous system which,
in turn, increases your heart rate, dilates your pupils, and shuts down digestion and
other non-critical bodily functions to prepare you for a "flight or fight" response. This
activation may have negative effects on your mind's interpretation of pain and thus
can have serious impacts on not only your sensitivity to pain but also your response

to surgery. You are in a state of "fight or flight" and thus take pain seriously, becoming hyper aware of it.

Expectations and beliefs set by commercial advertisements on TV and in magazines promise instant cures from pain and disease which may be far from the truth. You may go into surgery expecting an instantaneous cure, but, after surgery, realize that recovery may take longer. Thus, your expectations are disappointed, and your pain is worse (as in "This isn't something I was expecting"). Other psychosocial factors that may strongly influence the perception of pain are a past history of abuse, unemployment, financial struggle and ineffective coping skills (2). Why this is the case is currently not known, but likely relates again to your overall level of stress and how that level of stress affects the activation of your autonomic system.

In contrast, the idea of self-efficacy strongly predicts success in dealing with pain. Self-efficacy is the belief that you can function despite pain, distract yourself from pain and successfully obtain a desired outcome (see case 2 above). You believe pain is something natural that you can use to your advantage, and it's your body's way of telling you there is a problem or that you are healing. Suddenly pain is your friend and an agent to guide your recovery. Pain then is no longer scary and doesn't result in added stress because you are in control.

If this is not your regular way of looking at this, there are ways to arrive at this state of mind and practice it. In the section below on Psychological Treatments for Improved Resilience you will find a few ideas.

The Impact of Depression on Health and Surgical Outcome

In my experience, depression and anxiety have a profound impact on how a patient will interpret pain.

Considering the profound impact your psychological makeup has on the brain's interpretation of pain, it should come as no surprise that mood disorders not only negatively impact your health but also the success of surgery. Depression and anxiety cause you to overinterpret pain in a condition known as catastrophizing. Catastrophizing means you always expect the worse and so any pain can mean doom. This psychological interpretation makes any pain worse because it's associated with negative feelings. Studies have shown depression and anxiety to be one of the most predictive factors in how good your health is (3). Depression hinders healing and can even result in worse outcomes with therapy (4). In patients undergoing an amputation, depression and catastrophizing were associated with the development of phantom limb pain (5).

Psychological distress directly impacts the outcome of spine surgery, and many patients with depression and anxiety are at higher risk for dissatisfaction with spine surgery (6). Patients with depressive symptoms (in this study, those who scored less than 45 out of 100 on the Mental Component of the Short-Form 12 Health Survey, a scoring system to rate depression) have been shown to have worse outcomes and overall less improvement with lumbar (low back) fusion surgery (7).   Moreover, cervical (neck) spine patients with mood disorders who undergo elective spine surgery have worse outcome scores and tend to receive more opioid medications that increases the risk of dependence and pain sensitivity (see chapter 20 on opioid narcotics). Lumbar spine patients with mood disorders have worse outcome scores before and after surgery compared to those who do not (8).

What does this boil down to: Two patients have the same surgery for the same condition. One does well because he or she has a positive attitude, the other doesn't because of depression or other mood disorder. Your mind is this powerful.

How do you know if you are suffering from depression or anxiety?

Depression and anxiety are both clinical diagnoses set forth by the Diagnostic and Statistical Manual for Mental Disorders. Unfortunately, both depression and anxiety are very prevalent in society and especially so in those suffering from spinal disorders. Depression is characterized by symptoms of a low mood, inability to sleep (insomnia), low energy, poor concentration, an inability to enjoy things once thought to be joyful, thoughts of worthlessness, etc.

An accurate screening tool used to diagnose depression is the Patient Health Questionnaire–9 (PHQ-9) (9). It is scored from 0 to 27 with a score greater than 10 indicating depression. It may be useful to score yourself to determine if you are suffering from depression. If the score is ≥10 or major depression, please seek the services of a psychologist, therapist, or other mental health worker prior to any surgical intervention.

Psychological Treatments for Improved Resilience

Understanding that your mental state, stress levels and social issues will impact your perception of pain is the first step. The second step is to try to do something about it. There are several mental health therapies that have been shown to be effective for the treatment of low back pain, and, in general, reducing overall pain. Of course, like other non-operative modalities these should be done under the supervision of a treating physician.

stress reduction

Stress is your mental reaction to emotional strain or pressure. Your body principally reacts to stress by releasing the hormone cortisol which in short bursts can be useful but in chronic situations can be very detrimental to your health, leading to issues with healing, cardiovascular disease, and mental illnesses such as depression. There are many ways to reduce stress, but some simple and proven stress reduction techniques include getting enough sleep and performing daily exercise, taking time to be with loved ones and pursuing enjoyable hobbies.

Patient Health Questionnaire-9 (PHQ-9)(10)
Scoring:

A score greater than 10 is considered major depression

Over the past 2 weeks, how often have you been bothered by any of the following?	Not at all	Several Days	≥Half of the Days	Almost every day
Feeling down, depressed, or hopeless	0	1	2	3
Trouble falling or staying asleep, or sleeping too much	0	1	2	3
Feeling tired, or having too much energy	0	1	2	3
Little interest in doing things	0	1	2	3
Trouble concentrating on things	0	1	2	3
Moving so slow others have noticed, or the opposite, being more fidgety than normal	0	1	2	3
Thoughts that you would be better off dead, or by hurting yourself	0	1	2	3
Feeling bad about yourself, that you are a failure	0	1	2	3
Poor appetite or overeating	0	1	2	3
Total				

Ensuring you are getting enough sleep is paramount as it's hard to battle a psychological disorder if you are exhausted. Ensure your sleep hygiene is top notch by reducing screen time close to bed, keeping the temperature in your room cool, and making sure you have a comfortable mattress. Many spine patients have a hard time knowing what position is best for sleeping. There is no proven best practice but either sleeping on your side with a pillow beneath the legs or on your back with pillow beneath your knees will keep the spine in a good neutral position.

Daily exercise is also a great way to keep stress at bay. There is a whole chapter devoted to exercise; however, in brief, daily walking can be a low impact way to get in your exercise. Plan to walk at least 30-40 min 4-5 days a week. If you can plan a walk in a hilly area where there is exposure to nature this can be an excellent way not only to stay healthy but to reduce stress. Invite a loved one or friend for added stress reduction benefit (11).

cognitive behavioral therapy (CBT)

Cognitive behavioral therapy is a technique used by psychologists and therapists to identify and alter harmful or negative thoughts or beliefs regarding pain and disability—so called cognitive errors. For example, some patients may become fixated on their pain, generating an anxious state that increases hypervigilance for pain, thus making pain worse. Another patient may interpret a pain in the foot as evidence that the whole body is dying which then gets translated into full body pain by the mind.

The most common cognitive errors focus on misconstrued expectations (I must be pain-free to enjoy my life), negative projections (I will always be in pain) and pain misinterpretation (this foot pain means I am dying). CBT helps to break this mental cycle by focusing on positive thoughts and promoting healthy behavior. CBT may help you set realistic expectations about pain and how pain is treated and has been shown to help relieve low back pain (12). CBT also helps break behaviors which reinforce pain such as anticipation and avoidance of pain and will teach you to engage in activities you enjoy and to self-soothe.

mindfulness-based stress reduction (MBSR)

This type of therapy focuses on a type of meditation in which you focus on increasing awareness of your body. This trains you to accept moment-to-moment experiences such as pain, difficult emotions, and discomfort. MBSR has also been shown to improve low back pain (13,14).

Preparing Yourself Psychologically for Surgery

Aside from potentially being painful, surgery is a stressful, anxiety-provoking event in a patient's life. You may spend the weeks leading up to the surgery worrying about the procedure. You may panic at times and despair at others. Going to the hospital which is unfamiliar to you and seeing all the medical equipment and medical personnel is also scary. Patients often worry about the risks of surgery and what could go wrong.

Ultimately these behaviors get in the way of helping yourself heal by getting the procedure you need. Having a warm relationship with your surgeon is critical to help alleviate these worries. Many patients have anxiety because they do not get to spend enough time with their surgeons. Make sure you get to know your surgeon and get all your questions answered. Have a good understanding of what the procedure will entail, and why it will help you heal. It has been shown that patients who make more informed decisions prior to total knee replacements actually have superior outcomes and less regret (15). The more you understand the process, the more prepared you will be and the less anxiety you will have.

Make sure you know the schedule, where you are going to go for your tests and keep a list of things you need to accomplish before your surgery. Make sure you read information on your procedure (such as that contained in this book) and attend a class if your hospital offers one. There is risk in everything we do from crossing the street to riding in a car. Understand that while there is always a risk something can go wrong in surgery, it is rare that if something does go wrong, your medical team cannot correct course and still get you a great outcome. Similarly, surgery is often painful, but there are dozens of pain medicines and other treatments available to ensure your pain is tolerable.

The more you educate yourself on the problem and the surgical solution, the more you will be in control of your medical care and the less fear and anxiety you will have (16).

Develop a Plan to Deal with Your anxiety Related to Surgery

- **Figure out what aspects of surgery are worrisome to you and discuss these with your care team and your surgeon.**

- **Worry time: have a period of 20-30 minutes a day when you are allowed to worry. For the rest of the day, you are not allowed to worry. Worrying all**

day will place you under too much mental stress and ultimately lead to a worse outcome.

- **Exercise and sleep regularly to decrease your stress levels.**

- **If you find your anxiety and worrying unmanageable, seek the help of a mental health professional.**

Conclusion

Everyone experiences pain a little differently. Some hardly notice it while others have a pathological relationship with pain. Ultimately pain is either heightened or dampened depending on your mental state. Poor mental states such as depression, anxiety, and stress all decrease your tolerance for pain. Fortunately, there are strategies such as stress reduction cognitive behavioral therapy and mindfulness therapy which can help increase your pain threshold and turn pain from an enemy into an ally.

Frequently Asked Questions

- **I need surgery, but my fear is preventing me from having it. What should I do?**

Some fear can be a good thing. Fear keeps us from making some dangerous decisions and away from situations which could be harmful. Surgery can lead to a conundrum where you know it may benefit you, but you are afraid of the actual experience. I think a healthy fear of surgery is a good thing. Just don't let it get out of control. You really should not have surgery unless you absolutely need it. If your fear is greater than your pain, perhaps you are not ready to have surgery yet. On the other hand, if you have evaluated the options and decided that you need to move forward with a procedure, don't let your fear prevent you from doing something that can make a huge positive impact in your life. Surgery for the most part is very safe, and most surgeons are well-trained and very capable. Nowadays pain can be managed well with many different medications. Use fear as a guide, but don't let it control you.

References

1.   Vranceanu AM, Barsky A, Ring D. Psychosocial Aspects of Disabling Musculo-skeletal Pain: J Bone Jt Surg-Am Vol. 2009 Aug;91(8):2014–8.

2.	Tunks ER, Crook J, Weir R. Epidemiology of Chronic Pain with Psychological Comorbidity: Prevalence, Risk, Course, and Prognosis. Can J Psychiatry. 2008 Apr;53(4):224–34.

3.	Moussavi S, Chatterji S, Verdes E, Tandon A, Patel V, Ustun B. Depression, chronic diseases, and decrements in health: results from the World Health Surveys. The Lancet. 2007 Sep;370(9590):851–8.

4.	Hill JC, Lewis M, Sim J, Hay EM, Dziedzic K. Predictors of Poor Outcome in Patients With Neck Pain Treated by Physical Therapy: Clin J Pain. 2007 Oct;23(8):683–90.

5.	Richardson C, Glenn S, Horgan M, Nurmikko T. A Prospective Study of Factors Associated With the Presence of Phantom Limb Pain Six Months After Major Lower Limb Amputation in Patients With Peripheral Vascular Disease. J Pain. 2007 Oct;8(10):793–801.

6.	Sivaganesan A, Khan I, Pennings JS, Roth SG, Nolan E, Oleisky ER, et al. Why are patients dissatisfied after spine surgery when improvements in disability and pain are clinically meaningful? Spine J. 2020 Jun;S1529943020307890.

7.	Stull JD, Divi SN, Goyal DKC, Bowles DR, Reyes AA, Bechay J, et al. Preoperative Mental Health Component Scoring Is Related to Patient Reported Outcomes Following Lumbar Fusion. Spine. 2020 Jun 15;45(12):798–803.

8.	Jiménez-Almonte JH, Hautala GS, Abbenhaus EJ, Grabau JD, Nzegwu IN, Mehdi SK, et al. Spine patients demystified: What are the predictive factors of poor surgical outcome in patients after elective cervical and lumbar spine surgery? Spine J. 2020 Jun;S1529943020307713.

9.	Levis B, Benedetti A, Thombs BD, DEPRESsion Screening Data (DEPRESSD) Collaboration. Accuracy of Patient Health Questionnaire-9 (PHQ-9) for screening to detect major depression: individual participant data meta-analysis. BMJ. 2019 Apr 9;365:l1476.

10.	Kroenke K, Spitzer RL, Williams JB. The PHQ-9: validity of a brief depression severity measure. J Gen Intern Med. 2001 Sep;16(9):606–13.

11.	How to Reduce Stress | Psychology Today [Internet]. [cited 2022 Jul 4]. Available from: https://www.psychologytoday.com/us/blog/hide-and-seek/201702/how-reduce-stress

12.	Henschke N, Ostelo RW, van Tulder MW, Vlaeyen JW, Morley S, Assendelft WJ, et al. Behavioural treatment for chronic low-back pain. Cochrane Back and Neck Group, editor. Cochrane Database Syst Rev [Internet]. 2010 Jul 7 [cited 2020 Jul 8]; Available from: http://doi.wiley.com/10.1002/14651858.CD002014.pub3

13.	Cramer H, Haller H, Lauche R, Dobos G. Mindfulness-based stress reduction for low back pain. A systematic review. BMC Complement Altern Med. 2012 Dec;12(1):162.

14.	Cherkin DC, Sherman KJ, Balderson BH, Cook AJ, Anderson ML, Hawkes RJ, et al. Effect of Mindfulness-Based Stress Reduction vs Cognitive Behavioral Therapy or Usual Care on Back Pain and Functional Limitations in Adults With Chronic Low Back

Pain: A Randomized Clinical Trial. JAMA. 2016 Mar 22;315(12):1240–9.

15.   Sepucha KR, Vo H, Chang Y, Dorrwachter JM, Dwyer M, Freiberg AA, et al. Shared Decision-Making Is Associated with Better Outcomes in Patients with Knee But Not Hip Osteoarthritis: The DECIDE-OA Randomized Study. J Bone Jt Surg. 2022 Jan 5;104(1):62–9.

16.   Brant CS. Psychological Preparation for Surgery. Public Health Rep. 1958;73(11):9.

Chapter 29

The Bottom Line, Do I Need Surgery?

Summary

The decision to have spine surgery should be made carefully. Ultimately there are several factors which drive surgeons to operate on elective cases (cases that are not emergencies). The relief of pain is probably the most common reason patients and surgeons decide to pursue spine surgery. However, the pain should be not easily manageable with simple remedies such as physical therapy and over-the-counter medications. Surgery should not be considered if the pain is something you can ultimately live with, assuming the problem isn't one that will be progressive. Spinal cord compression or progressive spinal deformities are other reasons to operate, sometimes even if the patient is asymptomatic. Finally, neurologic dysfunction, particularly weakness or paralysis of a limb, is an indication for surgical decompression if the results of tests match the symptoms and the physical exam. Ultimately, the decision to have surgery is your own, as it's your body, so try and make an informed one with your surgeon as a guide.

Case

Ms. Tomato is a 52-year-old architect who has had a lumbar disc herniation for several years, causing her severe back pain and leg pain (sciatica). She found temporary relief with some epidural steroid injections but no matter what she does, the pain just keeps coming back and getting worse. She doesn't really have any weakness but does suffer from some numbness which is irritating. She is terrified at the thought of having surgery, as she knows people for whom "it didn't go well" and other doctors had told her to avoid surgery if possible. But now her life has been destroyed by the pain. She can no longer exercise which she used to enjoy, and her work has been affected. She decides to have a microdiscectomy after a discussion of the risks and benefits with her surgeon. She is discharged from the hospital the same day and after 12 weeks of outpatient therapy is now back to life 100%. She has no pain and no limitations. She wonders why she didn't have the procedure done earlier.

Introduction

Nobody wants to think about the possibility of having spine surgery. That is the point of the above story, the patient was quite nervous about having a procedure, but made her decision based on the severe symptoms she was experiencing. When faced with the consequences of severe pain, disability, and neurologic dysfunction (inability to use parts of your body due to nerve damage) surgery may be worth it. But in between crushing disability and mere inconvenience lies a huge gray zone where surgery may or may not be worth it. So, what's the bottom line? In this chapter we provide some guideposts to help you figure that out and to help make the discussion with your doctor more meaningful.

In my opinion the decision to undergo elective spine surgery comes down to preserving your quality of life such that you can live without any major dysfunction. In this regard there are five factors to consider when deciding about spine surgery: 1. How much pain are you having; has it gotten to the point where you cannot live with it anymore? 2. Is there the possibility that your life will get much worse without surgery? 3. Do you have neurologic impairment with loss of motor strength, sensation, bowel, or bladder function? 4. What is the chance the proposed surgery will help, and what are the risks? 5. Does the proposed surgery mesh with your value system (are you ok having metal implants in your body? Are you terrified at the thought of surgery for any reason)?

Pain

Before you consider surgery, ask yourself: Is your pain manageable? I have had countless patients walk into my office who were told somewhere that they need spine surgery. When they see me, they list the numerous problems their MRI report shows and various vague complaints. I then ask them a simple question, is your pain bad enough for you to consider surgery? They typically answer: "well, no. my pain is not that bad, and I can control it with some simple medicines and activity choices."

In cases where the pain is minor there needs to be another pressing issue (see below) to recommend surgery. There are many things that can be dramatically wrong with your spine on X-ray that are perfectly fine to live with because they are not causing you severe pain. Radiologists are incredible doctors who analyze every small aspect of your X-rays and scans and are required to document exactly what they see. Don't let a lengthy radiology report scare you into needing surgery without talking seriously about it with your surgeon.

You must also remember spine surgery is painful. Sometimes you need to go through some pain to cure the pain you are having—but not for minor aches. Thus, I generally only recommend spine surgery to treat incapacitating pain. The degree of your pain is sometimes what determines the need for surgery. For example, in the case of lumbar herniations, many will resolve in weeks to months. So why do surgery on them? The answer is some patients have such severe pain they simply cannot wait that long. For others, the pain never got better despite waiting. For these patients, surgery can be a godsend. But if your pain is manageable, why go through the additional pain and risk of surgery when the problem may simply get better on its own or isn't that bad to begin with.

Is there a chance your problem will get worse without surgery?

In this section we discuss the most common reasons to undergo surgery in the spine and their overall prognosis with and without surgery.

Stenosis

Stenosis just means there is narrowing of a tubular space. For example, arterial stenosis occurs when plaque builds up in an artery clogging them up. In the spine we use the term to describe narrowing of the spinal canal and resulting compression of the nerve roots and spinal cord.

Disc herniations (herniated/ruptured discs) may cause stenosis, and sometimes displaced disc material compresses nerve roots or spinal cord. Another cause of stenosis is simply aging: over time the vertebrae lose the elastic cushioning between them and the smooth cartilage that covers them. Your body reacts by generating bone spurs that can narrow the spinal canal and result in compression on your nerves. This can result in pain, weakness, numbness or all three.

Just because you have mild stenosis doesn't mean you should immediately have surgery—stenosis should be quite significant before surgery is recommended. Furthermore, just because you have stenosis, if you do not have significant symptoms, you may not require surgery. In the lumbar spine the development of stenosis can take decades and the nerves have time to adjust. Thus, stenosis occurring in the lumbar spine can be an indication to have surgery if it is symptomatic as surgery can readily relieve the symptoms but does not absolutely need to be treated in every patient depending on their circumstances. However, this may not be the case for the thoracic or cervical spines (upper back or neck respectively), as stenosis in these areas can cause permanent damage to the spinal cord and may be an indication for surgery even without significant symptoms. Just because a radiology report says you have stenosis does not necessarily mean you need surgery.

Nonetheless, overtime most degenerative stenosis (stenosis caused by old age) will only get worse. It could be that you may develop symptoms in the future. Cervical and thoracic stenosis similarly only get worse with time. Depending on your symptoms and how severe your stenosis is, this fact may help guide your decision for surgery.

Instability

When two bones move abnormally with respect to one another this is called instability. Instability can result from degeneration or "wear-and-tear," or from trauma, tumor, or infection. In the spine, instability can result in "dynamic stenosis" when one vertebra moves on the other resulting in nerve or spinal cord compression. Once instability starts in the spine it just tends to get worse as the bony and ligamentous anatomy that once held the spine together no longer work. Instability can also cause neck or back pain.   Instability is readily treated with surgery and can be a good reason to have a spine procedure.

Progressive Spine Problems

There are certain spine conditions that if not treated will tend to get dramatically worse. While this is not an exhaustive list, fractures, infections, tumors, spinal cord compression and major spinal deformity are some examples that come readily to mind. Spinal cord compression in many cases is asymptomatic but progresses in an insidious way. For example, if your spinal cord is pinched or compressed in the cervical spine (the neck), over time as you move your neck around it causes more and more spinal cord damage resulting in a serious condition known as cervical myelopathy (see chapter 5). This is one of the main "MRI findings" where I might offer treatment once it reaches a certain degree regardless of symptoms. This is because once spinal cord function is lost, there may be no getting it back so in my opinion it's better to take a prophylactic approach, especially if the surgery is minimally invasive. In some cases of spinal cord compression, the symptoms can also be very slow in onset, so slow you may not even notice it.

Though not all fractures and infections of the spine need to be treated, there are cases where things will obviously become worse if not treated. Abscesses which occur in the spinal canal known as an epidural abscess can cause progressive problems from nerve or spinal cord compression and should be evacuated. Fractures which compromise the integrity of the spine tend also to just get worse and should be treated to prevent deformity, neurologic dysfunction, or chronic pain from developing.

In cases of spinal deformity, there are some which will keep getting worse over time only making treatment more difficult. Scoliosis once it reaches a certain degree will only continue to progress. Although the progression is usually not rapid, by doing nothing you can easily paint yourself into a hole later in life where, with each year passing, your deformity and disability are progressing, and surgery is riskier.

For these reasons it's better to deal with these problems sooner rather than later. Moreover, if you have a fracture where there is progression of the deformity or any issue in the spine that is visibly getting worse, it's better to try and get on top of the problem when it's not as serious rather than waiting for the problem to become a complicated issue.

Neurologic Disorders (your body doesn't work right because your nerves are damaged)

Few experiences are as scary as the feeling of becoming paralyzed or losing strength. This typically occurs in the spine because of compression either of nerve roots or of the spinal cord. If the neurologic problem is progressive, meaning it seems to be getting worse with time, then it's better to strike while the iron is hot to stop it from getting worse. Because, as stated above, once it's lost, there is nothing in modern medicine which can readily bring it back. If you start to notice your arm or leg becoming weak and it seems to be getting worse, its best to seek the attention of a trained spine surgeon for an evaluation.

Similarly, numbness generally represents a loss of nerve function. Some numbness can be minor, such as a numb toe that may not bother you. On the other hand, if your entire leg is numb this could indicate a serious problem. Its best to describe your problem to your surgeon and learn whether surgery may help alleviate the numbness.

What is the chance the proposed surgery will help? What are the risks?

It is important to have a conversation with your surgeon about whether the proposed surgery will help your problem, and what are the estimated chances it will be successful (keep in mind no surgeon can predict with absolute 100% certainty if a surgery will be successful). There are many factors which go into this estimation (What condition you have, the severity of your disease, its location, your age, etc.) so a lot will depend on what your surgeon thinks. Most surgeons won't offer surgery if it has a slim chance of working, but in some cases, patients may be so fed up with pain, or disability, they may still want to pursue surgery even if the chances of improvement are slim.

It's also important to discuss the risks of the procedure. I explain to my patients that all surgeries have a cost in terms of risk and recovery time. A surgery may be beneficial for you, but if the risks are so high that a complication is all but guaranteed you must think hard before moving forward. Furthermore, be sure the recovery time is something that you can deal with. Will you need to be off work for a prolonged period? Will you be ok living with the restrictions a surgeon may put on you in the post-operative period?

I devote an entire chapter to surgical and medical complications in spine surgery to help you better understand these risks (chapter 30 and 31). In brief, surgical procedures have inherent (come with the territory) surgical risks but if you are very sick or elderly there may be additional risks inherent to your overall medical condition. Discuss these risks with your surgeon so you understand what the price will be.

Values and Understanding of Surgery

Ultimately in a non-emergency setting it is your choice to have surgery because it is your body. Your surgeon may suggest a particular procedure or treatment, but you should be comfortable with the decision to move forward. Does it sound like something that is worth it to you to go through? Studies have shown that the more engaged the patient is in the decision-making process the increased chance of satisfaction with surgery. What does being engaged mean? There is no strict definition, but I think it means having a basic understanding of your condition, and the proposed risk and benefits of treatment (see the chapter 27 on preparing for surgery on informed consent). There is often a disconnect between the values, expectations and understanding of a problem between the patient and the surgeon.

Thus, it is important to discuss your values and expectations with your surgeon, so he or she may have the opportunity to clarify any misconceptions (1).

I have created basic surgical decision guides so that my patients can have a better overview of how to make informed choices regarding spinal procedures. See below.

Conclusion

Sometimes the decision to undergo surgery comes down to common sense. Think carefully about your symptoms. Are they symptoms you can live with? Or would you rather not have to deal with them? Pain and neurologic dysfunction are two experiences most people would rather not live with if given the choice. There are some conditions that should be treated regardless of your symptoms, such as severe spinal cord compression and/or progressive deformity, but these are thankfully rare.

Frequently Asked Questions

- **I have a chronic disc herniation in my back that causes me to have back and leg pain. I have been offered surgery but have been getting epidural steroid shots which take the pain away, so I don't really notice it. However, I'm worried about getting these shots repeatedly. When is the right time to have surgery to treat my problem?**

    I think getting an occasional epidural steroid shot is fine but using them for a prolonged period (over 6 months) is probably not a good idea. Steroids weaken the bone and can have other side effects. Moreover, they can just mask the pain while your problem progresses. It may be worth considering surgery if your symptoms are significant enough that you are requiring multiple shots regularly to treat your pain. This is a judgment call that you will have to make with your surgeon.

References

1.   Alokozai A, Lin E, Crijns TJ, Ring D, Bozic K, Koenig K, et al. Patient and Surgeon Ratings of Patient Involvement in Decision-Making Are Not Aligned. Journal of Bone and Joint Surgery. 2022 May 4;104(9):767–73.

Figures:

Lumbar Surgery Decision Aid: Dr. Katsuura's Guide for a Big Decision

Symptoms which may prompt you to consider lumbar surgery:

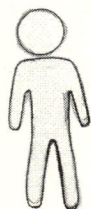

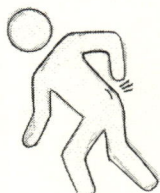

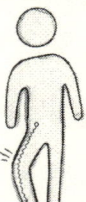

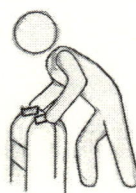

Low back pain | Sciatica/ leg pain | Leg Numbness/ tingling | Leg weakness | Inability to walk long distances

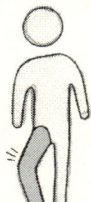

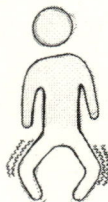

Treatments to consider before surgery: May try these individually or in combination

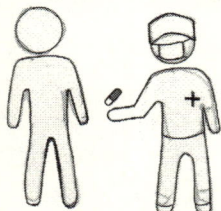

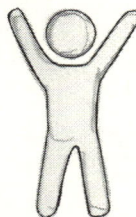

NSAIDS/ Pain medications | Physical therapy | Injections | Sometimes you just get better with time

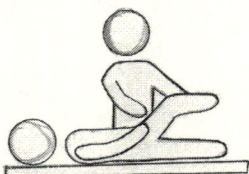

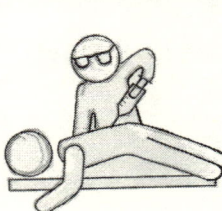

Things to consider about surgery: Sometimes surgery speeds recovery but know this:

Surgery has risks: for example scarring around nerves, infection (may require another surgery for washout), medical complications (like having a heart attack), nerve damage resulting in new weakness, pain or numbness.

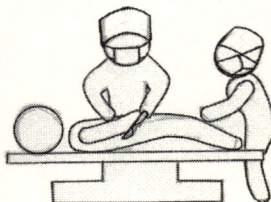

There is a chance surgery won't take away your symptoms. Some symptoms may improve while others may not (numbness/weakness). Even if you get better, you may have other issues in the future.

In some cases, you can typically decide to have surgery at a later date with no ill effects.

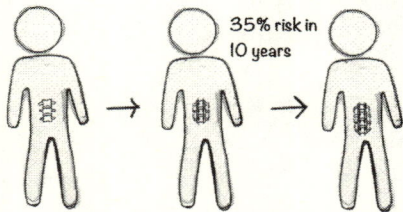

35% risk in 10 years

Decompressions may need to be **revised to fusions** in the future | Fusions may need to be **extended or revised in the future** | There are post-op restrictions: no bending lifting or twisting. | Share in decisions!

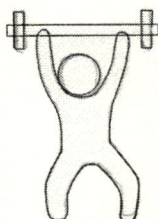

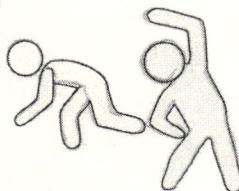

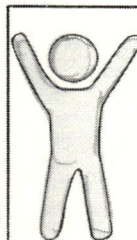

Lumbar surgery decision guide. Trying to assimilate all the factors that go into the choice to undergo a procedure can be difficult. Here you can see in cartoon format some things you should consider about lumbar surgery.

Cervical Surgery Decision Aid: Dr. Katsuura's Guide for a Big Decision

Symptoms which may prompt you to consider cervical surgery: surgery can treat these

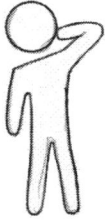

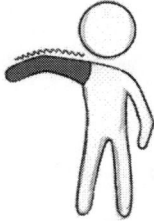

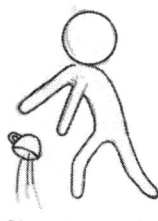

Neck pain | Arm pain, numbness, weakness | Imbalance | Clumsiness, loss of dexterity | Incontinence | Inability to walk/ paralysis

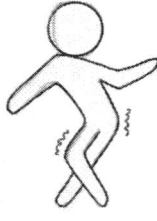

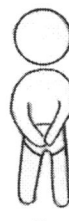

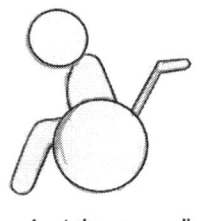

Treatments to consider before surgery: May try these individually or in combination

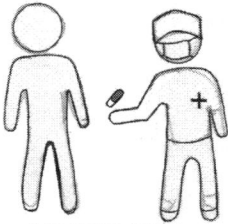

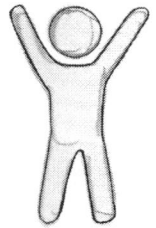

NSAIDS/ Pain medications | Physical therapy | Injections | Sometimes you just get better with time

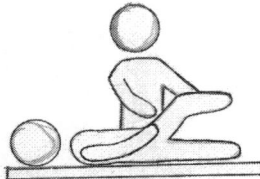

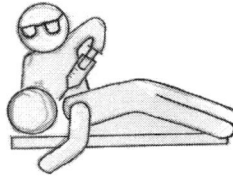

Things to consider about surgery: Sometimes surgery speeds recovery but know this:

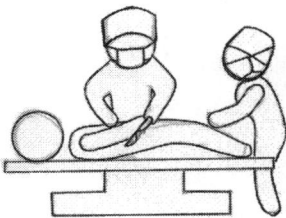

Surgery has risks: for example scarring around nerves, infection (may require another surgery for washout), medical complications (like having a heart attack), nerve/spinal cord damage resulting in new weakness, pain or numbness.

There is a chance surgery wont take away your symptoms. Some symptoms may improve while others may not (numbness/weakness). Even if you get better, you may have other issues in the future. Surgery is used in some instances to prevent further neurological decline, but can't improve damage that has already occurred.

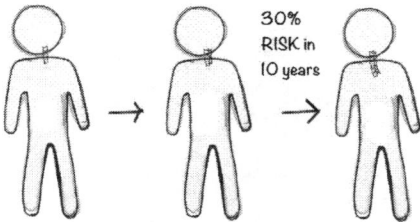

30% RISK in 10 years

Decompressions may need to be **revised to fusions** in the future

Fusions may need to be **extended or revised in the future**

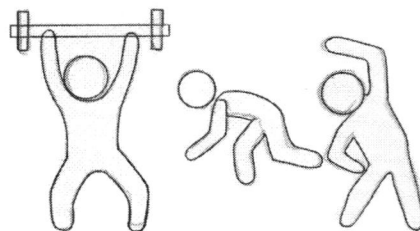

There are post-op restrictions: no bending lifting or twisting.

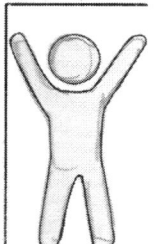

Share in decisions!

Cervical surgery decision guide. Here you can see in cartoon format some things you should consider about cervical surgery.

Chapter 30

What Are the Risks of Spine Surgery?

Summary

Every surgery is a risk-benefit analysis. This means that patients and surgeons alike should try to ensure the benefits of the operation outweigh the risks. However, the potential benefit from the surgery and the risks involved are independent of one another and so must be analyzed separately. Just because a spine surgery has a chance of helping you, if the risks are higher than the proposed benefit, it may not be worth it. Risks to spine surgery are numerous and can include anything from paralysis from neurologic injury, problems due to wrong-site surgery, complications from positioning, dural tears, bleeding, death, as well as any number of medical conditions. Some risks can be predicted, while others cannot. Even if a surgery has potential benefit, if the risks are insurmountable it still makes the procedure a bad idea.

Case

Ms. Orange is a 65-year-old and has bad spinal stenosis adjacent to a previous lumbar fusion that was done about 10 years ago. The stenosis is causing severe leg pain, weakness and numbness. For almost a decade after her first spinal

fusion she has done well, but this problem has been getting worse for about a year now. She is otherwise healthy. After discussing with her surgeon, they decide that a revision (a second surgery to correct issues from a first surgery) is the best course of action and the surgeon discusses that revision surgeries carry an increased risk. Sure enough, during the procedure Ms. Orange suffers a dural tear (a cut on the tissue that covers the spinal cord) with a cerebrospinal fluid leak, which is repaired. After the procedure she is kept on bed rest for several days but unfortunately starts to develop headaches that are quite severe when she stands up. After 5 days in the hospital, the surgeon thinks that the repair may still be leaking and decides to take her back to the operating room. In surgery he finds that the repair didn't hold, and this time decides to use a patch to fix the leak. After this procedure Ms. Orange notices an immediate improvement in her headaches. She is discharged from the hospital and states her leg and back pain are improved after having the surgery and she has no other issues.

Introduction

Before each surgery that I do, I review the risks of the procedure with the patient and family. For some patients this is just a formality, for others it is a serious discussion about the realities of something going wrong. The purpose of this conversation is always the same: to prepare the patient mentally and to help him/her understand that surgery always has some level of risk involved. There are an unlimited number of variables that determine whether someone will have a good or bad outcome with surgery. In elective surgery (surgery for a non-emergent condition/non-emergency), surgeons are trained to select safe cases with low-risk profiles. In non-elective surgery (surgery for emergencies or conditions that will result in a poor outcome without urgent intervention) we learn to live with the risks to save lives and preserve limb and function.

Understanding the risks prior to stepping foot in the operating room is empowering for the patient. You are more educated and thus more certain that the decision to have surgery is the one right for you. I tell my patients that the reality of something major going wrong is usually low but not impossible. If there is a high probability of something going wrong, or you aren't sure that surgery is worth the risk, you should pause and consider if surgery is the best option for you.

It's important to understand that the risks of surgery are independent of the chance surgery will be successful. Make sure you talk to your doctor carefully about the chances the surgery will help the pain or problem you are having. Then talk to him separately about the risks of surgery—that is, what can go wrong. As a surgeon I make calculations daily in my mind. I look at the patient, try to assess how great the problem is, then weigh that against the potential risk that what I do to them will cause harm. If the benefits seem to outweigh the risks, we move forward with surgery. If they don't, we stop and have a hard conversation.

This chapter is meant to paint in broad strokes the most feared complications in spinal surgery, with the understanding that the risk to all patients from various procedures cannot be summarized or predicted. Two of the major risks of spine surgery, infection and hardware complications, the latter often resulting in pseudoarthrosis (when bones fail to fuse together after a spinal fusion), are discussed separately in their own chapters (chapter 14 and chapter 31). If you are looking for a comprehensive list of medical complications associated with spine surgery, look up the first article listed in this chapter's references; this article by Lee et al provides a nice overview with incidence rates (1).

Surgical Risks

nerve root / spinal cord Injury

One of the most feared complications in spine surgery is paralysis—loss of motor function to part or all your body. If a nerve root is injured/irritated during surgery, weakness in an isolated arm or leg can occur. If the spinal cord is injured during surgery, partial or complete paralysis may be the outcome. Spinal cord injury in the thoracic spine causes paraplegia (loss of function below the waist) and in the cervical spine, quadriplegia (total loss of motor function below the neck). When this occurs during surgery it is known as "iatrogenic" which means it resulted somehow from the surgery itself. Iatrogenic spinal cord injury may result from unwanted compression of the spinal cord during surgery, a drop-in blood pressure, over-correction of a spinal deformity or even from mispositioned hardware or spinal instruments. Luckily, the incidence of complete paralysis is extremely rare in surgery performed by those trained specifically in spinal care.

In a large series examining the rate of spinal cord injury in elective surgery cases there were 3 cases of quadriplegia out of 12,903 cases of elective cervical surgeries. The rate also varies depending on the complexity of pathology and surgery being performed. For example, in routine cervical spine surgery the incidence of spinal cord injury can range from 0% to 0.3% whereas complex deformity procedures can have rates as high as 1.7% to 18% (2). Complicated cervical deformity surgery can even have a neurologic complication rate as high as 18% (3). The risk of nerve injury is higher in revision surgery (a second procedure to correct issues from a previous surgery) because normal anatomy is disrupted, making the nerves more difficult to identify and protect (4).

Fortunately, the prognosis (predicted outcome) of iatrogenic spinal cord or nerve root injury is good, with upwards of 90% recovery rate. However, recovery tends to be slow, taking anywhere from around 6 months to over a year.

Spinal cord and nerve root monitoring technology (neuromonitoring) has been developed to decrease the incidence of iatrogenic neurologic injury. Spinal cord monitoring works by sending electrical impulses up and down the spinal cord and monitoring the response either in the brain (sensory) or in the limbs (motor). Somatosensory-evoked potentials (SSEPs) are used to monitor the sensory system of the spinal cord and work by sending electrical signals from the limbs to the brain, where the signals are picked up by electrodes placed in the brain. Motor-evoked potentials (MEPs) work in the opposite way—they stimulate the brain to produce a muscle contraction in the arms and legs.

Spinal cord monitoring is typically performed by a neurophysiologist or neuro tech, who actively monitors the signals during surgery for any abnormalities and alerts the surgeon when there are changes. This can allow the surgeon to actively react to any emerging problems in the spinal cord and hopefully prevent permanent damage. The most common scenario occurs during deformity correction when a large change in the shape of the spine causes decreased blood flow to the spinal cord. This can result in a neuromonitoring alert that can allow the surgeon to decrease the amount of correction he is trying to achieve.

Neuromonitoring is unfortunately far from full proof. In many cases of severe cervical stenosis, neuromonitoring will not function correctly because the spinal cord is not functioning correctly. In these types of cases the surgeon is essentially "flying blind." Furthermore, at times neuromonitoring alerts occur during surgery and the patient wakes up unaffected. Finally, it is possible for nerve root and spinal cord injury to occur during surgery without neuromonitoring giving any indication of a problem. Thus, neuromonitoring is simply a tool for surgeons to use— it does not prevent all catastrophic neurologic injuries nor is it entirely accurate.

wrong site surgery

Wrong site surgery can happen in many different surgical fields but is an especially easy mistake to make in spine surgery. This is because many of the spinal segments look very similar—or identical—to surgeons' eyes. (A segment here refers to two vertebrae and the disc between them.) L3-4 doesn't look much different from L4-5 under the microscope. But surgery on the wrong location obviously will not help the patient and could do harm. The incidence of this happening is estimated to be around 0.3% to 5% of cases and can lead to significant distress in both patient and surgeon (5).

Wrong level surgery is more common in minimally invasive type procedures where the opening of the tissue beneath the skin is kept to a minimum; this approach makes it more difficult for the surgeon to confirm that he/she is on the right level. Thankfully, spine surgeons are very highly trained in how to prevent this. They double and triple check the levels (a level is a single vertebra or a single intervertebral disc) using X-ray, and as a result, wrong site surgery is becoming less and less common. It is important to understand that your surgeon may expose (approach and prepare to work on) the wrong area of the spine, known as wrong exposure; this is very common and not harmful. This is because spinal segments are very close together and you can easily move up or down in any given surgery. Once the surgeon gets down to the spine, he/she will place a marker and check, using X-ray, to confirm the levels.

You can also help prevent wrong level surgery. Be involved in the informed consent process, taking the time to check the levels yourself. Double confirm with your surgeon prior to the surgery what levels are planned. Have him/her write the levels on your back in permanent marker.

problems related to keeping the body immobile in the prone position for a long time

Spine surgery is typically performed in the prone position, meaning you are on your stomach with your back up so the surgeon can work on you.

Most spine surgeons use a frame that has pads around the chest and pelvis to allow your abdomen to be free. Your surgeon will ensure all your bony prominences are well padded; however, despite all precautions, complications can still occur. Even with the use of pads, the length of time the skin tissue is pressed against this frame by the body's bony weight can sometimes result in pressure ulcers or skin breakdown. This is more likely when the surgery takes a long time and when the patient is elderly.

Your face is usually cradled in a foam harness to keep pressure off your eyes. Nevertheless, it is still possible to have some pressure on the eyes that, in rare cases, can result in blindness. You should let your surgeon known if you have a history of retinal detachment, ischemia, or glaucoma, all of which increase the risk of blindness. Moreover, being in the prone position with your face in the foam harness for several hours can cause severe facial swelling such that you may not even recognize yourself for a few hours after surgery. It is possible to have peripheral nerve injury or compression that can result in new numbness or weakness—those symptoms are usually temporary (6).

dural tears/ cerebral spinal fluid (CSF) leaks

As described in earlier chapters the spinal cord, cauda equina and nerve roots are encased in thin, water-tight membranous tissues known as the meninges. Collectively the meninges are comprised of the outer dura mater (dura), and the inner arachnoid and the pia mater. The dura is the main layer that is clinically relevant as it is the tough (dura for durable) layer. The meninges also contain the cerebrospinal fluid (CSF), a crystal-clear liquid that bathes the spinal cord. You make about half a liter (500cc) of CSF a day, of which about a total volume of 150cc bathes the spinal cord and brain at any point in time. The dura may become thinned from compressive disease and, when operating around the spine, tears can easily occur allowing the CSF to leak out (7). Dural tears are one of the most common adverse events in spine surgery.

Dural tears occur at varying rates, depending on the surgery anywhere from 3-17%. Revision surgery carries an even higher risk of dural tears because the dura can be scarred and easily ruptured (8). There are several risk factors for dural tears, including calcification (ossification) of the tissues surrounding the dura (the ligamentum flavum and the posterior longitudinal ligament) increasing age, and severity of stenosis (narrowing of the spinal canal). Dural tears can lead to other complications such as CSF fistula (where spinal fluid continues to drain through the skin), pseudo meningocele (where CSF forms a pocket under the skin), and even meningitis (an infection of the CSF). Meningitis in the CSF is not like a viral meningitis and luckily is treatable.

Most dural tears can be repaired in surgery, and thus are inconsequential to the patient. A large study comparing the outcomes of patients with and without dural tears showed dural tears did not have a significant impact on the overall patient outcome (9).

If a dural tear occurs during surgery, it is typically repaired using suture and a special glue called Duraseal® or Tisseal®. A special patch from a collagen matrix, fascia or a fat graft may also be used to reinforce the repair. Because the CSF is a column of fluid, to aid healing you may be kept on bed rest after a dural tear, so that excessive hydrostatic pressure is not put on the repair. Despite an adequate repair, continued leaking can occur in 5-10% of tears and may require re-exploration.

Once it is determined that it is safe for you to become upright again, your clinical team may slowly elevate your bed and have you try walking. Common symptoms of a persistent CSF leak are severe headache, particularly when becoming upright, aversion to light (photophobia), nausea, dizziness, or clear fluid drainage from the wound. If these symptoms persist it may be necessary to return to lying on your back. Your surgeon may determine it is best to return to surgery to explore the wound and try to do further repairs of the dura.

Occasionally it is possible to develop a delayed CSF leak even remotely after surgery. In such cases you may be ok for weeks but then start to have symptoms of CSF leak and require a second surgery to repair it (10).

major hemorrhage

Almost all the major arteries of the body are near the spine and thus are at risk during spine surgery. Major hemorrhage in spinal surgery can occur when one of the main arteries of the body is punctured or lacerated and can be life-threatening. The most common scenario for major hemorrhage occurs when approaching the spine from the front of the body, specifically with an anterior abdominal approach for a lumbar fusion. When the surgeon approaches the spine going through the abdominal area, he/she must directly manipulate the inferior vena cava or common iliac vein which increases the chance of puncturing or cutting it.

For these reasons when spine surgeons perform an anterior abdominal approach, they typically do so with an assisting vascular or general surgeon who can immediately repair an injury. An injury to the inferior vena cava can occur in upwards of 3% of cases when the surgeon approaches the lumbar spine from the front, through the abdominal region (11). Luckily even though the risk of major hemorrhage is high, death is not common, and damaged veins and arteries can typically be repaired by a vascular surgeon. In cases where a high amount of blood loss can be anticipated, surgeons can have transfusion blood available, use a device called cell-saver which recycles your blood so that it can be reinfused, and have vascular (blood vessel) surgeons available to help stop the bleeding.

Medical Risks

death

Death cannot be predicted, but luckily it is a rare occurrence in elective surgery— somewhere between 0.03% to 3%. There are many factors which play into this but simply the older and sicker you are and more complicated your surgery will be, the greater the risk of death from any cause. It is important to have frank discussions about this with your spine surgeon to understand where on the risk-reward spectrum you fall. A small procedure with obvious benefit, may be worth performing even if you are elderly and sick. However, it may be better to live with your problem rather than die trying to undergo a complicated surgery required to treat your spine. Each of these decisions must be made on an individual basis between patient and surgeon.

blood clots: deep venous thrombosis (DVT) and pulmonary embolism

Blood clots in the leg or deep venous thromboses (DVT) occur when the blood moving through your leg veins slows down and congeals to form a clot. It's critical to realize there is a difference between veins and arteries. Arteries leave the heart and have high pressure thanks to your pumping heart. Blood clots in the arteries do not result in DVT but instead result in ischemia (loss of blood flow) which is much more dangerous. However, because arteries have high pressure and fast flow, clots are less common. Veins, on the other hand, are responsible for bringing blood back to your heart from your body. Veins are low pressure and slow flow. They do not have a mechanical pump driving the motion of blood but instead rely on your muscles to contract and push blood back. Thus veins are more prone to clots.

You may have heard of patients having blood clots from hip surgery. People who undergo hip surgery are at increased risk for DVT because of inflammation and lack of mobility. It's hard to move and get out of bed because of pain when your hip is broken and so your now inactive muscles do not pump blood back to the heart. Venous blood is allowed to pool and congeal and creates a perfect environment for a DVT to form. Blood clots occur in spine surgery for the same reasons—inflammation and the lack of mobility—but at much lower rates compared to hip surgery. A large meta-analysis on the topic showed the overall rate for DVT in elective spine surgery to be around 2% (12).

An isolated DVT may cause swelling, redness, and pain in your calves. A quick ultrasound test may be performed to detect them. Isolated DVTs are painful but generally do not cause serious harm. They are treated with blood thinners and resorb over time. However, if the clot breaks free and travels into the lungs (known as a pulmonary embolism or PE) it can be serious. Small PEs are inconsequential and treated similarly to DVTs, but larger clots can get stuck in the great arteries of the lungs and can be fatal. In spine surgery blood clots are also hard to treat with anticoagulants (blood thinners) since blood thinners can cause excessive bleeding in the wound. Bleeding in the wound can result in a compressive hematoma (a collection/pool of blood outside a blood vessel) that be catastrophic to neural or other vital structures. So, the spine surgeon must walk a careful line between too much clotting and too little.

Some risk factors for DVT in spine patients are a history of previous DVT, spinal cord injury, severe multisystem trauma, and an active malignancy. Furthermore, there are some surgical- related risk factors such as large deformity corrections, spinal fusions greater than 4 levels, or a combined anterior posterior surgical approach (that is, surgery that requires approaching the spine from both the front and the back) (13).

cardiac problems

Major adverse cardiac events (MACE) consist of new arrhythmias (abnormal heart beats) that require intervention, myocardial infarction (heart attack) or ischemia (loss of blood flow) (14). Spine surgery can precipitate MACE due to blood loss and long surgical times that put stress on the heart. The revised cardiac risk index (RCRI) has been used to estimate the risk of MACE in thoracic, abdominal and orthopedic surgery but may underestimate the risk in spine surgery, particularly if a fusion of more than 3 levels is performed (15,16).

The incidence of MACE in multilevel spinal fusions has been estimated to be around 9% (15). If you are high risk and are planning to undergo a high-risk surgery such as a lumbar fusion of more than 3 levels, having a cardiology consult prior to surgery is recommended.

gastrointestinal problems

Nausea is common after general anesthesia, occurring in 10-30% of patients (17). This is typically related to use of inhaled anesthetics (sevoflurane and isoflurane) and narcotic medicines. Nausea can be reduced by limiting narcotic medicines. Antiemetics such as a scopolamine patch, dexamethasone, and ondansetron (Zofran®) may also be used to reduce symptoms.

Antiemetics to Treat Nausea			
Name	Mechanism	Dose	Side effects
Ondansetron (Zofran®)	Serotonin antagonist	4mg IV every 8 hours	Prolonged QT on EKG (Indicates an electrical problem in one of the heart's ventricles)
Dexamethasone	Steroid anti-inflammatory	4-8mg IV	Wound issues, infection, osteoporosis
Scopolamine patch	Anticholinergic	1.5mg transdermal for 24 hours	Confusion, agitation, dry mouth, burry vision, urinary retention

Your gastrointestinal system (GI) is constantly moving such that food and liquids can make their way through the digestive tract. Sometimes following surgery your GI system undergoes a shock that causes it to stop moving, resulting in gut dysmotility causing severe constipation. This is known as a paralytic ileus and can occur after spine surgery, especially if the surgery is a large lumbar reconstruction approached from the front, through the abdomen (18). The incidence of Ileus is estimated to occur in around 5% of spine cases. Ileus can be further worsened by electrolyte imbalances, inflammation, lack of mobility, and narcotic medications such as morphine, oxycodone, hydrocodone, hydromorphone, and tramadol, all which cause constipation.

Ileus typically manifests with bloating of the abdomen, no passage of gas, no bowel motions and nausea/vomiting. Ileus can be quite uncomfortable and is treated with time and supportive measures including fasting and possibly the insertion of a nasogastric tube which helps decompress the stomach. Obviously, narcotics need to be limited in this scenario as they only worsen the problem.

neurologic problems

After major surgery, delirium and accelerated dementia can occur in the elderly, because of anesthesia. The elderly are more sensitive to narcotic and anesthetic medicines because of a reduced ability to excrete them from the body. Elderly patients who already suffer from dementia, delirium, or sun downing (becoming confused when the sun goes down) are at even higher risk for worsening post-operative delirium and dementia. Typically, post-operative delirium resolves once the anesthesia and narcotics have worn off. Please see chapter 34 on surgery in the elderly for greater detail about this topic.

Stroke occurs when the blood flow to the spinal cord or brain gets disrupted long enough for neural tissue to die, resulting in paralysis, cognitive issues, difficulty speaking or loss of sensation. Stroke can occur because of blood clots or existing vascular blockages that are worsened by surgery.

respiratory problems

Most spinal surgeries are performed under general anesthesia. General anesthesia is induced with medications that decrease respiratory drive, meaning that you will not breathe independently. These include a combination of sedative-hypnotic drugs such as Propofol, ketamine, halogenated gases (Sevoflurane or halothane), and opioid narcotics. Furthermore, most general anesthetics require some form of chemical paralysis during intubation such as succinylcholine, vecuronium or rocuronium, all which stop breathing. As a result, general anesthesia requires endotracheal intubation which means a plastic tube is placed in the airway to ensure you can breathe during the surgery through a ventilator.

Normally when you take a breath your diaphragm sucks in air through the airway. Ventilators do not recreate a normal respiratory environment but instead push air into the lungs (called positive pressure ventilation). Respiratory problems can occur because of positive pressure ventilation and intubations.

Prolonged intubation: If your surgery is prolonged your lungs may need time to adjust back to regular breathing and you may need to remain intubated after your surgery.

Upper airway obstruction: Blockage of the upper airway is a serious problem and can result if the airway goes into spasm (laryngeal spasm) or from external compression. In anterior cervical surgery, where you approach the cervical spine from the front of the neck, the airway is not only intubated but manipulated, sometimes causing swelling and hematomas (a collection of congealed blood). Either swelling or a hematoma can block the airway, which can result in suffocation. This is a medical emergency and typically requires decompression of the hematoma and reintubation. Luckily this problem is rare, occurring at a rate of 2-5% in most anterior cervical cases and, with careful monitoring, can be easily treated (19).

Atelectasis: Atelectasis occurs when some of the small air sacs in your lungs known as alveoli collapse because of positive pressure ventilation and secretions. This is usually asymptomatic but occasionally can result in symptoms of low-grade fever in the several days after surgery. It's treated by regular use of your incentive spirometer (a small device that trains you to take deep breaths).

The incentive spirometer is a device which measures how fast and deep you are breathing—incentivizing you to take good deep breaths and re-expand collapsed sections of your lungs. It consists of a flexible mouthpiece that is attached to a chamber containing a piston that can show how much air you move in a breath and a separate smaller chamber with a small ball that measures flow. To use the incentive spirometer, place the mouthpiece in your mouth and inhale deeply trying to get the piston to go as high as possible while keeping the small flow ball between the indicator arrows. If the ball is too high or too low, it means you are breathing too fast or too slow respectively. Once you get the piston as high as you can, hold your breath for 10 seconds and then slowly exhale. Repeat 10 times.

Aspiration: Healthy individuals have a reflex that prevents food and liquid from going down the windpipe when they swallow. However, when you undergo general anesthesia, you are not breathing independently and do not have that reflex to call upon, which means that until you are intubated, your airway is not protected from a reflux of stomach contents. In the time span between anesthesia taking effect and intubation, the airway is not protected, and any vomiting of gastric contents can go down the airway resulting in an aspiration. If vomit goes down into the airway it can result in a pneumonia because your bile contains bacteria that are not present in the lungs and can set up an infection or irritation of the lungs (pneumonia or pneumonitis). Therefore, you are required to fast (no eating or drinking) prior to surgery (typically for 6 to 8 hours), which dramatically decreases the risk of aspiration.

urologic problems

Urination occurs via a complicated neurological reflex that is regulated by your sympathetic and parasympathetic nervous systems (the autonomic nervous system responsible for unconscious regulation of the body). This reflex can become slowed or inactivated by the combination of surgery and anesthesia, as well as by the medications used to control pain after surgery. This can result in post-operative urinary retention (POUR) which can occur at a rate of anywhere from 9-70% (20). In spine surgery the incidence is around 18% (21). POUR is much more common in men and in those with increased age. Certain drugs such as anticholinergics (scopolamine, for example, which is sometimes given post-op to prevent nausea), beta blockers (metoprolol), which treat high blood pressure, anesthetics, and narcotics all increase the risk of POUR. POUR can lead to urinary tract infections and damage to the bladder and kidneys.

POUR is typically diagnosed in a patient who is unable to void, using an ultrasound scan of the bladder. If the scan shows a certain residual (remaining) volume of 500-600 cc urine after voiding, a catheter may need to be placed to drain the bladder and prevent injury to the kidneys. This may be done in an "in-and-out" technique where a catheter is inserted just for temporary drainage, or the catheter may be left in place (22). If several catheterizations are required with continued urinary retention, a catheter may be left in place, sometimes for up to a week or two.

Several medications may be used to treat POUR. Tamsulosin, an Alpha-1-adrenergic antagonist that helps the bladder sphincter and the prostate relax, is typical.

Typical Medication to treat POUR			
Name	Mechanism	Dose	Side effects
Tamsulosin (Flomax ®)	Alpha 1 antagonist inhibits smooth muscle contraction Or Relaxes bladder muscles	0.4mg daily may be increased to 0.8mg daily after 2 weeks	Orthostatic hypotension (low blood pressure on standing up) Floppy iris syndrome, which can affect cataract surgery

Conclusion

If you have made it through this chapter, you may be very nervous about surgery. I spend a good deal of my day discussing this material with patients. It's not enjoyable but it serves a purpose: being upfront and letting people make their own choices. The reality is surgeons take extraordinary measures to lower risk and ensure surgery is safe. Technology, science, and medicine keeps evolving to improve outcomes. Most surgeons are perfectionists who thrive on ensuring the process seamless for their patients. They have trained years and excelled on countless tests to do what they do.

As you consider whether surgery is for you, remember that many potential medical problems occur without any surgery at all, especially in an elderly population. Daily, you know you could get in a terrible car wreck tomorrow. Does that stop you from driving?

In fact, every decision for elective surgery requires an analysis of the risks and of the benefits. This chapter lays out the risks. Many of the other chapters in this book lay out the benefits. It is for you—with the help of your surgeon—to decide: Do the benefits outweigh the potential risks?

Frequently asked questions

• **I think I am too old for surgery, should I even consider it?**

This is a tough question to answer. There is no age where I say you are too old. What is more important is how healthy you are—or rather your "physiological age." I see people in their 90s who are physiologically 60 and people in their 60s who are physiologically 90. If you are healthy there is no real reason why you shouldn't be able to have elective surgery.

References

1.   Lee MJ, Konodi MA, Cizik AM, Bransford RJ, Bellabarba C, Chapman JR. Risk factors for medical complication after spine surgery: a multivariate analysis of 1,591 patients. Spine J Off J North Am Spine Soc. 2012 Mar;12(3):197–206.

2.   Daniels AH, Hart RA, Hilibrand AS, Fish DE, Wang JC, Lord EL, et al. Iatrogenic Spinal Cord Injury Resulting From Cervical Spine Surgery. Glob Spine J. 2017 Apr;7(1 Suppl):84S-90S.

3.   Kim HJ, Yao YC, Shaffrey CI, Smith JS, Kelly MP, Gupta M, et al. Neurological Complications and Recovery Rates of Patients With Adult Cervical Deformity Surgeries. Glob Spine J. 2020 Nov 23;2192568220975735.

4.   Pateder DB, Kostuik JP. Lumbar nerve root palsy after adult spinal deformity surgery. Spine. 2005 Jul 15;30(14):1632–6.

5.   Palumbo MA, Bianco AJ, Esmende S, Daniels AH. Wrong-site Spine Surgery. J Am Acad Orthop Surg. 2013 May;21(5):312–20.

6.   DePasse JM. Complications associated with prone positioning in elective spinal surgery. World J Orthop. 2015;6(3):351.

7.   Espiritu MT, Rhyne A, Darden BV. Dural Tears in Spine Surgery: Am Acad Orthop

Surg. 2010 Sep;18(9):537–45.

8.   Khan MH, Rihn J, Steele G, Davis R, Donaldson WF, Kang JD, et al. Postoperative Management Protocol for Incidental Dural Tears During Degenerative Lumbar Spine Surgery: A Review of 3,183 Consecutive Degenerative Lumbar Cases. Spine. 2006 Oct;31(22):2609–13.

9.   Nakajima K, Nakamoto H, Kato S, Doi T, Matsubayashi Y, Taniguchi Y, et al. Influence of unintended dural tears on postoperative outcomes in lumbar surgery patients: A multicenter observational study with propensity scoring. Spine J. 2020 Jun;S1529943020307907.

10.   Khazim R, Dannawi Z, Spacey K, Khazim M, Lennon S, Reda A, et al. Incidence and treatment of delayed symptoms of CSF leak following lumbar spinal surgery. Eur Spine J. 2015 Sep;24(9):2069–76.

11.   Fantini GA, Pappou IP, Girardi FP, Sandhu HS, Cammisa FP. Major vascular injury during anterior lumbar spinal surgery: incidence, risk factors, and management. Spine. 2007 Nov 15;32(24):2751–8.

12.   Glotzbecker MP, Bono CM, Wood KB, Harris MB. Thromboembolic disease in spinal surgery: a systematic review. Spine. 2009;34(3):291–303.

13.   Eskildsen SM, Moll S, Lim MR. An Algorithmic Approach to Venous Thrombo-embolism Prophylaxis in Spine Surgery: J Spinal Disord Tech. 2015 Oct;28(8):275–81.

14.   Brunelli A, Varela G, Salati M, Jimenez MF, Pompili C, Novoa N, et al. Recalibra-tion of the revised cardiac risk index in lung resection candidates. Ann Thorac Surg. 2010 Jul;90(1):199–203.

15.   Carabini LM, Zeeni C, Moreland NC, Gould RW, Hemmer LB, Bebawy JF, et al. Predicting Major Adverse Cardiac Events in Spine Fusion Patients: Is the Revised Cardi-ac Risk Index Sufficient? Spine. 2014 Aug;39(17):1441–8.

16.   Gualandro DM, Puelacher C, LuratiBuse G, Llobet GB, Yu PC, Cardozo FA, et al. Prediction of major cardiac events after vascular surgery. J Vasc Surg. 2017 Dec;66(6):1826-1835.e1.

17.   Koivuranta M, Läärä E, Snåre L, Alahuhta S. A survey of postoperative nausea and vomiting. Anaesthesia. 1997;52(5):443–9.

18.   Yilmaz E, Benca E, Patel AP, Hopkins S, Blecher R, Abdul-Jabbar A, et al. What Are Risk Factors for an Ileus After Posterior Spine Surgery?-A Case Control Study. Glob Spine J. 2021 Jan 12;2192568220981971.

19.   Fountas KN, Kapsalaki EZ, Nikolakakos LG, Smisson HF, Johnston KW, Grigorian AA, et al. Anterior cervical discectomy and fusion associated complications. Spine. 2007;32(21):2310–7.

20.   Baldini G, Bagry H, Aprikian A, Carli F. Postoperative urinary retention: anes-thetic and perioperative considerations. Anesthesiology. 2009 May;110(5):1139–57.

21.   Lee MJ, Hacquebord J, Varshney A, Cizik AM, Bransford RJ, Bellabarba C, et al. Risk factors for medical complication after lumbar spine surgery: a multivariate analy-

sis of 767 patients. Spine. 2011 Oct 1;36(21):1801–6.

22.   Luke J G, Peter A G, Hiba A, Nipun S, Burshtein J, Burshtein A, et al. The Effect of Bladder Catheterization Technique on Postoperative Urinary Tract Infections Following Primary Total Hip Arthroplasty. J Arthroplasty. 2020 Jan;S0883540320300760.

Figures:

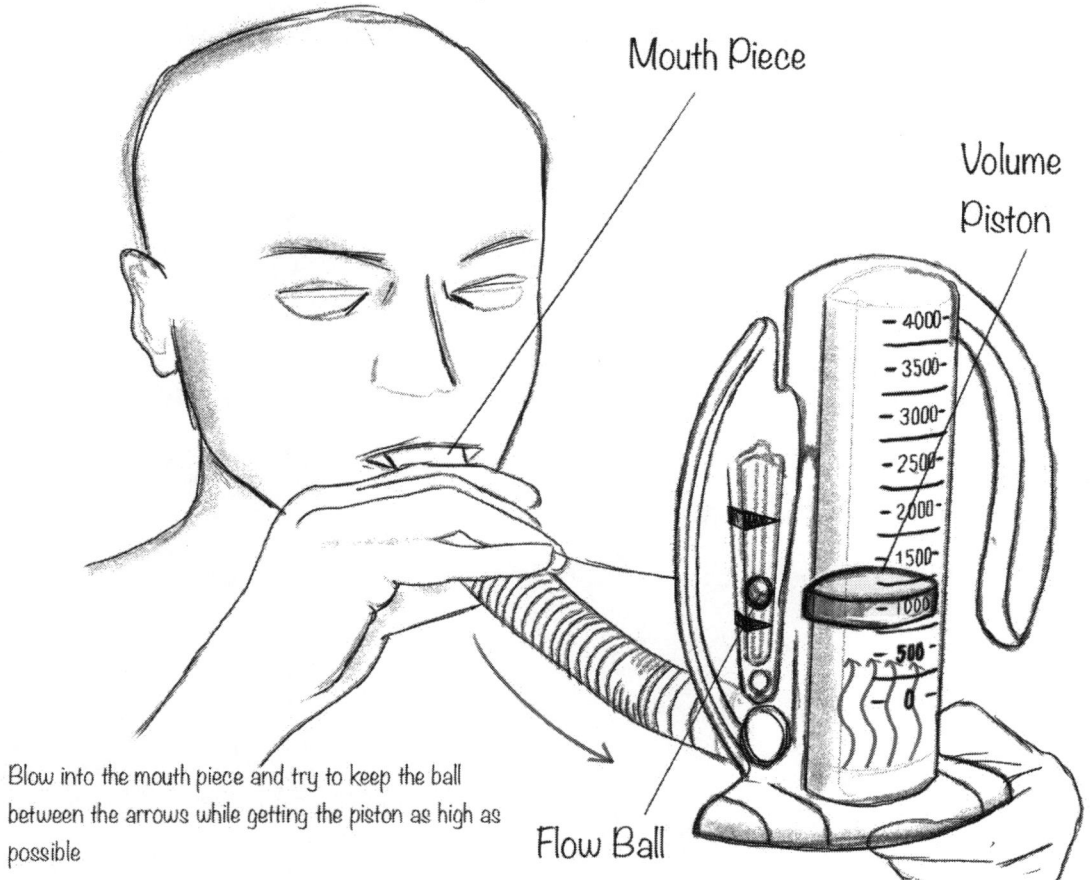

The Incentive Spirometer

Mouth Piece

Volume Piston

4000
3500
3000
2500
2000
1500
1000
500
0

Blow into the mouth piece and try to keep the ball between the arrows while getting the piston as high as possible

Flow Ball

Incentive spirometer. The incentive spirometer is a device designed to help your lungs expand after undergoing anesthesia. It can measure the rate and volume of your expiration.

Chapter 31

The Changing Spine: Understanding Why Sometimes One Surgery to Fix the Spine Leads to Another Surgery—Revision Surgery and Spinal Deformity

Summary

The need for a revision can be common in spine surgery compared to other surgical disciplines. Revision surgery may be necessary because of recurrence of stenosis, a new stenosis at another level, infection, failure of a fusion to heal (pseudoarthrosis) or a problem with alignment. Revision surgery and spinal deformity go hand in hand. Fusion surgery used to realign the spine creates a rigid segment that can cause wear and alignment issues in the non-fused spine down the road. Sagittal plane deformity (a deformity that occurs from front to back) is different from scoliosis (a coronal deformity which occurs from side to side) but is more debilitating than scoliosis because it affects your ability to stand upright. The full mechanics of how this works are yet to be completely understood.

Case

Mr. Tan is a 55-year-old male with down syndrome who unfortunately has had multiple previous spinal surgeries. They each seem to help for a short period of time but eventually his back pain and leg pain always return. He has lost touch with his most recent spine surgeon and because of his developmental delay his medical care has been fragmented. When he came to see me, he had a signifi-cant deformity of his low back causing his whole trunk to stoop to the side and forward. His X-rays show his two previous fusions have failed to heal and the hardware is breaking apart. To fix his spine requires a complicated revision surgery, including a procedure called an osteotomy to cut a portion of his ver-tebrae out so that his spine can be straightened. Surgery takes 7 hours, and the patient requires a 6-day hospital stay, but he walks straight now without any pain.

Introduction

Revision surgery is any surgery that occurs after an initial surgery on the same area. Revision surgery can be performed either because the first surgery was not successful or caused a new problem or because the initial problem has spread and now requires more work. Unfortunately, revision surgery is common after a primary spine operation and as many as 30% of patients over 30 years of age are likely to undergo revision surgeries (1,2). It is a reality for many who undergo a spine procedure and is worth understanding. Revision surgery typically is not a result of the previous surgery itself, but rather the progression of the spinal degenerative disease. This chapter will discuss revision surgery and spinal deformities (other than scoliosis) as the two can go hand in hand. Before reading this chapter, it may be useful to read the chapters on decompression and fusion surgery (chapters 36 and 37) to have a better understanding of the science and theory behind spine surgery.

Also, as a quick review, the terms segment and level can be used interchangeably, and, depending on the discussion, can refer to an individual vertebra OR can refer to two adjacent vertebrae and the disc between them. For example, in the section below on adjacent level degeneration, the terms level and segment are used interchangeably and refer to a single vertebra above or below the site of the first surgery. However, when the spinal fusion itself is being discussed, (as in the pseudoarthrosis section), and I talk about a level or a segment, I am referring to two adjacent vertebrae (in this case with the disc between them being removed).

Revision surgery

Revision surgery treats spine problems that occur in a spine that has already undergone at least one spine surgery. The spine is an incredibly complex organ system and sometimes it can be difficult to predict how it will react to surgery, which can result in the need for revisions. I spend a lot of time in my practice discussing the risk of a revision surgery following a primary operation. This second surgery can be a related to or independent of the initial surgery. Some common problems which are typically independent of the index (first) procedure are: recurrent herniations, post-laminectomy disease and adjacent level degeneration, all discussed below. Some common problems which can be related to the index (first) surgery are failure of fusion or pseudoarthrosis, or malalignment of the spine. Revision surgery tends to be more complicated than primary surgery with longer hospitalizations and risk of post-op adverse events (3). Nonetheless, this does not necessarily mean the eventual outcome should be worse (4). Specific risks and outcomes, however, are related to the type of surgical problem and proposed treatment. So, let's explore several different problems which cause a need for revision surgery.

reherniations

Disc reherniations are defined as a reherniation (protruding out again) of disc material at the site of a previous discectomy (a procedure that removes protruding disc material). For the problem to be classified as a reherniation, typically there is a period after the first discectomy in which symptoms improved. In the case of a reherniation, usually a second piece of disc material has been pushed out from the disc space and is now compressing the same nerve in the same or different manner as the original disc fragment. Unfortunately, this is one of the most common complications of a microdiscectomy (see the chapter 39 on lumbar discectomy) and can occur in anywhere from 4-15% of patients (5,6).

Some patient risk factors have been implicated in recurrent disc herniations including diabetes, smoking, obesity, and manual labor employment (5,7). Revision discectomy is the most commonly used treatment in this scenario and has been shown to be close to if not just as effective as primary discectomies (8). However, reports do exist of patients not doing as well after the second discectomy as after the primary procedure (9). Unfortunately, even after removing a disc for the second time, it may occur a third time! In these scenarios, most surgeons would choose to perform a spinal fusion, which would prevent any more recurrences (7).

post-laminectomy disease

A laminectomy is a surgical procedure that removes all or part of the thin arch of the vertebra called the lamina. In a small percentage of cases (around 2-11%) spinal instability may occur following a laminectomy (6,10). Spinal instability typically occurs in a patient with previous scoliosis or spondylolisthesis (where one vertebra slips forward onto the vertebra below it) but can occur even in a normal spine. In some patients, the narrowing of the spinal canal is so severe, the removal of some bone (laminectomy) is necessary to take pressure off the pinched nerve. However, if too much bone is removed it can cause a new problem—the spine becomes unstable, meaning the vertebra are no longer linked tightly and move with laxity (too easily) (11). This can be asymptomatic or the instability can result in worsening foraminal stenosis (the holes where the nerve roots exit the spine narrow), causing pinched nerve roots so even through the central area is decompressed the patient continues to experience pain (12). You may ask why you were not fused in the first place? Although a fusion may be the first choice for some surgeons, decompression alone is generally better tolerated by patients with a faster recovery, and so many surgeons will first want to see if decompression alone can take care of the problem.

adjacent level degeneration

Unfortunately, adjacent level degeneration, where the vertebra above or below a spinal fusion is wearing down (observed by radiographic evidence), is a very common problem in spine surgery. In fact, the occurrence of this kind of degeneration is estimated to be as high as 26% in lumbar fusions and 32% in cervical fusions within 5-10 years of surgery (13). Thankfully, the rate of actual symptomatic disease is much lower (around 9-17% after lumbar fusions and around 3% after cervical fusions) (14).

Why does adjacent segment disease occur? The answer is unclear and heavily debated among spine surgeons. While it makes sense to think that spinal fusions directly cause adjacent segment disease, the true relationship is likely more complex and related to the natural progression of spinal degeneration (14). It turns out that the rates of adjacent segment degeneration occurring after fusion procedures and after decompression procedures of the spine are very similar. However, spinal fusions in many studies have been shown to increase the biomechanical load on adjacent segments which may predispose them to early wear. I like to tell patients adjacent segment degeneration happens as a combination of the natural wearing down of discs and the increased biomechanical stresses exerted on the adjacent discs by the fusion. Several risk factors have been implicated, including being a younger age at time of fusion, genetics, preexisting degeneration, obesity, and osteoporosis (13). Fortunately, there are multiple treatment options to treat adjacent segment disease, all which have very good outcomes (15,16).

pseudoarthrosis

Spinal fusions are intended to artificially join two vertebrae via a bony union. This process occurs in a fashion similar to when bones heal back together after being broken. For example, when you break your arm, you go to the doctor, and he will usually put on a splint or cast so that the bones cannot move, and they heal together in the correct position. Spinal fusions work in a similar way: the disc is removed, and bone graft is placed between vertebrae such that they can grow together by the body's own healing process (see chapter 37 on spinal fusions). Pseudoarthrosis means false joint, that is, pseudoarthrosis is an area (a fused spinal segment) that is not supposed to have motion across it but does. Simply put, a pseudoarthrosis after spinal surgery means that the original spinal fusion did not work, and the area where surgery occurred did not heal together (fuse) as intended. Over time if the spinal fusion does not heal together, the hardware which acts as a splint for your vertebrae may fail—either breaking itself or breaking through the bone. This is because there is motion across the segment, and no hardware is meant to prevent motion forever.

While the risk for pseudoarthrosis (also known as non-union) may be high in certain instances (up to 50%), luckily many patients are asymptomatic and only a small fraction actually require a return to the operating room (1-2%) (17,18). When pseudarthroses do become symptomatic, they typically cause localized pain, and a return of the original symptoms that required the fusion such as leg pain, numbness, and weakness. Common patient risk factors for pseudoarthrosis are smoking, obesity, diabetes, vitamin-D deficiency, hypothyroidism, chronic steroid use, osteoporosis, and other chronic illnesses (17,19). Revision surgery is generally indicated for symptomatic pseudoarthrosis. Your surgeon may decide to try a different method to fix the problem and get the bone to heal, but even after such surgery it is possible to have a second pseudoarthrosis. Thus, it is critical to make sure you reduce any risk factors you may have, for example, stopping smoking, getting better control of your diabetes, correcting any vitamin deficiencies or treating hormonal issues (18,20).

Spinal Deformity (other than scoliosis): Flat Back and Proximal Junctional Kyphosis

The reason that I combine the topic of spinal deformity with revision surgery is that they can often occur together. For example, the spine may decompensate (fail to function) after a laminectomy or fusion surgery, which, in turn, creates a spinal deformity. The spine may be fused in a less than optimal position resulting in deformity. Spinal deformity can also occur independently of previous spinal surgery.

flat back

As discussed in the chapter on scoliosis (chapter 7), spinal deformity is very debilitating. Perhaps one of the most common causes is scoliosis (when you have a curve in the spine from side to side); however, there are other causes of spinal deformity such as fractures, infection, tumor, and osteoporosis. While the side-to-side curve and rotation of scoliosis can be quite painful, perhaps even more debilitating is a deformity in the spine occurring from front to back—or so-called sagittal plane deformity (20,21). As mentioned in the spine basics chapter (chapter 1) the lumbar spine naturally bends backward (lordosis) and one of the most common forms of deformity outside of scoliosis is the loss of this lordosis, resulting in a flattening of the back (so called flat back). Flat back is so debilitating because it makes standing upright difficult (22,23). Your muscles need to pull extra hard to compensate for the way your flat back makes you tilt forward. This leads to serious back pain and back muscle spasm. The muscles supporting your spine also fatigue quickly, making walking difficult for prolonged periods. To compensate and be able to look forward, patients with a flat back will bend their knees, crane their necks and tilt through their hips, all of which, over time, are very painful and put undue stress on the body.

Sagittal plane deformities such as flat back can occur because of degeneration of the spine, ankylosing spondylitis (spontaneous fusion of the spine), factures, infection, and tumors. However, one of the largest causes of spinal deformity is malalignment from an earlier spinal fusion (21). In the old days, when a spine surgeon performed a spinal fusion, he or she didn't have the sophisticated instruments we have now. As a result there were many sagittal plane deformities created in the 70's and 80's; however, it still occurs now from time to time for a number of reasons (24).

When flat back occurs spine surgeons typically do a lot of planning, looking at your X-rays and trying to figure out how best to correct the deformity. Often the correction will require an osteotomy (removing a wedge of the spine) and then a spinal fusion to keep the spine locked in that position. While this surgery is very complicated and often dangerous, the improvement in a patient's quality of life can be staggering (25). But you need to decide, is your pain terrible enough to warrant going through a major surgery that has a high incidence of complications? Some may be able to get by with an occasional epidural injection or with exercises to stay fit.

proximal junctional kyphosis (PJK)

Proximal junctional kyphosis (PJK) is a phenomenon that occurs in a fused spine and in some ways is the opposite of flat back. In its simplest terms proximal junctional kyphosis or PJK is a break down at the top of a rigid spinal fusion, which results in the patient's trunk and neck pitching forward. When a sagittal plane deformity is corrected (for example, a flat back is given lordosis) sometimes the body wants to return to its original pitched forward configuration. In other words, one deformity is corrected, but the body is used to being deformed and tries to return to that deformed configuration.

PJK can result from fracture, hardware failure, or both, as the mobile portion of the spine above the fusion pitches forward on the rigid fusion. The cause for this is heavily debated but has been attributed to several factors, such as the type of fusion, the degree of surgical deformity correction, age of the patient, and obesity (26,27). The rate of PJK in the adult spinal deformity population is unfortunately quite high (around 20%); however, the rate requiring treatment or return to the operating room is actually only a small percentage (1.4%) (26). Frustratingly, to date there have been no proven strategies to prevent PJK and, even if surgically corrected, PJK may recur (26,28).

Most PJK occurs within the first year of surgery and in some cases can be progressive. PJK may be asymptomatic but can result in back pain, disability, and other neurological symptoms. Luckily, if required, PJK can be treated with revision surgery, usually to extend the fusion higher in the spine with good outcomes (29).

Conclusion

Revision surgery is complicated and psychologically difficult for patients. Common reasons for revision surgery include reherniation of a disc as well as wear of the level above or below a previously treated spinal segment. While revision surgery is riskier than primary surgery the outcome can be just as good as primary surgery. Sagittal plane deformity, which occurs front to back in the spine (compared to the side-to-side deformity of scoliosis) has many causes, including an earlier fusion that has moved your lower back into a pitched forward position (flat back). Both flat back and PJK (in which the patient's neck and trunk pitch forward) can require further revision surgery.

Frequently Asked Questions

- **I had surgery for my back, and it generated more problems for me, how is this possible?**

   Spine surgery is extremely complex with an unlimited number of factors that can affect the outcome. Even now it is very difficult for surgeons to predict how your unique body will react over a long period of time to a change in biomechanics brought about by the addition of a fusion, decompression, or new prosthesis. Thus, most good spine surgeons are very careful in the cases they select for surgery—not all back problems are correctable with an operation. Unfortunately, even in the best hands, for known or unknown reasons, some people develop problems much faster than others would and can require a revision. It is important to work closely with your surgeon to meet your goals as the path through revision spine surgery can be difficult.

+   **How long will it be before I need a revision surgery?**

That is dependent on the type and extent of your spine surgery, the overall health of your spine and your age. You may never need a revision surgery. Roughly 30% of spinal fusion patients may need a second surgery within 30 years.

References

1.   Pitter FT, Lindberg-Larsen M, Pedersen AB, Dahl B, Gehrchen M. Revision Risk After Primary Adult Spinal Deformity Surgery: A Nationwide Study With Two-Year Follow-up. Spine Deformity. 2019 Jul;7(4):619-626.e2.

2.   Burkhardt BW, Grimm M, Schwerdtfeger K, Oertel JM. The Microsurgical Treatment of Lumbar Disc Herniation. 2019;9.

3.   Diebo BG, Passias PG, Marascalchi BJ, Jalai CM, Worley NJ, Errico TJ, et al. Primary Versus Revision Surgery in the Setting of Adult Spinal Deformity: A Nationwide Study on 10,912 Patients. Spine. 2015 Nov;40(21):1674–80.

4.   Fu L, Chang MS, Crandall DG, Revella J. Comparative Analysis of Clinical Outcomes and Complications in Patients With Degenerative Scoliosis Undergoing Primary Versus Revision Surgery: Spine. 2014 May;39(10):805–11.

5.   Dower A, Chatterji R, Swart A, Winder MJ. Surgical management of recurrent lumbar disc herniation and the role of fusion. Journal of Clinical Neuroscience. 2016 Jan;23:44–50.

6.   Aihara T, Endo K, Sawaji Y, Suzuki H, Urushibara M, Kojima A, et al. Five-year Reoperation Rates and Causes for Reoperations Following Lumbar Microendoscopic Discectomy and Decompression: SPINE. 2020 Jan;45(1):71–7.

7.   Shepard N, Cho W. Recurrent Lumbar Disc Herniation: A Review. Global Spine Journal. 2019 Apr;9(2):202–9.

8.   Patel MS, Braybrooke J, Newey M, Sell P. A comparative study of the outcomes of primary and revision lumbar discectomy surgery. The Bone & Joint Journal. 2013 Jan;95-B(1):90–4.

9.   Nolte MT, Basques BA, Louie PK, Khan JM, Varthi A, Paul J, et al. Patients Undergoing Revision Microdiskectomy for Recurrent Lumbar Disk Herniation Experience Worse Clinical Outcomes and More Revision Surgeries Compared With Patients Undergoing a Primary Microdiskectomy: Journal of the American Academy of Orthopaedic Surgeons. 2019 Sep;27(17):e796–803.

10.   Ahmad S, Hamad A, Bhalla A, Turner S, Balain B, Jaffray D. The outcome of de-

compression alone for lumbar spinal stenosis with degenerative spondylolisthesis. Eur Spine J. 2017 Feb;26(2):414–9.

11.   Suzuki K, Ishida Y, Ohmori K. Spondylolysis after posterior decompression of the lumbar spine: 35 patients followed for 3-9 years. Acta Orthopaedica Scandinavica. 1993 Jan;64(1):17–21.

12.   Inui T, Murakami M, Nagao N, Miyazaki K, Matsuda K, Tominaga Y, et al. Lumbar Degenerative Spondylolisthesis: Changes in Surgical Indications and Comparison of Instrumented Fusion With Two Surgical Decompression Procedures. SPINE. 2017 Jan;42(1):E15–24.

13.   Hashimoto K, Aizawa T, Kanno H, Itoi E. Adjacent segment degeneration after fusion spinal surgery—a systematic review. International Orthopaedics (SICOT). 2019 Apr;43(4):987–93.

14.   Hilibrand AS, Robbins M. Adjacent segment degeneration and adjacent segment disease: the consequences of spinal fusion? The Spine Journal. 2004 Nov;4(6):S190–4.

15.   Kepler CK, Hilibrand AS. Management of Adjacent Segment Disease After Cervical Spinal Fusion. Orthopedic Clinics of North America. 2012 Jan;43(1):53–62.

16.   Louie PK, Haws BE, Khan JM, Markowitz J, Movassaghi K, Ferguson J, et al. Comparison of Stand-alone Lateral Lumbar Interbody Fusion Versus Open Laminectomy and Posterolateral Instrumented Fusion in the Treatment of Adjacent Segment Disease Following Previous Lumbar Fusion Surgery: SPINE. 2019 Dec;44(24):E1461–9.

17.   Leven D, Cho SK. Pseudarthrosis of the Cervical Spine: Risk Factors, Diagnosis and Management. Asian Spine Journal. 2016;10(4):776.

18.   Hofler RC, Swong K, Martin B, Wemhoff M, Jones GA. Risk of Pseudoarthrosis After Spinal Fusion: Analysis From the Healthcare Cost and Utilization Project. World Neurosurgery. 2018 Dec;120:e194–202.

19.   Hills JM, Khan I, Archer KR, Sivaganesan A, Daryoush J, Hong DY, et al. Metabolic and Endocrine Disorders in Pseudarthrosis: Clinical Spine Surgery. 2019 Jun;32(5):E252–7.

20.   Glassman SD, Bridwell K, Dimar JR, Horton W, Berven S, Schwab F. The impact of positive sagittal balance in adult spinal deformity. Spine. 2005;30(18):2024–9.

21.   Leveque JCA, Segebarth B, Schroerlucke SR, Khanna N, Pollina J, Youssef JA, et al. A Multicenter Radiographic Evaluation of the Rates of Preoperative and Postoperative Malalignment in Degenerative Spinal Fusions: SPINE. 2018 Jul;43(13):E782–9.

22.   Enomoto M, Ukegawa D, Sakaki K, Tomizawa S, Arai Y, Kawabata S, et al. Increase in Paravertebral Muscle Activity in Lumbar Kyphosis Patients by Surface Electromyography Compared With Lumbar Spinal Canal Stenosis Patients and Healthy Volunteers: Journal of Spinal Disorders & Techniques. 2012 Aug;25(6):E167–73.

23.   Lafage V, Schwab F, Skalli W, Hawkinson N, Gagey PM, Ondra S, et al. Standing balance and sagittal plane spinal deformity: analysis of spinopelvic and gravity line

parameters. Spine. 2008 Jun 15;33(14):1572–8.

24.   Doherty, JH. Complications of fusion in lumbar scoliosis. J Bone Joint Surg Am. 1973;55(438).

25.   The Spinal Deformity Study Group, Smith JS, Shaffrey CI, Berven S, Glassman S, Hamill C, et al. IMPROVEMENT OF BACK PAIN WITH OPERATIVE AND NONOPERATIVE TREATMENT IN ADULTS WITH SCOLIOSIS. Neurosurgery. 2009 Jul 1;65(1):86–94.

26.   Kim HJ, Iyer S. Etiology and Risk Factors for Proximal Junctional Kyphosis and Proximal Junctional Failure. Journal of the American Academy of Orthopaedic Surgeons. 2016;24(5):9.

27.   Lee J, Park YS. Proximal Junctional Kyphosis: Diagnosis, Pathogenesis, and Treatment. Asian Spine J. 2016;10(3):593.

28.   Kim HJ, Wang SJ, Lafage R, Iyer S, Shaffrey C, Mundis G, et al. Recurrent Proximal Junctional Kyphosis: Incidence, Risk Factors, Revision Rates and Outcomes at 2 year minimum follow up. SPINE. 2019 Aug;1.

29.   Kim YC, Lenke LG, Bridwell KH, Hyun SJ, You KH, Kim YW, et al. Results of Revision Surgery for Proximal Junctional Kyphosis Following Posterior Segmental Instrumentation: Minimum 2-Year Postrevision Follow-Up. SPINE. 2016 Dec;41(24):E1444–52.

Figures:

Proximal Junctional Failure

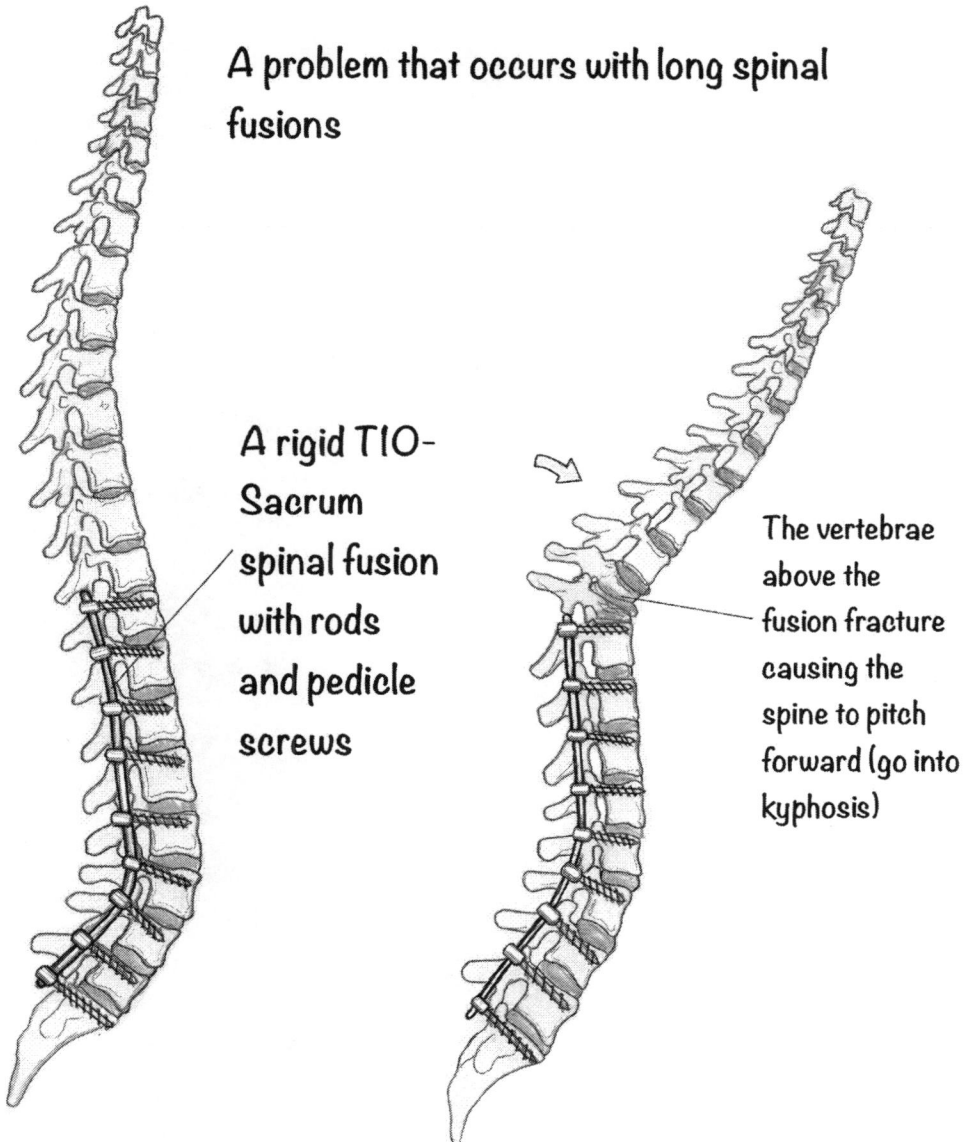

A problem that occurs with long spinal fusions

A rigid T10-Sacrum spinal fusion with rods and pedicle screws

The vertebrae above the fusion fracture causing the spine to pitch forward (go into kyphosis)

PJK. Proximal junctional kyphosis (PJK) occurs when there is break down at the top of a spinal fusion causing the upper portion of the spine to angulate forward (go into kyphosis). PJK typically is typically the result of fracture or other hardware failure at the topmost level. This is thought to occur because of a change in the biomechanics of the spine creating a rigid to mobile junction.

Normal Fusion Vs Pseudoarthrosis

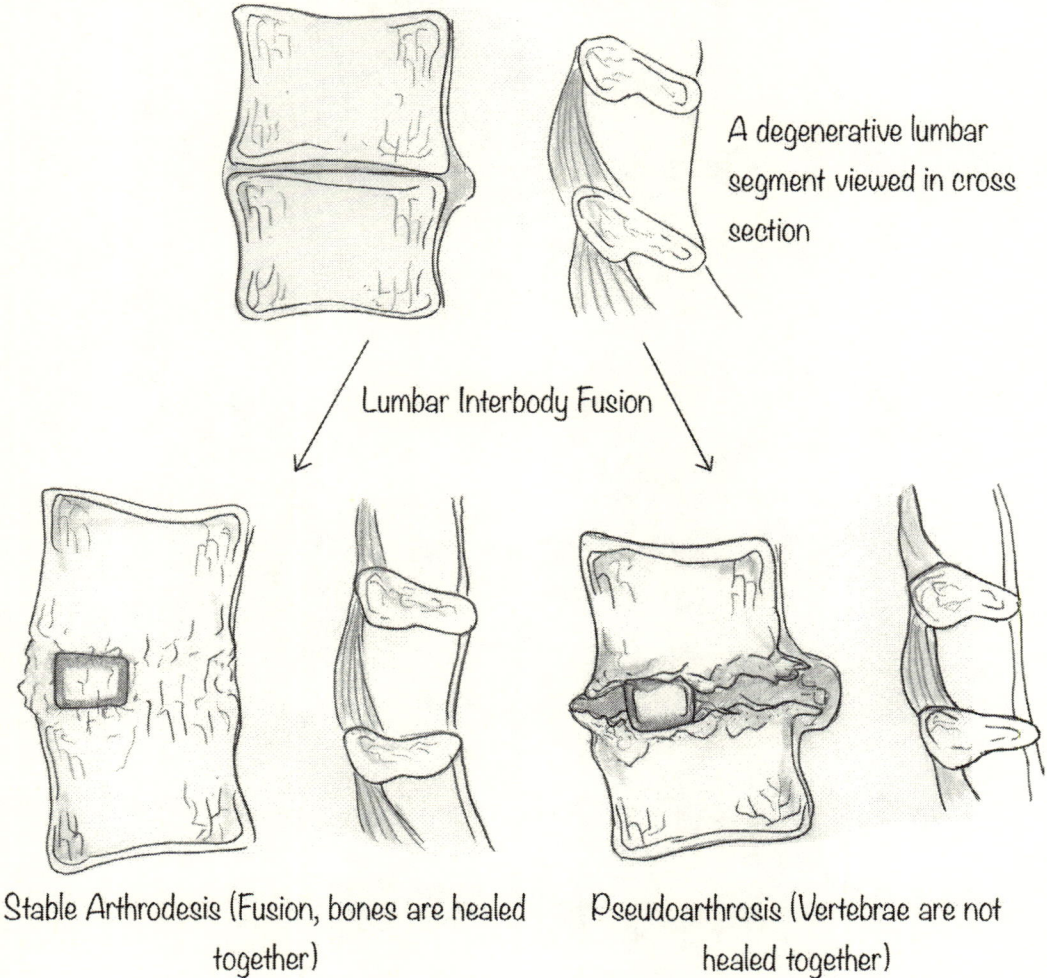

A degenerative lumbar segment viewed in cross section

Lumbar Interbody Fusion

Stable Arthrodesis (Fusion, bones are healed together)

Pseudoarthrosis (Vertebrae are not healed together)

Pseudoarthrosis. The goal of a surgical fusion is to have two or more vertebrae grow together (Left). A pseudoarthrosis (also known as a false joint or non-union) occurs when bony healing fails to unite two surgically prepared vertebrae (right). A pseudoarthrosis may be asymptomatic or may cause back pain. On the left, the bone grows around the intervertebral cage.

Chapter 32

Managing Bleeding in Spine Surgery: Anticoagulant and Coagulant Therapies

Summary

In spine surgery there exists a balance between too much bleeding and too much coagulation (clotting). Too much bleeding leads to hemorrhage, anemia and even hematomas which can compress the spinal cord and nerves. Too much coagulation can lead to deep venous thromboses (a blood clot in a vein) and pulmonary embolisms that can be fatal. To manage these risks, medicines known as anticoagulants and coagulants are used to thin or thicken the blood, respectively. Timing the administration of these drugs is critical to optimize your outcome. Patients who have known risk factors for blood clots or who are high cardiovascular risks may need to be on anticoagulants to thin their blood around their procedure. Others who are at high bleeding risk because of blood thinners may need to hold their medication prior to surgery.

Case

Mr. Red is an 80-year-old gentleman who is taking Eliquis® (a blood thinner) for atrial fibrillation (a condition of the heart that can cause fatal blood clots). He is scheduled to have a posterior cervical decompression and fusion for severe cervical stenosis that has been affecting his motor function. Prior to surgery, his surgeon notes that he is on the blood thinner and gives his cardiologist a call to express his concerns. He is worried that if he does the surgery while the patient is still on Eliquis® Mr. Red may be at risk of developing a hematoma in the neck which could pinch off his spinal cord causing paralysis. The cardiologist instructs the patient to stop his Eliquis® 5 days before the surgery to allow it to clear from his system. During surgery, although there is bleeding, it is not excessive, and the surgeon uses a substance called Floseal® to limit the blood loss. The surgeon restarts medication 7 days after the surgery.

Introduction

When you sustain a cut or scrape the body has natural mechanisms to seal the wound and stop the bleeding. This process is known as hemostasis or coagulation and involves two biological systems: platelets and a family of proteins in the blood known as the coagulation cascade.

Platelets are small cells present in the bloodstream which become activated anytime there is tissue damage. They work to patch leaking vessels by aggregating, meaning they become very sticky and shingle together to create a temporary patch. If platelets are the bricks to repair a damaged vessel, the coagulation cascade is the mortar. The coagulation cascade is a family of proteins which are also present in the blood, and when blood vessel damage occurs, these proteins start an enzymatic chain reaction to turn the blood from a liquid to a solid clot, blocking the leak. If you did not possess these two systems, every time you had a cut you would just continue to leak blood indefinitely.

Coagulation is a delicate balance. During surgery, coagulation is critical to keep bleeding from becoming hemorrhage. But too much coagulation and you end up with abnormal blood clots (thrombus) in vessels that cause problems. Thrombi may travel to the lungs causing a pulmonary embolism (PE). Pulmonary embolisms clog blood flow through the lungs and can range from asymptomatic to fatal. To manage this balance, doctors use drugs that can either anticoagulate (thin) the blood to prevent clot formations or cause the blood to coagulate (clot) in a controlled fashion to reduce blood loss during surgery.

Anticoagulants

Anticoagulants are drugs, also known as blood thinners, which interfere with (antagonize) the normal clotting processes in the blood. They do this by blocking the function of platelets or clotting factors. Anticoagulants are used to prevent clots from forming in the blood stream and are commonly used if you have a history of coronary artery disease (CAD), stroke, atrial fibrillation, venous thromboembolism, or a heart valve replacement (see glossary for more on these conditions). Anticoagulants are important regarding spine surgery for two opposite reasons: first, prior to your procedure you may need to stop taking anticoagulants to ensure you do not bleed excessively during surgery, and, secondly, after your procedure you may need to start taking anticoagulants to prevent blood clots from forming in the lungs and legs.

types of anticoagulants

Anticoagulants are categorized according to how they work and whether they can be administered orally or require injection.

The heparins are the prototypical injectable anticoagulants. Unfractionated heparin is an old and still commonly used anticoagulant. It is advantageous as it has a rapid onset, is quickly eliminated from the body, and has a reversal agent (protamine sulfate). Low molecular weight heparin is derived from unfractionated heparin through a chemical process making the heparin molecule smaller yet still therapeutically active. Unlike unfractionated heparin, it can safely be used in the outpatient setting and has minimal risk of heparin-induced thrombocytopenia (HIT), a side-effect of heparin where your platelets are depleted. Low molecular weight heparin has no reversal agent.

Oral anticoagulants include the direct thrombin inhibitors, warfarin (coumadin®), and antiplatelet medications. Direct thrombin inhibitors interfere with the thrombin-clotting molecule. They have a rapid onset, and may be administered orally, unlike the heparins. There is no reversal agent.

Warfarin is an old medicine which interferes with vitamin-K synthesis, which is crucial for clotting. Because warfarin must be carefully titrated to reach a certain threshold in the blood and monitored weekly by measuring the INR (international normalized ratio), it is not commonly used anymore.

Finally, antiplatelet medicines are drugs that interfere with platelet function and aggregation. These include drugs such as aspirin, and clopidogrel (Plavix®). Once taken, they render all platelets in your body useless such that it takes at least 7 days for your platelet population to rebuild—there is no reversal.

how to manage anticoagulants prior to surgery

Surgeons must balance the risk of a thromboembolism with the risk of bleeding during surgery. (Thromboembolism occurs when a blood clot has traveled from one part of the body to another where it blocks a blood vessel.) Spine surgery has a high risk of bleeding. Bleeding is problematic not just because of the amount (spinal fusions usually have moderate blood loss) but also because bleeding can form a compressive hematoma (blood pooling outside the blood vessel) that can be bad for the spinal cord and nerves. Thus, in most cases anticoagulation medication must be stopped prior to surgery. Patients who have a high risk of thromboembolism, such as those with a mechanical heart valve, coronary artery disease, recent DVT/PE (deep venous thrombosis/pulmonary embolism), or atrial fibrillation, require careful management to balance the risk of blood clot formation with excessive bleeding during surgery that can result from the presence of anticoagulants in your system. Usually, the medical doctor who prescribes you these medicines will coordinate with the surgeon to plan to interrupt your anticoagulation prior to surgery and may use an alternative shorter acting medicine to "bridge you" to your procedure. managing antiplatelet medicines before surgery

Antiplatelet medications permanently disable the body's current supply of platelets. In a normal person it takes 10 days to replenish your platelet supply and may take even longer in the elderly. Your body needs platelets to stop bleeding, so these medications should be stopped about 10 days before any operation. However, your body produces platelets constantly and you regain 50% of your platelet function in 5-7 days which is sufficient for clotting purposes (1). Certain patients may stay on their antiplatelet medications, especially if they have a heart condition such as coronary artery disease or a history of cardiac stents where stopping the medicine could be dangerous. This decision should be carefully made with your cardiologist and spine surgeon who can best assess the risks (2).

 In a major study evaluating the effects of aspirin on non-cardiac surgery, patients who were taking aspirin 100mg were found to have a higher bleeding risk but not a decreased risk of death from a vascular complication suggesting maintaining your aspirin may have dangers without significant benefit (3). Antiplatelet medications such as Clopidogrel (Plavix) are more potent anticoagulants and should be stopped at least 7 days prior to elective surgery whereas 81mg of aspirin may be continued on a case by case basis (4). Patients who may benefit from continued aspirin therapy are those with cardiac stents or bypass, or previous DVT/PE.

Other medications and supplements that are not used as anticoagulants may also have an antiplatelet effect and thus should be considered prior to surgery. Like aspirin, non-steroidal medications (NSAIDS such as ibuprofen, Toradol, diclofenac, meloxicam, naproxen) should also be stopped prior to surgery as they all exhibit some antiplatelet activity. While there are differences in the time you need to wait until you can have elective surgery with these medications, a safe rule is to wait 10 days, like aspirin.

Anticoagulation Medications

Drug name	Mechanism	Length of Action (Half Life)	Should be Stopped X days Prior to Surgery (2,10)	When Can Be Resumed After Surgery
Parenteral (Non-Oral) Anticoagulants (IV, IM or SC—given intravenously, intramuscularly, or subcutaneously)				
Unfractionated Heparin	Antithrombin 3 (AT-3) antagonist	1-1.5 hours	4 hours if IV—intravenous 10 hours If SC—beneath the skin	2-4 days minimum
Low Molecular Weight Heparin Enoxaparin (Lovenox®)	Antithrombin 3 (AT-3) antagonist	5 hours	24 hours	2-4 days minimum 1 day if HIGH RISK
Fondaparinux (Arixtra®)	Direct Factor Xa inhibitor	17 hours	4 days	1 day
Oral Anticoagulants				
Warfarin	Antagonist of Vitamin K synthesis (inhibiting Vitamin K epoxide reductase, thus blocking factors II, VII, IX and X)	20-72 hours	minimum 5 days prior to surgery. INR should normalize prior to surgery (needs to be less than 1.4)	2-4 days minimum
Rivaroxaban (Xarelto®)	Factor Xa Inhibitor	5-9 hours	3 days minimum (may be longer if you have kidney issues)	3 days minimum
Apixaban (Eliquis®)	Factor Xa Inhibitor	8-15 hours	3 days minimum (may be longer if you have kidney issues)	3 days minimum

post-operative management

Following surgery, your anticoagulation medications will need to be resumed, but only after a safe interval (usually at least 36 hours) to minimize the chances of bleeding occurring at the surgical site. In spine surgery, this can be particularly problematic as hematomas (collections of blood outside of blood vessels in the surgical wound) may cause compression on the nerves and spinal cord. The risk of a hematoma must be balanced against the risk of a deep venous thrombosis.

While the rate of a deep venous clot forming is lower post-spinal surgery than in other areas of orthopedics, its occurrence varies dramatically depending on the type of spine surgery and can be anywhere from 0.3% to 30% (5). Certain risk factors increase the risk of a DVT such as a history of venous thromboembolism, atrial fibrillation, history of cancer or active malignancy, spinal cord injury, or serious trauma. Certain surgical procedures also carry an increased risk of DVT, such as extensive instrumented lumbar fusions involving more than 4 levels and combined anterior and posterior lumbar approaches (5).

Risk for DVT: Repurposed from Eskildsen et al (5).			
	Low Risk	Moderate Risk	High Risk
Patient-related DVT Risk	• No Comorbidities	• Smoking • High BMI 30kg/m2 • CHF • ASA >3	• History of VTE • Malignancy • Spinal Cord injury • Multisystem trauma
Surgical Procedure-related VTE Risk	• Lumbar Decompression	• Posterior Lumbar Fusion	• Extensive Posterior thoracolumbar fusion (>4 levels) • Combined anterior posterior thoracolumbar fusion
Neurological Risk from Bleeding	• No decompression • Nerve root decompression	• Lumbar central canal decompression	• Cervical or thoracic spinal cord decompression • Excessive bleeding intraoperatively

BMI is body mass index, CHF is congestive heart failure, ASA is a physical assessment test to evaluate surgery readiness, VTE is venous thromboembolism

In general, after a surgery the risks of a DVT/PE and the risks of a bleeding complication must be balanced carefully with anticoagulation therapy (6). Compression stockings and pneumatic sequential compression devices (SCD) are simple ways to prevent lower extremity blood clots and facilitate circulation but do not increase the risk of bleeding (5). SCDs appear to be more important at preventing blood clots than compression stockings but both are useful in spine surgery because they do not increase the risk of bleeding (7). Anticoagulant medications reduce the risk further, and may also be considered (8). Again, the surgeon must weigh the risk of a clot against the risk of an epidural hematoma—bleeding into the surgical site that can cause devastating neurologic compression. In the neck and upper back, compression of the spinal cord from a hematoma may result in paralysis. Thus, your surgeon may avoid using an anticoagulant after your surgery if it was performed in either the neck or upper back.

If anticoagulation medication (chemoprophylaxis) is warranted, it is typically used for 4 to 6 weeks after the operation, although an agreed upon duration does not exist in spine surgery (9). Most surgeons will wait at least 36 hours after surgery to start anticoagulation to reduce bleeding risk but depending on the risk-benefit ratio may wait even longer (up to 7-10 days to start or resume anticoagulation) (9).

Anticoagulation Medications Continued				
Drug name	Mechanism	Length of Action (Half Life)	Should be Stopped X days Prior to Surgery (2,10)	When Can Be Resumed After Surgery
Oral Anticoagulants Continued				
Aspirin	Antiplatelet (inhibit thromboxane A2 by blocking COX enzymes)	3 hours	7 days minimum (10 days preferred) in high-risk cases may be safe to continue through surgery at low doses (81mg) especially if for a high-risk patient (stents/CAD) and a low-risk procedure such as uninstrumented spine surgery. (10)	7 days unless significant cardiac risk
Clopidogrel (Plavix®)	Antiplatelet (inhibits P2Y12)	6 hours	7 days minimum (10 days preferred)	7 days unless significant cardiac risk
INR stands for international normalized ratio, CAD means coronary heart disease				

inferior vena cava (IVC) filters

Inferior vena cava (IVC) filters are small wire cages which are placed in the IVC—one of the great vessels which returns venous blood from your body to your heart. IVC filters are used to block peripheral blood clots from getting into the lungs and causing a pulmonary embolism. Filters are placed into the IVC because when you get a blood clot, it needs to travel through your IVC to get to the lungs. Strictly speaking, IVC filters do not prevent blood clots, but can stop a fatal PE from occurring by blocking large blood clots from entering your lungs. In spine surgery, chemical anticoagulation with a blood thinner may not be possible due to the risks from bleeding as described above. IVC filters are used to prevent catastrophic blood clots in patients who are high risk for a blood clot (morbid obesity, history of a blood clot, malignancy, proposed surgery lasting more than 6 hours), and may be recommended by your surgeon. Possible complications to consider are migration, infection, and vessel injury with the filter. Most modern filters can be removed once they are no longer needed (11).

Bleeding Management

Blood loss from spine surgery may vary from a thimbleful to multiple liters, depending on the extent of the procedure. In major spine surgery, the amount of blood loss used to be a limiting factor to what a surgeon could accomplish. Now there are new technologies which help minimize bleeding during even major spinal reconstructions. These advances have been profound in spine surgery, opening treatments for cases which were once hopeless.

hemoglobin

Red blood cells, which are the major cell type in your blood, are jam-packed with an iron-containing molecule called hemoglobin (Hb for short). This molecule binds oxygen in oxygen-rich environments (lungs) and releases it in oxygen-poor environments (your peripheral tissues). Without oxygen your tissues become choked off and die. Hemoglobin levels differ depending on age and sex and are typically measured in a complete blood count (CBC) test. A hemoglobin level less than 12g/dl in women and less than 13g/dl in men is considered anemic, or having a low hemoglobin level (4). In instances of blood loss, anemia can put significant stress on your heart and lungs; thus, hemoglobin levels should be optimized prior to surgery. A low hemoglobin level is also a strong predictive factor that you will need a blood transfusion following major surgery, where your hemoglobin levels may drop to less than 7g/dl. In patients with a history of cardiovascular problems such as coronary artery disease, transfusion should be performed when Hb is less than 8g/dl.

If your hemoglobin levels are low, your surgery may be delayed allowing for correction. During this time, you should discuss with your internal medical doctor what the possible cause of the anemia is. Critical to rule out are unknown cancers such as colorectal carcinoma. While not all cases are correctable, iron deficiency is the most common cause and is easily replenished with oral iron supplementation for 6 weeks.

Erythropoietin (EPO) is a naturally occurring protein which is secreted from the kidney and stimulates the bone marrow to produce more red blood cells. It is famously used by elite cyclists as a blood doping method to increase performance during demanding cardiovascular competition. For surgeons wishing to raise the hemoglobin levels of their patients, the most common regimen of EPO is 40,000 IU, injected subcutaneously every week in the 4 weeks leading up to surgery. It has been shown to increase hemoglobin levels and reduce the requirement of allogenic blood transfusion; however, it is associated with certain risks such as DVT (12).

hemophilia

Rare patients have a deficiency in their clotting proteins (known as hemophilia), which makes them prone to excessive bleeding. Certain questionnaires have been developed to screen for those at increased risk for bleeding during surgery. If you answer yes to any of the following you should tell your doctor prior to surgery:

- **Have you ever consulted a doctor or received treatment for prolonged or unusual bleeding (such as nosebleeds or minor wounds)?**

- **Do you experience bruises/hematomas larger than 2 centimeters without trauma or severe bruising after minor trauma?**

- **Have you ever experienced bleeding into a joint, muscle, or central nervous system?**

- **After a tooth extraction have you ever experienced prolonged bleeding requiring medical/dental consultation?**

- **Have you ever experienced gastrointestinal bleeding?**

- **Have you experienced excessive bleeding during or after surgery?**

- **Is there anyone in your family who suffers from a coagulation disease (such as hemophilia or von Willebrand disease)**

- **For female patients**

  - Have you ever consulted a doctor or received a treatment for heavy or prolonged menstrual periods (for example, contraceptive pill or iron)

  - Did you experience prolonged or excessive bleeding after delivery?

Prior to surgery you may also undergo a laboratory coagulation panel test which measures the ability of your blood to form a clot. Tests such as the international normalized ratio (INR), partial thromboplastin time (PTT) and prothrombin time (PT) are examples of tests of coagulation but are by no means comprehensive (4).

during surgery

There has not been conclusive evidence that either general (affecting entire body) or spinal anesthesia is superior for reducing bleeding in surgery (4). Nonetheless, how your blood pressure is managed during spine surgery is critical for managing blood loss. For example, in most cases, during the exposure (when the surgeon is dissecting down to the problem area) blood loss can easily be avoided. This is done with careful surgical technique, but blood loss can also be reduced by keeping the patient's blood pressure low (called hypotensive anesthesia). Hypotensive anesthesia is not for all patients, however, and this is a decision which your surgeon and anesthesiologist will make together carefully.

Cautery (burning tissue to seal it) is also used to stop small vessels from bleeding to keep the surgical bed very dry.

Nonetheless, there are certain areas in spine surgery for which cautery will not work, namely bleeding from vessels around the spinal canal (epidural bleeding) and bleeding from bone. To stop the bleeding in these situations, hemostatic agents such as recombinant thrombin, gelatin sponges (Gelfoam®), regenerated oxidized cellulose (Surgicel®) and gelatin-thrombin matrices (Floseal®, Surgiflo®) are commonly employed in spine surgery. Thrombin is a molecule of the coagulation cascade which promotes clot formation. Originally thrombin was obtained from cows (bovine thrombin) however this was associated with the occasional development of antibodies against Factor V, which lead to life-threatening hemorrhage. Since then, human-derived thrombin has been developed which greatly reduces the incidence of this immune reaction (13,14). Gelfoam® is a gelatin sponge which also promotes coagulation and acts as a pressure barrier to stanch (tamponade) bleeding as it is extremely absorbent. The gelatin is typically obtained from porcine (pig) or bovine sources and dissolves naturally in the body within 4-6 weeks.

Floseal® and Surgiflo® are commonly used gelatin-thrombin matrices which have been shown to dramatically reduce bleeding in spine surgery and to be very safe in randomized, controlled trials (15). These products function by combining the best aspects of both gelatin and thrombin. The gelatin is delivered as small granules which can conform to and plug small bleeding surfaces and the thrombin then helps to seal off the area. Like standalone Gelfoam®, these products are absorbed in 4-6 weeks and are very safe for use. The one safety caveat for the use of gelatin is that it can cause a serious allergic reaction in patients allergic to gelatin and other porcine and bovine products. Please alert your doctor if you are allergic to gelatin.

Probably one of the biggest modern advances in orthopedic surgery is the use of tranexamic acid (TXA) to stabilize clots and reduces bleeding. TXA is an antifibrinolytic, a medicine that promotes blood clotting by inhibiting tissue plasminogen (a protein that breaks down clots). Most commonly, TXA is administered intravenously but may also be instilled into the surgical wound itself (although so-called topical TXA has not been as well-studied to date). The use of TXA has been shown to dramatically reduce the need for blood transfusions following orthopedic surgery (4). The use of this drug has been shown to be very safe; however, there are some concerns in very high-risk cardiac patients that it may precipitate an ischemic event. TXA is usually dosed based on your weight at a dose of 10mg/kg, which typically lasts 3 hours. You may get a subsequent infusion of TXA at 1mg/kg/hour. At very high doses of 100mg/kg, TXA has been associated with seizure.

blood recycling

In modern operating rooms a technique known as cell-salvage may be employed. This technique takes the blood a patient lost during the procedure and reinfuses it directly back into the patient. Cell-salvage uses a machine known as a cell-saver that collects, anticoagulates and washes the blood prior to packaging it for reinfusion. Cell-salvage is typically most useful in cases where there will be blood loss greater than 0.5 liters and has been shown to reduce the need for blood transfusions. In fact, use of a cell-saver can reduce the need for transfusion 54% (4). If you are having a small procedure, cell-salvage will not be useful as the blood loss will not be high enough to yield a reinfusion. Following your surgery it is also possible to recirculate your blood collected from a drain; however, this has not been shown to reduce the need for a transfusion (16).

Conclusion

Anticoagulation and blood loss management are complicated subjects and require expertise to manage. Decisions about blood thinners should be made carefully by your physicians. I believe a working understanding of how this works is important for patients, but it is important to leave some decisions up to your surgeon and medical doctors who can best guide you. The most useful thing a patient can do is alert a surgeon that they are on blood thinners and ask when they should start or stop them around surgery.

Frequently Asked Questions

- **I will not accept blood transfusion for religious reasons. Will I still be able to have safe surgery.**

    In most cases it is rare to require a blood transfusion and so it will be perfectly safe to have surgery. In high-risk cases where high blood loss is possible, for those who do not consent to the use of blood transfusion, hemostatic agents, blood alternatives and even blood recycling are possible. You should make sure to talk to your surgeon before surgery regarding your preferences for receiving blood transfusion.

References

1. Craig, Chad. Aspirin and Spine Surgery. Spineline. 2016 Sep;

2. Epstein NE. When to stop anticoagulation, anti-platelet aggregates, and non-steroidal anti-inflammatories (NSAIDs) prior to spine surgery. Surgical Neurology International. 2019 Mar 26;10:45.

3. Devereaux PJ, Mrkobrada M, Sessler DI, Leslie K, Alonso-Coello P, Kurz A, et al. Aspirin in Patients Undergoing Noncardiac Surgery. New England Journal of Medicine. 2014 Apr 17;370(16):1494–503.

4. Palmer AJR, Gagné S, Fergusson DA, Murphy MF, Grammatopoulos G. Blood Management for Elective Orthopaedic Surgery. Journal of Bone and Joint Surgery. 2020 Sep 2;102(17):1552–64.

5. Eskildsen SM, Moll S, Lim MR. An Algorithmic Approach to Venous Thrombo-embolism Prophylaxis in Spine Surgery: Journal of Spinal Disorders and Techniques. 2015 Oct;28(8):275–81.

6. Pirkle S, Cook DJ, Kaskovich S, Bhattacharjee S, Ho A, Shi LL, et al. Comparing Bleeding and Thrombotic Rates in Spine Surgery: An Analysis of 119 888 Patients. Global Spine Journal. 2019 Dec 26;219256821989629.

7. Ferree BA, Wright AM. Deep venous thrombosis following posterior lumbar spinal surgery. Spine. 1993 Jun 15;18(8):1079–82.

8. Glotzbecker MP, Bono CM, Wood KB, Harris MB. Thromboembolic disease in spinal surgery: a systematic review. Spine. 2009;34(3):291–303.

9. Bono CM, Watters WC, Heggeness MH, Resnick DK, Shaffer WO, Baisden J, et al. An evidence-based clinical guideline for the use of antithrombotic therapies in spine surgery. The Spine Journal. 2009 Dec;9(12):1046–51.

10. Porto GBF, Jeffrey Wessell D, Alvarado A, Arnold PM, Buchholz AL. Anticoagulation and Spine Surgery. Global Spine Journal. 2020 Jan;10(1_suppl):53S-64S.

11. Craig C. Inferior Vena Cava Filters and Spine Surgery. Spine Line. 2017;

12. Zhao Y, Jiang C, Peng H, Feng B, Li Y, Weng X. The effectiveness and safety of preoperative use of erythropoietin in patients scheduled for total hip or knee arthroplasty: A systematic review and meta-analysis of randomized controlled trials. Medicine. 2016 Jul;95(27):e4122.

13. Bowman L, Anderson C, Chapman W. Topical Recombinant Human Thrombin in Surgical Hemostasis. Semin Thromb Hemost. 2010 Jul;36(05):477–84.

14.	Doria C, Fischer CP, Wood CG, Mark Li P, Marra S, Hart J. Phase 3, randomized, double-blind study of plasma-derived human thrombin versus bovine thrombin in achieving hemostasis in patients undergoing surgery. Current Medical Research and Opinion. 2008 Mar;24(3):785–94.

15.	Renkens KL, Payner TD, Leipzig TJ, Feuer H, Morone MA, Koers JM, et al. A Multicenter, Prospective, Randomized Trial Evaluating a New Hemostatic Agent for Spinal Surgery: Spine. 2001 Aug;26(15):1645–50.

16.	Nemani VM, Kim HJ, Mina CA, Sheha ED, Ross T, Boachie-Adjei O. Postoperative Blood Salvage and Autotransfusion for Adult Spinal Deformity: A Randomized Controlled Trial. Spine. 2020 Sep 15;45(18):1247–52.

Figure:

Bleeding and Clotting

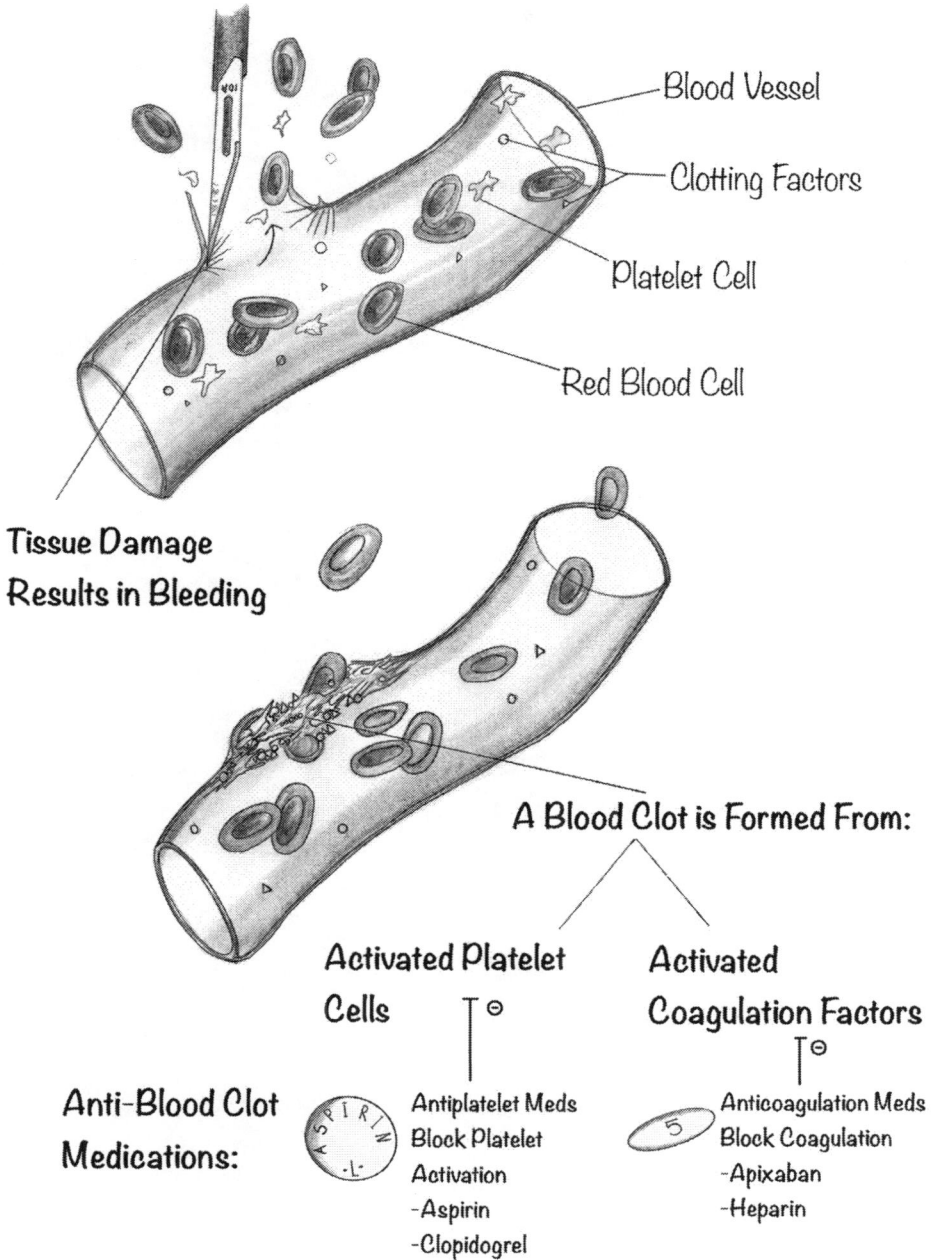

Blood Vessel

Clotting Factors

Platelet Cell

Red Blood Cell

Tissue Damage
Results in Bleeding

A Blood Clot is Formed From:

Activated Platelet
Cells

Activated
Coagulation Factors

Anti-Blood Clot
Medications:

Antiplatelet Meds
Block Platelet
Activation
-Aspirin
-Clopidogrel

Anticoagulation Meds
Block Coagulation
-Apixaban
-Heparin

Bleeding and Clotting. A blood vessel carries blood which contains red blood cells, platelets and clotting factors (such as thrombin). When tissue damage occurs (top left corner), blood can leak out of the vessel. A blot clot formed from platelets and clotting factors seals off the damage and stops the bleeding (Middle). Blood clot formation can be inhibited by antiplatelet or anticoagulation medications (Bottom).

Chapter 33

A Brief Introduction to Anesthesia

Summary

Anesthesia is a critical component of spine surgery and may differ significantly from anesthesia used in other areas of orthopedics and medicine. Unlike other areas of orthopedics where regional nerve blocks are common, general anesthesia is still the main form of anesthesia used in spine surgery. General anesthesia is very safe, but it's important to tell your anesthetist about any previous adverse history with anesthetic agents. In addition to giving you the medicine used to keep you asleep during the procedure, the anesthetist will also manage your IV lines and an air tube to give you oxygen, as well as help with your pain control after the procedure.

Case

Mr. White is a 70-year-old gentleman who is undergoing a spinal procedure. He arrives at the hospital and is seen by the anesthesiologist in the preoperative area. There Mr. White discusses that he generally does well with anesthesia, but the last time he had it he woke up with some nausea. The anesthesiologist discusses that they will be using an intravenous (IV) Propofol drip to keep

him unconscious during the procedure and explains that Mr. White will need an arterial line for monitoring his blood pressure and a Foley bladder catheter for monitoring his urine output. All this will be done while Mr. White is unconscious so he will feel no pain or discomfort. After the procedure, the surgeon places a local nerve block around the area of the wound to decrease pain. The anesthesiologist also gives Mr. White some Zofran, a powerful antiemetic, as he is waking up, to help prevent the nausea he experienced last time. In the post anesthesia care unit (PACU), Mr. White is sore but feels well with little pain or nausea.

Introduction

In most cases, you will meet your anesthesia provider on the day of surgery. Recent improvements in anesthesia allows for more complicated spinal cases to be done safely. Anesthesia for spine surgery differs from other specialties because there are unique challenges to spine surgery. There can be significant blood loss, prolonged time in the operating room (OR), challenges in positioning the patient in a way that doesn't stress tissues immobilized for that prolonged time, and difficulty with pain control. Luckily, improved anesthesia protocols have made spine surgery very safe, even in difficult cases.

The Night Before Surgery

It is critical to remember that, if you have eaten recently, anesthesia cannot be provided. This is because there is a chance you could aspirate when you are given anesthesia. Aspiration means you regurgitate something down your windpipe while unconscious, and that can result in a serious pneumonia. For this reason, anesthesia is generally not given for elective cases if you have eaten in the past 6-8 hours and most facilities will instruct you to be "N.P.O." which is an abbreviation for the Latin nil per os meaning nothing by mouth. Usually, it is ok to take your medicines with small sips of water but ask the hospital staff first. I have seen many cases delayed or canceled because the patient couldn't resist that early morning breakfast before surgery.

Not Allowed within 8 hours of surgery
Eating solid food
Milk or dairy
Juices/drinks (except a small sip of water to take medications if necessary)

You should try to go to bed early if possible because the hospital will often require you to be there early in the morning, often several hours in advance of your procedure, to check in.

Talking with Your Anesthesiologist Before Surgery

Your anesthesiologist will typically come to talk to you before the procedure—this is often the first time you will meet the anesthesiologist. He/she will ask you about your medical history. At this point it's important for you to bring up any issues with previous anesthesia experiences you may have had, such as a prolonged wake-up time, excessive bleeding, nausea, or blood pressure issues. You should also tell your anesthesiologist about any allergies you have—especially to antibiotics, latex, soybean oil, or egg yolk (which may prevent the use of Propofol, a common anesthetic agent), and any history of allergy to halothane or succinylcholine. Also tell your anesthesiologist about any medical problems, and any problems with your eyes or teeth. This is because loose teeth may be vulnerable during the intubation period, and your eyes will need to be covered shut.

You should also let him/her know if you or any of your family members have ever had a condition known as malignant hyperthermia, a severe reaction to certain drugs used for anesthesia. It is important to discuss certain religious preferences that may impact your anesthesia care, such as letting them know your preference on receiving blood products if necessary. It is critical to discuss any recreational drug and alcohol use with your surgeon and anesthesiologist as this can significantly affect your anesthesia.

Your anesthesiologist will perform a quick exam listening to your lungs and examining your mouth. If you have any dental issues or use dentures, it's important to let the anesthesiologist know.

He/she will generally then discuss the anesthetic plan with you, and have you sign an informed consent document that states you agree to allow to have anesthesia performed on you and are aware of the risks. In general, anesthesia is very safe, with a risk of death like flying on a commercial airline. It is estimated that one death may result directly from anesthesia in 100,000 cases of surgery. You may be given some pain medication (Tylenol and gabapentin) prior to your procedure, which has been shown to help decrease your pain and nausea following surgery (1). Finally, your anesthesiologist may provide some sedative medication to help you relax before rolling into the operating room.

Types of Anesthesia

Anesthesia may be categorized as either "general anesthesia" or "regional" or "local anesthesia." In the case of general anesthesia, you are completely unconscious and are unable to breathe on your own. Your airway must be protected with an endotracheal tube (ET tube) and a ventilator machine is used to regulate your breathing. In local anesthesia you are given a nerve block which prevents the pain from reaching your brain. In some instances, you may additionally be given a light sedation known as Monitored Anesthesia Care or MAC during which you are still very relaxed and unaware of the procedure. Most spinal surgery is performed using general anesthesia because it is safer, well-tolerated, and there are no adequate nerve blocks to fully anesthetize the spine (2). Smaller cases such as kyphoplasty may be done using local anesthesia and a MAC.

Anesthesia Considerations for Spine Surgeries (3)		
Classification of Procedure	Example Procedures	Anesthesia Considerations/ Requirements
Interventional Procedures (Minimally Invasive)	Kyphoplasty Biopsy	MAC anesthesia (Light sedation)
Minor Spine Surgery (Estimated blood loss (EBL) < 100cc)	1-2 Level Anterior Cervical Discectomy and Fusion (ACDF) ≤2 Level Decompression	General anesthesia 1 intravenous (IV) set-up
Major (EBL 100-1000cc)	3-4 Level ACDF 1-3 Level Anterior Lumbar Interbody Fusion (ALIF) or Extreme Lateral Interbody Fusion (XLIF) 1-2 Level Transforaminal Interbody Fusion (TLIF) 1-2 Level anterior posterior (AP) Fusion	General anesthesia Arterial line (Thin catheter inserted into an artery) 2 IV set-ups Foley catheter
Complex (EBL 1000cc-10L)	6-18 Level Fusions >3 level anterior posterior fusion Pedicle subtraction osteotomy (PSO) Corpectomy/Vertebral resection	General anesthesia Arterial Line 2 IV set-ups Central catheter Foley Catheter
See glossary for brief descriptions of these procedures.		

General anesthesia is accomplished with the use of either inhaled anesthetic agents or IV anesthetic agents. The IV agents such a Propofol and Remifentanil are generally preferred because, unlike inhaled agents, they do not interfere with neuromonitoring of the spinal cord. Inhaled agents may be used at the tail-end of procedures because Propofol takes time to come out of your system. When only IV medications are used for anesthesia it is known as total intravenous anesthesia (TIVA) which has been associated with less post-operative nausea and vomiting (1). Opioids are used sparingly during surgery because they cause nausea, oversedation, and increase the risk of gastrointestinal upset after the procedure.

Recently more local anesthesia is being used in spine surgery, not as the primary means of anesthesia, but to help with post-operative pain control. This can be accomplished by injecting numbing medicine directly into the wound, or by blocking the nerves supplying the surgical area, or even with neural axial anesthesia such as an epidural or spinal block. Erector spinae muscular blocks, where the muscles around the spine are numbed, have come into vogue recently and seem to be helpful in decreasing some pain in lumbar spine surgery but as of this writing are not proven effective (4,5). In large reconstructive type cases, spinal and epidural blocks may also be used for post-operative pain control, but their use must be balanced against the need for an accurate neurological exam. If an epidural blockade is performed and there is a new post-operative neurologic deficit, it's hard for the surgeon to know whether the block or some effect from the surgery is the cause.

Airway Management

In most cases of spine surgery, general anesthesia is used with endotracheal intubation, meaning an artificial airway is placed down the mouth. Usually, intubation is performed by extending the neck (chin pointing up) and inserting an instrument known as a rigid laryngoscope into the mouth (don't forget to mention any loose teeth to your anesthesiologist). In certain cervical spine cases endotracheal intubation requires special instruments such as a fiberoptic laryngoscope which allows the anesthesiologist to intubate you without manipulation of your neck. It is important to let your anesthesiologist know if your neck is stiff or if you have cervical problems. In long or extensive cases, even after the surgery is finished, you may remain intubated overnight to ensure there are no complications with your airway. This is a possibility your anesthesiologist may discuss with you prior to surgery.

Lines (IVs)

Lines are small catheters, also known as IVs, that are placed in your blood vessels and used to perform multiple tasks such as drawing labs, giving medicine/fluid and even monitoring. Most IVs are placed into the veins. The anesthesiologist may place an arterial line— a small catheter that is placed in the radial artery of the wrist (on the thumb side) and allows real-time monitoring of your blood pressure (as opposed to a blood pressure cuff which can only monitor your blood pressure intermittently). In cases where significant blood loss is expected a central line may be placed. A central line is a large IV that can allow rapid administration of fluid and or blood products. It is placed into one of the great vessels of the body such as the inferior jugular vein (in the neck), the subclavian vein (under the collarbone) or femoral vein (in the thigh).

Urinary (Foley) Catheters

When you are unconscious you obviously cannot go to the bathroom on your own. For this reason, a small soft rubber tube known as a Foley catheter may be placed into the bladder through the urethra. Although this sounds uncomfortable, it is usually done after you have gone to sleep and is very well tolerated. The use of Foley catheters makes sure your bladder is decompressed throughout surgery and that you do not have an accident, while also allowing your anesthesiologist to monitor your fluid status (how much fluid is leaving your system).

Post-operative Anesthesia Care Unit

Before you know it, your surgery will be over, and you will be transferred to the post-operative anesthesia care unit (PACU). Here you will be monitored by a specialized nurse and your anesthesiologist as you awake from sedation. In the PACU you will be provided with oxygen by a mask until you are fully conscious. Your vitals will be closely monitored to ensure you are breathing normally and your blood pressure and heart rate are normal. Your nurse will help to control your pain with pain medicines.

Post-operative nausea and vomiting (PONV) is, unfortunately, common after general anesthesia and can be very uncomfortable. This can be more common in women, and patients with a history of motion sickness. The use of nitrous oxide in surgery can also increase the risk of PONV. Your nurse will use antiemetic medications such as ondansetron (Zofran®) to help treat this.

Once you are fully alert and awake, your vital signs have been stable for at least 30 minutes, your pain is reasonably under control and you can tolerate some clear liquids, you will be safe for discharge from the PACU either to home or to your hospital room.

Conclusion

Anesthesia has evolved significantly and will only continue to improve. In spine surgery, general anesthesia with Propofol is the most used method. Local blocks are used, but mainly for pain control after the procedure. General anesthesia requires the use of a breathing tube. This chapter provided only the most basic information about anesthesia but will allow you to converse more fluently with your provider and to better get your questions answered.

Frequently Asked Questions

- **You talk about putting all these "lines" into my body, but when will they be removed?**

    IV lines are useful throughout your hospital stay for giving you fluids and medicines. Thus, some IV lines from surgery will be left in place after surgery and removed prior to your discharge home. IV lines are typically only good for a few days and may need to be replaced if you are still needing one during a prolonged hospitalization. Arterial lines are generally removed once the need for close blood pressure monitoring is no longer necessary. Urinary catheters are generally removed once the procedure is over but may be left in place overnight in larger procedures, so you do not have to try and "run" to the bathroom when your back is quite sore.

References

1.   Gan TJ. 4th Consensus Guidelines for the Management of Postoperative Nausea and Vomiting. :117.

2.   Khanna P. Anesthetic considerations in spine surgery: What orthopaedic surgeon should know! Journal of Clinical Orthopaedics and Trauma. 2020;7.

3.   Guidelines for the intraoperative management of patients undergoing spine surgery - Ether - Resources for Anesthesia Research and Education - Stanford University School of Medicine [Internet]. [cited 2021 May 26]. Available from: http://ether.stanford.edu/policies/spine_surgery.html

4.   Singh S, Chaudhary NK. Bilateral Ultasound Guided Erector Spinae Plane Block for Postoperative Pain Management in Lumbar Spine Surgery: A Case Series. J Neurosurg Anesthesiol. 2019 Jul;31(3):354.

5.   Goel VK, Chandramohan M, Murugan C, Shetty AP, Subramanian B, Kanna RM, et al. Clinical efficacy of ultrasound guided bilateral erector spinae block for single level lumbar fusion surgery: A prospective, randomized, case-control study. The Spine Journal. 2021 Jun;S1529943021007798.

Chapter 34

Spine Surgery in the Elderly

Summary

As you age, spinal degeneration, and the potential need for spinal surgery increases. However, you also become more sensitive to anesthesia and more likely to experience possible complications. Surgery and anesthesia may trigger cognitive decline and other complications, including death. These are more likely to occur in long complicated procedures and with use of narcotic medicine. While this should give you pause, if you are elderly but healthy it should not necessarily stop you from having a procedure that could make your life more comfortable. Spine surgery can be very well-tolerated in the elderly, particularly small procedures. Your medical team will attempt to plan your surgery to limit the invasiveness and duration to make it as safe as possible.

Case 1

Mr. Gray is an 85-year-old gentleman who is losing the ability to walk and use his arms. He was diagnosed with severe cervical stenosis that was causing spinal cord damage. His health was already failing in other areas as he

had diabetes, high blood pressure, atrial fibrillation, and a history of a heart attack. Surgery was not elective in his case, and he underwent a long cervical decompressive procedure. After the case, he required opioid pain medicines as his pain was severe and he became confused and delirious. Over several days his confusion resolved and he was noted to have dramatic improvement in his overall motor function. Even so, his family noted he was not as sharp as he was before the procedure and had a harder time with his memory.

Case 2

Mrs. Red is an 80-year-old lady who has severe spinal stenosis and leg pain every time she walks. Otherwise, she is in great shape, and does water aerobics 4 times a week, although recently this has become difficult. She doesn't take any medications aside from a baby aspirin for prophylaxis against heart attacks and a multivitamin with high vitamin D. After discussion with her surgeon, she elects to have a minimally invasive lumbar decompression. The surgery is fast, and she recovers immediately. She spends 3 nights in the hospital to ensure a good recovery but can go home on her own and remains active. Three months after the procedure her friends note she is more active than ever, and she is glad she didn't let her age stand in the way of getting a procedure that has helped her live a more pain-free life.

Introduction

The years following retirement are the ones we most look forward to—grandchildren, leisure, and finally having time to pursue the things we really enjoy. Life expectancy and activity levels continue to increase in the elderly population expanding the possibilities of this time of life. This is also when painful problems with the aging musculoskeletal system can arise in the spine: osteoporosis, fragility fractures, disc degeneration and arthritis. Sometimes these pains keep us from enjoying our best years and that which we have worked so hard for. Spine surgery can alleviate some of the pains that come from an aging spine, but many patients may wonder if it is safe at the advanced ages when you may need it most. In this chapter we examine the costs and benefits of spine surgery in the elderly.

But first, what defines elderly? Is it an age? A state of mind? A stage of physical and mental health? For the purposes of this chapter, which draws heavily on the results of numerous studies tracking how various age groups fare following spine surgery, elderly does not actually exist—various studies compare groups of patients younger than and older than 50, 65, 75, 80 plus. Being elderly is less determined by your number of years than your "physiological health," a term to describe the performance of your body and its number of diseases. Compare two cars of the same make and model: one is driven on dirt roads and does not have the proper maintenance, the other is stored in a garage, driven on good roads and has regular oil changes. Which one lasts longer? Similarly, a 50-year-old body with diabetes, heart conditions, osteoporosis and smoking related issues will behave more elderly than a 70-year-old one that is active and free of disease. Getting older in life does increase the chances of something going wrong—especially with some surgeries—but, with today's tools and expertise, for many, getting on in years has less impact on the results of surgery than you might think.

Surgery and the Aging Heart

As we age, the body loses its ability to cope with physiological extremes such as blood loss, hypoxia (not enough oxygen available to body tissues) and shifts in bodily fluids or electrolytes. The stresses of surgery on the aging body often invite such physiological extremes. For example, as you age your heart loses its ability to increase its heart rate to keep blood circulating in response to drops in blood pressure. The heart may be stiff resulting in an inability of the heart to relax when it is filling (diastolic dysfunction) resulting in a decreased pumping capacity. Thus, the aged heart cannot respond as well to the stress of blood loss during surgery as a younger heart and this can set off significant cardiac problems (1).

Problems with Giving Anesthesia to the Elderly

As we age, there is also deterioration in the biological systems the body uses to clear drugs and other toxins from the blood. Thus, the elderly are much more sensitive to anesthesia, and prolonged exposure to these chemicals can result in temporary or permanent damage to neural (nerve) tissue. Anesthesia may cause short-term delirium and long-term post-operative cognitive decline (POCD) in the elderly. Short-term delirium is characterized by fluctuating mental consciousness, and short-term impairment to cognition, memory, and perception ongoing for less than 7 days. In contrast, post-operative cognitive decline is like dementia, which includes long-term pathologic changes to concentration, memory, language, and social skills. The diagnosis of POCD typically requires the administration of a cognitive function test such as the Mini-Mental State Exam by a mental health professional. Many patients and families are concerned with the post-operative effects of general anesthesia and prefer to undergo regional anesthesia (such as a spinal block) but, unfortunately, in spine surgery regional anesthesia is rarely adequate. So, let's explore the incidence of POCD in both general and regional anesthesia.

In 1955 a study was performed on 1193 patients over the age of 50 who underwent a general anesthesia that showed about 10% of patients appeared to have permanent mental decline or post-operative cognitive decline (POCD) (2). Follow-up studies have corroborated these findings (3). Was this the result of general anesthesia? In a subsequent large randomized, controlled trial (International Study of Postoperative Cognitive Dysfunction) comparing general to regional anesthesia (anesthesia of just part of the body), interestingly there was no difference in the incidence of POCD. Based on these findings, the investigators concluded in their 2003 paper that it was not specifically the general anesthesia that was contributing to POCD but something else (4). This could be anything from the narcotics used to subtle physiologic changes that occur during surgery.

Those who already have abnormalities in cognition (such as patients with Alzheimer's), metabolic abnormalities (low sodium) or have had strokes are at greater risk for POCD and delirium. Anesthesia and surgery may precipitate or worsen already present mild dementia (5). Healthy elderly individuals do not experience POCD at the same rate as those who are unhealthy.

Anesthesiologists have techniques to make anesthesia safer for the elderly. Exposure to anesthesia should be limited both in duration and dose. Limiting medicines such as benzodiazepines and opioids that are the most harmful to cognitive function can result in less decline (6). Furthermore, using age- and weight-appropriate doses of pain medicine after surgery can reduce the rates of delirium and dementia. Regional anesthesia may also be combined with sedation to limit the amount of anesthetic medicines required (such as propofol, narcotics, and inhaled anesthetics). In spine surgery, this takes the form of local blocks such as field blocks or erector spinae blocks (the erector spinae are the long muscles on either side of the spine.) Following surgery, moving and even doing some exercise can help prevent POCD (7).

Lumbar (Low Back) Spine Surgery in the Elderly

Central canal stenosis, that is, the narrowing of the spinal canal resulting in compression of the spinal cord and nerves, is the most common indication for surgery in the elderly and the number of decompression surgeries to fix this has been increasing every year in the U.S.(8). Unfortunately, lumbar stenosis (stenosis occurring in the low back region) is more likely to be severe in the elderly and non-operative conservative care less effective (9). Laminectomy (removing the thin part of a vertebra) is one of the surgeries that can relieve the pressure on the spinal cord and nerves caused by the stenosis. A laminectomy can yield dramatic improvement in pain and body function. This is true regardless of age and this surgery is not associated with an increased risk of complications up to eight decades of life (10–12). Nonetheless there are two factors which seem to influence complication rates in the elderly, namely the duration of the operation and how many other illnesses the patient has (13). Other factors such as depression also negatively impact outcomes in the elderly (14). Wound complications are also more common in the elderly (as high as 18%). Nevertheless, laminectomy is a small procedure which tends to be well tolerated by the elderly.

Unfortunately, laminectomy is sometimes insufficient to treat lumbar disorders and spinal fusion (a more invasive procedure) must be performed. Several studies have shown similar outcomes and complication rates between those older than 75 and those younger than 75 years who have undergone instrumented lumbar fusion (involving hardware implants) (15,16). However, other studies indicate spinal fusions can have increased rates of complications and requirements for blood transfusions in the elderly. In the Medicare population (greater than 65 years of age), mortality after spinal fusions can be up to 2 times higher compared to decompression alone (17). Is this different from what a younger population would experience? Unfortunately, this study only looked at those aged 65 years and older so no direct comparison to a younger cohort is available.

Elderly patients may have an increased risk of failing to heal the spinal fusion itself. Nevertheless, in one study, although patients older than 65 years had increased complications, the overall clinical outcomes from surgery were similar to those younger than 65 years of age (18). In a separate study, hospital stays for those older than 65 undergoing fusion were longer but the clinical outcomes were similar for those younger than 65 years (19).

So, how old is too old for lumbar spine surgery? There is no absolute cut-off age. Your overall health and the size of the planned surgery tend to matter more than your age. However, after 80-85 years of age, the risk of surgical complications and death following lumbar surgery are increased (20,21). That said, with modern spinal surgical techniques the risks associated with surgery can be greatly reduced. For example, one study of 50 patients undergoing minimally invasive decompression surgery in patients older than 75 years showed no complications and no mortality (22). In another study looking at minimally invasive multilevel lumbar fusions there was no difference in the rate of complications between those younger than 70 years and those older than 70 years of age (23).

Cervical (Neck) Spine Surgery in the Elderly

The cervical (neck) spine is another common area where degeneration occurs in older age. Like lumbar surgery, more and more elderly patients are undergoing cervical surgery every year. Being older than 65 years statistically increases the risk for complications in patients undergoing anterior cervical discectomy and fusion (ACDF) (a common surgery to decompress the spinal cord by removing a disc and then fuse two or more vertebrae together) (24). In a study of a large national database, patients older than 65 who underwent cervical discectomy were more likely to have at least 1 complication, (the most common being respiratory) than those younger than 65. Those who were older than 75 years of age also had higher odds of death within 30 days. Following cervical decompression and fusion, temporary complications such as inability to urinate, confusion, nausea and vomiting are common (25).

On the other hand, a laminoplasty procedure, which is a non-fusion procedure that decompresses the spinal cord, seems relatively safe in the elderly (26). This could be because laminoplasties are performed in a minimally invasive fashion from the back of the neck (instead of through the front as most cervical fusions are performed), does not require the same healing time as a fusion, and still accomplishes the goals of spinal canal decompression.

Elderly patients with neurologic dysfunction from cervical spinal cord compression (cervical myelopathy) do not have the same capacity to recover as younger patients, but are still able to regain some function after decompressive laminoplasty (27,28).

Why the Family of Elderly Spine Patients Is the Key to Success

Elderly patients have a hard time not only because of increased risk of overall complications, but because of multiple other reasons as well. Elderly patients may have difficulty communicating or understanding the doctor because they are hard of hearing. Some elderly patients may also have difficultly remembering aspects of a conversation with doctors or nurses. Post-operatively, getting to the store and caring for your own basic needs is more difficult for the elderly. For these reasons I find it very helpful when a younger family member accompanies the patient to office visits and is available around the time of surgery to help support the patient. A family member can also help the patient make good decisions regarding medical care. Ensuring a good plan to support your elderly family member get through his or her surgery is essential for success.

Conclusion

Elderly patients are more sensitive to surgery and anesthesia. The decision to have surgery must be carefully discussed with your surgeon and considered based on your overall health and the extent of the procedure. I believe it's important for other close family members to help with these decisions as well. Although not always possible, smaller less invasive procedures that limit blood loss and exposure to anesthesia should be favored in the elderly. It can be tempting to want a fix everything wrong in the spine, but in the elderly patient this may increase the risks from surgery an unacceptable amount. It could be that a small procedure will offer just as much relief without the need for extensive surgery or hospitalizations. Nonetheless, you should not let age deter you from procedures that could dramatically improve your quality of life. Most studies show that outcomes are just as good after spine surgery in the elderly as they are in younger patients.

Frequently Asked Questions

- **Is there a certain age after which surgery is not recommended?**

    No there is not. The decision on whether surgery will be safe is more based on your overall health than your numerical age.

References

1.   Levine WC, Mehta V, Landesberg G. Anesthesia for the elderly: selected topics: Current Opinion in Anaesthesiology. 2006 Jun;19(3):320–4.

2.   Bedford PD. Adverse cerebral effects of anaesthesia on old people. Lancet. 1955 Aug 6;269(6884):259–63.

3.   Steinmetz J, Rasmussen LS. Long-term Consequences of Postoperative Cognitive Dysfunction. 2009;110(3):8.

4.   Rasmussen LS, Johnson T, Kuipers HM, Kristensen D, Siersma VD, Vila P, et al. Does anaesthesia cause postoperative cognitive dysfunction? A randomised study of regional versus general anaesthesia in 438 elderly patients. Acta Anaesthesiologica Scandinavica. 2003;47(3):260–6.

5.   Cottrell JE, Hartung J. Anesthesia and Cognitive Outcome in Elderly Patients: A Narrative Viewpoint. Journal of Neurosurgical Anesthesiology. 2020 Jan;32(1):9–17.

6.   Bellou V, Belbasis L, Tzoulaki I, Middleton LT, Ioannidis JPA, Evangelou E. Systematic evaluation of the associations between environmental risk factors and dementia: An umbrella review of systematic reviews and meta-analyses. Alzheimers Dement. 2017 Apr;13(4):406–18.

7.   Northey JM, Cherbuin N, Pumpa KL, Smee DJ, Rattray B. Exercise interventions for cognitive function in adults older than 50: a systematic review with meta-analysis. Br J Sports Med. 2018 Feb;52(3):154–60.

8.   Ciol MA, Deyo RA, Howell E, Kreif S. An assessment of surgery for spinal stenosis: time trends, geographic variations, complications, and reoperations. J Am Geriatr Soc. 1996 Mar;44(3):285–90.

9.   Shabat S, Folman Y, Leitner Y, Fredman B, Gepstein R. Failure of conservative treatment for lumbar spinal stenosis in elderly patients. Archives of Gerontology and Geriatrics. 2007 May;44(3):235–41.

10.   Silvers HR, Lewis PJ, Asch HL. Decompressive lumbar laminectomy for spinal stenosis. Journal of Neurosurgery. 1993 May;78(5):695–701.

11.   Cloyd JM, Acosta FL, Ames CP. Complications and Outcomes of Lumbar Spine Surgery in Elderly People: A Review of the Literature: LUMBAR SPINE SURGERY IN ELDERLY PEOPLE. Journal of the American Geriatrics Society. 2008 Jul;56(7):1318–27.

12.   Karsy M, Chan AK, Mummaneni PV, Virk MS, Bydon M, Glassman SD, et al. Outcomes and Complications With Age in Spondylolisthesis: An Evaluation of the Elderly From the Quality Outcomes Database. Spine. 2020 Jul 15;45(14):1000–8.

13.   Wang MY, Green BA, Shah S, Steven Vanni DO, Levi ADO. Complications associated with lumbar stenosis surgery in patients older than 75 years of age. FOC. 2003 Feb;14(2):1–4.

14.   Adogwa O, Carr K, Fatemi P, Verla T, Gazcon G, Gottfried O, et al. Psychosocial Factors and Surgical Outcomes: Are Elderly Depressed Patients Less Satisfied With Surgery? Spine. 2014 Sep;39(19):1614–9.

15.   Okuda S, Oda T, Miyauchi A, Haku T, Yamamoto T, Iwasaki M. Surgical Outcomes of Posterior Lumbar Interbody Fusion in Elderly Patients. VO LUM E. :7.

16.   Cassinelli EH, Eubanks J, Vogt M, Furey C, Yoo J, Bohlman HH. Risk Factors for the Development of Perioperative Complications in Elderly Patients Undergoing Lumbar Decompression and Arthrodesis for Spinal Stenosis: An Analysis of 166 Patients. Spine. 2007 Jan;32(2):230–5.

17.   Deyo RA, Ciol MA, Cherkin DC, Loeser JD, Bigos SJ. Lumbar spinal fusion. A cohort study of complications, reoperations, and resource use in the Medicare population. Spine. 1993 Sep 1;18(11):1463–70.

18.   Glassman SD, Carreon L, Dimar JR. Outcome of Lumbar Arthrodesis in Patients Sixty-five Years of Age or Older: The Journal of Bone and Joint Surgery-American Volume. 2010 Mar;92(Suppl 1):77–84.

19.   Kilinçer C, Steinmetz MP, Sohn MJ, Benzel EC, Bingaman W. Effects of age on the perioperative characteristics and short-term outcome of posterior lumbar fusion surgery. Journal of Neurosurgery: Spine. 2005 Jul;3(1):34–9.

20.   Raffo CS, Lauerman WC. Predicting Morbidity and Mortality of Lumbar Spine Arthrodesis in Patients in Their Ninth Decade: Spine. 2006 Jan;31(1):99–103.

21.   Oldridge NB, Yuan Z, Stoll JE, Rimm AR. Lumbar spine surgery and mortality among Medicare beneficiaries, 1986. Am J Public Health. 1994 Aug;84(8):1292–8.

22.   Rosen DS, O'Toole JE, Eichholz KM, Hrubes M, Huo D, Sandhu FA, et al. Minimally invasive lumbar spinal decompression in the elderly: outcomes of 50 patients aged 75 years and older. Neurosurgery. 2007 Mar;60(3):503–9; discussion 509-510.

23.   Claus CF, Lytle E, Tong D, Bahoura M, Garmo L, Yoon E, et al. Elderly as a Predictor for Perioperative Complications in Patients Undergoing Multilevel Minimally Invasive Transforaminal Lumbar Interbody Fusion: A Regression Modeling Study. SPINE. 2020 Jun;45(11):735–40.

24.   Buerba RA, Giles E, Webb ML, Fu MC, Gvozdyev B, Grauer JN. Increased Risk of Complications After Anterior Cervical Discectomy and Fusion in the Elderly: An Analysis of 6253 Patients in the American College of Surgeons National Surgical Quality Improvement Program Database. Spine. 2014 Dec;39(25):2062–9.

25.   Radcliff K, Ong KL, Lovald S, Lau E, Kurd M. Cervical Spine Surgery Complications and Risks in the Elderly: SPINE. 2017 Mar;42(6):E347–54.

26.   Tanaka J, Seki N, Tokimura F, Doi K, Inoue S. Operative Results of Canal-Expansive Laminoplasty for Cervical Spondylotic Myelopathy in Elderly Patients: Spine. 1999 Nov;24(22):2308.

27.   Machino M, Ando K, Kobayashi K, Ito K, Tsushima M, Matsumoto A, et al. The Feature of Clinical and Radiographic Outcomes in Elderly Patients With Cervical Spondylotic Myelopathy: A Prospective Cohort Study on 1025 Patients. SPINE. 2018 Jun;43(12):817–23.

28.   Machino M, Yukawa Y, Hida T, Ito K, Nakashima H, Kanbara S, et al. Can Elderly Patients Recover Adequately After Laminoplasty? A Comparative Study of 520 Patients With Cervical Spondylotic Myelopathy: Spine. 2012 Apr;37(8):667–71.

Chapter 35

Orthopedic Surgery in the Era of Covid 19: Protecting Yourself From Hospital-Acquired Infection

Summary

COVID-19 otherwise known as SARS-COV-2 has had a profound impact on the basic hygiene protocols of the hospital. Many of these changes are common sense and make the hospital a safer environment for everyone. Some of these changes include a greater emphasis placed on telemedicine visits to decrease traffic through the hospital, strict hygiene protocols including mask wearing, hand washing, and social distancing. Access to the hospital is also now strictly regulated with mandatory temperature checks, and controlled visiting. Although many of these changes were brought about by COVID-19, it's important to remember there are many other scary bacteria and viruses (MRSA and C. Diff to name a few) spread in the hospital that can be decreased by the improved hygiene protocols COVID brought about. These changes have ensured greater sanitation of the hospital, benefitting both patients and healthcare workers.

Case

Mr. Brown is a 45-year-old businessman with a low back and sciatic problem. His problem unfortunately got worse during the COVID pandemic where most in-person appointments were canceled. Luckily, he was able to secure a visit with a local spine surgeon using telemedicine where he described his problems. The surgeon was able to review his imaging and do a basic physical exam online. Based on this, he recommended Mr. Brown come in for an in-person visit and a formal exam. Mr. Brown was concerned about visiting the hospital during the COVID pandemic, but he wore an N-95 mask and regularly sterilized his hands to protect himself. His surgeon confirmed he needed surgery and 1 week prior to his procedure he underwent a COVID rapid PCR test which was negative—this allowed him access to the hospital. Mr. Brown had his procedure and was never kept close to other patients, and all healthcare workers wore masks and exercised good basic hygiene. Things went well and he was discharged from the hospital. He did his follow-up visits using telemedicine, and only had to come in for a routine X-ray. Mr. Brown appreciated the attention to hygiene and felt safer than ever before in the hospital.

Introduction

Hospital-acquired infection (also known as a nosocomial infection), or an infection that you get from being in the hospital, is unfortunately not a new concept. Even before the emergence of COVID-19 (see below), there existed many pathogens which thrived in the hospital setting. Sick people come to the hospital with bad diseases and these diseases can spread to other patients. These include things like methicillin resistant staphylococcus aureus (MRSA), clostridium difficile (C. Diff) among others. Because of COVID-19, hospitals were forced to increase precautions which are also useful for addressing a variety of bad infectious diseases. In this chapter we focus on COVID-19 because of the profound change it has made to healthcare, but the concepts discussed are easily applicable to other bacteria and viruses.

Overview of hospital acquired infections

Millions of healthcare associated infections (HAI) occur in the United States per year and are responsible for tens of thousands of deaths (1). HAI can cause urinary tract infection, pneumonia, surgical site/wound infection, respiratory infection among other conditions. Bacteria and viruses are responsible for causing HAI and may be transmitted from patient to patient, or visitor to patient. Some of the pathogens that have arisen as serious threats include methicillin-resistant staphylococcus aureus (MRSA), vancomycin-resistant enterococcus (VRE), Clostridium difficile (C. diff) and COVID-19, but there are many others. These pathogens successfully survive on inanimate objects in the hospitals for long periods of time and thus are easily spread from person to person. They are not only difficult to eradicate from the hospital but are also very difficult to treat once they start an infection. In cases where patients become infected by one of these pathogens, contact precautions may be initiated to prevent the spread of the disease to others. This means the patient will be placed in isolation, and all entering the room must gown, glove and mask. Here is an overview of common hospital acquired infections:

Types of Hospital Acquired Infections				
Pathogen	Type of Organism	Types of infections	Sources of infection	Prevention
Methicillin-resistant staphylococcus aureus (MRSA)	Bacteria that is resistant to the antibiotic methicillin	Wound infection, endocarditis (a type of heart infection), sepsis (blood infection), soft tissue and bone infections (osteomyelitis)	Any object in contact with skin 50-80% of individuals are already colonized (have MRSA present in their skin and nasal tissue) (2)	Frequent hand washing with soap and water Patients are generally screened for MRSA colonization prior to surgical procedures. If found to be positive, they may be prescribed a nasal antiseptic called mupirocin and use a special body wash containing chlorhexidine. Alcohol based hand sanitizer
Vancomycin resistant enterococcus (VRE)	Bacteria that is resistant to the antibiotic vancomy-cin	Wound infection, endocarditis (a type of heart infection), sepsis (blood infection), soft tissue, intraabdominal and pelvic, and central nervous system infections	Surfaces (may persist for 4 months) Human colonization Health care worker transmission	Frequent hand washing especially after using bathroom or handling food Alcohol based hand sanitizer (3)
Clostridioides difficile (C. diff)	Bacteria	Diarrhea and infection of the colon (colitis)	Fecal contamination of the hands	Frequent hand washing with soap and water especially after using the bathroom (4)

Covid-19

The severe acute respiratory syndrome corona virus 2 (SARS-COV-2 aka COVID) is a ribonucleic acid (RNA) betacorona virus that was first identified in December of 2019 in Wuhan, China. The virus has had a profound impact on almost all areas of medicine, not only changing the ways doctors interact with patients, but also how patients can access the hospital. The SARS-CoV-2 virus is spread through direct contact with infected individuals—especially by inhaling droplets emitted from a cough or sneeze. The virus typically takes 2-12 days to incubate during which time you may be asymptomatic but able to transmit the virus to others. Masks, handwashing, and social distancing have emerged as simple ways to protect yourself and others, not just from COVID, but other respiratory infections as well.

Symptoms

The majority of SARS-COV-2 cases are mild and upwards of 30-40% of individuals may be asymptomatic, making transmission easy (5). However, severe disease can occur in 5% of cases with a mortality rate of 2.3% (6). Those of older age and with a higher burden of medical comorbidities (other medical conditions or diseases already present) seem to be at higher risk. The symptoms of the SARS-COV-2 are typical of the flu, namely fever (greater than 100.4°F/38°C), fatigue, cough, headache, sore throat, and congestion (7). Recovery is typically 2 weeks for mild cases and 6 weeks for severe cases.

Diagnosis

All symptomatic patients should be tested for SARS-COV-2. Furthermore, all patients being admitted to the hospital or those who have had contact with someone positive for SARS-COV-2 should be tested even if they are asymptomatic. This is to limit the spread of the virus to others, particularly frail patients in the hospital. There are many commercial tests available today to test for COVID-19. A common way to test for the SARS-COV-2 virus is using a reverse transcriptase polymerase chain reaction (RT-PCR)—a test that looks for viral genetic material (ribonucleic acid—RNA) in samples collected from your nose or mouth that are not present in healthy individuals. This test is highly accurate and false positives and negatives are rare (8).

Elective Surgery During the Pandemic

During the COVID lockdown only certain orthopedic procedures were performed both to minimize the risk to elective patients and to decrease the overall burden on the hospital system. Following the lockdown elective surgery was allowed but on a tighter scale, focusing on patients who were low risk medically (ASA 1-2), or high-risk for compromise from a delayed procedure (risk for increased pain or severe dysfunction). Although hospitals have mostly opened back up the operating rooms for all, these guidelines serve as a reminder that those with increased medical issues are more susceptible to infections in the hospitals.

Surgical procedures which were performed during the COVID lockdown effectively indicate the urgency of certain conditions (9):

- **Infection:**

    - Deep tissue or joint infection (native or prosthetic)

    - Wound infection

- **Spine:**

    - Fractures

    - Infections

    - Cerebrospinal (CSF) leak

    - Spinal column injury resulting in instability with or without symptoms.

    - Spinal Cord compression or cauda equina causing myelopathy or loss of neurological function

- **Trauma:**

    - Amputations

    - Compartment syndrome (painful, dangerous build-up of pressure within muscles)

    - Dislocations

    - Fractures that if left untreated may lead to loss of function or permanent disability.

    - Hematoma evacuation (draining pooled blood that is pressing against the brain, spinal cord, or organs)

    - Ligament injury

    - Open fractures

- Pathological fractures (a bone break caused by a disease)

- Penetrating injury to bone and joint

- Peripheral nerve injury or compression with severe symptoms

- Wound dehiscence (rupture of stitches that closed a wound)

- Tendon laceration (tear) or disruption (pulled apart or off the bone)

Basic precautions

The virus has transformed medical care across the country with many new protocols and safety precautions in place to decrease the incidence of transmission. These precautions have ushered in a new era of medical safety measures and are useful not only for protection against COVID, but other commonly transmitted diseases. The most basic measures include social distancing, improved and more frequent hand washing, masks and vaccination.

Social distancing means a minimum distance of 6 feet should be always maintained between you and others in the hospital. This includes waiting rooms. Using telemedicine is another way to practice social distancing and keep you out of the hospital. Telemedicine is simply a doctor's appointment performed online using a video chat platform. This practice has enjoyed an expanded role in medicine because of COVID and may take the place of your traditional new and follow-up doctor's appointments. Many patients have found that this is convenient, especially if they are traveling from far away. Most follow-up after surgery visits are just "check-ins" to see how you are doing and do not require a detailed physical exam. In some cases, these can be efficiently performed using telemedicine. Even if a physical exam is required, basic exams can be performed over a video chat and diagnoses usually do not change with in-person visits (10).

Handwashing and masks have become universally available in the hospital. Make sure you clean your hands before entering the hospital, and after touching any surfaces in the hospital. This is especially important before you touch any vulnerable family members who may be patients. Gel hand sanitizer is a great and fast way to accomplish this, and dispensers should be near most doorways in the hospital. However, nothing beats hand washing with soap and water, which should be performed upon entering and exiting any patient room.

At all times, your face and mouth should be covered by a surgical mask that does not have a vent. If you do not have one, the hospital will provide you with one. This helps to prevent transmission of aerosolized diseases and is also protective while you are visiting the hospital. Masks have been shown to reduce the risk of infection by nearly 70% in healthcare workers (11).

Vaccination is perhaps one of the best ways to limit spread of COVID-19 to your loved ones and other healthcare workers. At the time of this writing three pharmaceutical companies are offering vaccines: Moderna, Pfizer and Johnson and Johnson. Despite their rapid development, the vaccines approved for use in the United States have all undergone rigorous testing with a high safety standard no different from other vaccines and have a very high efficacy rate of preventing infection. For the latest information on vaccines please visit the CDC website: www. cdc.gov.

Access to the hospital

Access to the hospital has also changed dramatically. Visitors, patients, and staff entering the hospital are strictly monitored with a body temperature check and to ensure everyone is wearing a mask. If you are symptomatic (cough, fever, other respiratory symptoms) or have had contact with someone who is positive for COVID-19, you should declare that to the screening personnel (and not enter the hospital unless there is a serious reason).

The more people who come into the hospital, the more risk there is to both patients and staff; thus, family visitation may be restricted during certain periods. Special provisions may be made for parents accompanying minors, for those visiting family members close to dying or if there is a special language barrier that may be facilitated by a bilingual family member. If you are coming in for a procedure, you should try to limit as much outside contact as possible for 2 weeks prior to the procedure to decrease the risk of becoming sick and bringing it into the hospital.

Prior to undergoing your pre-operative testing (1-4 days prior to surgery) you should undergo a SARS-CoV-2 RT PCR test. This is done by specific medical personnel who insert a small swab into your nose. This should be done within 6 days of the procedure but may vary by hospital. Every hospital will have a different protocol for handling the results of the test. Typically, if your test is negative, you are allowed access to the hospital and your procedure.

If you are positive, your surgery may be canceled, and you will be asked to go into quarantine. If you are symptomatic with a positive test, as of this writing the CDC recommends 10 days of quarantine. If you are asymptomatic you will need to quarantine for 5 days (from the first positive test). Your swab may be repeated depending at the discretion of your surgeon. Following these recommendations can lead to excellent outcomes, with a reported 0% incidence of infection of patients or spread to health care workers (12). As is the case in most evolving situations, these recommendations are likely to change with time.

Conclusion

COVID changed the world in many ways, and healthcare was particularly affected. Nonetheless, many of these changes were positive and have led to improved safety protocols in the hospital. COVID taught us about the importance of basic hygiene practices that are easy to follow and should be routine in the hospital setting. Keeping the hospital clean ensures you will have the safest possible visit.

Frequently Asked Questions

- **How easy is it to get a bacterial or MRSA infection in the hospital?**

The presence of MRSA in the hospital setting varies from 1% to 40%, depending on the geographic location (13). The overall rate of surgical site infection in spine surgery is around 3%, of which MRSA is responsible for about 22% (14). MRSA is brought into the hospital not just from people with active MRSA infections but also from people who are colonized by MRSA without knowing it—meaning they have the bacteria living on their skin and in their nostrils, but it does not cause symptoms. Most patients are tested for MRSA in their nostrils prior to admission for elective surgery and even possibly treated with an antiseptic such as mupirocin that is applied topically in the nose. Thankfully, MRSA transmission in the hospital is easily prevented with the precautions outlined above, including mask wearing, social distancing and hand washing.

References

1.   McFee RB. Nosocomial or Hospital-acquired Infections: An Overview. Dis Mon. 2009 Jul;55(7):422–38.

2.   Turner NA, Sharma-Kuinkel BK, Maskarinec SA, Eichenberger EM, Shah PP, Carugati M, et al. Methicillin-resistant Staphylococcus aureus: an overview of basic and clinical research. Nat Rev Microbiol. 2019 Apr;17(4):203–18.

3.   VRE in Healthcare Settings | HAI | CDC [Internet]. 2019 [cited 2022 Jul 24]. Available from: https://www.cdc.gov/hai/organisms/vre/vre.html

4.   CDC. C. diff germs are carried from person to person. [Internet]. Centers for Disease Control and Prevention. 2021 [cited 2022 Jul 24]. Available from: https://www.cdc.gov/cdiff/prevent.html

5.   Oran DP, Topol EJ. Prevalence of Asymptomatic SARS-CoV-2 Infection?: A Narrative Review. Ann Intern Med. 2020 01;173(5):362–7.

6.   Bajema KL, Oster AM, McGovern OL, Lindstrom S, Stenger MR, Anderson TC, et al. Persons Evaluated for 2019 Novel Coronavirus - United States, January 2020. MMWR Morb Mortal Wkly Rep. 2020 Feb 14;69(6):166–70.

7.   Guan W jie, Ni Z yi, Hu Y, Liang W hua, Ou C quan, He J xing, et al. Clinical Characteristics of Coronavirus Disease 2019 in China. N Engl J Med. 2020 Feb 28;NEJMoa2002032.

8.   Lieberman JA, Pepper G, Naccache SN, Huang ML, Jerome KR, Greninger AL. Comparison of Commercially Available and Laboratory-Developed Assays for In Vitro Detection of SARS-CoV-2 in Clinical Laboratories. J Clin Microbiol. 2020 Jul 23;58(8).

9.   Sarac NJ, Sarac BA, Schoenbrunner AR, Janis JE, Harrison RK, Phieffer LS, et al. A Review of State Guidelines for Elective Orthopaedic Procedures During the COVID-19 Outbreak. J Bone Jt Surg. 2020 Jun 3;102(11):942–5.

10.   Iyer S, Shafi K, Lovecchio F, Turner R, Albert TJ, Kim HJ, et al. The Spine Physical Examination Using Telemedicine: Strategies and Best Practices. Glob Spine J. 2020 Aug 5;2192568220944129.

11.   Li Y, Liang M, Gao L, Ayaz Ahmed M, Uy JP, Cheng C, et al. Face masks to prevent transmission of COVID-19: A systematic review and meta-analysis. Am J Infect Control. 2021 Jul;49(7):900–6.

12.   Zorzi C, Piovan G, Screpis D, Natali S, Marocco S, Iacono V. Elective Orthopaedic Surgery During COVID-19: A Safe Way to Get Back on Track. JBJS Open Access. 2020;5(4):e20.00084-e20.00084.

13.   Voss A, Milatovic D, Wallrauch-Schwarz C, Rosdahl VT, Braveny I. Methicillin-resistant Staphylococcus aureus in Europe. Eur J Clin Microbiol Infect Dis Off Publ Eur Soc Clin Microbiol. 1994 Jan;13(1):50–5.

14.   Zhou J, Wang R, Huo X, Xiong W, Kang L, Xue Y. Incidence of Surgical Site Infection After Spine Surgery: A Systematic Review and Meta-analysis. Spine. 2020 Feb 1;45(3):208–16.

Chapter 36

Spinal Decompression: Taking Pressure Off the Spinal Cord and Nerve Roots Directly (by Removing Tissue) or Indirectly (by Realigning the Spine)— Laminectomy and Foraminotomy

Summary

Decompression of the spine is a general term used to describe a surgical procedure to treat spinal stenosis. Stenosis simply implies a narrowing of the spinal canal that can result in compression of nerves and the spinal cord. Decompression can be performed either directly or indirectly. Direct decompression means that the surgeon, under direct visualization, removes offending structures that are compressing nerves. The most common direct decompression procedure is a laminectomy, wherein part of the arch of the vertebra is removed allowing the surgeon access to the spinal canal. Indirect decompression means that the surgeon is realigning the spine to unkink or unpinch nerves; this typically requires a spinal fusion. Indirect decompression is particularly useful if there is a dynamic component to the stenosis, meaning the stenosis gets worse with motion between vertebrae.

Case

Ms. Yellow is a 75-year-old retired photographer that now enjoys trips to the beach to take pictures of birds. She normally is an avid walker but recently she has noted that she can't walk very far and every time she tries, she develops shooting pain in her legs. Her back otherwise feels fine. She is diagnosed with spinal stenosis and a surgeon recommends a minimally invasive decompression since her problem predominantly affects a single spinal level. He explains that he will make a small hole in the lamina (a laminotomy) through which he will remove compressive structures. She undergoes the procedure and spends one night in the hospital. Her back is sore initially, but this goes away within several weeks and there is a dramatic improvement in her overall walking capacity and pain levels. She now can take long hikes to the beach and even carry a backpack full of photography equipment.

Introduction

To understand spinal decompression, we need to review what the term stenosis means. Stenosis just means something is narrowed. So, the term spinal stenosis means there is a narrowing or stricture in the spinal canal. When the spinal canal is narrowed, it results in compression of the nerves or the spinal cord which can cause symptoms. Compression of the nerves can result in pain, weakness, or numbness of the extremities. Compression of the spinal cord can cause more sinister symptoms such as loss of balance, urinary and bowel incontinence, and increasing loss of manual dexterity.

Spinal decompression is a grab-all term for a procedure which relieves stenosis or pressure on the nerves in the spine. It is mostly performed by removing whatever is compressing the nerve and causing pain. As discussed in a previous chapters (chapters 3, 7 and 8) there can many different issues that can cause compression in the spinal canal, but the most common structures that compress the spinal cord are herniated discs, thickened ligaments, and bone spurs. However, compression may also be the result of a kink or collapse in the spine such as from a fracture, which can be relieved by realigning the spine.

Laminectomy

Probably the most common procedure used to accomplish spinal decompression is the laminectomy. In a laminectomy the arch of the vertebra, called the lamina, is removed, unroofing the spinal canal. The lamina itself rarely causes compression, but performing a laminectomy allows you access to remove whatever is causing the compression, for example, a thickened ligament, cyst, or a bone spur. Basically, a laminectomy is like taking the manhole cover off a pipe allowing you to clear out the tree roots that have caused a clog. Laminectomy is a term which just means part of the lamina is removed. If just a small portion of the lamina is removed, it's called a laminotomy or partial laminectomy. Occasionally in severe or multilevel stenosis the entire lamina of each vertebra involved may be removed. As described above, If the entire lamina is removed it's called a total laminectomy.

Most patients will wonder how a part of the vertebra can be removed without compromising it. The answer is that the lamina is not a load bearing structure and removing it does not usually destabilize the spine. In addition to this, laminectomies can be performed in many ways—some ways only remove a small amount of bone and have very little impact on the structural integrity of the spine. For example, in a typical single level (one vertebra) decompression only the inferior edge of the lamina is removed (known as a dome laminectomy) to allow access to the spinal canal.

Foraminotomy

A laminectomy is good at decompressing the spinal canal but does nothing to decompress the nerve roots as they exit the spine. To decompress a nerve root the surgeon needs to create more space in the corridor where the compressed (pinched) nerve root exits the spine; this corridor (or opening) between two adjacent vertebrae is known as a foramen. Thus, the surgical procedure that enlarges that corridor is called a foraminotomy. Foraminotomies are commonly done in the lumbar spine and in the cervical spine and include removal of a portion of the facet joint (the joint between vertebrae where movement occurs).

Indirect Decompression: Unkinking the Spine

When stenosis of the spinal canal results from malalignment of the spine, decompressing the spinal canal usually doesn't require removing bones or ligaments. The spine simply needs to be realigned in the proper shape to restore the normal canal diameter. This is known as an "indirect decompression." It means that a decompression is achieved without performing a laminectomy to clean out the spinal canal. The most typical deformity resulting in malalignment is a slipped disc or spondylolisthesis. This occurs when a disc space collapses (for example, because of disc degeneration) and a vertebra shifts forward, resulting in a kink in the spinal canal that causes stenosis. Restoring height to the disc space shifts the spine back into the proper position and removes the kink. Thus, a decompression is accomplished without ever opening the spinal canal. Surgeons can accomplish an indirect spinal decompression through a procedure known as spinal fusion, where the bones are realigned and joined together with rods and screws. Also, collapsed discs can be replaced with spacers that restore height and allow the spine to return to normal position.

The foramen can also be indirectly decompressed. Sometimes when the disc space collapses, the foramen can also decrease in size causing stenosis. Reconstructing the disc space with a graft spacer recreates the original size of the foramen and can decompress the nerve as it exits without the need for a foraminotomy. Sometimes the spinal canal and the foramen are both stenotic; sometimes it is just one or the other.

Lumbar Laminectomy (Removing the Lamina in a Low Back Vertebra)

What are the varieties of lumbar laminectomy? Laminectomies are generally used to treat lumbar stenosis that is causing leg pain radiating from the back (lumbar radiculopathy or sciatica). A complete laminectomy is useful when the stenosis causing the compression encircles the spinal canal. In contrast, as described above, a laminotomy is useful for taking out a herniated disc on one side. A full laminectomy generally requires a longer recovery time than a hemilaminotomy because the full laminectomy requires more resection (tissue cut out), which makes the surgery take longer, and, also, a full laminectomy removes more bone.

The most common indication for a laminectomy is spinal stenosis. This can be treated with either a formal open decompression with removal of the lamina, or through a minimally invasive approach.

In an open approach, a midline incision is made over the back, the midline ligaments and parts of the spinous processes are removed, and usually the portions of the top and bottom laminae (so, for example, the top of the L5 lamina and the bottom of the L4 lamina for a L4-5 decompression) are removed including the tissue in between. If there are multiple levels of stenosis the lamina in the middle may need to be completely removed.

In minimally invasive laminectomy, a hemilaminotomy is performed on one side only, which gives the surgeon access to the spinal canal. From this access point the ligamentum is cleaned out from within the spinal canal, without need to disrupt the spinous processes or the dorsal ligaments. It's a more elegant way of performing the decompression, but much more technically demanding and time consuming.

Studies have shown that both approaches are safe and effective for decompression of the spine so it really comes down to what your surgeon thinks is best for you (1).

Cervical Laminectomy (Removing the Lamina from a Neck Vertebra)

Cervical laminectomies work in a very similar way to those performed on the lumbar spine. However, in contrast to lumbar laminectomies, cervical laminectomies are not as commonly done as a standalone procedure because of the risk of what is called post-laminectomy kyphosis (2,3). This condition occurs when the removal of the lamina and surrounding structures cause the head to sag forward. This is more likely to happen in the neck than in the low back. To avoid that, cervical laminectomies are often combined with a cervical fusion especially at multiple levels. Please see the chapter 43 on posterior cervical fusion.

Nonetheless, single- or two-level cervical laminectomies can be performed in certain patients without significant disruption and are very well-tolerated (2). They can be an easy answer for treating cervical stenosis in patients who may not tolerate a fusion surgery well and have a very quick recovery.

Conclusion

Decompression of the spine can be accomplished in many ways but most commonly refers to a procedure called a laminectomy. This procedure has been performed safely for decades and can result in great relief of leg pain or arm pain from pinched nerves.

Frequently Asked Questions

- **If the lamina is removed, what will be protecting my spinal canal?**

     The lamina is a bony casing that protects the spinal canal, so when it is removed people often wonder what is left to protect the sensitive nerves and spinal cord within. The spinal canal is deep within the body and not vulnerable to injury from superficial pressure. Furthermore, the area will scar over after your surgery which gives more protection. Theoretically the spinal canal is more vulnerable, but in practice, injury just does not happen. It's not possible to get bumped on the back or neck after surgery and suffer a neurologic injury.

References

1.   den Boogert HF, Keers JC, Marinus Oterdoom DL, Kuijlen JMA. Bilateral versus unilateral interlaminar approach for bilateral decompression in patients with single-level degenerative lumbar spinal stenosis: a multicenter retrospective study of 175 patients on postoperative pain, functional disability, and patient satisfaction. J Neurosurg Spine. 2015 Sep;23(3):326–35.

522 The Spine Encyclopedia

2.   Kim BS, Dhillon RS. Cervical Laminectomy With or Without Lateral Mass Instrumentation: A Comparison of Outcomes. Clinical Spine Surgery: A Spine Publication. 2019 Jul;32(6):226–32.

3.   Kaptain GJ, Simmons NE, Replogle RE, Pobereskin L. Incidence and outcome of kyphotic deformity following laminectomy for cervical spondylotic myelopathy. Journal of Neurosurgery: Spine. 2000 Oct 1;93(2):199–204.

Figures:

Different Lumbar Decompressions/Laminectomies

Lumbar vertebra from behind:

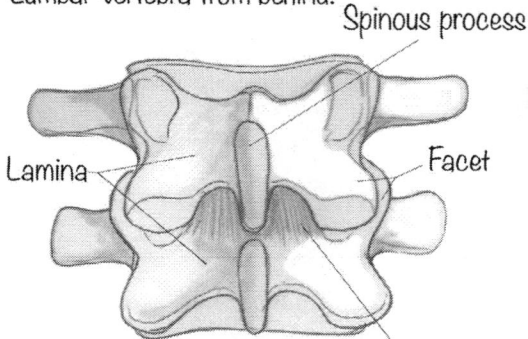

Spinous process

Complete Laminectomy:

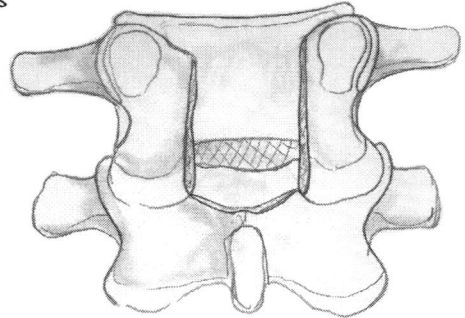

Lamina

Facet

Hemilaminotomy:

Ligamentum flavum

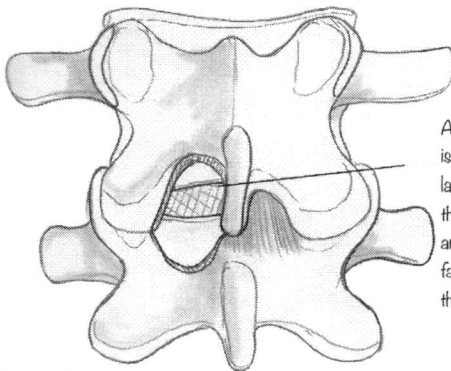

Hemilaminotomy and Foraminotomy:

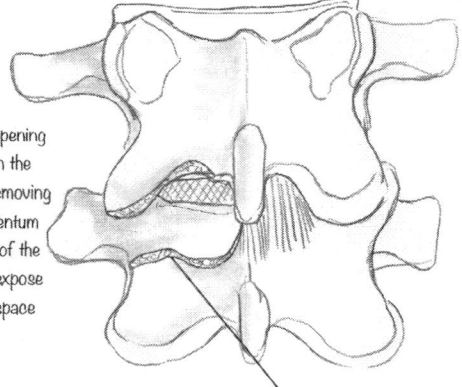

A small opening is made in the lamina, removing the ligamentum and part of the facet to expose the disc space

Dome Laminectomy:

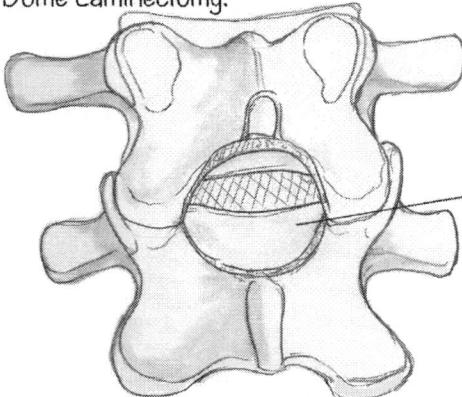

The facet is completely removed to decompress the foramen

The top and bottom portions of the lamina and ligament are completely removed

Laminectomy. Beginning at the top left is a back view of a typical lumbar vertebra. Top right shows a complete laminectomy—the entire lamina has been removed. Middle left shows a hemilaminotomy, performed by removing one side of the superior and inferior lamina as well as the connecting ligamentum flavum. A foraminotomy involves performing a hemilaminotomy as well as removing part or all the facet joint (middle right). A dome laminectomy is performed by removing both sides of the lamina (bottom left).

Chapter 37

Spinal Fusion, Bone Graft Technology and Bone Morphogenic Protein (BMP)

Summary

Spinal fusions, otherwise known as spinal arthrodesis (Greek: arthro-joint, desis- to bind), are procedures which join two or more vertebrae together surgically. This is done to stabilize the spine in a locked position such that one vertebra cannot move against another, thus removing any abnormal motion. Spinal fusion can also be used to hold the spine in the correct shape if it has collapsed. Common indications for this type of surgery include instability of the spine or deformity caused by degeneration, tumor, infection, fracture, or an aggressive decompression procedure. Spinal fusions are accomplished with the use of bone grafts that help bridge the two bones together. Bone grafts can either come from your own body (an autograft), a cadaver (allograft) or from a synthetic source. Bone grafts are combined with a scaffolding known as spinal instrumentation that consists of screws, rods, and cages to hold the spine together as it heals. There are many different implants and techniques available to surgeons and patients, and the science behind them continues to expand at a rapid rate.

Case

Mrs. Silver is a 75-year-old retired social worker who has severe lumbar steno-sis with a spondylolisthesis (slipped disc) at L4-5 incapacitating her from back and leg pain. Every step she takes is painful, and she has made the decision to seek treatment. She meets with her spine surgeon who suggests a lumbar fusion using a posterior lumbar interbody cage or a PLIF cage. The surgeon explains that in addition to placing two titanium cages into the disc space to help reconstruct the height she has lost from disc collapse, he will use some bone morphogenic protein (BMP) to perform a posterior lateral fusion or so called 360° fusion. To help the bone graft heal he will also place pedicle screws into the spinal vertebrae linked together with a rod. Using this approach, he thinks he will be able to perform a full decompression and relieve her of both back and leg pain. The procedure is successful, and Mrs. Slivers pain is great-ly relieved. She follows up with her surgeon who monitors the progress of the fusion healing with X-rays. At one year after surgery the surgeon declares her fusion totally solidified and tells Mrs. silver to go live her life without worry.

Introduction

Spinal fusion is a common procedure in spine surgery and involves the process of surgically joining two adjacent vertebrae, so they no longer move relative to one another. This is accomplished with the use of bone graft to stimulate the vertebrae to grow together and fixation hardware to brace the bones as they heal. Think of bone graft as concrete and the fixation hardware as the rebar or scaffolding. The hardware holds things together as the bone graft heals into a solid structure. Spinal fusion may also be referred to as spinal arthrodesis which comes from the Greek arthro (joint) and desis (to bind).

Spinal fusions were originally developed for the treatment of spinal tuberculosis which destroys the vertebra and results in significant deformity and pain. The doctor who pioneered the spinal fusion, Dr. Russell Hibbs, was originally blackballed by orthopedic associations because of his radical idea that fusing two vertebrae together in the spine could be helpful. History always has a way of rectifying injustice. Now, the number of spinal fusions performed only continues to increase each year as the baby boomer population ages. Spinal fusions are now used to treat many different wide-ranging conditions, including spinal degeneration, infection, fractures, progressive deformity, tumor, and spinal instability.

Spinal fusions can stabilize the spine and correct any deformity that may be causing pain. Disc spaces that are collapsed are reconstructed to the appropriate height and any angular deformity is corrected and locked into a good position. In other joints in the body, such as the knee and hip, arthrodesis or fusion is rarely performed because there are good joint replacement options. While joint replacement options exist in the spine, the indications for their use are very narrow and, frankly, the technology is still developing. Each of the 24 vertebra is, to some degree, a motion segment of the spine, so immobilizing a few of them still allows sufficient spinal movement. Therefore, fusing some vertebrae is very well tolerated.

Why Spinal Fusion Gets a Bad Rap

Most patients will not like the thought of having two of their vertebrae joined with rods and screws, but spinal fusion can be an incredibly powerful tool to treat pain. However, if you don't need a spinal fusion and get one, you will probably not be happy. This is like a getting a total knee replacement in a knee that is perfectly normal—you will notice the difference between what you could do before and after if the knee was not originally causing pain. Spine surgeons are generally very careful about recommending spinal fusions because it is a big procedure with many risks.

Spinal fusions are only useful for specific spinal conditions and, as stated above, are used primarily to treat deformity and instability. This includes instability arising from performing such an extensive decompression of your spine that the required removal of bone or ligament renders the spine unstable. Spinal fusions performed to treat back pain due to degenerative disc disease are where people get into trouble. A spinal fusion will give you back pain—at least temporarily, and so, if the source of your back pain is not clear, having a spine fusion is like trying to treat a viral infection with penicillin (penicillin is only effective against bacteria). If you are considering having a spinal fusion for a bad disc or for nonspecific back pain, you may want to reconsider or at least talk it over carefully with your surgeon.

The Basics of Spinal Fusion Biology

Bones are composed of cells which live in a hard mineral matrix. Spinal fusions heal in a similar way to a broken bone. When a bone breaks, blood vessels at the site of the break bleed and form a hematoma (a pool of blood) to which stem cells (cells which lack a specific function but can become functional cells like muscle or bone) migrate and, once there, differentiate into (change into) bone-forming cells. These cells form a soft bone (callus) that slowly turns it into hard normal bone. When you break a bone, a cast may be placed to stabilize the bone and allow it to heal. This makes intuitive sense. It's hard to imagine a bone healing if it can flop around, just as it would be hard to imagine gluing two pieces of wood together without securing them with a clamp.

A spinal fusion works by creating an environment where two bones can heal together. This typically requires two elements: bone graft (that serves as glue) and stability provided by some sort of fixation device (that serves as a clamp). In modern spine surgery screws, rods, plates, cages, and hooks hold bones together and give them the stability to heal. Sounds medieval, but spine surgeons are experts at placing this hardware in a safe way that is becoming increasingly less painful.

The bone graft material is infiltrated by your own bone-forming cells and gradually the graft turns into normal bone. This process is biologically complicated and takes upward of a year to obtain full strength. The fixation devices provide the stability to hold the bones in place until the bone graft is solid and are only intended to support the spine for a short period of time. They will not resist motion independent of a solid fusion for more than a few months. If the bone graft fails to heal, it becomes a pseudoarthrosis (or false joint) which is a painful condition and may require a second surgery to remove and replace the hardware.

Bone Graft

Bone graft can come from many sources and ideally has three major properties: osteoinduction, osteoconduction and osteogenesis. These are complicated medical terms but are important to understand, so I will explain each in turn:

- **Osteoinduction: This is the process by which stem cells turn into bone-forming cells. This requires chemical signals such as bone morphogenic protein which tell the cells to activate bone-forming genes. The ideal bone graft contains these signaling molecules.**

- **Osteoconduction: This refers to the ability of a bone graft to act as a matrix where the body's own new bone cells can infiltrate and take up residence. Think of osteoconduction as providing a good environment for attracting bone cells and allowing them to thrive. We tend to think of bone as inert, but this could not be further from the truth. Bone is a living organ system, housing numerous cell types in a complex mineral matrix with a rich blood supply. The cells in the matrix are what keep the bone healthy by constantly breaking down old parts and rebuilding new ones. A material with good osteoconduction is porous and similar in structure to the normal bone mineral matrix. A solid material, for example, would have poor osteconduction because there would be no way for cells to enter it.**

- **Osteogenesis: Osteogenesis refers to the capacity of living bone cells in the graft itself to reproduce. A good example of this would be bone graft**

from your own body which contains many bone cells. Other examples involve commercially available grafts that contain living bone cells.

No commercial products to date possess all three of the ideal bone graft properties of osteoinduction, osteoconduction and osteogenesis.

Bone grafts are classified based on where they come from. An autograft is bone graft obtained from a donor site in your own body (such as the iliac crest in the pelvis). An allograft (from the Greek allos, or other) is a bone graft from a cadaver (dead person) that has undergone processing to make it safe for implantation. In addition to autografts and allografts there are a variety of manufactured bone grafts made of synthetic materials.

autografts

In the past there were no other viable substitutes for autografts. For spinal fusions, large grafts could be cut out of the pelvis, which was painful. People often hurt more from the bone-grafting procedure than from the actual spinal fusion. In modern times autografts are used more sparsely and harvested through more minimally invasive means. Nonetheless, autografts remain the "gold standard" because there is no industry-produced material that matches it in osteoinduction, osteoconduction and osteogenesis (1).

There are two main places in the body where autograft is obtained during spine surgery. The first is the iliac crest, which some people may call the "hip bone" but has nothing to do with the hip. A better term would be the "waist bone" or pelvis. Minimally invasive approaches through small incisions are now used to obtain the graft. Nonetheless, obtaining autografts can still be painful, especially if the bone graft site is remote from the surgical site (for example, an iliac crest graft obtained for a cervical (neck) fusion). If the bone graft is obtained close to the site of surgery, you will hardly notice it because it will not be perceived as a separate pain. For example, bone graft obtained for a lumbar fusion is very well tolerated and generally is not even noticeable by the patient (2,3). There are risks involved in harvesting iliac crest graft such as neurologic injury, fracture, hematoma formation and infections. Sometimes, instead of obtaining formal structural graft, bone marrow from the iliac crest may be aspirated (withdrawn with a needle). Bone marrow contains osteoinductive and osteogenic properties, but does not have any solid osteoconductive structure and, therefore, must be combined with allograft.

The second place to obtain bone graft is from the area of surgery. When spine surgery is performed some bone is generally removed from the spine. This can be bone from the lamina that is removed during a decompression process or from other areas.

Vertebral bone is useful because it needs to be removed as part of the procedure anyway and still contains all the properties necessary to help form a fusion.

allografts

Allograft is bone obtained from a cadaver source that has been processed to remove any living cellular elements so that only the dead mineral matrix remains. Allografts go through a rigorous sterilization process to make them safe for implantation while retaining their mechanical properties. Unlike autografts, since only dead mineral matrix remains after this preparation process, allografts are strictly osteoconductive and serve mainly as scaffolds for your own bone cells to grow into. Overtime your body incorporates the allograft so that its matrix is populated with your own cells.

Because the tissue is processed and sterilized, there is little chance of immune rejection, as is possible with other transplants. Allografts are available as strong cortical struts, or as ground cancellous chips, both of which provide strength and a good environment for cell infiltration. Allograft is also available as demineralized bone matrix (DBM) which contains some growth factors/proteins that promote cellular migration but lack calcium. DBM has been shown to be very effective in promoting a fusion.

Allografts work well in spinal fusions and, unlike autografts, do not cause any complications at the donor site such as pain and scarring or even infection (1). However, there are some disadvantages such as the small risk of disease transmission (Hepatitis or Human immunodeficiency virus—HIV). The risk of these is miniscule— from 1/100,000 for hepatitis to 1/1,000,000 for HIV. Moreover, allografts are dead tissue and lack the osteoinduction or osteogenic properties found in autografts. However, to overcome this limitation allografts may be populated with a bone marrow sample from your pelvis containing cells capable of becoming bone cells (4).

synthetic bone grafts

Synthetic bone grafts derived from calcium have been created as an alternative to cadaver allografts. They are similar in consistency to native bone and are osteoconductive. Example compounds include hydroxyapatite, calcium phosphate and calcium sulfate. Unlike allografts, synthetic grafts have no risk for disease transmission. However, some preparations are known to cause wound drainage and may have poor strength.

There are several other synthetic compounds that are used as bone graft spacers, namely PEEK (polyetheretherketone) which is a non-absorbable plastic. PEEK is primarily used in cages, which are placed between two adjacent vertebrae after the disc between them has been removed. After being placed, the cages are packed with an allograft or autograft. Cages serve primarily as structural support and, in the past, did not have osteoinductive, osteoconductive or osteogenic properties. More modern cages have complex designs which make them osteoinductive and osteoconductive by reproducing the normal 3-dimensional structure of bone.

Bone Morphogenic Protein

The family of molecules known as bone morphogenic proteins (BMP) was discovered in the 1980s by the orthopedic surgeon Marshall Urist, who was looking for molecules to speed up bone healing in rabbits. BMPs are a family of naturally occurring designer proteins (numbered 1-8) that stimulate the formation of bone by signaling stem cells to become bone producing cells. This was obviously a useful discovery, not only for fracture healing, but also for spinal fusions.

Since their discovery, molecular extraction purification techniques have greatly improved, allowing us to use BMPs clinically. There are two main preparations that are used in surgery, recombinant human BMP-2 (rhBMP-2 and rhBMP-7). They are called "recombinant human" because they are derived from human genes and have less of a chance of generating an unwanted immune response.

While BMP is a very powerful and useful drug, like any medicine there can be side effects. One worrisome risk has been cancer. Although a hallmark study showed that BMP improved outcome scores and fusion rates by 12% when compared to traditional iliac crest bone grafting methods, cancer was more common in the BMP group (5). However, the fact that it was more common in one group does not necessarily mean a definitive conclusion on this point could be drawn. Encouragingly, later studies showed that there was no increased risk of cancer up to 3 years following the use of BMP in spinal fusions. In fact, the control arm (the group not receiving BMP) had a higher incidence of cancer (6). Recently, a large meta-analysis of 20 randomized controlled studies showed that lumbar fusions with rhBMP-7 had higher fusion success rates, better improvement in disability, lower reoperation rate compared to iliac crest bone graft, without significant difference in adverse events or cancer (7). At this point in time BMP has been in clinical use for around 40 years and it is well established as a non-carcinogenic substance.

BMP can cause side effects resulting from intense inflammation, including nerve irritation (radiculitis), seroma formation (a fluid collection), osteolysis (the breakdown of bone due to inflammation). The rate of these problems depends on how BMP is used. For example, BMP is no longer used in the anterior cervical spine because the swelling in the neck caused by BMP can be life threatening. The safety of BMP is not well established in women who may become pregnant or in women who may be nursing.

A final note about BMP is regarding its FDA (Food and Drug Association) clearance. The most popular preparation of BMP is called Infuse® which is produced by the corporation Medtronic. A common way for BMP to be used is to be packaged into an interbody cage to spur growth between two vertebrae. Currently the FDA has given a limited approval for BMP—it is to be used in conjunction only with cages produced by Medtronic for anterior lumbar interbody fusions (ALIF). There is nothing particularly special about the Medtronic cage that makes it more compatible with BMP—that's just how the patent for BMP was drawn up. Your surgeon may prefer to use BMP with other cages not produced by Medtronic which will not affect the efficacy of fusion. However, because the FDA has not specifically approved BMP use with other cages this practice is called "off-label use" of BMP, even though the function and technique is the same. Furthermore, any use of BMP in posterior lumbar and cervical fusions is considered "off-label" despite robust evidence that it is very safe (8–10). BMP functions independent of the type of cage used or location where it's applied.

gene therapy

In the future it may be possible to introduce the BMP gene into local tissues such that they produce local BMP and cause a robust fusion. However, this technology is science fiction currently. A certain amount of bone formation is a good thing, but one can easily imagine a situation where too much bone is formed without a good way to turn it off.

advanced materials and tissue engineering

Recently there have been many advances in the realm of material science and tissue engineering that have made contributions to spinal fusion surgery. Probably the most important of these is the design of implants that mimic the natural structure of bone such that native bone cells can easily incorporate into them and produce new bone. This is done through several techniques, the most powerful of which is 3D printing. In 3-D printing an implant is fabricated from scratch to mimic the 3-dimensional microstructure of bone (11). This technology has been used in total hip replacements to improve incorporation of implant surfaces of the hip cup into the bone of the pelvis. These advanced surfaces allow your own bone to grow into the implant, ensuring it will not come loose with time. Now this same technology can be used in spine surgery to enhance spinal fusions.

In the spine, 3D surface technology can transform an inert plastic or metallic graft into an implant capable of independently incorporating into the spine and creating a stable fusion. In other words, structural grafts become osteoconductive. Most spinal interbody cages that are used to reconstruct the disc space now incorporate advanced surfaces capable of having bone grow into them and thus becoming incorporated in the body.

Other advanced materials such as tissue scaffolds and hydrogels which mimic human tissues are in the experimental phase and not widely used (1).

designer cells

Bone grafts that contain living cells that can produce bone matrix are called osteogenic. The gold standard osteogenic graft is an autograft from the patient's own bone. Some surgeons, hoping to avoid the potential complications of taking an autograft, may use bone marrow aspirate (blood removed from the bone) obtained through a small needle and mix this with dry allograft. This combines the best of both worlds, populating a dry inert allograft with bone building stem cells (4).

There are currently also commercially available cellular bone matrices (CBMs) such as Osteocel® and Trinity® that contain stem and progenitor cells which are claimed to produce osteogenic properties. While products may be proven superior to traditional autograft and allograft in the future, there currently is not enough data to demonstrate advantage to their use (12).

Fixation Devices

If the bone graft is the mortar which helps a spine fuse, fixation devices are the scaffolds to hold everything in place. Fixation devices have also evolved considerably since the advent of the spinal fusion but continue to essentially consist of metallic devices that can anchor into the vertebrae and are connected with a rod. The anchors can be in the form of wires, hooks, or screws.

The most common fixation device used currently is the pedicle screw, which is inserted into the pedicle of the vertebra. Pedicle screws are safe to use because they are fully contained within bone and do not come into contact with the nerves or spinal cord. Pedicle screws are typically inserted on either side of a vertebra and are connected with rods to adjacent vertebrae. These devices thus support the spinal column and stop motion across a segment allowing the fusion to heal. There are many different brands and styles of pedicle screw, but all are in essence the same and have similar features.

An interbody cage (also known as a spacer), is a small device that is placed into the disc space between vertebrae to support the spine and promote a fusion. There are many different interbody cages available on the market but, again, all have similar properties. They come in different sizes and can help reconstruct a collapsed disc space.

Types of Spinal Fusions

There are many ways to perform a spinal fusion; however, the basic concept is to get the bone surface to bleed (a process known as decortication) and put bone graft between the areas you want to fuse. Getting the bone surface to bleed allows a good blood supply to the bone graft so it can heal. Spinal fusions may be instrumented, meaning they are done with the use of a pedicle screw or other fixation device, to stabilize the area, or they may be un-instrumented meaning just bone graft is used. Most spinal surgeons these days perform instrumented spinal fusions as it has been shown to increase the rate of a successful fusion; however, some surgeons still perform un-instrumented fusions. Un-instrumented fusions can be used in situations where adding metallic devices is not desirable or dangerous. The advantage of performing a un-instrumented fusion is that it can still stabilize the spine in a situation where it could be technically challenging to put in fixation devices.

Most spinal fusions are classified based on where the bone graft is placed. For example, a posterior spinal fusion is one which places the bone graft along the lamina and spinous processes, which lie on the back (posterior) side of the vertebra. A posterolateral spinal fusion is done when bone graft is placed along the sides of the vertebrae between and in contact with the transverse processes—they extend on either side of a vertebra. Anterior spinal fusions are accomplished by placing bone graft and interbody spacers in the disc space. There are several different ways to perform an interbody fusion which are discussed in chapter 41.

Conclusion

Spinal fusions are powerful procedures that when used for the right reasons can significantly improve your quality of life. There is a lot of complicated science that goes into accomplishing a fusion but, in essence, fusion is trying to get two bones to grow together. This is done to restore a collapsed or twisted spine to its natural shape or prevent abnormal grinding between vertebrae from causing pain. Currently, we use pedicle screws and rods to connect the vertebrae and a variety of bone grafts to help the gap between them grow together.

Frequently Asked Questions

- **Will a spinal fusion reduce my motion or mobility?**

The short answer is yes. Spinal fusions are designed to stop motion between vertebrae. However, most patients who need spinal fusions are so debilitated from pain they are not moving much to begin with. Spinal fusions can stop the pain and surprisingly, increase your function.

- **Will a spinal fusion cause the disc above to wear down faster?**

The discs above and below a spinal fusion tend to wear out over time—known as adjacent segment degeneration (ASD). Degeneration in and of itself is not problematic unless it causes symptoms. Symptomatic degeneration occurs at a rate of 16% every 10 years (13). Whether or not this is the result of the spinal fusion is not definitively proven (it could be that the disc above has just worn out). My personal belief is that a spinal fusion will cause accelerated degeneration of the segment above or below and this should be anticipated by spinal fusion patients.

References

1. Katsuura Y, Shafi K, Jacques C, Virk S, Iyer S, Cunningham M. New Strategies in Enhancing Spinal Fusion. HSS Jrnl. 2020 Jul;16(2):177–82.

2. Radcliff K, Hwang R, Hilibrand A, Smith HE, Gruskay J, Lurie JD, et al. The Effect of Iliac Crest Autograft on the Outcome of Fusion in the Setting of Degenerative Spondylolisthesis. J Bone Joint Surg Am. 2012 Sep 19;94(18):1685–92.

3. Sheha ED, Meredith DS, Shifflett GD, Bjerke BT, Iyer S, Shue J, et al. Postoperative pain following posterior iliac crest bone graft harvesting in spine surgery: a prospective, randomized trial. The Spine Journal. 2018 Jun;18(6):986–92.

4. Niu CC, Tsai TT, Fu TS, Lai PL, Chen LH, Chen WJ. A comparison of posterolateral lumbar fusion comparing autograft, autogenous laminectomy bone with bone marrow aspirate, and calcium sulphate with bone marrow aspirate: a prospective randomized study. Spine (Phila Pa 1976). 2009 Dec 1;34(25):2715–9.

5. Simmonds MC, Brown JVE, Heirs MK, Higgins JPT, Mannion RJ, Rodgers MA, et al. Safety and Effectiveness of Recombinant Human Bone Morphogenetic Protein-2 for Spinal Fusion: A Meta-analysis of Individual-Participant Data. Annals of Internal Medicine. 2013 Jun 18;158(12):877.

6. Kelly MP, Savage JW, Bentzen SM, Hsu WK, Ellison SA, Anderson PA. Cancer Risk from Bone Morphogenetic Protein Exposure in Spinal Arthrodesis: The Journal of Bone and Joint Surgery. 2014 Sep;96(17):1417–22.

7. Liu S, Wang Y, Liang Z, Zhou M, Chen C. Comparative Clinical Effectiveness and Safety of Bone Morphogenetic Protein Versus Autologous Iliac Crest Bone Graft in Lumbar Fusion: A

Meta-analysis and Systematic Review. Spine. 2020 Jun 15;45(12):E729–41.

8.	Kim HJ, Buchowski JM, Zebala LP, Dickson DD, Koester L, Bridwell KH. RhBMP-2 Is Superior to Iliac Crest Bone Graft for Long Fusions to the Sacrum in Adult Spinal Deformity: 4- to 14-Year Follow-up. Spine. 2013 Jun;38(14):1209–15.

9.	Bess S, Line BG, Lafage V, Schwab F, Shaffrey CI, Hart RA, et al. Does Recombinant Human Bone Morphogenetic Protein-2 Use in Adult Spinal Deformity Increase Complications and Are Complications Associated With Location of rhBMP-2 Use? A Prospective, Multicenter Study of 279 Consecutive Patients: Spine. 2014 Feb;39(3):233–42.

10.	Weinberg DS, Eoh JH, Manz WJ, Fakunle OP, Dawes AM, Park ET, et al. Off-label usage of RhBMP-2 in posterior cervical fusion is not associated with early increased complication rate and has similar clinical outcomes. The Spine Journal. 2022 Feb;S152994302200050X.

11.	Katsuura Y, Qureshi SA. Additive Manufacturing for Metal Applications in Orthopaedic Surgery: Journal of the American Academy of Orthopaedic Surgeons. 2020 Jan;1.

12.	Abedi A, Formanek B, Russell N, Vizesi F, Boden SD, Wang JC, et al. Examination of the Role of Cells in Commercially Available Cellular Allografts in Spine Fusion. 2020;102(24):10.

13.	Ghiselli G, Wang JC, Bhatia NN, Hsu WK, Dawson EG. Adjacent segment degeneration in the lumbar spine. J Bone Joint Surg Am. 2004;86(7):1497–503.

Figures:

Osteoconductive Graft

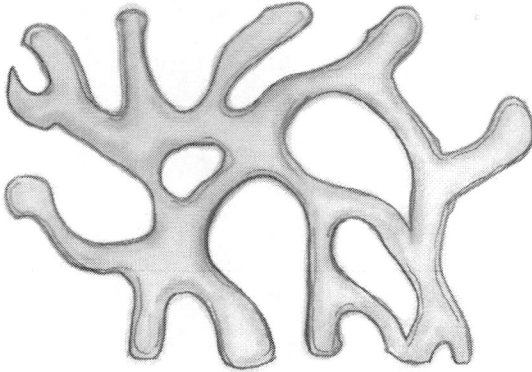

Mineral bone provides a scaffold for bone cells to populate

Osteogenic Graft:

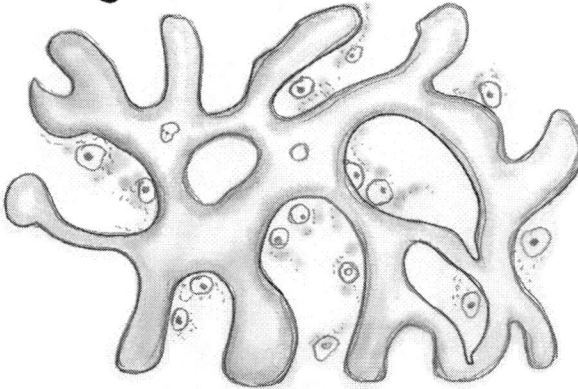

Bone grafts are called osteogenic when they contain cells which can produce bone

Osteoinductive Graft

BMP

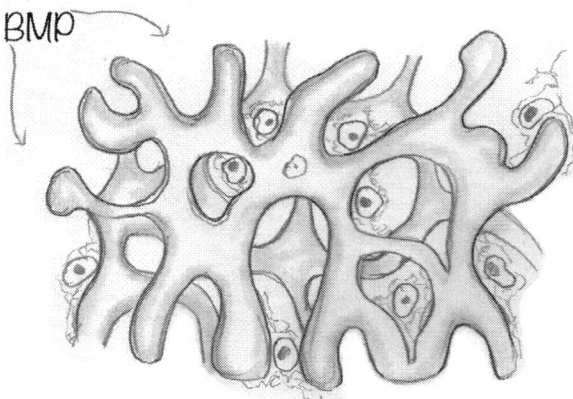

Bone grafts containing growth factors such as bone morphogenic protein (BMP) stimulate bone growth

Fusion biology. A basic bone graft is osteoconductive meaning that it can act as a substrate (place) for bone cells to grow into (top). An osteogenic bone graft is one that contains a cell population that can generate new bone (middle). An osteoinductive graft is one that contains cellular signaling molecules such as bone morphogenic protein (BMP) that can stimulate bone cells to produce bone (bottom).

Posterior Lumbar Fusions

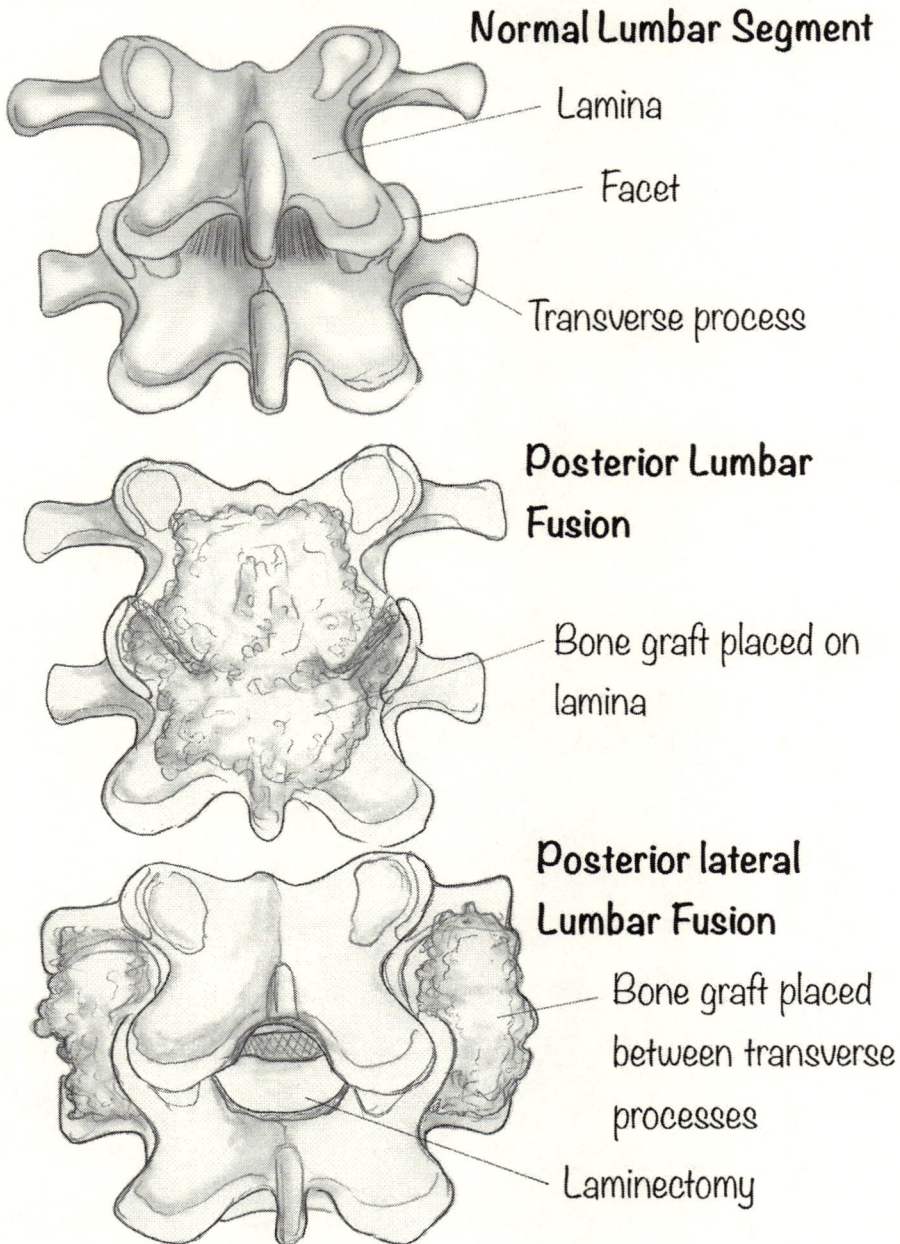

Normal Lumbar Segment

- Lamina
- Facet
- Transverse process

Posterior Lumbar Fusion

- Bone graft placed on lamina

Posterior lateral Lumbar Fusion

- Bone graft placed between transverse processes
- Laminectomy

Fusion basics. Spinal fusions may be performed by laying down bone graft directly on the lamina, known as a posterior spinal fusion (middle), or by placing bone graft between the transverse processes which is known as a posterolateral spinal fusion (bottom).

Chapter 38

How Surgeons Get to And Open The Spine to Fix the Problem: Open vs Minimally Invasive Spine Surgery, Lasers, and Other Spine Surgery Techniques

Summary

There is a huge effort currently being made to reduce the size of incisions in spine surgery and to make it more so-called "minimally invasive." Minimally invasive spine surgery is performed through multiple smaller incisions instead of the one larger midline incision that is used in traditional surgery (referred to as open surgery). To accomplish this minimally invasive approach, new retractors and imaging systems have been developed that allow the surgeon to access the spine in ways that were not previously possible. Ultimately, this all sounds good, but is this approach better in the long-term outcomes compared to more traditional approaches? I believe minimally invasive surgery has the power to enhance recovery; however, it certainly should not be applied to every spine case, as some patients are better served with a traditional approach. Currently there are no major long term outcome differences between minimally invasive and traditional spine surgery. Moreover, minimally invasive surgery is more technically demanding, and possibly riskier than open traditional surgery. Just because you hear of a new treatment which sounds amazing does not mean it has been thoroughly vetted and is superior to older treatments. In this chapter we examine the benefits and downsides of minimally invasive spine surgery

Case

Ms. Lavender is a very active 64-year-old psychologist who has an L4-5 spondylolisthesis (slipped disc) with severe central stenosis. She has done extensive research on various spinal techniques and has read up on minimally invasive ways to treat her problem. She saw one surgeon who recommended an L4-5 posterior spinal fusion with a transforaminal lumbar interbody fusion (TLIF) and formal decompression through an open posterior approach. She saw a second surgeon for another opinion who proposed performing a minimally invasive fusion known as XLIF with imaging-guided percutaneous screws. She prides herself on doing her research, and ultimately selects to have the minimally invasive approach as that seems like the most modern way of treating her problem. After the surgery she notices her, left quadriceps is significantly weaker than the other side which is explained to her as a normal part of the process. A repeat MRI scan is performed which shows some marginal improvement in her stenosis and slip. Her pain is improved somewhat but the weakness in her quad is worrisome. Her surgeon suggests she "give it more time," but her analytical mind is churning. Why is there residual stenosis? Ultimately after 6 months of therapy her strength in the quad improves and she feels better. She is satisfied with her surgery but wonders if the minimally invasive approach was worthwhile.

Introduction

The most common buzz words in spine surgery are "minimally-invasive spine surgery" or MIS. The idea behind minimally invasive surgery is to use smaller incisions to accomplish the same surgical goals as traditional approaches which require large incisions. This hopefully translates to a better surgical experience and speedier recovery. Patients often ask about MIS and whether they should have it. Minimally invasive spine surgery is a technique, and like other techniques described in this book, does not apply to everyone. Sometimes it can be advantageous and other times it can be detrimental. Minimally invasive surgery sounds more palatable to patients than traditional "open" surgery and at times can enhance recovery but, in other cases, it will make the procedure more difficult and may not get the job done.

In this chapter we discuss the concept of minimally invasive surgery, and other spine treatment buzz words. If you are looking for specifics about a particular procedure, please see the other chapters dedicated to individual techniques.

Some important reminders for this chapter: the term approach refers to how the surgeon accesses the spine. When spine surgeons talk about an anterior approach to the surgery, they are talking about performing surgery on a patient while the patient is lying face up (supine) and going through the front of the body. With a posterior approach, the patient is lying face down (prone) and the incision is made on the back. For a lateral approach the patient is sometimes lying face down and sometimes positioned on his/her side and the spine is accessed through the flank. The term exposure refers to how or how much the spine is exposed during surgery. Minimally invasive techniques all generally require less exposure than open techniques which require larger exposures.

Minimally Invasive Spine Surgery

Minimally invasive spine surgery (MIS) is really a grab-all term for many different techniques in spine surgery. The overarching theme of those who promote the surgery is that the procedure is accomplished through "smaller, non-muscle-splitting approaches" or put another way, percutaneously, that is, through small incisions in the skin. The goals of this approach are to avoid large open wounds that have a potential for infection and poor healing and to decrease muscle disruption which causes pain. Theoretically this should speed up the recovery and make the surgery itself easier to get through.

Traditional open surgery is done by making an incision through the midline of your back or abdomen and typically includes stripping the ligamentous structures and muscle off the bones to get access to the spine. The muscle is then pulled back to allow the surgeon access to the spine. This can increase soreness and pain following the surgery (1). The pain and soreness can be minimized by releasing the retractors every 1 hour of surgery for 5 minutes, but some surgeons do not do this. In contrast, minimally invasive techniques attempt to use small retractors and various other devices to accomplish spine surgery through small incisions without muscle stripping or destruction of the ligamentous complexes.

While this sounds amazing, the reality is somewhat different. Minimally invasive techniques dramatically reduce visibility of the spine, making the procedure more technically difficult and the chances of "incomplete" surgery higher. If a fusion is being performed, the surface area available for the fused bone to grow is also reduced. Minimally invasive techniques also require significant amounts of radiation from intra-operative computer tomography (CT) to guide instruments. The surgeon then uses computer navigation to assist in putting hardware in because there is no visibility. Because the surgeon is relying on computer technology to put in screws, if the computer is off, it can lead to major complications. Just like any computer system, it can malfunction or simply not work that day.

Smaller non-muscle splitting incisions are advertised in MIS, but this is a misnomer and misleading since traditional spine surgery is done generally without splitting the muscle and minimally invasive approaches are all done by splitting the muscle. A more accurate description would be "midline-preserving" surgery as MIS techniques all generally leave the middle ligamentous structures intact (the ligaments linking the spine together). The midline is preserved because most of the work is done from the side of the spine.

Despite all of this, MIS procedures can be performed through small incisions, require less anesthesia, and in some cases can be done on an outpatient basis. I use minimally invasive surgery in my practice and do believe it has its uses. The key to success is selecting the correct problem and the correct patient on whom to use these tools. Minimally invasive does not necessarily mean maximally effective. Some problems are more severe and do not benefit from half measures. Most spine procedures can be performed on a minimally invasive basis, but I believe some are better suited for this approach than others.

Minimally Invasive Lumbar Decompression

The first minimally invasive procedure to decompress the lumbar spine was the injection of a digestive enzyme (Chymopapain) into the intervertebral disc to dissolve disc herniations in a process known as "chemonucleosis." This practice is all but discontinued because frequently the medicine would spill out into the spinal canal, resulting in complete paralysis and severe allergic reactions—not good.

Similarly, some surgeons used lasers to debulk and disintegrate the intervertebral disc to decompress the nerves compressed by the herniated disc material. This was done in a minimally invasive fashion, where the laser was inserted in a "blind" fashion without a formal exposure. The idea was to use a high-powered laser which could burn through tissue to evaporate a disc herniation. The laser was inserted into the intervertebral disc and used to disintegrate it. Because this procedure was done in a "blind" fashion it had complications associated with heat injury to nerves and major blood vessels. The famous Laser Spine institute in Tampa Florida went bankrupt in 2019 after a wake of malpractice lawsuits and offering illegal incentives to patients such as transportation and hotels (2). Laser surgery is not performed in mainstream spine surgery currently.

Microscopes and endoscopes that can look into the spine through small incisions are the current iteration of minimally invasive surgery. Like arthroscopic surgery used in the knee and shoulder, in endoscopic spine surgery a small fiberoptic camera is placed into the spine to help magnify the surgical field and assist surgery. In contrast, microscopes are external to the surgery site but similarly help the surgeon see the nerves and discs better and thus help limit exposure of the spine. Small tubes and other more advanced retractor systems are used in conjunction with microscopes to allow a surgeon easy access through small incisions to a location that would once have required a larger open exposure. The use of tubes is considered a form of minimally invasive spine surgery. Currently there is no significant difference in clinical recovery or safety between the use of tubes to perform a microdiscectomy, and endoscopic surgery (3,4).

I believe that MIS concepts are best suited for decompression and less well-suited for fusion (as described below). In decompression surgery the goal is to remove offending structures with as little disruption of tissue as possible and MIS techniques do help accomplish this. In fusion surgery, the goal is ultimately to get two or more vertebrae to grow together which exposure and visibility of the spine help facilitate. Traditionally this has been done through an incision in the back and full exposure of the spine but as we will discuss below, there are now many new techniques that are marketed as minimally invasive to avoid this approach. Again, the overarching theme of minimally invasive procedures is that they are done in such a way as to reduce the pain from the initial surgery.

minimally invasive anterior lumbar fusion

Anterior (front) approaches are used to reconstruct the anterior column of the spine meaning, typically, any collapsed disc or damaged vertebra. This is accomplished with the implantation of a graft interbody spacer (placed between the large round vertebral bodies of two adjacent vertebrae). The spacer sits between the vertebrae in the disc space and promotes fusion between the bones. Anterior abdominal approaches are included in the grab-all term of minimally invasive spine surgery for several reasons. First, anterior approaches are generally well tolerated causing less pain than posterior approaches because there is less muscle splitting. Secondly, they accomplish the goals of decompressing the spine without having to open the spinal canal (see below).

Procedures that fuse vertebrae in the low back by placing an interbody spacer between two vertebrae are known as LIFs (lumbar interbody fusions). The anterior lumbar interbody fusion or ALIF is an example of this where the surgeon approaches the spine from the front of the body and uses a spacer as part of the fix. Others of this type which are gaining in popularity are the extreme lateral lumbar interbody fusion or XLIF (approaching the spine from the side of the body—more on this below) and the oblique lumbar interbody fusion or OLIF (approaching the spine through the obliques). Both the XLIF and OLIF are considered alternative anterior approaches. Anterior approaches were traditionally performed through major open abdominal and thoracoabdominal exposures but now can be done through small minimally invasive exposures.

Anterior approaches can also be done through a laparoscopic approach (performed with the aid of a camera, like how many intraabdominal approaches are performed, for example, gall bladder surgery); however, studies have shown that there is no real meaningful difference in symptom reduction between this and an open approach and the laparoscopic procedure requires many special instruments and is considerably more technically difficult. The complication rate with laparoscopic ALIFs have been noted to be at least 4 times higher than with a standard open approach. Today most ALIFS are performed through a small open incision in the abdomen in a minimally invasive fashion that is very well tolerated without the use of microscopes or endoscopes.

The XLIF procedure is done through a small minimally invasive incision through your flank and the surgeon carefully inserts a retractor onto the spine itself after moving the abdominal contents aside. This approach is very effective but requires the retractor system to be placed through the lumbar nerves, which can cause some problems. The advantage with the XLIF procedure is that it puts the great blood vessels at less risk than with an ALIF anterior approach. The disadvantage is that there is a potential for neurologic injury; however, this is rare and can be avoided with the use of an electrical stimulator that helps detect if nerves are near the retractor. Stretching the nerves of the lumbar plexus may result in groin numbness or weakness of the quadriceps. These problems are generally not encountered through an open posterior approach (approaching the spine from the back by making an incision at the midline) as the surgeon knows exactly where all the nerves are and how to avoid them. Finally, the XLIF approach cannot be readily used for the lower lumbar levels such L5-S1 and sometimes L4-5.

Critical to understand about minimally-invasive anterior lumbar fusions, is that they frequently rely on so called "indirect decompression," which simply means that instead of physically decompressing the nerves—usually by removing tissue, the decompression is achieved indirectly by restoring disc height and shape to the spine. Indirect decompressions can be effective in specific cases but can leave residual stenosis (part of the spinal canal still narrowed) compared to direct decompressions. Most of the time this is inconsequential, as the restoration of normal anatomy and stabilization of the spine is more than enough to dramatically improve symptoms.

minimally invasive posterior lumbar approaches

Most posterior lumbar spine surgery is done through an open surgical approach on your back. This requires a midline incision and for the muscles to be stripped off the spine and retracted. This allows the surgeon to place implants into the spine and perform fusion as well as decompression procedures. Retraction of the muscles in the midline is painful, and can interfere with the midline ligaments. The midline ligaments contribute to spinal stability but are less important to preserve in fusions as the hardware will fully support the spine. Minimally invasive posterior techniques were developed to allow decompression and instrumentation of the spine with less tissue disruption to the muscles, skin, and ligaments.

Pedicle screws are fixation devices used to connect two adjacent vertebrae to keep them from moving while they fuse together. In an open approach these screws are traditionally placed into the spine using anatomic landmarks that the surgeon sees and feels during the procedure. However, they may be placed "percutaneously" through the skin using image-guidance systems to help guide the screws into the correct spot without exposing the spine. Image guidance is a critical part of MIS surgery because the surgeon exchanges a large exposure where he can see anatomic landmarks for a small incision where a computer becomes the surgeon's eyes and helps place hardware.

Image guidance can be either fluoroscopy with X-ray or 3D navigation with an intra-operative CT scan. In fluoroscopy, X-ray images are used to direct the screws into the correct position without need for the surgeon to see the spine itself. In 3D navigation, an intra-operative CT is performed and fed into a computer system to build a real time model of the spine. This model is then referenced against an antenna device (known as an implanted array), which is fastened to the skeleton and tells the computer where the patient's bones are located in space. The surgeon can then use this model to target instruments into the spine based on a 3D video projection, somewhat like a videogame. In computer navigation, the instruments are all tagged and followed by a camera system that allows the surgeon to track the motion of the instrument relative to the spine in space.

3D Navigation is incredibly powerful but does have some downsides. If the antenna is moved slightly all measurements can be totally off and the surgeon can have no idea, he or she is putting screws in the wrong place. Because the incisions are all small, it is not possible to check based on actual surgical feedback and serious errors can occur which might not have occurred in traditional surgery.

Image-guided screws are placed through incisions located off midline. The incisions may be smaller, but two incisions need to be performed (one on each side). These procedures are technologically marvelous but require significantly increased radiation exposure for both the surgeon and the patient. Recently the technology has been advanced even further with the advent of robotically assisted pedicle screw placement. Here the surgeon no longer directs screws into the spine but instead relies on a robotic arm to help guide screws. This technology can be helpful in cases where there is significant deformity of the spine or where anatomic landmarks are non-existent.

The transforaminal lumbar interbody fusion procedure (TLIF), in which the surgeon approaches the site of decompression and fusion via the foramen (the opening in the spine where nerve roots exit), may be performed through a minimally invasive style. In a TLIF procedure the interbody device is placed in the disc space of the spine by removing one of the facet joints. The TLIF may be done through a traditional lumbar exposure or through a minimally invasive exposure using a tube.

Minimally invasive (MIS) TLIFS do reduce surgical trauma, but one must also consider the goals of the operation. The overarching goal is to create a stable healed fusion—so the 1- week recovery rate is less important than the overall long term recovery rate and durability of a procedure. Open TLIFS allow the placement of much more bone graft across a wider bone surface thus increasing the changes of successful fusion. MIS TLIFs rely entirely on fusion through placement of the graft cage. In a procedure which success is measured by fusion rate, I still prefer open exposures to ensure the job gets done to the best of my ability. Nonetheless, there is new long-term evidence that MIS and open TLIF procedures are essentially equivalent with slight improvement in short term recovery with the MIS TLIF (5).

Outcomes

Minimally invasive spine surgery has a lot of proposed benefits but many of these are theoretical. Most studies comparing minimally invasive surgery (MIS) to open surgery are of poor quality, and definitive conclusions cannot be drawn from them. However, there have been some several large studies which have compared the standard open approach to minimally invasive approaches.

MIS approaches have been linked to longer surgeries but less peri-operative narcotic pain medication requirements (6,7). What this means is that the surgeries do take longer to perform, but there may be less pain afterwards in the short peri-operative period. In a large meta-analysis comparing standard to minimally invasive lumbar decompression for lumbar spinal stenosis, MIS decompression had a significantly decreased rate of need for an eventual lumbar fusion, total reoperation, or subsequent spinal instability compared to open approaches (8). I believe this highlights the power for MIS for decompression surgery where minimizing soft tissue and bone trauma can be very important. For lumbar fusion procedures, a large meta-analysis comparing standard open to MIS posterior lumbar fusion showed no difference in reoperation rates, fusion rates, or surgical complications. There was a decreased medical complication rate with MIS approach (9). For fusion, MIS seems to be less important in the long term but may have some short-term gains.

Conclusions

Some surgeons think minimally invasive surgery is worthless, while others think it's a godsend. This really comes down to what the surgeon's experience is and how the surgeon was trained. Minimally invasive spine surgery can result in smaller incisions and a theoretical faster recovery. The ultimate outcomes tend to be similar between traditional open approaches and minimally invasive surgery and, having performed both, I would argue that the two are very similar in the end. I think it comes down to surgeon preference. If your surgeon thinks he can get the job done through a minimally invasive approach, then that is the way to go, but remember minimally invasive does not automatically mean maximally effective.

Frequently Asked Questions

• **Is it possible for a robot to put my screws in incorrectly?**

Yes. Although use of navigation and robotics decrease the incidence of screw malposition, major complications have occurred from technical errors in computer navigation and robotic-assisted surgery (10). In these cases, the surgeons blindly follow machine instructions and have no feedback on when something is going terribly wrong. Screws and hardware can end up in the wrong place causing serious problems. While the technology overall improves accuracy of screw placement, it's important to note that new technology is not always perfect and can't beat surgical training, experience, and intuition (at least not yet).

References

1.   Datta G, Gnanalingham KK, Peterson D, Mendoza N, O'Neill K, Van Dellen J, et al. Back pain and disability after lumbar laminectomy: is there a relationship to muscle retraction? Neurosurgery. 2004 Jun;54(6):1413–20; discussion 1420.

2.   Company TP. Tampa's Laser Spine Institute abruptly closes, lays off hundreds [Internet]. Tampa Bay Times. [cited 2021 Apr 20]. Available from: https://www.tampabay.com/business/tampa-based-laser-spine-institute-is-shutting-down-20190301/

3.   Gadjradj PS, Harhangi BS, Amelink J, van Susante J, Kamper S, van Tulder M, et al. Percutaneous Transforaminal Endoscopic Discectomy Versus Open Microdiscectomy for Lumbar Disc Herniation: A Systematic Review and Meta-analysis. Spine (Phila Pa 1976). 2021 Apr 15;46(8):538–49.

4.   Chen Z, Zhang L, Dong J, Xie P, Liu B, Wang Q, et al. Percutaneous transforaminal endoscopic discectomy compared with microendoscopic discectomy for lumbar disc herniation: 1-year results of an ongoing randomized controlled trial. Journal of Neurosurgery: Spine. 2018 Mar;28(3):300–10.

5.   Kwon JW, Park Y, Lee BH, Yoon SR, Ha JW, Kim H, et al. Ten-Year Outcomes of Minimally Invasive Versus Open Transforaminal Lumbar Interbody Fusion in Patients With Single-Level Lumbar Spondylolisthesis. Spine. 2022 Jun 1;47(11):773–80.

6.   Skovrlj B, Belton P, Zarzour H, Qureshi SA. Perioperative outcomes in minimally invasive lumbar spine surgery: A systematic review. World J Orthop. 2015 Dec 18;6(11):996–1005.

7.   Hockley A, Ge D, Vasquez-Montes D, Moawad MA, Passias PG, Errico TJ, et al. Minimally Invasive Versus Open Transforaminal Lumbar Interbody Fusion Surgery: An Analysis of Opioids, Nonopioid Analgesics, and Perioperative Characteristics. Global Spine J. 2019 Sep;9(6):624–9.

8.   Schöller K, Alimi M, Cong GT, Christos P, Härtl R. Lumbar Spinal Stenosis Associated With Degenerative Lumbar Spondylolisthesis: A Systematic Review and Meta-analysis of Secondary Fusion Rates Following Open vs Minimally Invasive Decompression. Neurosurgery. 2017 Mar 1;80(3):355–67.

9.   Goldstein CL, Macwan K, Sundararajan K, Rampersaud YR. Perioperative outcomes and adverse events of minimally invasive versus open posterior lumbar fusion: meta-analysis and systematic review. SPI. 2016 Mar;24(3):416–27.

10.   Shin BJ, James AR, Njoku IU, Härtl R. Pedicle screw navigation: a systematic review and meta-analysis of perforation risk for computer-navigated versus freehand insertion: A review. SPI. 2012 Aug;17(2):113–22.

Figures:

Traditional Open vs Minimally Invasive Spinal Fusion

OPEN TLIF (Transforaminal Lumbar Interbody Fusion): the spine is exposed completely and retractors are placed to hold muscle out of the way

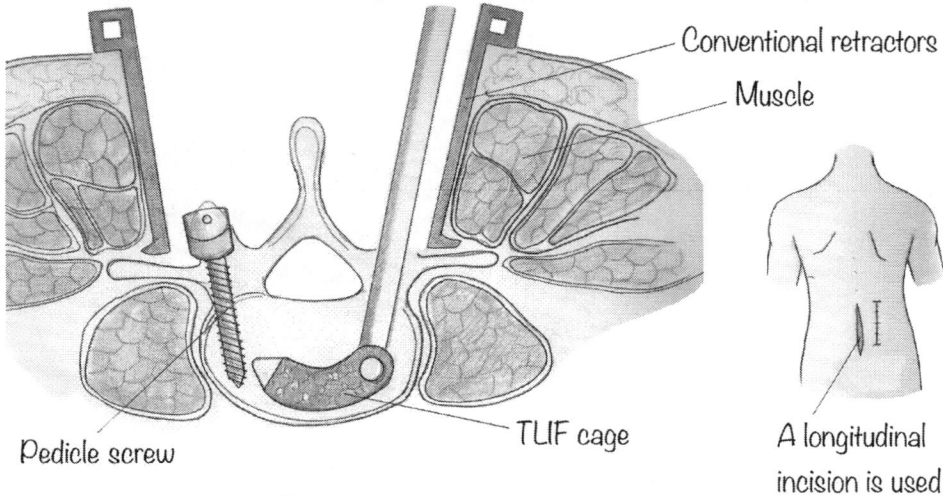

Conventional retractors

Muscle

Pedicle screw

TLIF cage

A longitudinal incision is used

MIS TLIF (Transforaminal Lumbar Interbody Fusion): instruments are placed percutaneously through the skin guided either by X-ray or CT.

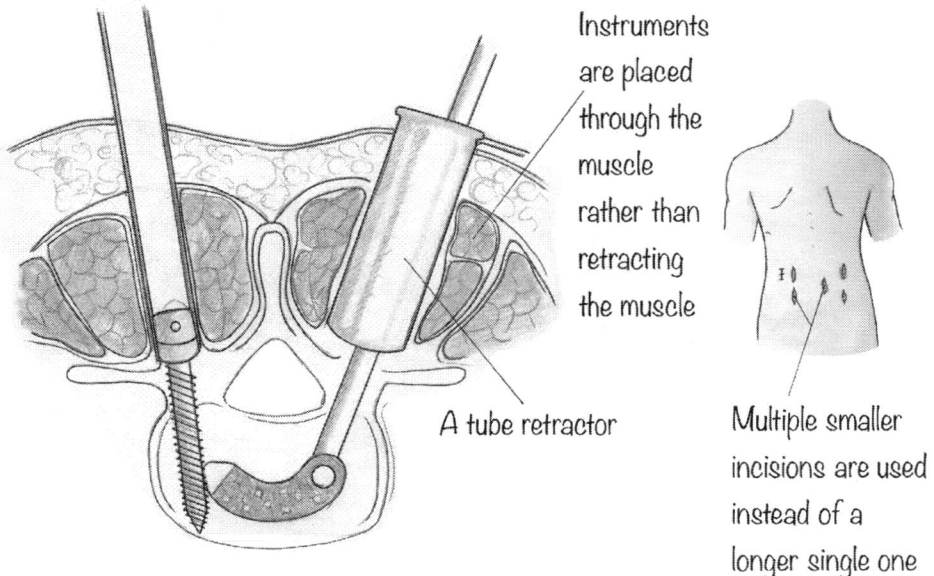

Instruments are placed through the muscle rather than retracting the muscle

A tube retractor

Multiple smaller incisions are used instead of a longer single one

TLIF (transforaminal lumbar interbody fusion procedure): open vs MIS. In an open TLIF, screws and an interbody spacer are inserted after performing a midline incision and retracting the muscles to the sides (top). In a MIS TLIF the screws and interbody spacer are inserted through small incisions in the muscle. Instead of one large incision there are several smaller ones (bottom).

Chapter 39

Removing a Spinal Disc Fragment That is Compressing a Nerve in The Low Back (Lumbar Discectomy)

Summary

The lumbar microdiscectomy is a very common, safe, and effective spinal procedure that is performed under visual magnification to remove a disc fragment compressing a lumbar nerve. A small opening in the spine (called a hemilaminotomy) is created to get access to the spinal canal and the nerves are retracted to allow the disc fragment to be removed. This can be done in many ways, including through a small open incision or through a minimally invasive approach with a tubular retractor, or even with the use of a fiberoptic endoscope. All approaches are very effective and different surgeons will have different preferences. Studies show that the outcomes are favorable to non-operative treatment and that good outcomes can be expected over the long-term in most patients. One of the most common complications Is reherniation, and so it is important to attend to your post-operative restrictions carefully.

Case

Ms. Pink is a 45-year-old marketing agent whose life has been put on hold by severe leg and back pain. She is typically very active and prides herself on her physical fitness. The pain started after a competitive tennis match; she was playing with her friends. Her whole leg and foot are numb and feel weak. She can't walk and even narcotic medicines can't touch the pain. Her surgeon recommends an epidural steroid injection which has no effect. She goes back and is desperate for surgery—even the thought of another week like this is hard to imagine. They decide to perform a microdiscectomy through a minimally invasive approach. The surgery takes about an hour-and-a-half, and she is discharged the same day. She thinks a miracle has occurred. Her pain is erased, and she can feel her leg again. She goes back to competitive tennis after 2 months of physical therapy. At 2 years after surgery, she is still feeling amazing, and looks back fondly on her surgery.

Introduction

The lumbar microdiscectomy is a common procedure used to treat leg pain or sciatica from a disc herniation compressing a nerve. Lumbar means located in the low back. The term "ectomy" means removal; a disc+ectomy means removal of the disc. The term micro means the surgery is performed through a small incision with the use of microscope or loupe magnification. Typically, a lumbar microdiscectomy is used to treat a herniated disc that has been pressing on a nerve in the low back and causing leg pain and has failed to get relief from non-operative treatments for at least 6 weeks.

A herniated disc is a disc whose jellylike center has escaped through a "tear" in its hard outer shell. When the escaped disc material presses against a nerve, you will know it! Usually after 6 weeks of non-operative treatments such as physical therapy, anti-inflammatory medications, and/or steroids, the pain from a herniated disc will have subsided. If after 6 weeks you have failed to get relief, a microdiscectomy may be in order if the pain is too much to deal with. In cases of progressive neurologic problems such as weakness or numbness or severe unrelenting pain, the microdiscectomy may be performed before the 6-week waiting period has passed.

What Is Involved in a Microdiscectomy?

A typical microdiscectomy is performed through a small incision, usually 2-3 cm (2.54 cm = 1 inch), made over the problematic spinal segment. Muscle tissue is spread to expose the lamina and spinous process on the symptomatic side of the body. A small tube retractor is inserted which allows the surgeon to access the spine.

A powerful microscope is then used to allow the surgeon to see down into the spine. To access the disc and spinal canal, a small opening is made in the bottom part of the lamina, a procedure known as a hemilaminotomy. A ligament that joins adjacent vertebrae, called the ligamentum flavum, is removed, which exposes the nerve and aids in decompression. The nerve and thecal sac (the lining that encases the spinal cord, nerves, and holds the cerebrospinal fluid (CSF)) are moved aside to expose the disc herniation and disc space. The disc fragment may be freely expressed and extracted or may require a small incision in the disc called an annulotomy. Any free fragments of disc are generally removed to decrease the risk of reherniation.

The two main techniques used to perform a microdiscectomy are "open" and "minimally invasive." The major differences between the two are the types of incisions made and the kind of retractor used. In an open approach, a larger midline incision is used, the spine is exposed on one side and a spreading retractor is inserted. In the minimally invasive technique, a smaller tube retractor is passed through the muscle. There are advantages to either technique and which one is used often depends on what your surgeon is comfortable with. As someone who performs both, I can say the differences between the two techniques are academic and the main concern for you as the patient is that your disc fragment is removed as safely as possible. Some say that there is a faster recovery with a microdiscectomy, but it has not been proven definitively (1).

What to Expect After a Microdiscectomy

Microdiscectomy is usually done in the outpatient setting, meaning that after a period of observation you can go home. If you have poor health, or the surgery was unexpectedly complicated, you may stay a night or two in the hospital. In most cases there is a dramatic relief of your leg pain, but you may have some incisional pain at the site of the procedure. If you are expecting a dramatic relief in your weakness or numbness you may be in for disappointment. Nerve damage is unpredictable, and you may have residual numbness or weakness that can take months to go away, if ever. You will not require any bedrest and should be able to walk after the procedure if you were able to do so before.

Recovery After a Microdiscectomy

The major concern following microdiscectomy surgery is reherniation of the disc, which is defined as having a period of symptom relief followed by sudden recurrence of your leg pain or numbness. Reoperation for a recurrent disc may be required in upwards of 9% of cases, with those at younger age more at risk (2). The symptoms may be the same as they were before surgery or may differ slightly. Currently there is no good way to prevent a disc herniation from recurring; however, common sense tells us that a reherniation is more likely to occur when higher forces are exerted across the spine during recovery. Thus, following your operation, you should not perform any vigorous activities that might cause a reherniation, such as lifting heavy objects of bending sharply at the waist.

You may start formal physical therapy 4-6 weeks after surgery. Rehab that starts immediately after surgery is no more effective at improving the prognosis than that which starts 4-6 weeks after surgery. Furthermore, there is no significant difference between a rehab program that is supervised versus one that is unsupervised, meaning one you do on your own may be just as effective as one you do with a therapist (3). Nonetheless, you do not get to just sit around after lumbar disc surgery. For the first 4 weeks you should get up and walk at least twice a day. The distance will vary depending on your overall cardiovascular health. Your doctor may recommend some gentle nerve glide exercises (see below) Once you are healed enough (around 4-6 weeks), you may be able to begin an exercise program where you work on your core strength.

Nerve glide exercises that help the nerves remain mobile after a decompression procedure.

- **Laying down on your back, gently pull your heel from an extended position towards your buttock, sliding the heel on the bed until your knee is bent, then reextend. Repeat on the other side and do a total of 10 reps on each side.**

- **Laying down on your back, have a family member or friend elevate your heel off the bed and gently bend your knee until your hip and knee are both at 90 degrees. Repeat on the other side for a total of 10 reps on each side.**

Outcomes

The success rate is very high for correctly indicated microdiscectomies. A large clinical trial comparing surgical versus non-operative treatment of lumbar disc herniations was the Spine Patient Outcome Research Trial (SPORT). This trial showed that surgically treated disc herniations had greater improvement in clinical symptoms up to 4 years out compared to those treated non-operatively (4). Long term outcomes are very favorable for lumbar microdiscectomies and most patients (around 70%) remain pain free up to 30 years following their procedure (5).

As stated above, one of the most common complications is reherniation of a new fragment of disc even if the primary fragment is removed. Other potential complications include wound infection, hematoma, and dural tears (a tear in the lining that encases the spinal cord, causing CSF to leak out). Nerve root damage or irritation is very uncommon but can also occur.

Conclusion

The lumbar microdiscectomy is one of the most common and most successful procedures in spine surgery. With modern techniques, this procedure can be done safely in an outpatient setting and with just a small incision. I have seen this procedure literally whisk away pain. In the correct patient, it can safely reduce pain with only minimal recovery.

Frequently Asked Questions

- **Can the surgery be performed using an endoscopic camera instead of a microscope?**

    Yes, this is possible, and while some centers specialize in this, it has not proven superior to conventional microscopic surgery. The use of the camera allows the incision to be slightly smaller but makes the surgery overall more difficult and requires pressurized fluid to be put in your spine. In some instances, this has caused temporary headache and other neurologic problems. While the technical advances are interesting, they have not been widely adopted as of this writing. Furthermore, just as the differences in outcome between an open and minimally invasive discectomy are insignificant, the differences in outcome between an endoscopic discectomy and microdiscectomy are also likely to be insignificant. A key area where endoscopic surgery seems promising is in the treatment of nerve root compression in the foramen as opposed to the central spinal canal (6).

- **Will there be increased risk to my back with the thecal sac (containing CSF) exposed?**

    No, this is generally not a concern; there is a thick, soft tissue sleeve still covering and protecting the lumbar spine.

- **If the disc is removed, what is providing the cushion between vertebrae?**

    If the disc is removed entirely, the bone of the vertebrae will come into contact and may cause problems. Thus, typically only the herniated portion of the disc is removed as well as any loose fragments, leaving most of the disc intact. These fragments are already "biomechanically useless" and serve no further function other than to cause you pain; thus, removing them does no harm. No further functional loss will occur from removing such fragments.

- **Will my spine degenerate further with removal of the bone and disc?**

Spinal degeneration is an ongoing problem regardless of whether surgery is performed. Long term outcome studies show that most people will have good results up to 30 years after the procedure and suffer no ill consequences.

- **What's the difference between the thecal sac and the dura (that can experience tears)?**

The thecal sac is another term for the membranous dura mater that holds the spinal fluid, nerves, and spinal cord.

References

1.   Rasouli MR, Rahimi-Movaghar V, Shokraneh F, Moradi-Lakeh M, Chou R. Minimally invasive discectomy versus microdiscectomy/open discectomy for symptomatic lumbar disc herniation. Cochrane Database Syst Rev. 2014 Sep 4;(9):CD010328.

2.   Abdu RW, Abdu WA, Pearson AM, Zhao W, Lurie JD, Weinstein JN. Reoperation for Recurrent Intervertebral Disc Herniation in the Spine Patient Outcomes Research Trial: Analysis of Rate, Risk Factors, and Outcome. SPINE. 2017 Jul;42(14):1106–14.

3.   Oosterhuis T, Costa LO, Maher CG, de Vet HC, van Tulder MW, Ostelo RW. Rehabilitation after lumbar disc surgery. Cochrane Back and Neck Group, editor. Cochrane Database of Systematic Reviews [Internet]. 2014 Mar 14 [cited 2020 Dec 29]; Available from: http://doi.wiley.com/10.1002/14651858.CD003007.pub3

4.   Weinstein JN, Lurie JD, Tosteson TD, Tosteson ANA, Blood EA, Abdu WA, et al. Surgical versus nonoperative treatment for lumbar disc herniation: four-year results for the Spine Patient Outcomes Research Trial (SPORT). Spine. 2008 Dec 1;33(25):2789–800.

5.   Burkhardt BW, Grimm M, Schwerdtfeger K, Oertel JM. The Microsurgical Treatment of Lumbar Disc Herniation. 2019;9.

6.   Butler AJ, Alam M, Wiley K, Ghasem A, Rush III AJ, Wang JC. Endoscopic Lumbar Surgery: The State of the Art in 2019. Neurospine. 2019 Mar 31;16(1):15–23.

Figures:

Lumbar Microdiscectomy

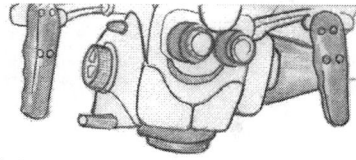

High powered dissecting microscope

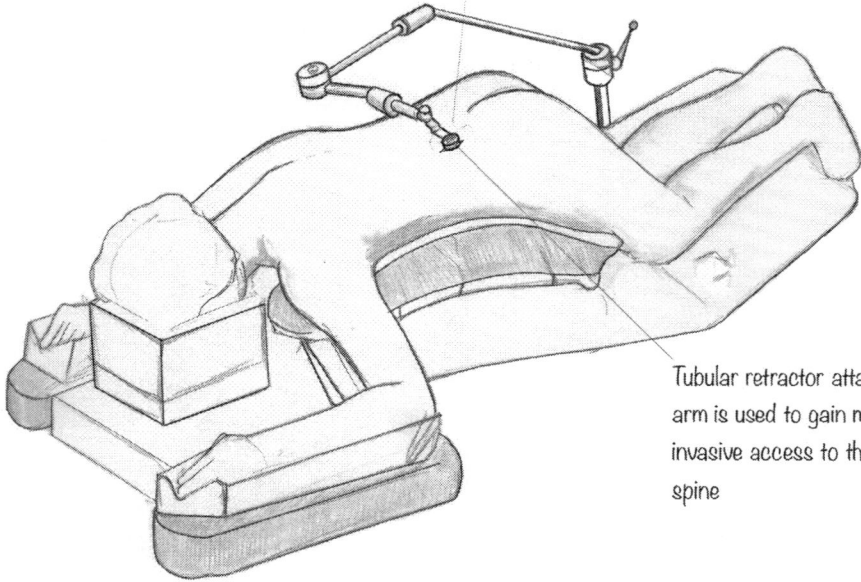

Tubular retractor attached to an arm is used to gain minimally invasive access to the lumbar spine

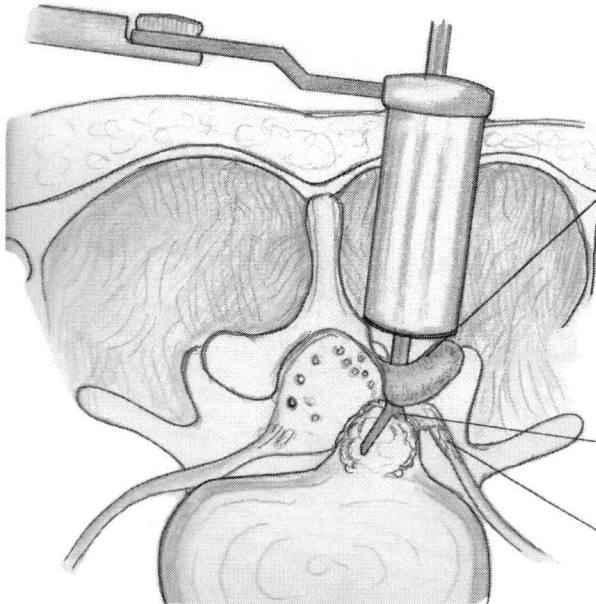

A small opening in the bone called a laminotomy is made to gain access to the spinal canal

A grasper device is used to remove the disc herniation

A compressed nerve root

Microdiscectomy. A microdiscectomy is performed with the patient lying in the prone position (on the stomach) using a high-powered microscope (top). A tube retractor can be used to access the spine and remove the disc in a minimally invasive fashion as viewed in this cross section (bottom).

Chapter 40

How Surgeons Remove a Damaged Disc in the Neck and Restore the Cervical Spine to Good Function— Anterior Cervical Discectomy and Fusion (ACDF)

Summary

The anterior cervical discectomy and fusion (ACDF) procedure is one of the most common surgical procedures to treat herniated or degenerative discs pinching nerves or the spinal cord in the neck. An ACDF procedure involves removing the intervertebral disc, decompressing the spinal cord, and placing a graft spacer to help reconstruct the disc space. A metal plate is then applied to stabilize the bones allowing them to fuse, but some spacers are "stand-alone" and do not require this. The surgery is very well-tolerated but there are some common adverse effects such as swallowing problems, hoarseness, and neck stiffness. In most cases this goes away with time or is something that you can live with. Rarely there can be catastrophic complications such as spinal cord injury, visceral organ injury, or compressive hematomas resulting in airway obstruction. The long-term outcomes are very good for ACDFs with about 90-95% good outcomes reported up to 10 years.

Case

Ms. Green is a 50-year-old homemaker who has been suffering from severe right arm pain and weakness for 2 years. Nothing seems to work, she has tried steroids, pain medications and physical therapy. In addition to the pain, she notices weakness in her grip, and trouble pushing with her arm. Her hand and thumb are numb, and it seems to get worse when she turns her head. She makes an appointment to see a spine surgeon who recommends an ACDF at C5-6 and C6-7 for herniated discs that are pinching on the nerve roots. She decides to have the procedure and the day after surgery immediately feels her arm pain is resolved. She notes some difficulty with swallowing after the procedure, but this gets better over the course of the week to the point where she can eat solid food easily. Her doctor has her wear a brace for 6 weeks after the procedure. Now she is about a year out and has no neck or arm pain. Her arm strength is back to normal.

Introduction

Anterior cervical discectomy and fusion (ACDF), similar to lumbar microdiscectomy, is both one of the most commonly performed and one of the most successful procedures in orthopedic surgery (1). For this reason, it is a work-horse approach for treating a multitude of cervical spine problems. As stated in the name of the procedure, an ACDF is performed through the front (anterior) of the neck (cervical) to remove a troublesome disc (discectomy) and replace it with a graft of some type to get the bones to grow together or fuse (fusion). Following placement of the graft a thin metal plate is typically applied to secure the two or more vertebrae together, although stand-alone grafts are also available that do not require the use of a plate.

Anterior cervical discectomy and fusion procedures are performed to relieve compression of the spinal cord and nerve roots from herniated discs but may also be used in trauma, and tumor surgery. A portion or all of the vertebra (the vertebral body) may also be removed; this is called a corpectomy. Relieving the pressure on the spinal cord in the neck can improve symptoms of imbalance and loss of dexterity, while decompressing the nerve roots can relieve pain, numbness, and weakness of the upper extremities.

Pressure on the spinal cord in the neck can result in a syndrome known as cervical myelopathy, with symptoms of general weakness, imbalance, incontinence, and loss of manual dexterity. Pressure on the nerve roots located in the neck can cause cervical radiculopathy (a pinched nerve in the neck) with symptoms of weakness, numbness, tingling and pain in the extremities. Both these conditions may be treated by an anterior cervical discectomy and fusion (ACDF). ACDFs can be done at a single level (here a level is two adjacent vertebrae and the disc between them) or multiple levels, depending on the degree of disc degeneration. They are among the most successful and well tolerated procedures in orthopedics.

The Anterior Approach to the Cervical Spine

Surgery done through the front of the neck (anterior) is a favorite of spine surgeons because it can be done with minimal pain to the patient. The anterior approach is accomplished through a small horizontal (sometimes vertical) incision placed in a skin crease. No major muscles are cut, but the airway and esophagus are retracted to expose the spine.

Discectomy, Grafting and Plating

Once the spine is exposed, the disc is carefully removed, and the interbody spacer of choice is inserted to prop open the disc space. The disc is typically removed using a small device known as a curette. Once the disc is removed the spinal cord is exposed by removing the posterior longitudinal ligament. At this point the spine surgeon looks at the thecal sac (the lining that encloses the spinal cord and holds the cerebrospinal fluid (CSF)) and can make sure the nerves are decompressed. A graft which recreates the dimensions of a healthy disc is inserted and helps rebuild the normal shape of the neck.

When this surgery was pioneered by Ralph Cloward, a surgeon from Hawaii, he initially inserted wedges of bone from the pelvis. Now there are many different commercially available grafts which make the procedure more effective and tolerable. For example, graft spacers are available in titanium, carbon fiber, a plastic called PEEK, and cadaver allograft bone, all of which work reasonably well. The choice of graft is up to your surgeon. Opening the disc space causes the foramen (the space where nerve roots exit from the spine) to open as well, decompressing the nerves (see chapter 38 on indirect decompression).

Interbody grafts typically have a hollow area that is filled with either autograft (bone graft from the pelvis, or local bone graft collected from drilling), or some form of synthetic graft that stimulates healing. Following placement of the graft, a metal plate is applied to the front of the bone with screws. Cervical plates are made from titanium and are low profile so that they do not take up much space in the neck.

stand-alone implants

As stated above most cervical plates are thin (1-2 mm) but they still take up some space in the neck and do press against the esophagus. For this reason, stand-alone interbody grafts have been developed which incorporate anchoring screws into the interbody spacer device inserted between the vertebrae. These devices, which are also known as zero-profile devices, have the benefit of taking up no added space in the front of the cervical spine. However, stand-alone constructs have been associated with an increased risk (up to 30%) of pseudarthrosis (failure to fuse) compared to standard plate and cage constructs (2). Thus, I mainly use these grafts for certain situations where the chances of pseudoarthrosis are low.

Post-op

Some surgeons use a brace after surgery to provide additional support for the first few weeks of the fusion. It's not absolutely essential for single level cervical fusions, but it's a decision best left to your surgeon (3). There are some adverse events to watch out for after an anterior cervical procedure such as difficulty swallowing, hoarseness, loss of mobility in the neck, failure of the vertebrae to fuse and some very rare complications, all discussed below.

difficulty swallowing

Difficulty swallowing (dysphagia) is a very common occurrence after an ACDF, occurring in about 50% of patients in the first month following surgery and higher in patients with 3-4 level fusions (4). The cause is likely due to multiple factors and could be related to plate thickness, retraction of the esophagus and the local nerves, swelling, change in alignment of the cervical spine and scarring. In most cases, dysphagia resolves within a month of surgery, but in a small handful of patients may persist and become permanent. To help prevent this from occurring steroids may be used either intravenously or locally in the wound to decrease inflammation and prevent swelling. Drinking ice cold liquids such as smoothies after surgery may also be helpful to reduce inflammation and ease swallowing.

hoarseness

Hoarseness (dysphonia) can occur following an anterior cervical procedure because of retraction of the recurrent laryngeal and superior laryngeal nerves that supply motor and sensory function to your vocal cords. If you are a professional singer, announcer, teacher, or someone who relies on your voice to draw an income, you should discuss the chances of this occurring prior to surgery. ACDF may not be the correct approach in these cases. Hoarseness is generally temporary, but in rare cases can become permanent.

loss of motion of the neck

Cervical fusions are designed to stop motion between vertebrae. In a person with a lot of mobility in their neck this may result in neck stiffness. While 1-level fusions do not result in perceptible change, 2- and 3- level fusions will result in increasing stiffness. Certain professions that require a lot of head tilting and angulation of the neck (surgeons, photographers, dental hygienists) may have difficulty with a multilevel cervical fusion.

Nonetheless, in most cases, ACDF procedures are performed on degenerated necks that already lack motion. Patients with significant degeneration in their spines will not notice an appreciable difference in neck motion and may feel as if they have more motion because of reduced pain.

pseudoarthrosis

As discussed in previous chapters, sometimes the vertebrae fail to fuse together. This is called a pseudarthrosis, non-union or "false joint." Pseudarthroses are for the most part asymptomatic in the cervical spine but in rare cases can result in neck pain. The more levels that are fused the greater the chance of a pseudoarthrosis. Even if a pseudoarthrosis is detected within a year after surgery, most go on to fuse over the course of 2 years (5). However, if you are very symptomatic you may require revision surgery which is usually a "back up" posterior cervical fusion. While the rate of nonunion ranges from 13-32% in ACDFs, many of these are asymptomatic and do not require further surgery (6).

rare but potentially devastating complications

Anterior cervical fusions are performed by moving essential structures around in the neck. This includes the airway, the esophagus, and the major arteries and veins of the neck. Injury to any of these structures is possible, but rare in trained hands. In some cases, a hematoma (a pool of mostly clotted blood) can develop and obstruct the airway. This is a medical emergency and must be addressed immediately to preserve life with an evacuation of the hematoma, sometimes done at bedside. Thus, most patients undergoing ACDFs are kept in the hospital overnight for observation, even if they feel great.

Outcomes

So, if you made it this far, you may be wondering why on earth people go through with these procedures. The reason is that ACDFs are well tolerated and enjoy a very high success rate for treating cervical pain and radiculopathy with long term (10 year) successful outcomes approaching 92-95% for reduction in arm pain, numbness and weakness (7–9). Similar results are reported for treatment of cervical spinal cord compression and myelopathy with this procedure.

Conclusion

The anterior cervical discectomy and fusion procedure is a tried-and-true treatment for a multitude of cervical spine problems. The most common complications are difficulty swallowing and some hoarseness, but these generally resolve with time. The ACDF has a good track record with excellent long term outcomes.

Frequently Asked Questions

- **What can happen after 10 years? I heard the disc above and below can "wear out."**

    Yes, this can happen. Whether it happens because of the fusion or because of natural aging of the disc is a matter of debate. As the fusion and patient gets older there is increased chance of needing another procedure done either above or below the fusion. Revision ACDFs are more dangerous and technically demanding because of scar formation from the first procedure but are still quite manageable in expert hands.

- **What about a disc replacement? Isn't this better?**

    This is a complicated question and I devote an entire chapter to it. Please see the chapter 44 on cervical disc replacement.

References

1.   Fountas KN, Kapsalaki EZ, Nikolakakos LG, Smisson HF, Johnston KW, Grigori-an AA, et al. Anterior cervical discectomy and fusion associated complications. Spine. 2007;32(21):2310–7.

2.   Gandhi SD, Fahs AM, Wahlmeier ST, Louie P, Possley DR, Khalil JG, et al. Radiograph-ic Fusion Rates Following a Stand-alone Interbody Cage Versus an Anterior Plate Construct for Adjacent Segment Disease After Anterior Cervical Discectomy and Fusion: SPINE. 2020 Jun;45(11):713–7.

3.   Overley SC, Merrill RK, Baird EO, Meaike JJ, Cho SK, Hecht AC, et al. Is Cervical Bracing Necessary After One- and Two-Level Instrumented Anterior Cervical Discectomy and Fusion?

A Prospective Randomized Study. Global Spine Journal. 2018 Feb;8(1):40–6.

4.   Bazaz R, Lee MJ, Yoo JU. Incidence of Dysphagia After Anterior Cervical Spine Surgery: A Prospective Study. Spine. 2002 Nov;27(22):2453–8.

5.   Lee DH, Cho JH, Hwang CJ, Lee CS, Cho SK, Kim C, et al. What Is the Fate of Pseudarthrosis Detected 1 Year After Anterior Cervical Discectomy and Fusion?: SPINE. 2018 Jan;43(1):E23–8.

6.   Crawford CH, Carreon LY, Mummaneni P, Dryer RF, Glassman SD. Asymptomatic ACDF Nonunions Underestimate the True Prevalence of Radiographic Pseudarthrosis. Spine. 2020 Jul 1;45(13):E776–80.

7.   Engquist M, Löfgren H, Öberg B, Holtz A, Peolsson A, Söderlund A, et al. A 5- to 8-year randomized study on the treatment of cervical radiculopathy: anterior cervical decompression and fusion plus physiotherapy versus physiotherapy alone. Journal of Neurosurgery: Spine. 2017 Jan;26(1):19–27.

8.   Bohlman HH, Emery SE, Goodfellow DB, Jones PK. Robinson anterior cervical discectomy and arthrodesis for cervical radiculopathy. Long-term follow-up of one hundred and twenty-two patients. J Bone Joint Surg Am. 1993 Sep;75(9):1298–307.

9.   Heidecke V, Rainov NG, Marx T, Burkert W. Outcome in Cloward Anterior Fusion for Degenerative Cervical Spinal Disease. Acta Neurochirurgica. 2000 Mar 15;142(3):283–91.

Figures:

Cervical Spine Degeneration:

A view of the cervical
spine from the front
(anterior)

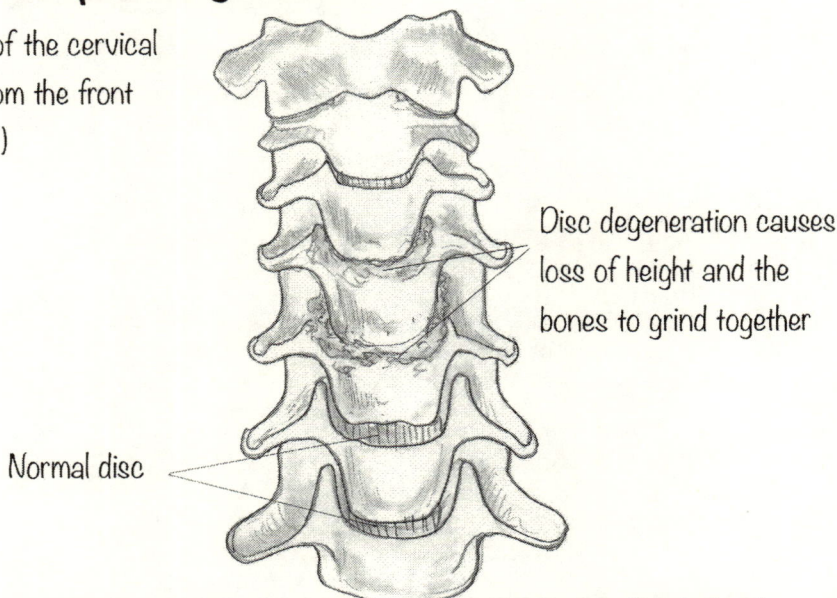

Disc degeneration causes
loss of height and the
bones to grind together

Normal disc

Anterior Cervical Discectomy and Fusion (ACDF)

Front view:

Side view:

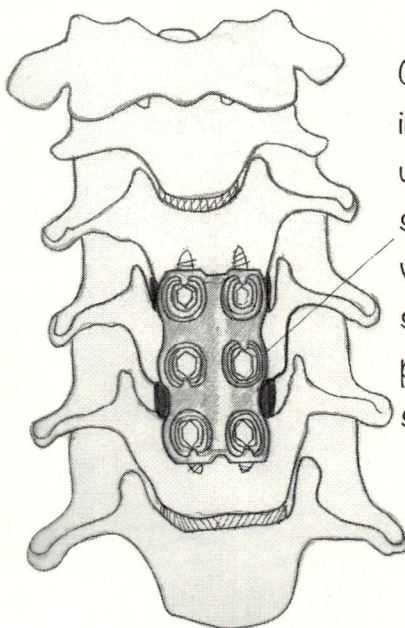

Cages are
inserted in the
wornout disc
spaces and the
vertebrae are
stabilized by a
plate and
screws

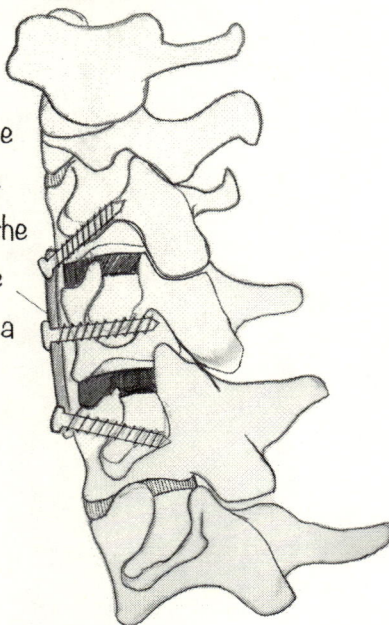

ACDF. The cervical vertebrae undergo degeneration at the C3-5-disc spaces (top). A cervical fusion and plate can be used to stabilize and decompress the degenerated segments (bottom left and right).

Chapter 41

When Fixing the Spine in the Low Back Requires Fusing 2 Vertebrae: Lumbar Spinal Fusion

Summary

Lumbar fusions are procedures which surgically join two or more vertebrae together in the lower back. There are many ways to accomplish this, but the basic principles are the same: bone graft is placed around the vertebrae to help them grow together while screws, rods and cages are used to hold the bones in place. Lumbar fusion is a powerful treatment commonly used to treat spinal deformity, stenosis, instability, and many other conditions. Lumbar fusions are often performed with spinal decompression and represent one of the most common spinal operations in the world.

Nowadays, fusion techniques known as lumbar interbody fusions (LIFs) are commonly employed. These techniques use a spacer cage filled with bone graft and insert it into the disc space. This helps reconstruct the disc space to its original dimensions, stabilize the vertebrae so they no longer move and ultimately help the bones fuse. The various types of lumbar interbody fusions are so named based on the direction through which the spacers are inserted into the body. Anterior lumbar interbody fusions (ALIFs) are performed through the front of the spine while transforaminal lumbar interbody fusions (TLIFs) are performed through the back of the spine. Extreme lateral interbody fusions (XLIF) are performed through the flank. Each technique has advantages and disadvantages and what will work well for one person may not work well for another.

Case

Mrs. Pink is a 50-year-old female who has an old back injury and has had multiple lumbar fusions to treat it. She initially had two TLIF procedures at L4-5 and L5-1. Unfortunately, she developed adjacent segment disease and had a stand-alone lateral interbody fusion (XLIF) performed at L3-4, meaning there was a graft-filled cage inserted but no posterior screws placed at this level. When she came to her surgeon, her back was in bad shape, and she had a pseudoarthrosis at L5-S1 and L3-4 and her hardware was breaking in both places because the fusions had failed to heal. She had chronic pain and was desperate for help. Her surgeon removed her non-union at L5-S1, replacing her TLIF cage for a wide ALIF cage. This required opening her abdomen and retrieving the TLIF cage from the disc space. Her surgeon then performed a revision fusion from L2 to her pelvis, removing the entire old hardware and spanning all the old non-union spots. After the surgery she noted immediately improved stability and less pain in her back, despite an extensive revision. Even today 2 years from surgery she is still happy all the problem spots were fixed and has minimal pain aside from some occasional aches.

Introduction

Lumbar spinal fusion is a procedure that surgically connects two or more lumbar vertebrae to get them to grow together to become a single bone. Another term commonly used is lumbar arthrodesis: arthro (Greek for joint) + desis (Greek for binding or fixation). Currently, we accomplish this with pedicle screws that act as anchors in the vertebrae and are linked by rods. Bone graft, either from a cadaver (allograft) or from your own body (autograft) is then used to promote bony bridging between the vertebrae. Occasionally synthetic grafts such as bone morphogenic protein (BMP) may be used as well. If you are interested in learning more about grafts, please see the chapter 37 on spinal fusion basics. Having screws and rods implanted into your spine is a scary concept, but, in the right patient, can dramatically reduce pain.

Who Can Benefit from a Lumbar Fusion?

Spinal fusions are performed thousands of times a year across the United States. Currently lumbar spinal fusions are used to correct deformity such as scoliosis (a curved spine) or spondylolisthesis (a slipped vertebra). They may also be used to treat spinal instability resulting from surgical decompression, trauma, or infection. Finally, a lumbar fusion may be used to treat foraminal stenosis (tightening of the bony tube through which the spinal nerves exit the spinal canal) which cannot easily be accomplished with decompression alone.

Who Should Not Get a Lumbar Fusion?

Lumbar spinal fusions are not good at treating low back pain resulting from painful degenerated discs (discogenic low back pain). And you do not need a lumbar fusion just because you throw your back out and a radiologist notices some degenerative disc disease. The reality is lumbar fusions will only help specific conditions. You may want to have a lumbar fusion to relieve the pain your worn-out discs are giving you, but there is no guarantee it will help you. Lumbar spinal fusions themselves create back pain and can aggravate your problem if not used correctly.

Lumbar spinal fusions also have risk. The surgeon puts rods and screws right around the spinal cord and nerve roots. If your bone quality is poor or you have bad osteoporosis the screws may not hold well in the bone (like trying to put screws into rotten wood). This is another reason osteoporotic compression fractures are rarely treated with spinal fusions. Any number of things can go wrong, so this procedure is for you only if it is reasonably likely to solve your problem.

Technique

Lumbar fusions are based on the concept that bone graft placed between the vertebrae can heal into new bone and bridge the segment turning two vertebrae into a single vertebra. The bone for the bone graft may be obtained from a cadaver or from your own body (typically your pelvis which has ample bone). The vertebral segments which are being fused are decorticated (the dense outer layer of bone is roughened and removed) to allow for a good healing surface. The bone graft is then placed either on the lamina (an interlaminar fusion), between the transverse processes (a posterolateral fusion), in the disc space (an interbody fusion) or a combination of these.

There are many ways to perform a lumbar fusion which come from the long history of scientific advancement. Lumbar fusions may be "instrumented" or done "in situ." An in-situ fusion is an older style of surgery where bone graft is placed in the spine and allowed to heal "in situ" or in place, without changing the alignment of the spine. Despite being an older technique, in-situ fusions are still performed by surgeons with success because putting instruments in the spine has added risk. If you don't need a major correction, an in-situ fusion may be all you need.

In an instrumented fusion, metallic implants (typically rods and screws) are used to fixate the spine and hold it in position while the bone graft heals and hardens. These implants can realign deformities and stop instability. The most common instrument used in the spine is the pedicle screw which is inserted carefully down the corridor of bone known as the pedicle of the vertebra (the two pedicles of a vertebra, one on each side, connect the lamina to the vertebral body). Pedicle screws were developed in the 1980s and were held in low regard for a period, with large class-action lawsuits filed against surgeons in the 1990s for using pedicle screws. Nonetheless, these lawsuits turned out to be frivolous and the pedicle screw is now the gold standard instrument used in spinal fusions.

Types of Interbody Fusions

Within the category of instrumented lumbar fusions are a subcategory called lumbar interbody fusions (LIF). In a LIF, a device known as a cage (also known as an interbody device or spacer) is inserted between the two vertebrae in the disc space after a complete discectomy (removal of the disc) has been performed. The cage itself is a hollow structure that can be filled with bone graft allowing it to become incorporated into the spine. This allows the load across the vertebrae to stay balanced and the two vertebrae to grow together. Interbody fusions dramatically increase the rate of successful fusion compared to a standard posterolateral only fusion and have made lumbar fusions more reliable (1).

There are several types of lumbar interbody fusions named according to the direction through which the graft is inserted into the spine. These include the anterior lumbar interbody fusion (ALIF), posterior lumbar interbody fusion (PLIF), transforaminal lumbar interbody fusion (TLIF), and extreme lateral lumbar interbody fusion (XLIF). Now there is even an oblique lumbar interbody fusion (OLIF), although this is similar in concept to an ALIF. Each approach has different benefits and risks.

Anterior Lumbar Interbody Fusion (ALIF): an ALIF is performed through an anterior approach through the abdomen either by going around the abdominal cavity (retroperitoneal) or through the abdominal cavity (transperitoneal). This approach requires the surgeon to work around the great blood vessels of the body (the abdominal aorta and the inferior vena cava) and thus is typically performed with a vascular or general co-surgeon. Although devices now exist so that the ALIF can be done in a stand-alone fashion, the standard procedure is to back up the cage with posterior screws and rods. Thus, in addition to going through the stomach to place the cage, an ALIF surgery requires a separate approach from the back to insert the posterior screws.

ALIFs have several advantages; they allow a wide graft to be placed and are effective at restoring disc height, which may be lost due to collapse. ALIFs are effective procedures because they allow a large graft to be placed, thus increasing fusion capacity. This is the procedure Tiger Woods underwent—after multiple spinal decompressions—that allowed him to return to dominate the Masters Golf Tournament in 2019.

ALIFs also have disadvantages. The risks of performing the anterior approach are greater than the posterior approach and are described below. ALIFS require two incisions typically and may even be done in a staged fashion where the ALIF is done one day and the posterior screws another day, necessitating a longer hospital stay. The ALIF is typically done with two surgeons which also means two bills, and in some cases the assisting surgeon may be "out of network" resulting in a dramatic increase in cost because insurance will not cover his fees. Recent legislation has sought to curtail this practice.

While most ALIF cases are quite successful, the procedure does have a specific set of potential risks. The most feared of these complications is an intra-operative vascular laceration (cutting) of one of the great vessels or branches. This most commonly occurs around the inferior vena cava or the veins that drain into it (the common iliac vein, the iliolumbar vein) and may occur in anywhere from 2-6% of cases (2,3). As these cases are typically done in conjunction with a vascular access surgeon, the vast majority can be repaired immediately, but still may result in significant blood loss. As this procedure does occur in the abdomen, it is rare but possible to have an injury to one of the visceral structures (bowel, kidney, ureter). Furthermore, as the operation takes place in the abdomen, you may have difficulty moving your bowels following the operation (called an ileus). This typically improves in 7 days. Hernias may occur around the incision at a rate of 1%, which may require a revision operation to fix. Finally, in the anterior lumbar spine run a group of nerves called the sympathetic plexus, and damage to these nerves can cause swelling, temperature changes in the leg, and, in men, even retrograde ejaculation (during orgasm semen enters the bladder instead of exiting the penis). These problems typically improve within 6 months in virtually all cases (2).

Transforaminal Lumbar Interbody Fusion (TLIF): a TLIF is performed through a posterior (from the back) approach and the cage is inserted through a channel created by cutting out a facet joint. This allows safe access to the disc space while completing a discectomy and foraminal decompression at the same time (See foraminotomy in the glossary). An older style of interbody fusion called a PLIF (posterior lumbar interbody fusion) that some surgeons still use, is like the TLIF;

however, the passage of the cage is less oblique and does not require the entire removal of the facet joint.

TLIFs are advantageous because they can easily be performed through a standard posterior approach and do not need a separate incision or surgery. They are faster, and require less hospitalization because they can be done in a single setting without the need for two approaches and separate surgeries (4).   The incidence of dramatic vascular complications is much lower than in ALIFs.

The main disadvantage of a TLIF is that a smaller graft must be used compared to that of an XLIF of an ALIF. The access point is smaller in a TLIF which limits the size of the graft that can be placed. Thus, you may not get as much height restoration or correction of spine alignment as you will in an ALIF. Moreover, because the grafts are smaller, they have increased risk of collapse and pseudoarthrosis (non-union) compared to ALIF and XLIF.

Extreme Lateral Lumbar Interbody Fusion (XLIF)/aka Direct Lateral: an XLIF cage is inserted through a small incision on your flank. It is also called the trans-psoas approach because the cage must be inserted through the psoas muscle, which is a hip flexor that attaches to the side of your spine. This procedure can generally be performed through a small incision with a tubular retractor and thus is called "minimally invasive" by many surgeons.

XLIF has a blend of the advantages of a TLIF and an ALIF. Like the ALIF, it offers a nice cage size but, unlike an ALIF, it does not require a major open abdominal surgery to do it. The fusion rates are excellent and because, like the TLIF, it can be performed through a small incision, the recovery time is speedy.

However, the XLIF cannot be performed safely at all lumbar levels, especially at L5-S1 and sometimes L4-5, which are the most common levels that require fusion. At L4-S1, the great vessels and nerves are near the XLIF access channel and thus you run the risk of major complications. Like the ALIF, an XLIF is backed up with screws that are inserted from posterior. Thus, an XLIF, as with the ALIF, also requires two separate incisions and requires a change in position during the surgery: the cage is inserted with you on your side and then you are flipped prone (facing down) for screw insertion from the back.

So called "single-position surgery" is used in some centers where the graft and screws are all placed with you positioned on your side, but this is not done universally. XLIF still has all the dangers of an ALIF (vascular and bowel injury) but, unlike an ALIF, can also cause significant injury to the lumbar plexus. The lumbar plexus is the collection of nerves that originate from the lumbar spine and course through the psoas muscle. When retractors are placed through these nerves the stretch applied can irritate them. This can result in quadriceps muscle weakness and can be permanent.

Stand-alone Fusion

When a surgeon fuses two vertebrae by going in from the front to place an interbody cage but does not add pedicle screws (that are placed by going in from the back), it is called a stand-alone fusion. This type of approach relies on the inherent stability of the cage implant to provide a mechanical environment that is capable of fusing. The advantages of this approach are that the procedure is faster and does not include the complications of a dual front-back surgery. The obvious concern with this is that there may not be enough mechanical stability to generate a successful fusion. A large meta-analysis reviewing stand-alone lateral fusions suggest that the average fusion rate with a stand-alone lateral approach is 85% (5).

Minimally Invasive Lumbar Spine Fusions

Minimally invasive surgery (MIS) generally refers to surgery that is not performed through a standard midline incision but instead is accomplished through multiple smaller peripheral incisions with the use of special retractors (tools that can hold back tissue to enable a better view). The advantage to this approach is that there is greater preservation of the soft tissue envelope and back muscles and thus faster healing and recovery. For a lumbar fusion this generally means the pedicle screws are inserted "percutaneously," meaning through small peripheral incisions made through the skin, using either X-ray or CT-Guidance. The interbody cage— such as is used with an XLIF— is placed through a tube or small retractor.

Having surgery via a minimally invasive approach sounds good in theory and there have certainly been incredible advances in the technology to make MIS spine surgery feasible. Nonetheless, there has not been definitive evidence that MIS results in superior long term outcomes (6). In lumbar fusions where the goal is to achieve a stable solid arthrodesis (fusion), having a wide exposure is actually very beneficial to make sure you can put a large amount of bone graft in the surgical bed and ensure all the bony surfaces are prepared properly. It also ensures complete decompression of the nerves. Performing the surgery through small incisions limits the amount of tissue disruption but also the space for bone graft placement and visualization of the spine. MIS also limits the amount of manipulation you can perform to reduce deformities and correct alignment. Finally, MIS requires the judicious use of radiation in the form of either fluoroscopy or X-ray. Despite this, MIS surgery has been associated with faster recovery in the early period, a decreased risk of infection and possibly less risk of readmission and so is worth discussing with your surgeon.

What to Expect Post Op

You will typically have a certain degree of back pain from the surgical incision following a lumbar spinal fusion; however, in most cases you will be able to get out of bed and walk the day of surgery. You may have a small drain which prevents fluid from building up at the site of surgery. In some instances, you may be required to wear a brace following fusion.

Some of your symptoms may be improved immediately. However, it is important to remember that a spinal fusion takes about 1 year to fully mature. Typically, your surgical pain will last for about 4-6 weeks after the procedure and gradually subside thereafter, but your fusion will still be improving for about a year. During this healing time it is important to maintain your restrictions of no bending, lifting, or twisting.

Pseudoarthrosis (Non-Union)

In a small percentage of patients, a pseudoarthrosis, otherwise known as a non-union, may occur. A pseudoarthrosis occurs when the bone graft fails to heal the two vertebrae together. In these cases, the hardware may eventually start to loosen and can cause pain because they are only designed to hold the spine in place for a matter of months. Pseudoarthroses are diagnosed with a CT scan or X-ray that show that that the bones have not healed. This sounds scary, but strangely the majority of pseudoarthroses will do fine and do not require more surgery (7). A fibrous nonunion, meaning that the segment is joined together with scar tissue may occur instead of a bony fusion. Fibrous nonunions are invisible to CT and X-ray but can still stabilize the spine and prevent symptoms from occurring. However, if the hardware is loose, you may require revision to keep the screws from migrating into dangerous places.

Adjacent Segment Disease

Fusions are well tolerated in the spine because the spine is a chain, and, like a chain, if you lock two segments it will still move relatively normally. However, this motion occurs because the other segments move more to compensate. A fusion of a single segment of the spine will take a fraction of your motion away but the reason you do not notice this is that the other segments compensate by moving MORE. This is the theory behind a phenomenon known as adjacent segment disease, a condition where the segments near a spinal fusion break down. The true cause of adjacent segment disease is unknown and could also possibly be related to the natural breakdown of non-fused segments. It's hard to blame the fusion when your other untreated discs are already bad and wearing down; however, I have seen many cases where the level just above or below the fusion goes bad and requires a reoperation. The process of symptomatic breakdown has been estimated to occur in 16% of patients at 5 years and 36% at 10 years (8).

Hardware Failure

A spinal fusion generally involves placing hardware (screws and cages) into the spine. If the bone is weak, sometimes the hardware can pull out (think of putting a screw into rotten wood). This is more common in patients who have osteoporosis or low bone mineral density. In cases of osteoporosis, screws do not get as much purchase, and cages tend to subside (collapse into the vertebral body) (9). If you have severe osteoporosis, you may not be a candidate for a spinal fusion.

Conclusion

Selecting a lumbar fusion technique is a very complicated decision and depends on many factors, including your own unique anatomy, your spinal problem, your bone density, age, and what your surgeon's preferences are. Ultimately what matters about a fusion is that it heals and accomplishes the surgical goals of stability and decompression. Most of the different techniques will work well, including uninstrumented fusions, which are the oldest forms of lumbar fusions. Selecting the correct approach for you is up to your surgeon, but you should understand the pros and cons between the various techniques.

Frequently Asked Questions

- **Will I lose my mobility after a lumbar fusion?**

    Lumbar fusions are designed to stop motion between vertebrae so yes, some loss of motion is expected. However spinal fusions are generally performed in very degenerative levels that may not be moving much to begin with and thus fusing these segments will not be very noticeable. However, as more levels are incorporated into a fusion there will be a gradually increasing loss of motion. Most patients who undergo a 1 or 2 level lumbar fusion do not report a change in their ability to perform activities of daily living. Patients who have 3 or 4 segments/levels fused do report limitations in their activities. For example, those with 3 level fusions do report difficulty with activities like cutting toenails and squatting down. Four level fusion patients have more difficulty with things like putting on a jacket, getting out of bed and taking a bath (10).

References

1.   Levin JM, Tanenbaum JE, Steinmetz MP, Mroz TE, Overley SC. Posterolateral fusion (PLF) versus transforaminal lumbar interbody fusion (TLIF) for spondylolisthesis: a systematic review and meta-analysis. Spine J. 2018 Jun;18(6):1088–98.

2.   Mobbs RJ, Phan K, Daly D, Rao PJ, Lennox A. Approach-Related Complications of Anterior Lumbar Interbody Fusion: Results of a Combined Spine and Vascular Surgical Team. Glob Spine J. 2016 Mar;6(2):147–54.

3.   Fantini GA. Access related complications during anterior exposure of the lumbar spine. World J Orthop. 2013;4(1):19.

4.   Dorward IG, Lenke LG, Bridwell KH, O?Leary PT, Stoker GE, Pahys JM, et al. Transforaminal Versus Anterior Lumbar Interbody Fusion in Long Deformity Constructs: A Matched Cohort Analysis. Spine. 2013 May;38(12):E755–62.

5.   Manzur MK, Steinhaus ME, Virk SS, Jivanelli B, Vaishnav A, McAnany S, et al. Fusion rate for stand-alone lateral lumbar interbody fusion: a systematic review. Spine J. 2020 Jun;S1529943020307877.

6.   Heemskerk JL, Oluwadara Akinduro O, Clifton W, Quinones-Hinojosa A, Abode-Iyamah KO. Long-term clinical outcome of minimally invasive versus open single-level transforaminal lumbar interbody fusion for degenerative lumbar diseases: a Meta-Analysis. Spine J Off J North Am Spine Soc. 2021 Jul 14;S1529-9430(21)00821-4.

7.   Gertzbein SD. Scoliosis Research Society. Multicenter spine fracture study. Spine. 1992 May;17(5):528–40.

8.   Ghiselli G, Wang JC, Bhatia NN, Hsu WK, Dawson EG. Adjacent segment degeneration in the lumbar spine. J Bone Jt Surg Am. 2004;86(7):1497–503.

9.   Formby PM, Kang DG, Helgeson MD, Wagner SC. Clinical and Radiographic Outcomes of Transforaminal Lumbar Interbody Fusion in Patients with Osteoporosis. Glob Spine J. 2016 Nov;6(7):660–4.

10.   Kimura H, Fujibayashi S, Otsuki B, Takahashi Y, Nakayama T, Matsuda S. Effects of Lumbar Stiffness After Lumbar Fusion Surgery on Activities of Daily Living. Spine. 2016 Apr;41(8):719–27.

Figures:

The "LIFs" (Lumbar Interbody Fusions

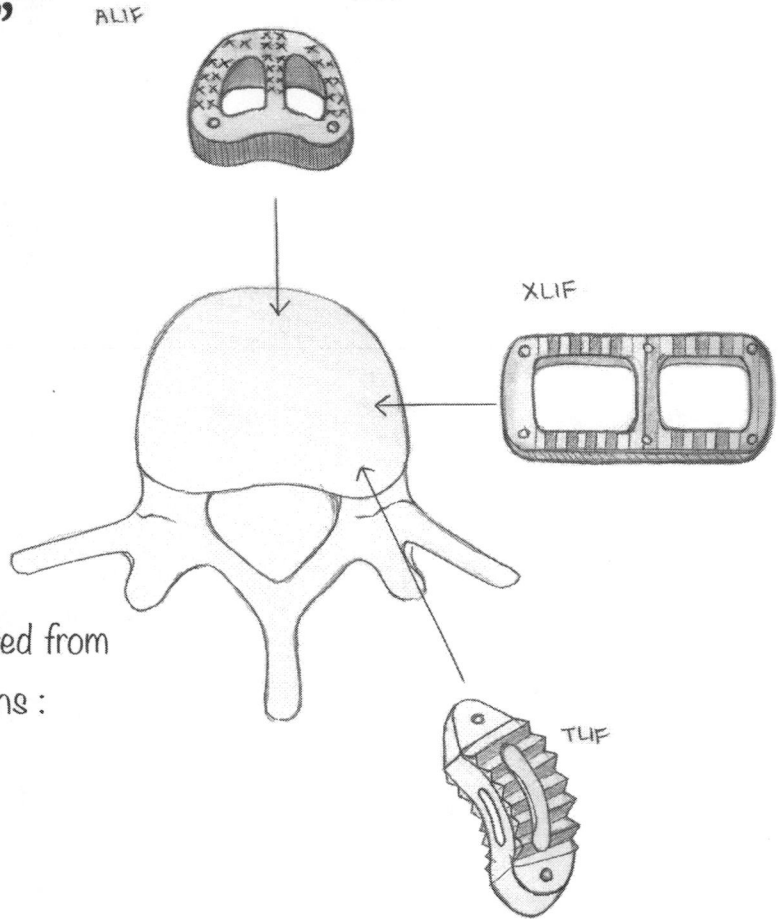

ALIF

XLIF

TLIF

Cages are inserted from different directions :
ALIF: Anterior
XLIF: Lateral
TLIF: Posterior

The LIFS. There are three main ways to perform a lumbar interbody fusion (LIF). The TLIF is done from the back, the XLIF from the side, and the ALIF from the front of the spine.

Transforaminal Lumbar Interbody Fusion (TLIF)

View from the back of spine:

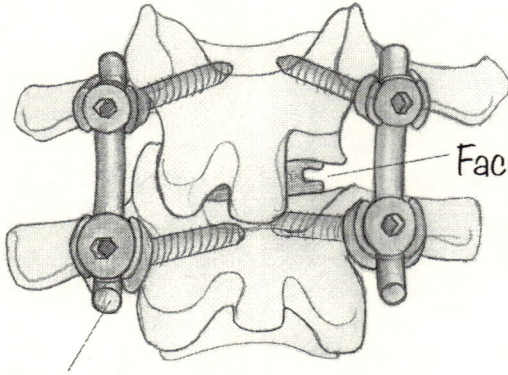

Standard TLIF cage:

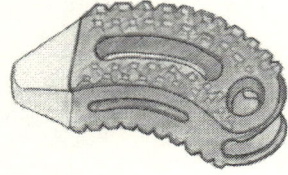

Facet is removed to insert cage

Disc material is removed

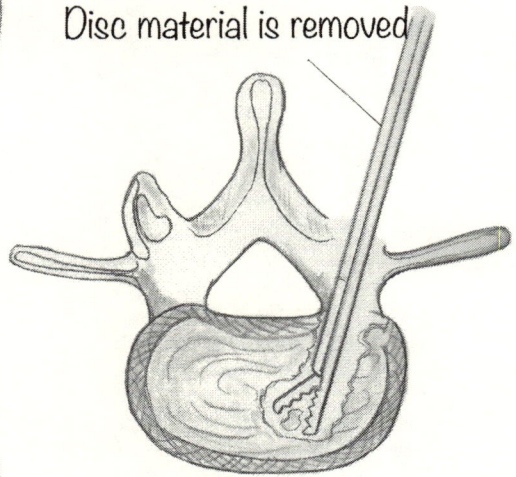

Pedicle screws with rod

View from the side of spine:

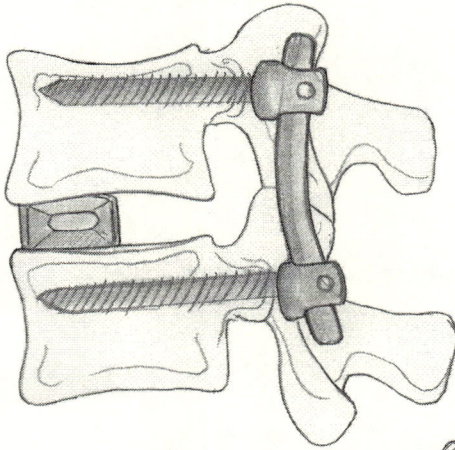

TLIF cage is inserted

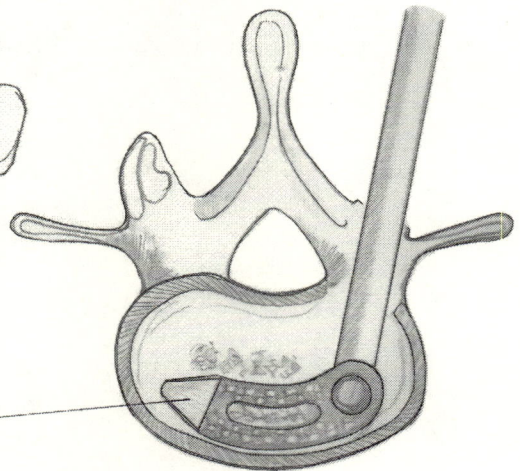

TLIF. A transforaminal lumbar interbody fusion (TLIF) is performed by removing the facet joint to create a channel to the disc, which is also removed. An interbody spacer filled with bone graft is inserted into the disc space and then stabilized with screws and rods.

Lateral Lumbar Fusion

Psoas muscle

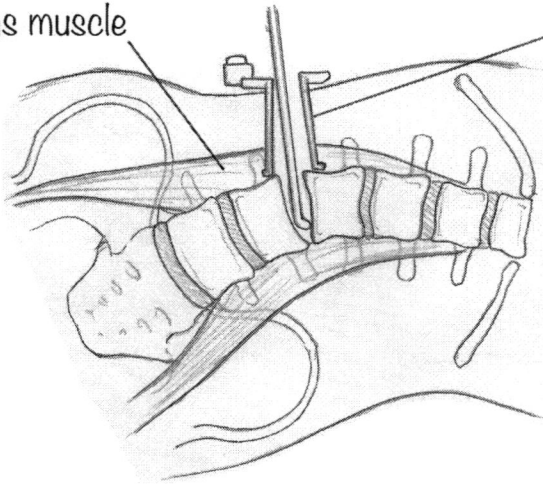

A retractor is placed through the side of the abdomen to access the spine

Cross Section of the Abdomen:

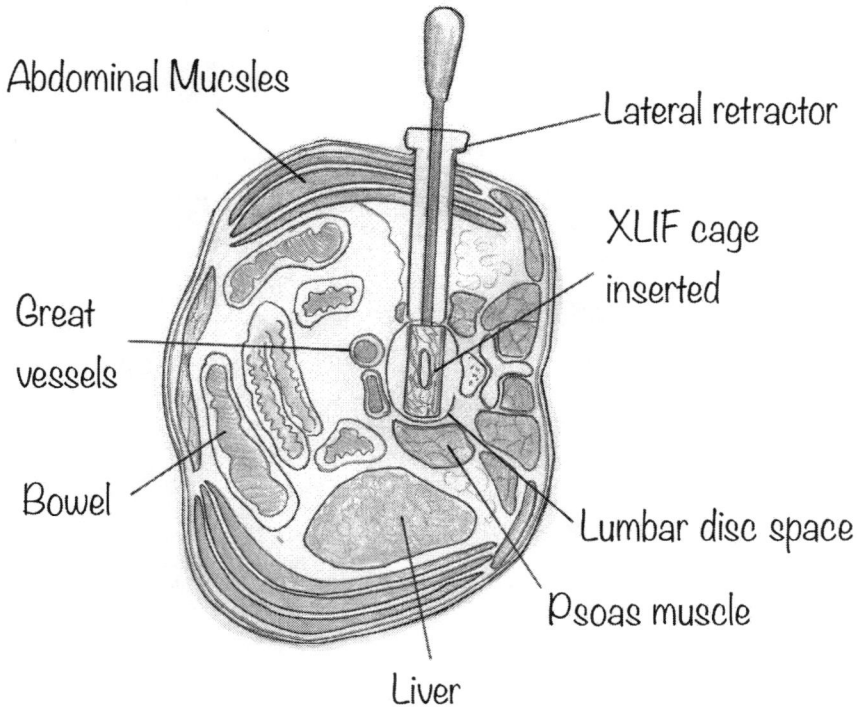

Abdominal Mucsles

Lateral retractor

XLIF cage inserted

Great vessels

Bowel

Lumbar disc space

Psoas muscle

Liver

XLIF How to: The extreme lumbar interbody fusion (XLIF) is performed through the side of the abdomen with the spine in a bent position (top). Cross section of the XLIF procedure. Note the organs, blood vessels and muscles in close vicinity. A retractor is used to access the spine (bottom).

Lateral Lumbar Interbody Fusion

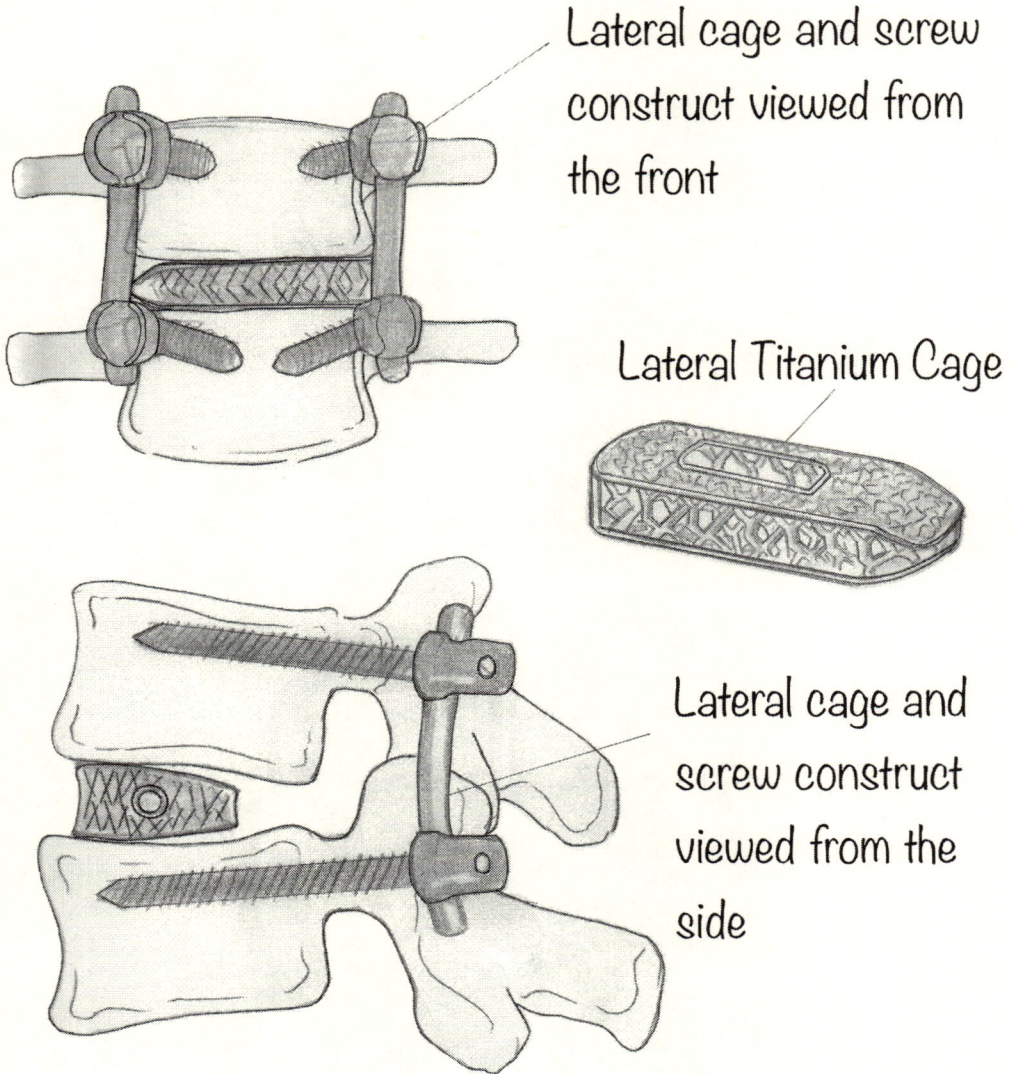

Lateral cage and screw construct viewed from the front

Lateral Titanium Cage

Lateral cage and screw construct viewed from the side

XLIF. In the XLIF procedure an interbody spacer is inserted from the side of the spine and typically stabilized by screws.

Anterior Lumbar Interbody Fusion (ALIF)

ALIF Cage with 3

screws

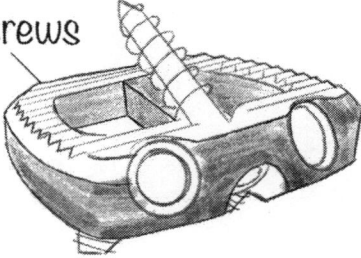

ALIF retractor

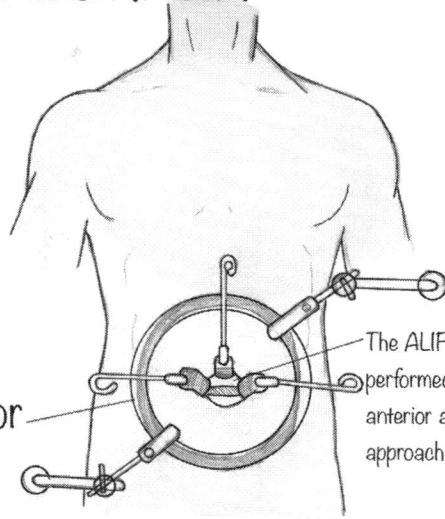

The ALIF procedure is performed through an anterior abdominal approach

The great arteries
must be retracted

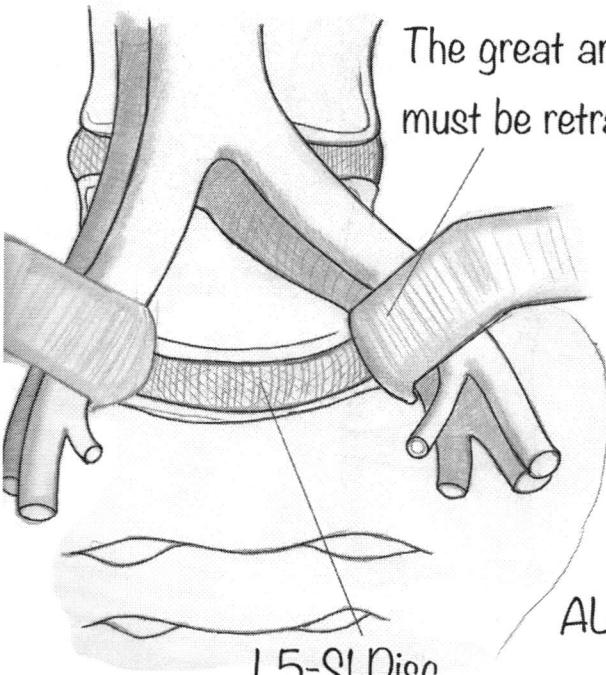

ALIF Cage is inserted

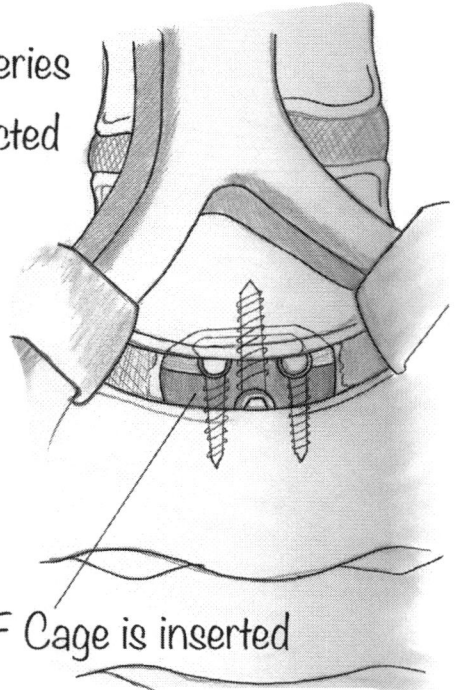

L5-S1 Disc

ALIF. Anterior lumbar interbody fusion (ALIF) is performed through an abdominal approach and requires retraction of the great vessels.

Chapter 42

Scoliosis and Deformity Correction Surgery

Summary

Adult and pediatric spinal deformities are corrected using posterior (approaching through the back) instrumented spinal fusions which use rods and screws to correct the curvature of the spine. While the main goals of the surgery are to stop the progression of deformity and to ease pain, substantial correction of the deformity, cosmetics and posture may also be possible. If the curve is flexible, rods and screws may be all that are necessary, but if the spine is rigid, more advanced procedures called osteotomies, where the bones are literally cut to loosen up the spine, may be performed. The overall complication rate for these procedures can be high in some situations, but the pay-off for patients who are in chronic pain and disfigured from spinal deformity may be equally rewarding.

Case

Ms. Black is a 56-year-old female who has had 3 failed spinal surgeries. She had two previous lumbar fusions from L2-5 that left her back flat and now she is in chronic pain and constantly feels "pitched forward". After failure of different

non-operative treatment plans, she finally decides It's time to try surgery again. Since her spine is already fused and not flexible, her surgeon recommends that the current hardware be removed, and a posterior column osteotomy (PSO) be performed that will rebuild her normal spinal curvature. New hardware extending from T10 to her pelvis will be inserted. During the procedure a nerve root that was scarred from the previous surgery is injured which results in some weakness when Ms. Black wakes up. However, she notes that her posture is dramatically improved, and it does not take as much energy for her to stand upright. Overtime her weakness in her foot improves and she heals well. Today she is doing great after her procedure but notes that her back certainly isn't what it once was. She has significant stiffness and cannot tolerate long car rides or flights very well as she starts to get achy. Some basic activities like tying her shoes are difficult, but the tradeoff for decreased pain and improved posture are worth it to her.

Introduction

Pediatric and adult spine deformity surgery ranks amongst the riskiest procedures in spine surgery but the benefit to patients can be tremendous. With the use of spinal instrumentation, surgeons can reshape the spine, reducing pain and disfigurement, while improving ambulation and general function.

There are several reasons why deformity procedures are challenging. They often require large open surgical exposures that have high blood loss. Big deformity corrections can also place the nerve roots and spinal cord at risk because of the stretch of those tissues caused by the change of shape in the spine. Instrumenting the deformed spine with screws is also more challenging as regular anatomic landmarks are not as reliable. The complication rates in some spinal deformity procedures can be upward of 35% (1).

Nonetheless, the goals of the surgery are to halt and improve the deformity which may be progressive, to help restore a good balanced posture which is critical for moving around and to improve pain levels. A surgeon typically will look to correct not only scoliosis but also kyphosis, thus restoring not only side-to-side balance but also your posture. These surgeries are only really contemplated after extensive non-operative care has failed. If there are no simple options, in many cases, surgery can be very beneficial at improving quality of life.

To understand spinal deformity correction it's helpful to review the basic configuration of the spinal vertebrae. The vertebra consists of an anterior (front) part and a posterior (back) part. The anterior part is the cylindrical vertebral body which is the major weight bearing portion of the spine. Every vertebra is connected to the vertebra above and below it by an intervertebral disc. That disc sits between the two vertebrae's vertebral bodies. The posterior part consists of everything else: the lamina, facet joints, spinous processes (this is the part you can feel with your fingers), transverse processes and pedicles and contribute to spinal stability and motion. Thus, anterior procedures focus on the vertebral body and discs, while posterior procedures focus primarily on the lamina, pedicles, and facets.

Basics of Deformity Correction

Scoliosis is corrected with instrumented spinal fusions performed through a posterior approach; screws and hooks act as anchors in the vertebrae and are connected with a rod that helps reshape the spine. A posterior spinal fusion is one that places bone graft in over the lamina and transverse processes to promote healing. Sometimes screws can be difficult to place into the spine and other devices are used, such as hooks that latch onto the spine or wires that tie onto the spine. A surgeon will make a midline incision (straight up and down the spine) to the levels of intended fusion, insert screws and rods and then place bone graft to help a bony fusion to occur. Placing a straight rod into a curved spine and attaching it to screws will help straighten it but other maneuvers may be necessary to mold the spine back into the correct shape. The surgeon can bend the rods to a specific shape, and manipulate the screws to move the vertebrae, thus bringing the spine back into position when the screws are connected. These maneuvers help contour the spine back into a more normal shape.

If spinal stenosis (a narrowed spinal canal that is causing nerve compression) is present along with the deformity, a decompression procedure may be done in conjunction with the fusion procedure. Anterior column fusions such as anterior lumbar interbody fusions (ALIFS), extreme lateral interbody fusions (XLIF) or transforaminal lumbar interbody fusions (TLIFS) may be done in conjunction with the posterior fusion procedure. These anterior grafts can be very helpful in restoring the shape of a collapsed disc space and thus restoring the overall shape of the spine.

Osteotomies

The extent of the surgery performed depends on what the deformity looks like and what it will take to get the spine in a straighter configuration. Pedicle screws and rods are very effective at bending the spine back into place but in certain instances this is not enough. If the spine is particularly rigid, even strong metallic rods will not be able to pull the spine back into place. In these cases, special cuts in the bone known as osteotomies are performed to make the spine less rigid or to dramatically change the shape of the spine. Once the cuts are made in the bone the surgeon can "lock" the spine into a certain position with pedicle screws and rods. Unfortunately, the spine becomes stiffer in adulthood and thus adult patients are more likely to need these more aggressive procedures compared to children.

Osteotomies come in many varieties, but all remove some bone to make the spine more flexible. There is a hierarchy of osteotomies ranging from small to large. Smith Petersen osteotomies involve removal of the facet joints to unlock the back of the spine. These are commonly used in adolescent scoliosis cases where the back tends to be flexible

The next level of osteotomies includes the so-called pedicle subtraction osteotomy and then the vertebrectomy.

The first technique is called the pedicle subtraction osteotomy (PSO) and involves cutting a wedge of bone out of the back of the spine (the lamina, pedicle, and spinous process) and the anterior column (the large round vertebral body). This is a very powerful procedure for recontouring the spine and is useful for correcting both coronal ((side to side) scoliosis) and sagittal (front to back) hunched forward, arched back) deformity. The next osteotomy up the ladder is the vertebral column resection (or VCR /vertebrectomy) where an entire vertebral segment is removed. Both procedures are typically reserved for very severe angular deformities in the spine and are most deployed in cases where there is a preexisting fusion that will not move without breaking the spine

These procedures are complex and risky but have major payoffs for patients with spinal deformities. Symptom relief is significant and lasting which is why, despite their risk, surgeons continue to perform the procedures. Most osteotomies involve increasing amounts of blood loss because when cuts are made in the bone, there tends to be bony bleeding that is difficult to stanch and so you may require transfusions after having this type of surgery. Because you are manipulating the shape of the spine there is increased risk for neurological injury. Overall, there is a high complication rate with osteotomy-type procedures—as high as a 35% major complication rate (1).

Corpectomy

Sometimes, when most of the deformity is in the front of the spine in the vertebral body, an anterior procedure called a corpectomy is performed where the vertebral body is removed from an anterior (front) or lateral (side) approach. Then a large cage spacer is inserted to maintain the integrity of the anterior column and to help a bony fusion to occur. This procedure is typically backed up with the placement of posterior pedicle screws and rods and are thus called anterior-posterior procedures, meaning the surgeon approaches the spine both through the front and through the back, which typically requires a change of position for the patient during the surgery.

Corpectomies are frequently used to treat fractures, infections, and tumors, which tend to destroy the anterior part of the spine.

Possible Complications

Even the most experienced spine deformity surgeons cannot completely avoid complications in this type of surgery. Complications may be something minor, like a urinary tract infection, or could be major such as hardware failure or need for revision surgery. Nerve root or spinal cord injury is particularly feared in this these types of procedures and, unfortunately, are common (upwards of 15% of cases) \(1).

Recovery After a Deformity Surgery

Recovering from a spinal deformity surgery can be long and challenging. You can expect to spend at least 4-8 days in the hospital following a major spinal reconstruction and even a few nights in the intensive care unit (ICU). These procedures can take anywhere from 4-12 hours, depending on what is being done, and so it's not uncommon to keep patients intubated overnight after the surgery to avoid any airway complications. Following this you will typically start your physical therapy to regain your independent ambulation (walking) and eventually will be discharged home.

Even after you are discharged to home your recovery may be lengthy and it may not be until 3-4 months after the procedure that you are feeling recovered. Luckily, you get to enjoy the benefits of deformity correction immediately and your posture should be significantly improved.

Outcomes

So far, we have talked a lot about what can go wrong in deformity surgery. I think this is appropriate considering the risks of these aggressive procedures. But what about the ultimate outcome? Deformity surgery is quite rewarding as you can transform someone who is crippled from a spinal deformity and make them able to stand and walk normally again. Spine surgery societies such as the Scoliosis Research Society (SRS) and the International Spine Study Group (ISSG) have shown in large studies that people with spine deformity actually do better with surgery than continued conservative care and that deformity surgery has a major positive impact on quality of life (2,3). Talk about the risks and benefits with your surgeon but if your life is significantly compromised from spinal deformity, surgery is certainly an option.

Conclusion

Deformity surgery in the spine is serious and risky but has the potential for huge payoffs in terms of improved posture, function, and pain. It's important you understand that in a fair proportion of cases, something may go wrong. It may be something small or something large but is usually something that your surgeon can help you get through with supportive measures and won't impact your long-term outcome.

Frequently Asked Questions

- **How does osteoporosis impact spinal deformity surgery?**

    Spine deformity surgery relies on the use of screws and rods to manipulate your spine into a correct posture. Thus, the strain on the screws is even higher than in surgery for basic degenerative conditions. Poor bone quality can significantly increase complication rates because the screws have less holding power in the more porous bone (again, think about putting a screw into wet and rotten wood). Osteoporosis should be treated prior to spine surgery with a bone building osteoporosis medicine to give the surgery the best chance of success.

References

1.   Auerbach JD, Lenke LG, Bridwell KH, Sehn JK, Milby AH, Bumpass D, et al. Major Complications and Comparison Between 3-Column Osteotomy Techniques in 105 Consecutive Spinal Deformity Procedures: Spine. 2012 Jun;37(14):1198–210.

2.   Ailon T, Smith JS, Shaffrey CI, Kim HJ, Mundis G, Gupta M, et al. Outcomes of Operative Treatment for Adult Cervical Deformity: A Prospective Multicenter Assessment With 1-Year Follow-up. Neurosurgery. 2018 Nov 1;83(5):1031–9.

3.   Smith JS, Shaffrey CI, Berven S, Glassman S, Hamill C, Horton W, et al. Operative Versus Nonoperative Treatment of Leg Pain in Adults With Scoliosis: A Retrospective Review of a Prospective Multicenter Database With Two-Year Follow-up. Spine. 2009 Jul;34(16):1693–8.

Figures:

Pedicle Subtraction Osteotomy (PSO)

A compressed vertebra creates a deformity in the spine. The lines represent a planned resection

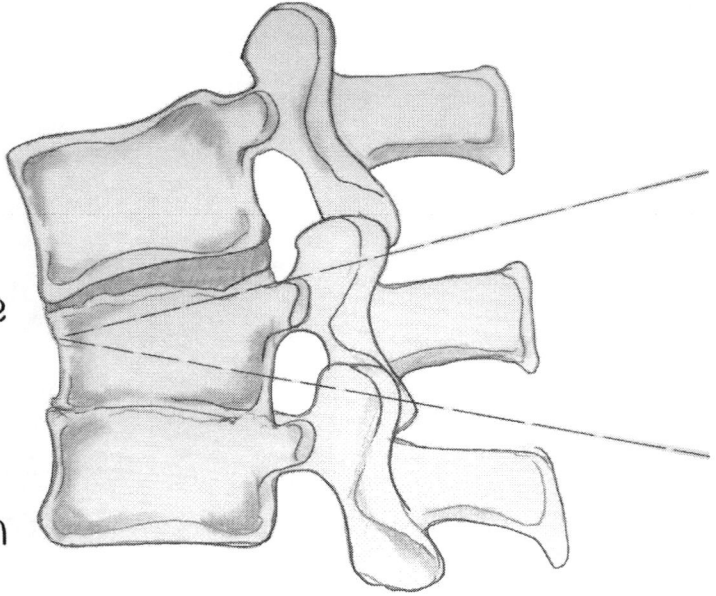

The bone is resected allowing for correction of the deformity, which is secured with screws

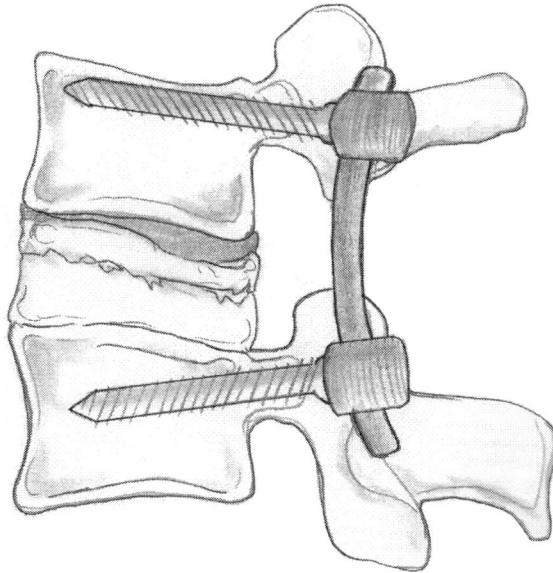

PSO. A planned pedicle subtraction osteotomy (PSO) used to correct a kyphotic segment of the spine. Resection means to surgically remove (top). The osteotomy removed a wedge of the spine and is stabilized by posterior rods and screws (bottom).

Chapter 43

Procedures to Fix Stenosis in the Neck: Laminectomy, Fusion With Laminectomy, and Laminoplasty

Summary

Stenosis is a narrowing of the spinal canal that causes the spinal cord to be compressed, often causing pain or neurologic symptoms in the extremities. Cervical procedures can treat stenosis as well as other diseases either through the front or back of the neck. Going through the back of the neck, known as the posterior approach, requires a vertical incision in the neck and requires the muscles to be moved to the side. The posterior approach is favored in cases where an anterior approach may be difficult or dangerous, such as if there has been a previous anterior surgery that has resulted in scarring, obscuring vital structures. The posterior approach is safe since there are no major vital organs in the back of the neck to work around. For this reason, the posterior approach is favored when multiple spinal levels require treatment—doing multiple levels through the front of the neck results in increased risk of complication. The downside is that the posterior approach can be

more painful than an anterior approach because it requires the neck muscles to be
retracted.

There are three primary posterior procedures to treat stenosis: a laminectomy alone,
a laminectomy + posterior fusion, and a laminoplasty. A laminectomy removes the
arch of bone covering the back side of the spinal cord (the lamina). A fusion joins the
bones with rods and screws so that they grow together. A laminoplasty is a motion
preserving procedure where a small metal plate is used to create a door-like opening
in the lamina to make more space in the spinal cord.

Case

**Mr. Orange is a 76-year-old male who has noticed that his balance and manual
dexterity have been rapidly deteriorating. His doctor recommends a cervical
MRI which shows severe multi-level stenosis crushing his spinal cord. He has
several other medical problems, including a previous heart attack, diabetes,
and asthma. He has minimal neck pain but cannot shake the feeling that his
body is "losing power." When he comes to me, I explain to him that the signals
coming from his brain are not reaching the body because of the stenosis in his
neck. His neck alignment is good and considering his many medical problems
we decide to do a laminoplasty from C2-7. Following the surgery, he notes
improved power in his arms and legs and that his balance is improved. His
wounds heal rapidly with minimal pain. He is pleased as his neck motion remains like before surgery, with minimal pain, and he does not need to undergo
the prolonged recovery process he would have had with a fusion surgery.**

Introduction

A posterior approach means your surgery will be performed through the back side of
your neck, through a vertical incision. Posterior approaches provide a safe corridor
to access the spinal canal to perform a decompression of the spinal cord and/or
fusion of the vertebrae because, unlike the anterior approach, which approaches the
spine from the front of the neck, there are no vital structures here. In the anterior
neck, there are major arteries and veins, nerves, your trachea, and esophagus. In the
posterior spine there is mainly muscle, making the chance of a major complication
much lower. Posterior approaches give the surgeon access to the posterior parts of
the spine: the lamina, the spinous process, and the facets. For example, sometimes
a compressed spinal cord can be unpinched by enlarging the surrounding area
with a laminectomy (removal of the lamina or arch of bone on the back side of
the vertebrae), which opens the canal and takes the pressure off the spinal cord
(decompresses it). Similarly, an individual nerve root may be decompressed with

a foraminotomy (a procedure that makes a small opening over the nerve, thereby taking the pressure off it).

There are a variety of technical reasons your surgeon may perform your surgery through the back of the neck, rather than the front. If you have had previous neck surgery through the front, the anterior approach is more dangerous because scarring makes vital structures clump together and hard to identify and dissect (cut) through without causing injury. If you have a condition known as ossification of the posterior ligament where calcium builds up in the front of the spinal canal, anterior surgery is also risky. Finally, posterior approaches work better if multilevel decompressions (more than 3 levels, that is, more than 4 consecutive vertebrae) are required. A level (or segment) consists of two adjacent vertebrae and the disc between them, for example, C3-4. So, a posterior approach would be well suited to treat C3-7 stenosis.

Posterior approaches have different side effects than anterior approaches (1). They tend to be more painful and there is a small increased risk of infection. However, the benefits of the posterior approach are that there is little chance of dysphagia (difficulty in swallowing), airway issues, or other complications that can result from the manipulation of the airway and esophagus that is required with an anterior approach.

The posterior approach to the cervical spine is a work horse for treating multilevel spinal cord compression or stenosis (narrowed spinal canal). There are three main procedures available: decompression (laminectomy), laminectomy combined with a fusion, which uses rods and screws, and a hybrid type procedure called a laminoplasty. Laminoplasty uses a metal plate to prop up the lamina to take pressure off the spinal cord but helps maintain stability of the spine because the bone is not removed as it is in a laminectomy. It is a hybrid procedure because it combines the best parts of a laminectomy alone and a laminectomy with fusion. All these procedures are used to treat spinal cord compression. In this chapter we explore the differences between the procedures and some guiding evidence.

The Posterior Approach

As stated above, a posterior approach is performed through a vertical incision behind the neck. There is a surgical plane that can be used to expose the spine without cutting any muscles (although the muscles are retracted (pulled aside), which can be painful). To gain access to the higher levels of the cervical spine your hair may need to be trimmed—not always a stylish cut—but will quickly grow back after the procedure. You may have some temporary numbness in the back of the neck from the exposure because the nerves supplying the skin can be disrupted.

Laminectomy

A laminectomy is the surgical removal of the posterior arch of the vertebra called the lamina. Think of this as taking the top off a clogged pipe so it can be cleaned. Removing the lamina allows the surgeon to relieve whatever is causing pressure on the spinal cord. An isolated laminectomy (without fusion) may be performed for 1- or 2-level disease and is a relatively simple procedure with a quick recovery. Laminectomies alone are not typically done for greater than 2-level procedures (involving more than 3 consecutive vertebrae) because multiple laminectomies increase the risk of destabilizing the spine and can result in a change in your neck posture. Thus, in patients with more than 2 levels of stenosis, laminectomies may be either combined with a posterior cervical fusion procedure or with a laminoplasty (both described below). Laminoplasty is a favorite of mine for elderly patients (older than 70 years) and young patients (less than 40 years) who may not tolerate a fusion very well. Cervical laminectomies of 1-2 levels can be done quickly, with minimal tissue disruption and have a rapid recovery.

Posterior Cervical Fusions

In a posterior cervical fusion, screws are placed into the vertebrae and connected with rods and bone graft to get the vertebrae to grow together. These screws are named according to the location where they are inserted. In the cervical spine, the facet joints are made of blocks of bone known as the lateral mass and are adjacent to the spinal canal. Lateral mass screws may be inserted into the lateral mass very safely and provide an excellent anchor to connect the bones. Cervical vertebrae also have pedicles where pedicle screws may be inserted, but this is less commonly done because it's not as safe as lateral mass screws.

There are four main reasons to do a posterior cervical fusion and they all have to do with keeping the spine stable: A fusion is a good idea 1) if there is already instability (abnormal motion between vertebral bones) or spondylolisthesis (slipped disc) in the neck, 2) if the surgeon needs to back up, extend or support an existing anterior cervical fusion, 3) if there is deformity in the spine or 4) if the patient requires greater than 2 or 3 levels of decompression, in which case what the surgeon has to do to decompress the spine may actually cause it to become unstable. In all these cases, a decompression is typically done in conjunction with a fusion. The hardware serves to support the neck if a wide (removing more bone) laminectomy is performed and to stabilize segments.

Posterior cervical fusions are commonly used to deal with multi-level stenosis, trauma, tumor, or deformity. These procedures sound scary, but they are well tolerated and safe. Since the screws are covered by soft tissue, they are not readily noticeable to the patient.

Laminoplasty

Laminoplasty is a unique procedure that was designed to allow surgeons to perform multi- level decompressions without destabilizing the spine. The idea behind a laminoplasty is that instead of completely removing the lamina, it is hinged open like a door to create space in the spinal canal. This is done by cutting one edge of the lamina completely and creating a hinge on the other side by partially cutting it. The lamina can then be elevated which creates space in the spinal canal without completely uncovering the spine or destabilizing it. It also allows the muscles and soft tissues to reattach to the bone and keeps the spinal cord protected. The lamina is held open with a small metal plate that serves as a door jam. In a laminoplasty procedure the posterior approach is used; however, careful attention is paid to preserving muscular attachments.

The main benefits to a laminoplasty procedure are that the recovery is much faster than for a fusion and the motion of the neck is not lost. The downsides are that laminoplasty procedures are not good at treating neck pain and may even create it. A post-operative change in alignment of the neck known as post-laminectomy kyphosis frequently occurs with multilevel laminectomy and may also still occur with a laminoplasty at a rate of 7-10% (2). Despite laminoplasty being a motion-preserving procedure, as much as 25% of total motion may be lost as a result of scarring and further degeneration (2). Thus, laminoplasty procedures are not used in patients who already have alignment issues of the spine.

Nonetheless, laminoplasty is an effective treatment option for patients suffering from cervical myelopathy with multilevel compression; it is very well tolerated and combines the best of posterior cervical fusion and isolated laminectomy. The procedure has been studied for decades and long-term studies with 10 years of follow up show great improvement in function and satisfaction with the procedure (2). From my own experience, patients do very well with these procedures and do not have the same level of complications and side effects as a cervical fusion, but they are not useful for all patients.

Comparing the Procedures

The indications to use a posterior decompression and fusion of the cervical spine or a decompression with a laminoplasty are different and thus the procedures are not directly comparable. Nonetheless, when comparing the two procedures, studies have shown that laminoplasty is associated with less blood loss and a shorter hospital stay (3). Complication rates are similar between groups in the acute phase (the time immediately following surgery) and can include neurologic injury, infection and need for revision surgery. Over a longer term, posterior laminectomy and fusion has a higher complication rate than laminoplasty, with pseudoarthrosis (failure of the bone to fuse) as the primary difference.

In patients who have significant neck pain, fusions are generally preferred; however, fusions do not necessarily result in less neck pain over time. Fusion procedures have been reported to have superior neurologic outcomes over time (3).

Conclusion

When stenosis that is compressing the spinal cord occurs in only one or two levels, a simple laminectomy may be the best choice. However, in larger cases with multiple areas of compression, either a laminectomy + posterior fusion or a laminoplasty is typically chosen. Posterior cervical fusion with laminectomy and laminoplasty have similar outcomes but different indications and so it's important to discuss the rationale for choosing one or the other with your surgeon. Laminoplasty can only really be used in patients with good neck alignment and no existing instability. Laminoplasty is associated with a rapid recovery but may not be useful in every patient. Posterior cervical fusions take longer to heal and have more long-term complications but may be used to correct alignment and instability.

Frequently Asked Questions

- **If the bone is removed from my lamina, what is protecting the spinal cord?**

    While it is true that removing the lamina (laminectomy) removes the protective bone, because there is plenty of soft tissue around your neck over the spinal cord, it is very hard to injure it. In a laminoplasty procedure the lamina is left intact and still serves to protect the cord.

References

1.   Fehlings MG, Smith JS, Kopjar B, Arnold PM, Yoon ST, Vaccaro AR, et al. Perioperative and delayed complications associated with the surgical treatment of cervical spondylotic myelopathy based on 302 patients from the AOSpine North America Cervical Spondylotic Myelopathy Study. J Neurosurg Spine. 2012 May;16(5):425–32.

2.   Kawaguchi Y, Kanamori M, Ishihara H, Ohmori K, Nakamura H, Kimura T. Minimum 10-Year Followup After En Bloc Cervical Laminoplasty: Clinical Orthopaedics and Related Research. 2003 Jun;411:129–39.

3.   Lau D, Winkler EA, Than KD, Chou D, Mummaneni PV. Laminoplasty versus laminectomy with posterior spinal fusion for multilevel cervical spondylotic myelopathy: influence of cervical alignment on outcomes. Journal of Neurosurgery: Spine. 2017 Nov;508–17.

Figures:

Posterior Cervical Fusion/ Decompression

Cervical spine viewed from behind (posterior)

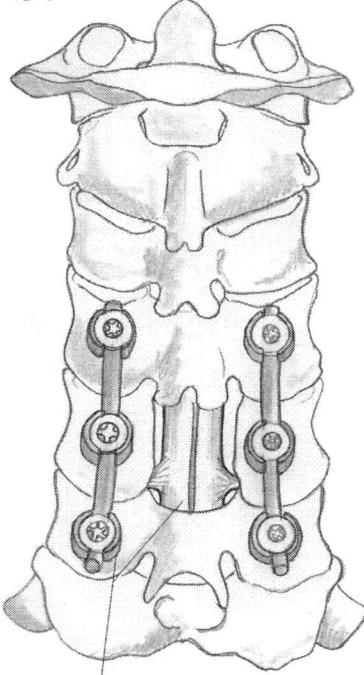

Cervical spine viewed from the side (lateral)

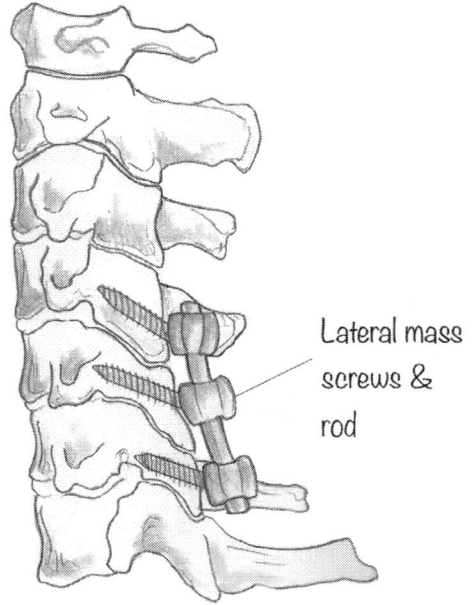

Lateral mass screws & rod

C4-C6 Posterior Fusion and C5 Laminectomy

Posterior cervical fusion. A posterior cervical fusion typically involves placement of screws into the lateral masses of the cervical vertebrae and performing a laminectomy (removal of lamina).

Cervical Laminoplasty

Cross sections of the cervical spine demonstrating laminoplasty:

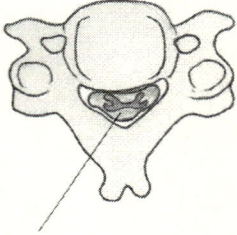 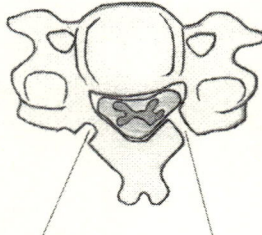 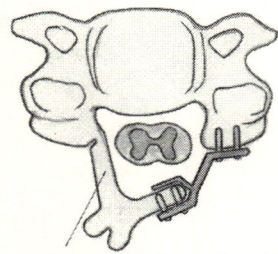

Spinal cord compression   Hinge cut   Trough cut   Lamina is hinged and held open by a small plate creating room for spinal cord

View of the cervical spine from behind (posterior):

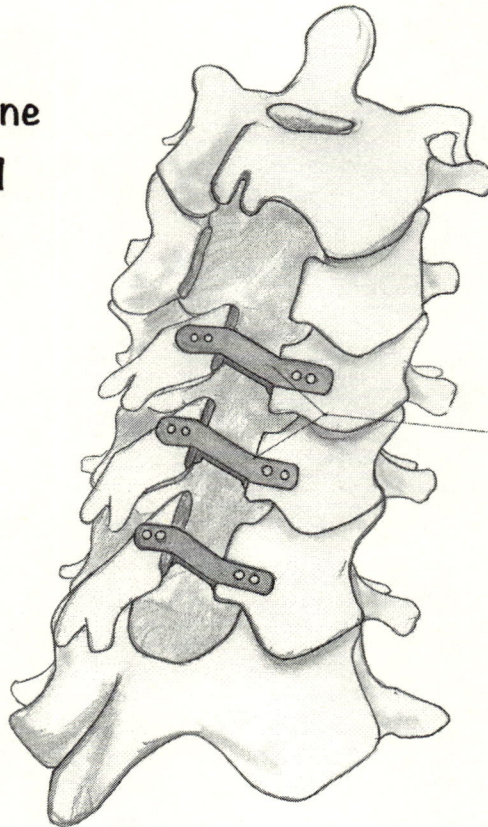

Laminectomy at C3 and C7 with laminoplasties at C4, C5 and C6

Cervical laminoplasty. A cervical laminoplasty procedure is used to generate more space in the spinal canal by opening the lamina up like a door and holding it open with a small plate(top). A C4-6 laminoplasty with laminectomies at C2-3 and C6-7 (bottom). The main advantage of the procedure is that it does not fuse the vertebrae and is thus motion preserving.

Chapter 44

Fixing Disease in the Neck While Preserving Neck Movement: Cervical Disc Replacement and Cervical Foraminotomy

Summary

While fusions are a work horse procedure that can be used to treat many problems in the neck, they result in the loss of motion. Cervical disc replacement (CDR), which uses a prosthesis to replace the native disc, is an alternative to fusion that can both treat disease and maintain motion. Scientific trials have shown that CDRs have improved results compared to fusions over the long term. Cervical foraminotomy is another option that can be useful for decompressing individual nerve roots. Both procedures have very specific indications and may not be used in all patients with neck problems. Unfortunately, many patients who want to avoid a fusion may be disappointed to find that they are not candidates for a CDR or foraminotomy. Both cervical foraminotomy and cervical disc replacement are known as motion-preserving procedures because they do not involve fusing any bones in the neck.

Case

Mr. Black is a 53-year-old businessman who had sudden onset of neck and arm pain while lifting weights. He also started to experience significant weakness of the arm and shoulder that occurred with numbness. He notices rapid atrophy of his chest and biceps muscles. He was diagnosed with a C5-6-disc herniation resulting in a pinched nerve in his neck that was causing his symptoms. Considering his young age and the fact that he was very healthy with little degeneration in his neck, I recommended cervical disc replacement. After the procedure his arm immediately regained strength and the pain was gone; however, some of his numbness remained. Over the course of a year, he fully regained all strength in his arm and the numbness eventually resolved. He is now stronger than ever and has no problems with his neck function.

Introduction

The neck is amazing because it is meant to allow you to have 180° motion to better observe the world around you. While fusion is an effective treatment method for many cervical diseases, it does remove motion from the spine and affects biomechanics. Fusing a level in the spine changes the way the neck moves and can put increased strain on the segments above and below the fusion. This leads to a 2.9% per year chance of future adjacent level degeneration, which will eventually require surgical treatment following the initial fusion surgery in the neck (1). Why this occurs is up for debate. It could be that this is part of the natural disease process where adjacent discs degenerate like the one that was treated. However, it is also thought that the rigid nature of a fusion causes increased stress on adjacent structures, resulting in a faster rate of degeneration.

When possible, motion-preservation surgery is desirable because it allows you to not only retain the natural way your neck moves, but also decreases the risk of further spine break down. Cervical disc replacement and the cervical foraminotomy are two common methods to decompress nerve roots and still retain neck motion. Disc replacement in the cervical spine, is more widely used than in the lumbar spine because it is easier to achieve better long-term outcomes and, in the right patient, can lead to amazing results.

Cervical laminectomy/laminoplasty are other motion-preserving procedures but are discussed in chapter 43.

Cervical Disc Replacement

Your neck has gelatinous discs between the vertebrae to allow motion. When things go wrong with the disc, the accepted treatment is for a spine surgeon to fuse the bones together with bone graft. Cervical disc replacement (CDR) also known as cervical disc arthroplasty (CDA) has become increasingly accepted as a motion-preserving alternative to cervical fusion, which has been the gold standard to treat disorders of the cervical spine for decades. The concept behind CDR is to remove the diseased disc and replace it with a prosthesis that helps recreate its normal motion. CDR is generally indicated for single-level disc disease, although two devices, the Mobi-C® and Simplify® are indicated for two-level degeneration.

Like fusions, cervical disc replacements are performed through an anterior (through the front) approach to the neck. The diseased disc is removed, and the spinal cord and nerve roots are decompressed. The disc is then replaced with a prosthesis that is designed to mimic the biomechanical properties of the native disc. CDR prostheses typically consist of a plastic-bearing spacer made from ultra-high-molecular-weight polyethylene (a plastic) sandwiched between two metal plates made from cobalt chromium alloy. These materials are like what is used in a total hip or knee replacement. The metal plates of the prosthesis bind to top and bottom of the vertebrae, ultimately growing into the bone and the plastic bearing glides between them allowing motion.

Cervical disc prostheses designs may either be a single piece or multipiece. In a single-piece prosthesis all components are linked together, while multipiece prostheses are composed of separate pieces inserted independently. The theoretical advantages and disadvantages between these two designs are just that—theoretical, as there have been no major clinical trials to compare the different types. Some prostheses incorporate a spongy center which allows for compression but again this has not been shown to be superior to other designs. There are many different models. Some are designed with little teeth to hold them in place. Others have specifically designed keels (like the keel on a boat) which are cut into the bones above and below and used to fixate the device. The metal plates are coated with a porous titanium-alloy spray surface which allows them to grow into the bony surfaces and thus become well fixed in place over time.

There are theoretical advantages to cervical disc replacement over fusion surgery. Biomechanical models have shown that a CDR reduces strain on the levels above and below by preserving motion at the diseased level (8,9). Recovery time is much faster with a CDR, and a lower profile prosthesis means fewer swallowing issues after surgery, which are common after fusion procedures (10). There are improved clinical outcomes and better satisfaction up to 10 years following surgery and a decreased risk of reoperation. Overall, there is robust evidence supporting both the use of cervical disc replacements and, in correctly chosen patients, its superiority to cervical fusion (see table above) (2,4–6).

MOST POPULAR CERVCIAL DISC REPLACEMENT (CDR) DEVICES			
Device name and Manufacturer	Design Features	Market Availability	Major Evidence/Randomized Controlled Trials (RCT) comparing disc replacement devices (CDR) with disc removal and fusion (ACDF)
BRYAN® Manufacturer: Medtronic	DESIGN: Single piece with polyurethane core Anchorage: Bony ingrowth	No, retired	Sasso et al (2017) (2): Prospective RCT comparing 23 CDR patients to 25 ACDF (disc removed and vertebrae fused) patients with 10-year follow-up: CDR showed improved clinical outcome scores, lower rates of revisions, compared to fusion.
M6-C® Manufacturer: Orthofix	DESIGN: Single piece with compression core and woven annulus (exterior) Anchorage: Teeth	Yes	Phillips et al (2021): Prospective RCT comparing 160 CDR patients to 189 ACDF patients with 10- year follow-up: Both ACDF and M6-C ® resulted in significant clinical improvement. There was lower use of opioids in the M6-C at 24 months compared to ACDF. Similar revision and complication rates between groups (3).
Mobi-C Manufacturer: Zimmer Biomet	DESIGN: Single piece with plastic polyethylene core Anchorage: Teeth	Yes	Radcliff et al (2017) (4): Prospective RCT comparing 225 two-level CDR patients to 105 two-level ACDF patients and 164 one-level CDR to 81 one-level ACDF with 7-year follow-up: Demonstrated clinical superiority of two-level CDR over ACDF and non-inferiority of single-level CDR to ACDF.

If it sounds too good to be true, you should remember that there are several limitations to the cervical disc replacement device. The indications for a CDR are strict and not everyone is a candidate. Firstly, the compression on your spine or nerve root must be coming from the disc, that is, the front part of the bones (anterior) rather than the back (posterior). A cervical disc replacement will not treat spinal stenosis originating from the back of the canal. As cervical disc replacements are motion-preserving, if you have significant neck pain from arthritis of the bones, a fusion is more appropriate. There are also intra-operative findings which may force a surgeon to abort and switch to a fusion in the middle of surgery. For example, cervical disc replacement requires careful positioning of the device using X-rays. In some individuals, adequate X-rays may be impossible to acquire and thus a fusion will need to be performed. If the graft cannot be implanted in a stable position, the surgeon may elect to perform a fusion instead, which can generally be made stable because of use of a fixation plate.

MOST POPULAR CERVCIAL DISC REPLACEMENT (CDR) DEVICES			
Device name and Manufacturer	**Design Features**	**Market Availability**	**Major Evidence/Randomized Controlled Trials (RCT) comparing disc replacement devices (CDR) with disc removal and fusion (ACDF)**
Prestige ST® **Manufacturer** Medtronic	**DESIGN:** Multipiece, metal on metal **Anchorage:** Screws to anchor to bone above and below	Yes	**Burkus et al (2014) (5):** Prospective RCT comparing 276 CDR patients with 265 cervical fusion patients with 7-year follow- up: CDR showed improved clinical outcome scores, lower rates of revisions compared to fusion.
Prodisc-C® **Manufacturer:** Centinel Spine	**DESIGN:** Multipiece (device is inserted piecemeal instead of as a single unit) **Anchorage:** Keel (central prong)	Yes	**Janssen et al (2015) (6):** Prospective RCT comparing 103 CDR patients with 106 cervical fusion patients with 7- year follow-up: Similar clinical outcomes between techniques. Markedly higher revision rates in the ACDF group.
Simplify® **Manufacturer:** Nuvasive	DESIGN: Multipiece, ceramic on polyetheretherketone (PEEK) bearing **Anchorage:** Small keel and titanium coated endplates	Yes	**Coric et al (2022) (7):** Prospective non-randomized multicenter trial comparing two level Simplify ® CDR and ACDF with 2-year follow-up. The Simplify ® showed improved clinical outcomes compared to ACDF with decreased revision rates

The most common problem preventing surgeons from performing a CDR is arthritis (or other degeneration or arthropathy) in the vertebral joints at the level of replacement. Arthritis in the neck causes bone spur formation as well as wearing down of the disc space and facet joints, which stiffens the motion of that segment. Disc replacements are very good for treating so-called "soft disc herniations" where there is not much degeneration of the bones outside of the disc. Unfortunately, this is a very rare scenario, and most cases of stenosis come along with a fair deal of arthritis. There are two main reasons degeneration is a problem. The first is that a significant amount of bone resection (cutting out) must be done to fully decompress stenosis resulting from degeneration, which can increase the chance the bones spontaneously fuse after the procedure.

The second is that if there is significant arthritis at the level of disease, maintaining motion may not be a good thing as it could result in increased pain. For young patients, CDR is preferable over fusion to help them maintain healthy discs but certainly CDR is not limited only to young patients. Older patients may also have great results from CDR so long as they meet the above criteria. As more and more studies on CDR come out, surgeons are using CDR far more frequently, allowing more and more people to benefit. Current restrictions (contraindications) that prevent you from having a CDR are listed in the table below.

Until recently CDR could only be used at single levels, but new devices have broken through barriers and shown excellent outcomes for multilevel indications. Hybrid constructs consisting of a fusion at one level and a cervical disc replacement at another may also be considered. This hybrid technique is commonly used and has been reported to have good outcomes but has not been studied with formal prospective randomized trials (10,11).

Contraindications to Cervical Disc Replacement
Significant degeneration of the disc or facet
Instability or spondylolisthesis
More than 50% loss of disc height
Osteoporosis
Ossification (calcification) of the posterior longitudinal ligament
Greater than 3 levels of disease
Significant spinal deformity
Metal allergy

There are certain risks with a CDR surgery some of which are like traditional fusion techniques. CDR still requires an anterior approach to the cervical spine and can result in injury to essential structures including the airway, nerves and esophagus. Thera are some complications which are unique to CDR. Despite being motion-preserving, the prosthesis can undergo ossification and become auto-fused. This has been reported to occur anywhere from 7% to 70% of cases depending on implant type and the patient. However, if ossification occurs it typically does not impact clinical results and even if the prosthesis completely fuses it will result in the same function a fusion procedure would provide. The opposite can also occur, where the implant fails to grow into the bone and can become displaced. This is generally a more serious complication and may warrant revision surgery.

Cervical Foraminotomy—Unpinching Nerves in the Neck

The cervical foraminotomy is a procedure which may be used to treat pinched nerves in the neck causing pain. As described in previous chapters, nerves exiting the spine are known as "nerve roots." They exit the spinal cord through a corridor in the vertebral bone known as a foramen and a foraminotomy makes this corridor larger. A cervical foraminotomy is performed through a small posterior (through the back) incision in the neck. A portion of the facet joint is carefully removed to enlarge the foramen, taking pressure off (decompressing) the nerve root that travels through it. Once this opening is created any bone spurs or soft disc herniations that may also be compressing the nerve root may be removed

Foraminotomies are used to treat radiating arm pain that originates from cervical nerve root compression known as radiculopathy. Cervical foraminotomy procedures are called motion-preserving because no fusion is performed. They may be used in similar situations to a cervical fusion or a cervical disc replacement.

Like cervical disc arthroplasty (replacement), cervical foraminotomy is not a work horse procedure like a fusion and can only be used in certain situations. If the pathology compressing the spinal cord or nerve root is in the middle of the spinal canal, a cervical foraminotomy will not work. What this means is that foraminotomies are only useful for treating problems occurring in the foramen, which is lateral to the spinal canal. Moreover, if your predominant symptom is neck pain or your arm pain occurs on both sides, a fusion surgery may be more appropriate.

Overall cervical foraminotomies have an excellent track record. In a large retrospective review of 162 single-level cervical foraminotomies with 5 years of follow-up, 95% had improvement in arm pain and neck pain (12). (A single level involves one vertebra whereas a 1-level procedure would involve two adjacent vertebrae.) In a large meta-analysis comparing cervical foraminotomy to CDR and cervical fusion, while all treatments resulted in significant improvement in symptoms and functional outcomes, cervical foraminotomy was associated with the lowest incidence of complications (13).

However, there are complications which are unique to cervical foraminotomy. Because a portion of the facet must be removed, there is a small chance spinal instability will develop after the surgery. This is estimated to occur in around 5% of cases. If this occurs a follow-up fusion surgery may be required. Also, the normal alignment of your neck may be changed by a cervical foraminotomy and result in what is called kyphosis or a forward posture of the neck which can occur in up to 20% of patients; however, this is usually asymptomatic.

Overall cervical foraminotomy is a good option for younger patients who may want to avoid fusion, have cervical spine problems which meet the indications for the procedure, and who are not candidates for cervical disc replacement.

Conclusion

Both cervical foraminotomy and cervical disc replacements are great procedures that can relieve neck and arm pain without the loss of motion. The catch is that these procedures will only work in a subset of patients who have relatively mild disease. In patients who have severe pathology, a cervical fusion is more appropriate. Deciding which procedure to have should be at the discretion of your surgeon.

Frequently Asked Questions

- **How much arthritis is too much for a cervical disc replacement?**

   Typically, if there is arthritis and bone spurs coming off the facet joint a cervical disc replacement should not be attempted. This is because this portion of the spine will not be treated by the prosthesis and the arthritis may be worsened or become inflamed from the increased motion provided by a CDR. Nonetheless, as the indications for CDR expand, more and more degrees of arthritis and bone spurs at the disc space are being tolerated by surgeons across the country. This means that some surgeons will not be dissuaded from performing a CDR if there are some small bone spurs that can be removed, and if the disc space is reasonably intact.

References

1.   Hilibrand AS, Carlson GD, Palumbo MA, Jones PK, Bohlman HH. Radiculopathy and Myelopathy at Segments Adjacent to the Site of a Previous Anterior Cervical Arthrodesis*. J Bone Jt Surg. 1999;81(4):519–28.

2.   Sasso WR, Smucker JD, Sasso MP, Sasso RC. Long-term Clinical Outcomes of Cervical Disc Arthroplasty: A Prospective, Randomized, Controlled Trial. SPINE. 2017 Feb;42(4):209–16.

3.   Phillips FM, Coric D, Sasso R, Lanman T, Lavelle W, Blumenthal S, et al. Prospective, multicenter clinical trial comparing M6-C compressible six degrees of freedom cervical disc with anterior cervical discectomy and fusion for the treatment of single-level degenerative cervical radiculopathy: 2-year results of an FDA investigational device exemption study. Spine J Off J North Am Spine Soc. 2021 Feb;21(2):239–52.

4.   Radcliff K, Davis RJ, Hisey MS, Nunley PD, Hoffman GA, Jackson RJ, et al. Long-term Evaluation of Cervical Disc Arthroplasty with the Mobi-C© Cervical Disc: A Randomized, Prospective, Multicenter Clinical Trial with Seven-Year Follow-up. Int J Spine Surg. 2017;11(4):31.

5.   Burkus JK, Traynelis VC, Haid RW, Mummaneni PV. Clinical and radiographic analysis of an artificial cervical disc: 7-year follow-up from the Prestige prospective randomized controlled clinical trial: Clinical article. J Neurosurg Spine. 2014 Oct;21(4):516–28.

6.   Janssen ME, Zigler JE, Spivak JM, Delamarter RB, Darden BV, Kopjar B. ProDisc-C Total Disc Replacement Versus Anterior Cervical Discectomy and Fusion for Single-Level Symptomatic Cervical Disc Disease: Seven-Year Follow-up of the Prospective Randomized U.S. Food and Drug Administration Investigational Device Exemption Study. J Bone Jt Surg. 2015 Nov;97(21):1738–47.

7.   Coric D, Guyer RD, Bae H, Nunley PD, Strenge KB, Peloza JH, et al. Prospective, multi-center study of 2-level cervical arthroplasty with a PEEK-on-ceramic artificial disc. J Neurosurg Spine. 2022 Apr 1;1–11.

8.   Dmitriev AE, Cunningham BW, Hu N, Sell G, Vigna F, McAfee PC. Adjacent level intra-discal pressure and segmental kinematics following a cervical total disc arthroplasty: an in vitro human cadaveric model. Spine. 2005 May 15;30(10):1165–72.

9.   Park DK, Lin EL, Phillips FM. Index and adjacent level kinematics after cervical disc replacement and anterior fusion: in vivo quantitative radiographic analysis. Spine. 2011 Apr 20;36(9):721–30.

10.   Laratta JL, Shillingford JN, Saifi C, Riew KD. Cervical Disc Arthroplasty: A Comprehensive Review of Single-Level, Multilevel, and Hybrid Procedures. Glob Spine J. 2018 Feb;8(1):78–83.

11.   Jia Z, Mo Z, Ding F, He Q, Fan Y, Ruan D. Hybrid surgery for multilevel cervical degenerative disc diseases: a systematic review of biomechanical and clinical evidence. Eur Spine J Off Publ Eur Spine Soc Eur Spinal Deform Soc Eur Sect Cerv Spine Res Soc. 2014 Aug;23(8):1619–32.

12.   Jagannathan J, Sherman JH, Szabo T, Shaffrey CI, Jane JA. The posterior cervical foraminotomy in the treatment of cervical disc/osteophyte disease: a single-surgeon experience with a minimum of 5 years' clinical and radiographic follow-up. J Neurosurg Spine. 2009 Apr;10(4):347–56.

13.   Gutman G, Rosenzweig DH, Golan JD. The surgical treatment of cervical radiculopathy: meta-analysis of randomized controlled trials.: SPINE. 2017 Jul;1.

Figures:

Cervical Disc Arthroplasty

Mobi-C®

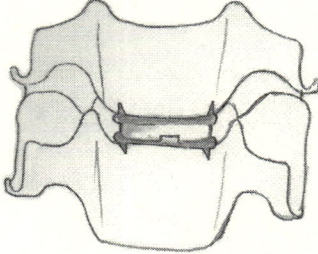
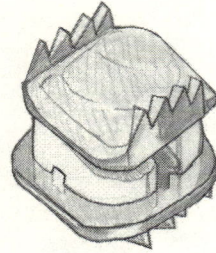

Prodisc-C®

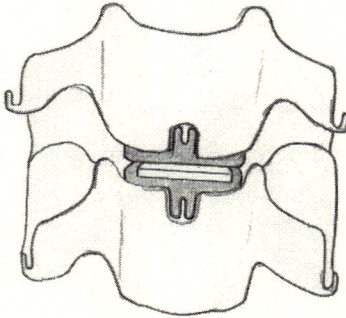
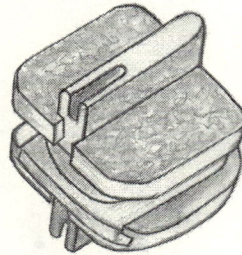

Bryan®

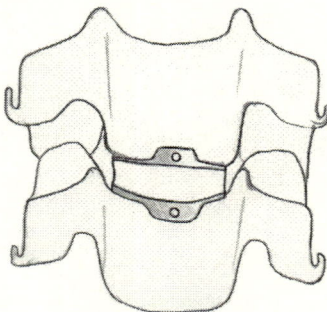
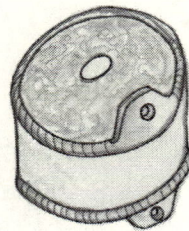

Cervical disc replacement. There are many different cervical disc replacement devices available. They differ by endplate design, core bearing and anchoring method. The three shown here are the Mobi-C®, the ProDisc-C® and the Bryan® (from top to bottom).

Cervical Foraminotomy

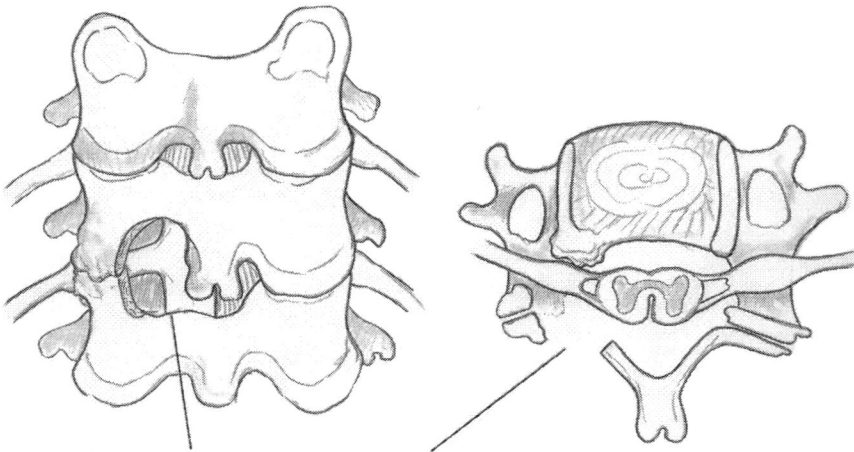

Back view of cervical vertebrae

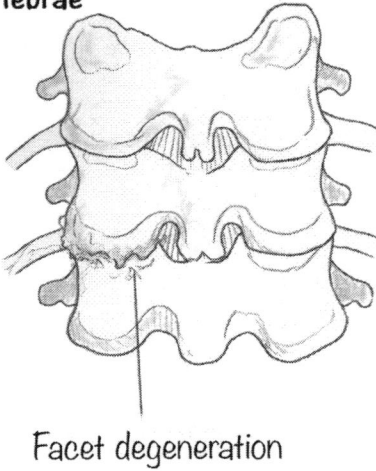

Cross section of cervical spine

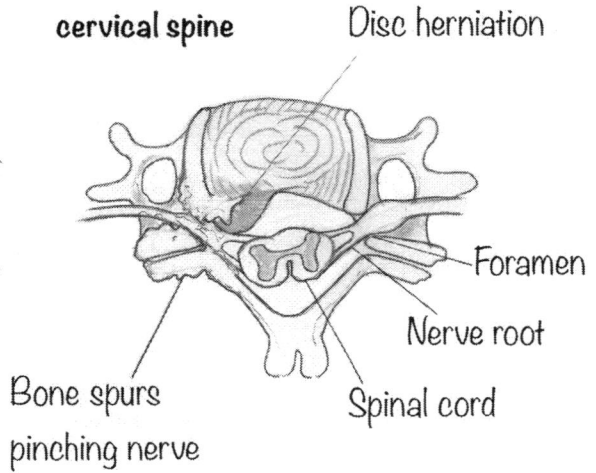

Disc herniation

Foramen

Nerve root

Bone spurs pinching nerve

Spinal cord

Facet degeneration

Foraminotomy

A small area of bone is removed to take pressure off of the nerve

Cervical Foraminotomy. A cervical foraminotomy is a procedure used to treat a compressed nerve in the neck (top). This is accomplished by removing part of the facet and lamina (bottom).

Chapter 45

Replacing a Disc in the Low Back to Relieve Low Back Pain—How and Who it is for: Lumbar Disc Replacement/Arthroplasty

Summary

Low back pain is a very common problem, and many patients are looking for a quick and easy fix. Lumbar disc replacement (LDR), where a degenerative disc is replaced with a biomechanical prosthesis, is a relatively new option for treating low back pain. It is enticing because it promises to replace a degenerative disc with a functional prosthesis, retain motion and take away the pain unlike a lumbar fusion (joining two vertebrae together surgically). Trials have shown that in properly selected patients, it is at least as good as a lumbar fusion and is beneficial in relieving symptoms of low back pain. However, there have been several of these devices which have been approved only to be retracted from the open market because of problems. Furthermore, it is hard to find patients who are good candidates that will benefit from the procedure and when the procedure does fail there are no safe bail-out options. Nevertheless, for those who meet the strict criteria to have an LDR performed it can be a beneficial procedure for easing back pain. If you are interested in this procedure, there are several things to consider. Your insurance may not cover it, and it may be necessary to pay cash to have it performed. Finally, not all spine surgeons perform the procedure, so you may have to travel to a specialty center to have it performed.

Case

Mr. Teal is a 66-year-old financier who has had 5 years of persistent low back pain. He has tried everything he can think of including several years of physical therapy, multiple injections and even a radiofrequency ablation procedure. He was seen by a spine surgeon and told that he has degenerative disc disease with one black disc at L5-1, but that there was really nothing to do about this. Determined to find a solution to his problem, he seeks out treatment at a center in Germany that specializes in lumbar disc replacement. A discogram is performed at this center that helps to confirm his pain is indeed arising from the black disc (as seen in his MRI) in his lumbar spine. He undergoes a single level LDR (lumbar disc replacement) and has improvement in his pain. Unfortunately, over time the device starts to migrate and lose its position in the spine. After several months the device is sticking into the abdomen and his surgeon recommends that a fusion be performed through the back of the spine. Unfortunately, because of scarring the device cannot be safely retrieved, although it does not seem to be causing any immediate harm to nearby structures. He undergoes a fusion, but this also fails, and the future is uncertain.

Introduction

The lumbar disc replacement (LDR) is a procedure designed to replace a degenerative disc with a prosthesis and has had a long and complicated history. Lumbar disc replacement, unlike cervical disc replacement, has not become totally mainstream in spinal surgery. The reason for this is that lumbar disc replacements have not had the same universal success that cervical disc replacements have enjoyed. There are more demands on a lumbar disc prosthesis because, unlike the cervical disc replacements which must only withstand the forces of the weight of the head, a lumbar disc replacement needs to support the weight of the entire torso. There is a certain subset of patients who may benefit from this procedure, but distinguishing them is difficult, and because the procedure is risky, many surgeons are not willing to perform them. Moreover, insurance will rarely approve the procedure. To understand why there is so much controversy over lumbar disc replacements or LDR, we need to understand a little about how the diagnosis process works.

The Black Disc

Lumbar disc degeneration and low back pain are very common problems in adults, affecting up to 70% of individuals (1). Lumbar disc degeneration can result in a phenomenon known as discogenic back pain, meaning the degenerative disc is the source of the pain. This type of pain generally occurs across the low back and may radiate to the SI joints bilaterally without many other distinguishing features. An MRI image may show a characteristic black disc (a healthy, well-hydrated disc is white in the center on MRI). Along with this there may be tears of the annulus fibrosis (the outer tough layer of the disc) and loss of disc height. The confusing thing about degenerative disc disease is that many asymptomatic people will also have similar findings and never go on to develop problems (2). This begs the question, if most black discs are asymptomatic who will benefit from an LDR?

Discography is a test to help confirm the diagnosis of discogenic back pain. In a discogram, contrast fluid is injected into the disc space to cause it to expand. If this reproduces the patient's pain or shows a tear in the annulus (indicated by a contrast leak or by the observation that the injection has no resistance, suggesting easy flow into the space) the test result is said to be "positive." A separate discogram test is also performed in an adjacent healthy disc to act as a control for the procedure. Ideally, the disc that is symptomatic would be positive, while the control disc would be negative, and the physician would know that the pain was originating from the degenerative disc. Unfortunately, this test has a very high false positive rate because the test itself is painful and can create pain in a totally normal disc (3). Even in patients with a positive test result, surgery may not result in significant pain relief (4,5). Discograms are controversial because of these reasons, yet they remain the single best test we have to confirm discogenic back pain (6).

Another way to test the disc is to inject numbing medicine after the saline. If the pain you are experiencing is then relieved by the injection of the medicine into the disc, this further indicates that the pain is indeed coming from that disc. Personally, this method makes more sense to me, but it is impossible to know how accurate it is as there are no other tests to compare it to.

Performing routine discograms has also fallen out of favor because it has been shown that injecting into the disc itself can cause damage and further degeneration.

Disc Arthroplasty

Lumbar disc replacement (LDR, also known as total disc arthroplasty TDA) is a procedure where the diseased lumbar disc is replaced with a prosthetic designed to mimic the function of a natural disc. LDR is performed through an anterior abdominal approach like the ALIF (anterior lumbar interbody fusion) approach and usually requires a vascular or general surgeon to help get access to the spine. The LDR concept was developed around the same time as the first total hip replacements. Early designs consisted of a stainless steel ball which was implanted between vertebrae and had many failures (7).

Since then, the design has advanced considerably to now look more like a normal lumbar disc. Modern arthroplasty designs have been approved by the FDA (Food and Drug Administration) for treatment of single level (one disc space) discogenic pain with the absence of spinal instability from L3 to S1 (8). Patients should have a positive response on discograms as discussed above and have failed 6 months of conservative therapy. Multilevel arthroplasties may be performed, but this is "off label" (not FDA-approved) and is typically done at surgeon discretion (9).

Currently the gold standard treatment for many low back spinal problems is a fusion procedure. This process removes the disc and causes two or more vertebrae to grow together, preventing motion at the diseased level. Lumbar disc replacement was designed to theoretically prevent some of the problems that occur following spinal fusions. For example, in an LDR, there is no need to wait for the bones to heal together, which may shorten the time to return to normal function. Moreover, there is no chance for the bones to fail to heal together (pseudoarthrosis), which may occur in many lumbar fusion cases. Also, spinal fusions may produce increased stress on segments adjacent to the fusion (the vertebra and its disc adjacent to the fused segment), which may cause them to break down prematurely (known as adjacent segment disease). This occurs at a rate of around 4% per year for 10 years and probably results because of the loss of mobility of the spine at the site of the fusion, requiring other adjacent segments to move more to compensate. Since an LDR functions more similarly to a native disc, it may reduce the occurrence of adjacent segment disease (10). However, this concept has not been solidly proven (11). Furthermore, over a longer period of time an LDR may become biomechanically similar to a fusion as many become gradually fused (12).

One of the main problems with disc arthroplasty is that it has many contraindications (reasons not to use it) and patients must be selected very carefully. There are many parts of the spine that can cause pain; these must be ruled out prior to disc arthroplasty since the procedure will not treat any diseased area of the spine other than a bad disc.

You are not a candidate for lumbar disc arthroplasty if you have:

- **Concurrent stenosis (narrowing of the spinal canal at the site or adjacent to the problem disc)**

- **Scoliosis**

- **Arthritis of the facet joints**

- **Osteoporosis or chronic steroid use**

- **Vertebral slips (spondylolisthesis) or damage to the pars bone (spondylosis)**

- **Symptomatic disc herniations causing nerve root irritation**

- **Obesity**

- **Previous lumbar fusion, fracture, or infection**

- **Pregnancy**

- **Age younger than 18 or older than 60 years**

Types of Arthroplasty Devices

The typical total disc prosthesis undergoes extensive testing in a biomechanical lab to ensure its strength and durability prior to approval by the FDA. There are several differently designed LDR devices on the market currently, but most arthroplasty devices consist of three main pieces: two metallic endplate pieces which connect with the vertebrae above and below and a central bearing piece which allows motion. Variations on this basic design (see table) include endplate structure and composition, bearing composition, and constraint between bearing and endplate anchorage, that is, how freely the bearing moves relative to the vertebrae endplates they connect to. The metallic endplates are typically coated with a special titanium finish that allows the host bone to grow into the implant and gives the device longevity.

LUMBAR DISC REPLACEMENT (LDR)

Device Name and Manufacturer	Design Features	History and Market Availability	Major Evidence/Randomized Controlled Trials (RCTs)
Charité® I Charité® II Charité® III (Named after the Charité hospital in Germany) Manufacturer: Depuy Synthes	Components: two metallic endplates (cobalt chromium molybdenum alloy) and a central core of plastic (polyethylene) that acts as the bearing, gliding between the metallic endplates Constraint: Unconstrained Anchorage: Teeth	Charité® I: Ultimately discarded due to migration of the device, replaced by Charité® II which had more surface area. Charité® I and II were never commercially available. The Charité® III is the modern version and was the first LDR implant approved by the FDA in 2004. Was removed from the market in 2012 due to significant complications such as subsidence (loosening and caving in of the implant into the vertebra), lack of long-term pain relief, adjacent segment degeneration. Also, its unconstrained design led to concerns of increased polyethylene wear. Market Availability: No	Blumenthal et al 2005: FDA RCT 304 patients ALIF (anterior lumbar fusion with spacer) vs LDR with 2-year follow-up. Charité® III was not inferior to lumbar fusion and did show shorter hospital stays and lower reoperation rates (13). Guyer et al 2009: FDA RCT of Charité ® vs ALIF with 133 Patients and 5-year follow-up. No differences in clinical outcomes (14). Lu et al 2015: Prospective study of 32 patients implanted with the Charité ® and had 11-year follow-up. 87% had acceptable outcomes. Reoperation performed in 2 patients. Disc height and range of motion increased significantly from initial levels in LDR patients (15).

Outcomes

In general, results from lumbar disc replacements are good. Randomized controlled trials have shown similar efficacy and complication rates between lumbar fusion and lumbar disc replacement in patients who are candidates for the LDR procedure. A large meta-analysis synthesizing 6 randomized control trials compared lumbar disc replacement to lumbar fusion in 1600 patients. LDR patients had improved clinical outcomes compared to lumbar fusion with a similar complication profile up to 2 years following surgery. Both groups had similar reoperation rates (22).

LUMBAR DISC REPLACEMENT (LDR) continued			
Device Name and Manufacturer	Design Features	History and Market Availability	Major Evidence/Randomized Controlled Trials (RCTs)
Prodisc L* Manufacturer: Centinel Spine previously Depuy Synthes	Components: two metallic endplates (cobalt chromium molybdenum alloy) and a central core of plastic (polyethylene) that acts as the bearing Constraint: Semi-constrained polyethylene core is fixed on inferior (lower) endplate Anchorage: Keels with Titanium plasma-sprayed finish	FDA approved in 2006. Had some design improvements on the Charité* to decrease subsidence (See above). Market Availability: Yes	Zigler et al 2007: FDA RCT comparing Prodisc L* to lumbar spinal fusion with 2-year follow-up. Improved clinical outcomes and pain compared to fusion at final follow-up(16). Siepe et al 2014: Prospective study of 201 patients implanted with the Prodisc L* with 5-to-10-year follow-up. 63% reported high satisfaction, 22% were satisfied and 13% were not satisfied. 7.2% revision surgery (17).
Maverick* Manufacturer: Medtronic	Components: two metallic endplates, each housing its own metallic bearing component Constraint: Semi-constrained Anchorage: Keels with Titanium plasma-sprayed finish	First used in Europe in 2006 and, in contrast to the Prodisc L* and Charité *, it has a two-piece metal-on-metal design. Some concerns that metal-on-metal design produces metallic debris and increased blood concentration of metal ions (18). Market Availability: Outside US only.	Gornet et al 2011: FDA RCT comparing the Maverick* to ALIF with 2 years follow-up. The maverick had superior outcomes at all post-op evaluations (19).

LUMBAR DISC REPLACEMENT (LDR) continued			
Device Name and Manufacturer	**Design Features**	**History and Market Availability**	**Major Evidence/Randomized Controlled Trials (RCTs)**
FLexiCore® Manufacturer: Stryker	**Components:** two metallic endplates, each housing its own metallic bearing component **Constraint:** Fixed **Anchorage:** Teeth with Titanium plasma-sprayed finish	**Market Availability:** No	**Sasso et al 2008:** RCT comparing the FlexiCore® (44 patients) to fusion (23 patients) with 2-year follow- up. FlexiCore® compared favorably to circumferential fusion (an ALIF plus posterior pedicle screws) (20).
ActivL® Manufacturer: Aesculap	**Components:** two metallic endplates (cobalt chromium molybdenum alloy) and a central core of plastic (polyethylene) that acts as the bearing **Constraint:** Semi-constrained **Anchorage:** Teeth with Titanium plasma-sprayed finish	FDA approval in 2015 **Market Availability:** Yes	**Yue et al 2019:** FDA Investigational Device Exemption. Non inferiority trial comparing the ActivL® (218 patients) to ProdiscL®(65 patients) or the Charité ® (41 patients) with 5 years of follow-up. The ActivL® was more effective at preserving range of motion and had a better safety profile than the other implants (21).
ALIF is Anterior Lumbar Interbody Fusion			

Complications

The main reported complications from first generation disc arthroplasty devices were related either to the approach (approaching from the front through the abdomen, which is standard to lumbar fusions) or related to degeneration of the facet joints. It is also possible for the implant to unexpectedly fuse by a process known as heterotopic ossification—a process where bone tissue grows in or on non-bone tissue or material causing loss of motion—spinal fusions depend on this process to succeed. However, if the disc implant fuses, it loses its ability to move like the regular spinal disc it replaces, which is obviously contradictory to the design and intent of the implant. Finally, if the implant fails to incorporate into the bony surface, it can migrate from its original position to a different location or subside (sink) into the bone on which it sits. Both complications may lead to early failure of the implant.

In a large database study of 52,000 patients who underwent LDR, a wound infection was the most common adverse event. The rate of subsequent surgery within the follow-up period was less for LDR compared to fusion and was around 5-6% at 5 years (23).

One of the main problems with LDR is that once implanted, there are no perfect revision strategies. Revising an anterior approach to the lumbar spine can be very dangerous, because of scarring around the great vessels, bowels and other visceral structures increases risk of inadvertent injury. Moreover, it is impossible to remove the LDR device from a posterior (through the back) approach. A fusion may be performed from a posterior approach to stabilize an anterior LDR device. However, this surgery may easily fail because the front of the spine is still unconstrained and can move because of the LDR device. Thus, this can lead to an even greater problem, where both anterior and posterior approaches have failed. There is no easy escape route from a failed LDR (11).

Conclusion

LDR has been on the market for almost 20 years at this point; however, it is still not widely adopted except for a few centers in the United States. In correctly indicated patients it seems at least comparable to lumbar fusion. It should be noted that despite the good literature supporting its use, there is a bias that exists in surgeons publishing this data, many of whom have ties to the industry producing these implants (24). Studies that have a financial conflict are more likely to produce favorable results. However, some may also argue that the centers with this bias also have a greater expertise with these devices, which may lead to improved results. In conclusion, LDR has shown promise to treat low back pain associated with degenerative lumbar disc disease. However, LDR does not represent a panacea, and the indications for a positive outcome are slim. To date only a few carefully selected patients will benefit in a meaningful way from this technology. Patients who may desire to be treated with the technology should avoid the impulse to think "I know better than the surgeon!"

Frequently Asked Questions

◆   Where are the specialty centers that specialize in LDR?

The one that comes easily to mind is the Texas Back Institute where much of the research on LDR has been performed. Other centers include the Hospital for Special Surgery in New York, and Rush Medical Center in Chicago.

References

1.   Andersson GB. Epidemiological features of chronic low-back pain. The Lancet. 1999 Aug;354(9178):581–5.

2.   Boden SD, Davis DO, Dina TS, Patronas NJ, Wiesel SW. Abnormal magnetic-resonance scans of the lumbar spine in asymptomatic subjects. A prospective investigation. J Bone Joint Surg Am. 1990 Mar;72(3):403–8.

3.   Carragee EJ, Alamin TF, Carragee JM. Low-Pressure Positive Discography in Subjects Asymptomatic of Significant Low Back Pain Illness: Spine. 2006 Mar;31(5):505–9.

4.   Smith SE, Darden BV, Rhyne AL, Wood KE. Outcome of unoperated discogram-positive low back pain. Spine. 1995 Sep 15;20(18):1997–2000; discussion 2000-2001.

5.   Carragee EJ, Lincoln T, Parmar VS, Alamin T. A Gold Standard Evaluation of the "Discogenic Pain" Diagnosis as Determined by Provocative Discography: Spine. 2006 Aug;31(18):2115–23.

6.   Madigan L, Vaccaro AR, Spector LR, Milam AR. Management of Symptomatic Lumbar Degenerative Disk Disease: Journal of the American Academy of Orthopaedic Surgeons. 2009 Feb;17(2):102–11.

7.   Abi-Hanna D, Kerferd J, Phan K, Rao P, Mobbs R. Lumbar Disk Arthroplasty for Degenerative Disk Disease: Literature Review. World Neurosurgery. 2018 Jan;109:188–96.

8.   Lin EL, Wang JC. Total Disk Arthroplasty: Journal of the American Academy of Orthopaedic Surgeons. 2006 Dec;14(13):705–14.

9.   Scott-Young M, McEntee L, Zotti M, Schram B, Furness J, Rathbone E, et al. Patient-Reported Outcome Measures After Multilevel Lumbar Total Disc Arthroplasty for the Treatment of Multilevel Degenerative Disc Disease: SPINE. 2020 Jan;45(1):18–25.

10.   Harrop JS, Youssef JA, Maltenfort M, Vorwald P, Jabbour P, Bono CM, et al. Lumbar Adjacent Segment Degeneration and Disease After Arthrodesis and Total Disc Arthroplasty: Spine. 2008 Jul;33(15):1701–7.

11.   Patel AA, Brodke DS, Pimenta L, Bono CM, Hilibrand AS, Harrop JS, et al. Revision Strategies in Lumbar Total Disc Arthroplasty: Spine. 2008 May;33(11):1276–83.

12.   Putzier M, Funk JF, Schneider SV, Gross C, Tohtz SW, Khodadadyan-Klostermann C, et al. Charité total disc replacement—clinical and radiographical results after an average follow-up of 17 years. Eur Spine J. 2006 Feb;15(2):183–95.

13.   Blumenthal S, McAfee PC, Guyer RD, Hochschuler SH, Geisler FH, Holt RT, et al. A Prospective, Randomized, Multicenter Food and Drug Administration Investigational Device

Exemptions Study of Lumbar Total Disc Replacement With the CHARITÉTM Artificial Disc Versus Lumbar Fusion: Part I: Evaluation of Clinical Outcomes. Spine. 2005 Jul;30(14):1565–75.

14.   Guyer RD, McAfee PC, Banco RJ, Bitan FD, Cappuccino A, Geisler FH, et al. Prospective, randomized, multicenter Food and Drug Administration investigational device exemption study of lumbar total disc replacement with the CHARITÉ artificial disc versus lumbar fusion: Five-year follow-up. The Spine Journal. 2009 May;9(5):374–86.

15.   Lu S bao, Hai Y, Kong C, Wang Q yi, Su Q, Zang L, et al. An 11-year minimum follow-up of the Charite III lumbar disc replacement for the treatment of symptomatic degenerative disc disease. Eur Spine J. 2015 Sep;24(9):2056–64.

16.   Zigler J, Delamarter R, Spivak JM, Linovitz RJ, Danielson GO, Haider TT, et al. Results of the Prospective, Randomized, Multicenter Food and Drug Administration Investigational Device Exemption Study of the ProDisc?-L Total Disc Replacement Versus Circumferential Fusion for the Treatment of 1-Level Degenerative Disc Disease. :8.

17.   Siepe CJ, Heider F, Wiechert K, Hitzl W, Ishak B, Mayer MH. Mid- to long-term results of total lumbar disc replacement: a prospective analysis with 5- to 10-year follow-up. The Spine Journal. 2014 Aug;14(8):1417–31.

18.   Zeh A, Planert M, Siegert G, Lattke P, Held A, Hein W. Release of Cobalt and Chromium Ions Into the Serum Following Implantation of the Metal-on-Metal Maverick-Type Artificial Lumbar Disc (Medtronic Sofamor Danek): Spine. 2007 Feb;32(3):348–52.

19.   Gornet MF, Burkus JK, Dryer RF, Peloza JH. Lumbar Disc Arthroplasty With MAVERICK Disc Versus Stand-Alone Interbody Fusion: A Prospective, Randomized, Controlled, Multicenter Investigational Device Exemption Trial. Spine. 2011 Dec;36(25):E1600–11.

20.   Sasso RC, Foulk DM, Hahn M. Prospective, Randomized Trial of Metal-on-Metal Artificial Lumbar Disc Replacement: Initial Results for Treatment of Discogenic Pain. Spine. 2008 Jan;33(2):123–31.

21.   Yue JJ, Garcia R, Blumenthal S, Coric D, Patel VV, Dinh DH, et al. Five-year Results of a Randomized Controlled Trial for Lumbar Artificial Discs in Single-level Degenerative Disc Disease: SPINE. 2019 Dec;44(24):1685–96.

22.   Wei J, Song Y, Sun L, Lv C. Comparison of artificial total disc replacement versus fusion for lumbar degenerative disc disease: a meta-analysis of randomized controlled trials. Int Orthop. 2013 Jul;37(7):1315–25.

23.   Eliasberg CD, Kelly MP, Ajiboye RM, SooHoo NF. Complications and Rates of Subsequent Lumbar Surgery Following Lumbar Total Disc Arthroplasty and Lumbar Fusion: SPINE. 2016 Jan;41(2):173–81.

24.   Guntin JA, Patel DV, Cardinal KL, Haws BE, Khechen B, Yoo JS, et al. The Influence of Conflicts of Interest on Outcomes in the Lumbar Disc Arthroplasty Literature: A Systematic Review. SPINE. 2019 Aug;44(16):1162–9.

Figures:

Lumbar Disc Arthroplasty Designs

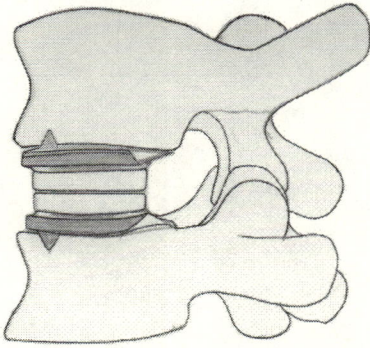

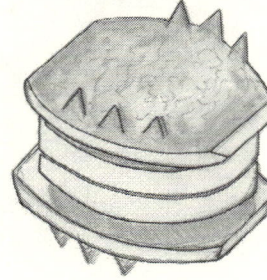

Charité®

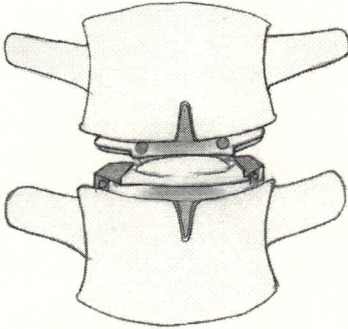

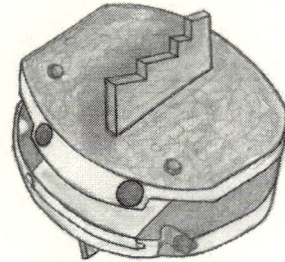

Prodisc-L®

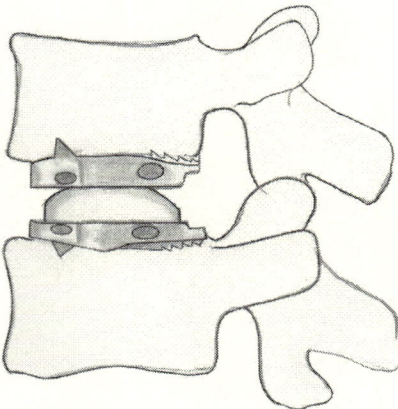

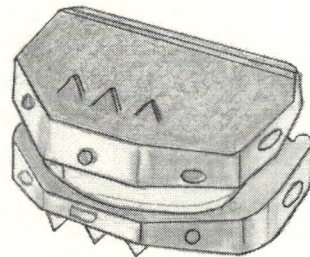

ActivL®

Lumbar disc replacement. Three common lumbar disc replacement prostheses including the Charite®, the Prodisc L® and the ActivL® from top to bottom.

Chapter 46

Treating Osteoporotic Fractures in the Spine With Bone Cement: Vertebral Augmentation—Kyphoplasty and Vertebroplasty

Summary

Osteoporotic compression fractures are very common and may range in symptom severity from asymptomatic to extreme incapacitating back pain. Patients who are suffering from severe back pain resulting from compression fractures may be candidates for a procedure known as cement augmentation or kyphoplasty. In a kyphoplasty procedure a bone cement known as polymethylmethacrylate (PMMA) is injected through a small needle into the vertebra to strengthen it and to prevent collapse. This procedure is best done within 6 weeks to 3 months from the injury and has been shown to be effective at treating pain from acute compression fractures. The procedure is not effective for chronic compression fractures that have already healed—typically those older than 6 months. Overall, the procedure is very safe but does have some potential risk such as cement embolization (explained below) and the movement of cement into the spinal canal. If one vertebra fractures, others may fracture as well, or even the same vertebra may re-fracture—this procedure does not prevent future fractures—so it's very important to have your osteoporosis treated in conjunction with a kyphoplasty.

Case

Ms. Grey is a 76-year-old female who was trying to lift a heavy vase 4 weeks ago and after hearing a pop in her back had sudden onset of back pain. At first, she didn't think anything of it, but over the course of several weeks it got to the point where she was totally incapacitated by the pain and decided to come into the emergency room. She was diagnosed with an L4 compression fracture, resulting from weak bones or osteoporosis. Because the patient was bedbound because of her pain, a kyphoplasty procedure was performed. She had immediate improvement in her pain after the procedure. There was no prolonged recovery, and she was discharged from the hospital the following day amazed that she would now walk again.

Introduction

Osteoporosis is a condition where the bones become thin and weak. Osteoporosis-related bone loss occurs at a rate of 3-5% /year from the age of 30 years (1), and accelerates particularly in women after menopause. This results in a gradual weakening of the bone that can lead to fractures of the spine. Typically, it takes a significant force to crack the bones of the spine, for example, a high-speed car accident. But when you have osteoporosis, fractures of this weak bone occur at low energies (such as a fall from standing or from minor incidents such as even sneezing or coughing) and are thus called insufficiency fractures—because the bone is insufficient in strength. Vertebral osteoporotic compression fractures (VOCF) are very common, occurring at an incidence of 700,000/year or once every 22 seconds worldwide. Women over age 50 years have a 25% risk of having at least one vertebral fracture and those over 80 have a 50% risk (2). Almost one third of women older than 65 will suffer from a vertebral compression fracture (3). Unfortunately, once you have a single VOCF, your chances of having another within the year increase about 7-fold.

When an insufficiency fracture occurs in the spine it is typically wedge-shaped, meaning that the front of the vertebra becomes angled and shortened. These fractures can cause severe back pain but are unlikely to cause neurological injury. The most common location for these fractures to occur is at the thoracolumbar junction (T10-L2).

Luckily, most of the time the pain from these fractures goes away with healing. Many fractures are unnoticed, and it may not be until later that the fracture is even diagnosed. When a fracture occurs, there is loss of the height of the vertebral body, and you get shorter! More worrisome is that if the fracture is asymmetric (anterior wedging) you start to stoop forward which can cause gastric and pulmonary problems. The first symptom of a VOCF may be a change in height or posture. When a VOCF occurs, many people assume the pain is just "old age" but VOCFs are serious sentinel events that can be a sign of failing health and are associated with an increase in mortality rate by roughly 30% (4). The overall 5-year survival is roughly half in those with VOCFs compared to age-matched healthy patients without fractures (2,5). Finally, VOCFs can have a significant impact on the overall quality of life for those few remaining years, causing many patients to be hunched over with severe chronic back pain (6).

How VOCF Symptoms Can Affect Your Life

Vertebral osteoporotic compression fractures often have symptoms of back pain that are usually self-limited, meaning they go away with time. However, some VOCFs are excruciating and require hospitalization and others continue to cause chronic pain that cause a patient to significantly lose mobility. The pain causes the patient to stay in bed, which can further accelerate bone deterioration (7). This pain can even become chronic if there are ongoing small micro fractures in the vertebra or kyphosis. Kyphosis of the spine (a stooped posture) results from the VOCF and causes pain both through muscle spasm and pressure from the ribs descending on the pelvis (8). As kyphotic deformity progresses, lung function may become compromised and depression may occur from loss of body image (9,10).

Treatment

Many VOCFs can be managed without surgery. Mild analgesics such as tramadol and Tylenol may be used to allow early activity. Once the pain is controlled, exercise can be used in the treatment of VOCFs. Programs should include a combination of muscle strengthening, balance, and walking. Back strengthening exercises can actually reduce the disfiguring slumping (kyphosis) of the spine that can occur and reduce pain from stretched ligaments that can occur as a result of deformity (11). Bed rest is not recommended because it can result in worsening of your osteoporosis and deconditioning. Intranasal calcitonin, a hormone that promotes bone strengthening, has been shown to help with the pain from VOCFs in randomized trials and may be used for 2-4 weeks (12). Bracing is not commonly used to treat VOCFs because of the negative effect it can have on the core muscles and lack of any scientific evidence that bracing works (13).

With osteoporotic compression fractures, conventional spine stabilization surgery with rods and screws is rarely used. This is because the bone is typically too weak to hold the hardware that is commonly used to fix broken spines. Instead, a procedure known as percutaneous cement augmentation was developed to help those with intractable pain. In this procedure a small needle is used to inject polymethylmethacrylate bone cement into the vertebral body (the crushed portion of the vertebra). This helps seal the fractures, thus relieving pain. Percutaneous just means the procedure is done through a small poke in the skin. Cement augmentation means the bone cement is used to shore up the broken vertebral body to prevent further collapse. There are two main types of cement augmentation: vertebroplasty and kyphoplasty. They are both indicated to treat the pain which occurs from VOCFs and to help patients debilitated and unable to walk, especially if non-operative treatment is failing (2).

Vertebroplasty refers to insertion of cement alone and is not as commonly used anymore. This is primarily because high profile studies showed it was not any more effective than a sham procedure (14). Even though these studies had critical methodological flaws and were not totally trustworthy, they did lead to vertebroplasty falling out of favor (2). Subsequently, a large meta-analysis proved cement augmentation to be superior to placebo with regard to pain relief and functional recovery (15). Kyphoplasty represents the evolution of the vertebroplasty procedure. With kyphoplasty, before the cement is inserted, the collapsed vertebra is expanded with a balloon to create a cavity to expand the crumpled vertebral shape back to normal. Restoring the shape of the vertebra is important because progressive deformity in the spine can result in increasing pain and other problems with the internal organs (1). Kyphoplasty attempts to restore some of this shape, although total restoration is impossible with this technique. In general, while both vertebroplasty and kyphoplasty procedures are effective for short- and long- term pain control, kyphoplasty has been shown to have superior results for improved function (16). Both procedures are done percutaneously, meaning through small poke incisions in the skin. The American Academy of Orthopedic Surgeons recommends kyphoplasty as an option to treat compression fractures (2).

If possible, kyphoplasty should be performed within 3 weeks to 3 months following a fracture. This allows the greatest chance at re-expansion of the vertebral shape (2,17). If the fracture is allowed time to heal no expansion will be possible. While the correct timing of surgery is hotly debated, there is evidence to support early surgical intervention within weeks of injury if the pain is not improved with simple conservative measures (18). If the pain is severe or there is progressive deformity of the spine, kyphoplasty may be performed acutely even within one week of injury (19). The short-term pain relief from vertebroplasty/kyphoplasty is excellent and can be upwards of 90% (20). Long-term relief also appears to be good; however, there is less evidence on this and some reports state the relief can taper off at 2 years (21). In a large randomized, prospective study comparing kyphoplasty to non-operative therapy with 2-year follow-up, kyphoplasty had superior clinical outcomes regarding back pain and quality of life (22).

A new type of kyphoplasty procedure using a titanium implantable vertebral augmentation device (TIVAD) may be used in lieu of a balloon to expand the collapsed vertebra. These are small metallic devices which are inserted into the vertebral body and act like car jacks to elevate the collapsed vertebra. They are more successful at restoring the shape of the vertebra compared to a balloon. This procedure is newer than balloon kyphoplasty but offers several advantages, both in terms of better restoration of vertebral shape and pain control and has been studied in major international trials (23). Newer procedures such as vertebral screw stinting, where metallic expandable balloons are implanted into the vertebra through small screws are showing promise in treating the most collapsed vertebra. This technique is promising because it can be used to stabilize fractures where traditional kyphoplasty may not offer much correction and prevents any cement leakage (a benefit over TIVAD). As of this writing this technology has yet to undergo randomized testing proving its superiority to traditional kyphoplasty (24).

Patients on blood thinners or who have a bleeding disorder (coagulopathy) are not candidates for surgery and should have these problems reversed prior to having the procedure. You should also let your surgeon know if you have any allergies to bone cement or contrast agents. In addition, pain shooting down your leg (radiculopathy) is not likely to be corrected with a kyphoplasty.

Complications of Cement Augmentation

In general, kyphoplasty is very safe, but does have some risks. Short-term complications may include fever and skin reactions at the injection site. One concerning adverse event from kyphoplasty is leakage of the cement into adjacent structures, most importantly, the spinal canal. Cement leakage or "extravasation" occurs very commonly but in most cases it is inconsequential. In rare cases, if the cement goes into a vital structure such as the spinal canal, it may be devastating. Cement leakage can occur anywhere from 30-70% of the time but is rarely consequential. However, in less than 1 % of cases, it can result in catastrophic spinal cord or nerve injury.

Embolization of cement is also possible, meaning that the cement or a chemical component of the cement travels to a distant part of the body through the blood stream and gets lodged there. Furthermore, as the cement is pressurized in the vertebra it may also push out or embolize fat or bone marrow that can have a similar effect. In very rare cases this can result in a fatal pulmonary, heart, or cerebral embolism (obstruction).

Kyphoplasty only treats individual vertebral bodies, but osteoporosis effects the entire spine. Therefore, it is possible to get new vertebral fractures adjacent to the one treated with kyphoplasty. It is also possible to re-fracture through or around the cement even after it has been placed (25).

After the Procedure

Following your procedure, your surgeon will generally want you out of bed as quickly as possible and to begin physical therapy. In general, kyphoplasty is performed as an outpatient procedure. This is to prevent deconditioning and other complications such as bed sores. Most importantly, you must have your osteoporosis treated. If you have had a single VCOF you should be started immediately on an anti-osteoporosis medication regimen to strengthen the rest of your bones and hopefully prevent collapse or another new fracture from occurring (see chapter 12 on osteoporosis).

Conclusion

Osteoporotic fractures can be extremely painful but are also signs of failing health and potentially even upcoming mortality. The patients with VCOFs are usually not good conventional surgical candidates because they have many health issues as well as very weak bones. Luckily kyphoplasty is a safe, effective, and minimally invasive approach to treating these fractures that have not responded to medical management.

Frequently Asked Questions

- **Is kyphoplasty an outpatient procedure?**

     Many kyphoplasties can be done as an outpatient procedure, depending on your overall health. This means you come into the hospital for your procedure and get to go home the same day. However, many kyphoplasties are performed on inpatients who are admitted to the hospital for pain and other reasons.

- **How long is the recovery from a kyphoplasty?**

     There is minimal recovery from a kyphoplasty procedure, and the benefit is usually immediate with considerable reduction in pain. There are no major wounds or grafts to heal and thus it is only slightly more painful than receiving a flu shot. You may experience some soreness in the area of surgery, but this should resolve within a day or two. If the procedure is successful, it's like turning off the pain switch. There generally is no need for post-op therapy other than just basic exercises to prevent deconditioning.

References

1.   Rao RD, Singrakhia MD. PAINFUL OSTEOPOROTIC VERTEBRAL FRACTURE: PATHOGENE-
SIS, EVALUATION, AND ROLES OF VERTEBROPLASTY AND KYPHOPLASTY IN ITS MANAGEMENT.
J Bone Jt Surg-Am Vol. 2003 Oct;85(10):2010–22.

2.   Savage JW, Schroeder GD, Anderson PA. Vertebroplasty and Kyphoplasty for the
Treatment of Osteoporotic Vertebral Compression Fractures: J Am Acad Orthop Surg. 2014
Oct;22(10):653–64.

3.   Riggs BL, Melton LJ. Involutional osteoporosis. N Engl J Med. 1986 Jun
26;314(26):1676–86.

4.   Kado DM, Browner WS, Palermo L, Nevitt MC, Genant HK, Cummings SR. Vertebral
fractures and mortality in older women: a prospective study. Study of Osteoporotic Fractures
Research Group. Arch Intern Med. 1999 Jun 14;159(11):1215–20.

5.   Cooper C, Atkinson EJ, Jacobsen SJ, O'Fallon WM, Melton LJ. Population-based study
of survival after osteoporotic fractures. Am J Epidemiol. 1993 May 1;137(9):1001–5.

6.   Oleksik A, Lips P, Dawson A, Minshall ME, Shen W, Cooper C, et al. Health-related
quality of life in postmenopausal women with low BMD with or without prevalent vertebral
fractures. J Bone Miner Res Off J Am Soc Bone Miner Res. 2000 Jul;15(7):1384–92.

7.   Krølner B, Toft B. Vertebral bone loss: an unheeded side effect of therapeutic bed rest.
Clin Sci Lond Engl 1979. 1983 May;64(5):537–40.

8.   Lyritis GP, Mayasis B, Tsakalakos N, Lambropoulos A, Gazi S, Karachalios Th, et al. The
natural history of the osteoporotic vertebral fracture. Clin Rheumatol. 1989 Jun;8(S2):66–9.

9.   Leech JA, Dulberg C, Kellie S, Pattee L, Gay J. Relationship of lung function to severity
of osteoporosis in women. Am Rev Respir Dis. 1990 Jan;141(1):68–71.

10.   Silverman S. The clinical consequences of vertebral compression fracture. Bone.
1992;13:S27–31.

11.   Pfeifer M, Sinaki M, Geusens P, Boonen S, Preisinger E, Minne HW, et al. Musculoskeletal Rehabilitation in Osteoporosis: A Review. J Bone Miner Res. 2004 Aug;19(8):1208–14.

12.   Lyritis GP, Tsakalakos N, Magiasis B, Karachalios T, Yiatzides A, Tsekoura M. Analgesic
effect of Salmon calcitonin in osteoporotic vertebral fractures: A double-blind placebo-controlled clinical study. :4.

13.   Kim HJ, Yi JM, Cho HG, Chang BS, Lee CK, Kim JH, et al. Comparative Study of the
Treatment Outcomes of Osteoporotic Compression Fractures without Neurologic Injury Using
a Rigid Brace, a Soft Brace, and No Brace: A Prospective Randomized Controlled Non-Inferiori-
ty Trial. J Bone Jt Surg. 2014 Dec;96(23):1959–66.

14.   Buchbinder R, Osborne RH, Ebeling PR, Wark JD, Mitchell P, Wriedt C, et al. A randomized trial of vertebroplasty for painful osteoporotic vertebral fractures. N Engl J Med. 2009
Aug 6;361(6):557–68.

15.   Pa A, Ab F, Wl T. Meta-analysis of vertebral augmentation compared with conservative treatment for osteoporotic spinal fractures [Internet]. Vol. 28, Journal of bone and
mineral research?: the official journal of the American Society for Bone and Mineral Research.
J Bone Miner Res; 2013 [cited 2020 Dec 2]. Available from: https://pubmed.ncbi.nlm.nih.

gov/22991246/

16.   Han S, Wan S, Ning L, Tong Y, Zhang J, Fan S. Percutaneous vertebroplasty versus bal-loon kyphoplasty for treatment of osteoporotic vertebral compression fracture: a meta-analy-sis of randomised and non-randomised controlled trials. Int Orthop. 2011 Sep;35(9):1349–58.

17.   Garfin SR, Yuan HA, Reiley MA. New technologies in spine: kyphoplasty and verte-broplasty for the treatment of painful osteoporotic compression fractures. Spine. 2001 Jul 15;26(14):1511–5.

18.   Son S, Lee SG, Kim WK, Park CW, Yoo CJ. Early Vertebroplasty versus Delayed Verte-broplasty for Acute Osteoporotic Compression Fracture?: Are the Results of the Two Surgical Strategies the Same? J Korean Neurosurg Soc. 2014;56(3):211.

19.   Hirsch JA, Beall DP, Chambers MR, Andreshak TG, Brook AL, Bruel BM, et al. Manage-ment of vertebral fragility fractures: a clinical care pathway developed by a multispecialty panel using the RAND/UCLA Appropriateness Method. Spine J Off J North Am Spine Soc. 2018 Nov;18(11):2152–61.

20.   Barr JD, Barr MS, Lemley TJ, McCann RM. Percutaneous vertebroplasty for pain relief and spinal stabilization. Spine. 2000 Apr 15;25(8):923–8.

21.   Grados F, Depriester C, Cayrolle G, Hardy N, Deramond H, Fardellone P. Long-term ob-servations of vertebral osteoporotic fractures treated by percutaneous vertebroplasty. Rheu-matol Oxf Engl. 2000 Dec;39(12):1410–4.

22.   Boonen S, Van Meirhaeghe J, Bastian L, Cummings SR, Ranstam J, Tillman JB, et al. Balloon kyphoplasty for the treatment of acute vertebral compression fractures: 2-year results from a randomized trial. J Bone Miner Res Off J Am Soc Bone Miner Res. 2011 Jul;26(7):1627–37.

23.   Noriega D, Marcia S, Theumann N, Blondel B, Simon A, Hassel F, et al. A prospective, international, randomized, noninferiority study comparing an implantable titanium vertebral augmentation device versus balloon kyphoplasty in the reduction of vertebral compression fractures (SAKOS study). Spine J. 2019 Nov;19(11):1782–95.

24.   Cianfoni A, Delfanti RL, Isalberti M, Scarone P, Koetsier E, Bonaldi G, et al. Minimally Invasive Stent Screw–Assisted Internal Fixation Technique Corrects Kyphosis in Osteoporotic Vertebral Fractures with Severe Collapse: A Pilot "Vertebra Plana" Series. :8.

25.   Liebschner MAK, Rosenberg WS, Keaveny TM. Effects of Bone Cement Volume and Distribution on Vertebral Stiffness After Vertebroplasty: Spine. 2001 Jul;26(14):1547–54.

Figures:

Kyphoplasty: Cement Augmentation

Vertebra accessed with a needle

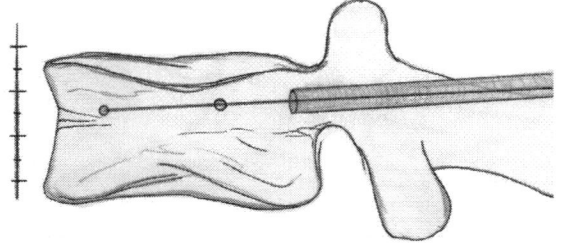

L3 compression fracture:

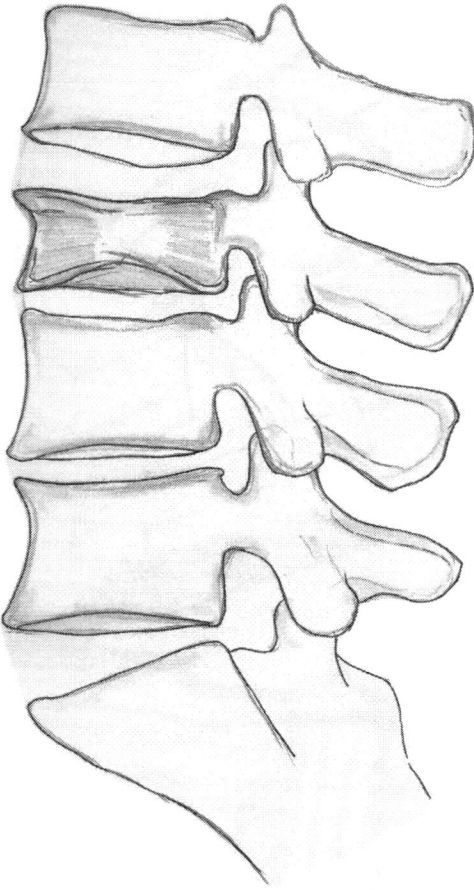

A special balloon is inserted and inflated

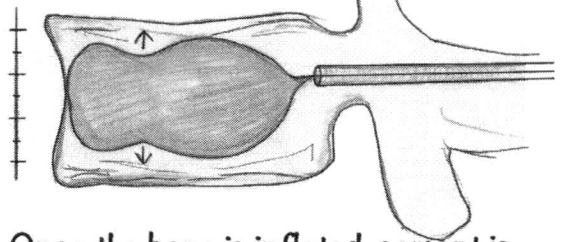

Once the bone is inflated, cement is injected

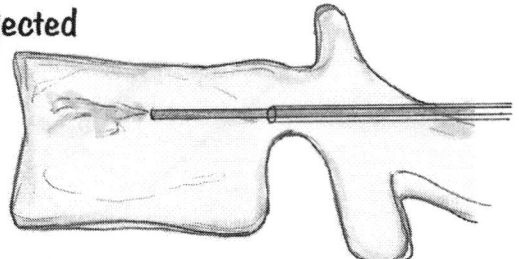

Cement stabilizes the fracture

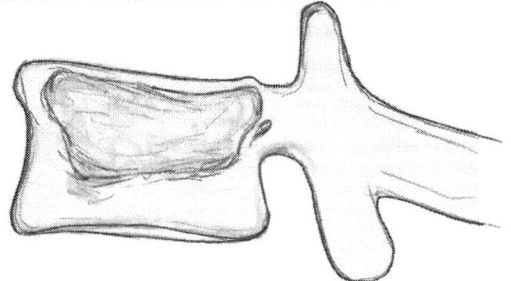

Kyphoplasty. The kyphoplasty is used to treat a painful vertebral compression fracture. A small cannula (thin tube) is used to gain access to the vertebral body (top right) through which a balloon can be inserted and inflated (second right). Bone cement is used to fill the vertebra (third and bottom right).

Chapter 47

Minimally Invasive Procedures for Lumbar Stenosis: Interspinous Process Devices and Techniques

Summary

Spinal stenosis is commonly caused by thickening of the ligament that connects two vertebrae together (the ligamentum flavum) in the back of your spinal canal. When you arch your back, this ligament kinks into the spinal canal worsening any existing stenosis. When you stoop your back forward, it unkinks, relieving stenosis. Therefore, patients with lumbar stenosis may feel better holding onto a shopping cart with their back forward. Interspinous spacers are devices that are inserted between the spinous processes or the lamina of the vertebrae to permanently jack them open, recreating a stooped forward posture at that level. There are many types of these devices on the market, some of which have a reasonable track record and, in most cases, can be inserted under local anesthesia. However, being put in a permanent kyphotic or "stooped" position is not good for your spine, and thus these devices are reserved for those who are in such poor health they will not tolerate anesthesia for a regular surgical decompression. While they may offer temporary pain relief (6 months), they do not provide lasting results and may worsen your condition in the long term.

The Spine Encyclopedia

Serious complications can still occur with these devices, just as in any other surgical procedure.

Case

Mrs. Tan is a 63-year-old retiree who had lumbar stenosis which caused her great leg pain and made it impossible for her to walk any distance and was treated with a Coflex® device at two levels at a clinic in Florida. This was done under local anesthesia, and she was "in and out." For a time, she had relief of her leg pain and was able to walk farther, but then started to develop increasing back pain by about 6 months. Her leg pain eventually came back after 2 years and was worse now than ever. She was evaluated and the Coflex® devices were found to be migrating into her spinal canal and rubbing on the nerves. Now she was in a complicated situation, where the devices needed to be removed so that a formal decompression and fusion procedure could be performed—a more complicated surgery than she would have needed initially had the Coflex® devices not been used. The devices were so close to the nerves they had eroded through the casing of the dura and there was leakage of spinal fluid during the removal process. This was repaired and the remainder of her surgery went well and now she has a successful spinal fusion. She improved greatly after having the devices removed.

Introduction

When degeneration occurs in the spine the disc space between the vertebrae collapses, allowing the posterior ligaments to buckle into the spinal canal, which causes the canal to narrow (stenosis). Interspinous and interlaminar devices are so named because they sit between the posterior bones of the vertebrae and act to hold them apart, theoretically relieving stenosis. There are many different devices available but are all touted as a percutaneous (done through a small poke in the skin) or "minimally invasive" method to treat lumbar stenosis. They are designed to avoid fusions and because they act as a support between the bones while preserving some motion of the vertebral segment, they proclaim to offer "dynamic stabilization." Because they only require a small incision and minimal dissection to implant, they tend to have less complications than a fully instrumented spinal fusion with pedicle screws and interbody implants in the short term. Moreover, they are popular because they can be done as outpatient surgery under local anesthesia. Because they are easy to implant, many non-surgeons such as pain management doctors attempt to put these in (see the chapter 26 on training in spinal surgery). Sounds good, right? Unfortunately, they also fail to fully address the problem of stenosis and can lead to difficult revision surgery scenarios which the treating physician will not likely handle without consulting a qualified spinal surgeon.

Interspinous Process Devices and Interlaminar Devices—Where, Why and How Do They Work?

First, where specifically is the interspinous process device implanted? The lumbar vertebrae all have spinous processes which are bony struts that extend out posteriorly from the lamina, the thin bone on the backside of each vertebra. The spinous process can be felt when you run your hand along your spine. Lumbar interspinous devices are designed to be inserted between these bony struts through a small incision in the back. Alternatively, they can be inserted deeper into the spine to sit between the lamina themselves. This is a small technical detail, but functionally accomplishes the same goal of blocking extension (arching backward) motion of the spine.

Second, why can they be used to treat pain? Lumbar (low back) degeneration starts with collapse of the intervertebral disc that results in loss of height between the two vertebrae. This can cause buckling of the ligamentous structures that hold the spine together; the buckling pinches the nerves in the spinal canal and causes pain. To relieve this pressure, you may naturally want to stoop over, moving your back forward as this unkinks the buckled ligaments. On the other hand, when you extend or arch your back this buckling worsens, causing a worsening of your symptoms. You may walk around in a flexed (stooped forward) posture to help keep the spinal canal open and avoid the pain. An interspinous device permanently places a spinal segment in this flexed posture, recreating this position of relief.

And, finally, what does the interspinous process device do? The interspinous process device is designed to "jack" open the posterior space of the spine (between adjacent spinous processes) and relieve some of this buckling; unfortunately, it keeps you in a permanent state of being "stooped forward." The device acts as a mechanical stop to prevent extension (bending back) of the segment and thus helps relieve some symptoms occurring with that motion. Some surgeons say it also reduces pressure on the disc and may help with low back pain but there are no studies confirming this.

The interspinous process device limits extension of the vertebrae (how much they can bend backwards) by acting as a door-jam between the spinous processes while still allowing flexion and bending. The procedure can usually be performed under local anesthesia. Many physicians who are not trained properly in surgery attempt to implant them.

Types of Devices

The X STOP® device was FDA-approved for use in patients greater than 50 years of age with pain resulting from spinal stenosis that is relieved with flexion (bending forward) and have undergone at least 6 months of non-operative management. It is contraindicated in cases of osteoporosis, scoliosis, or spondylolisthesis (slipped disc)—all of which are common in the elderly patient population they are intended to treat. It was removed from the market in 2015.

The Superion® InterSpinous Spacer is like the X STOP® device as it does not require a decompression and can function independently. This device is delivered through a small incision into the space between two adjacent spinous processes. The device has H-shaped wings that then open to attach to the spinous processes.

Coflex® is another FDA-approved interspinous process device but is implanted in conjunction with a decompression procedure and takes the place of a formal fusion. The device is designed to "extend the lifetime of a decompression procedure" or "replace the need for an instrumented fusion" with screws and rods. This concept is different from other interspinous process devices because it is done in conjunction with a decompression procedure. Because the device is done in conjunction with a decompression, they are more likely to be performed by a trained spinal surgeon. Coflex® is approved for one- or two-level stenosis and should only be used in patients who experience relief of leg pain with forward flexion of the back. It should not be used in patients with isolated back pain, prior fusion, or decompression at the surgical level, or in patients with fracture or instability of the spine.

Inter Spinous Process Devices			
Device Name/Manufacturer Name	Design Features	History and Market Availability	Major Evidence/Randomized Controlled Trials (RCT)
X STOP® Manufacturer: Medtronic	Components: Oval titanium spacer with two wings to hold it in place against the spinous process	FDA Approved: yes but, removed from market in 2015 for high complication rates	Zucherman et al (2005) (1): Prospective RCT comparing 100 X STOP® patients to 91 Non-op patients with 10 year follow up. X STOP® showed significant improvement in pain up to 2 years compared to non-op. 73% of patients were at least somewhat satisfied; however, there was a relatively low overall clinical success rate of 59%. There were 4 device-related complications including dislodgement, fracture and increased pain, and many patients experienced regression to baseline by 24 months. Significant bias limits the overall impact of this study.

Complications and Concerns

In general, permanent flexion of the spine is not good, as it causes you to stoop forward and may increase wear of the other segments of the spine. As someone who is concerned with restoring the normal shape to deformed spines, the concept of creating deformity for temporary relief doesn't make a lot of sense to me. Furthermore, there is significant concern that these devices are not durable, may migrate and cause more serious problems in the spine than what they are designed to treat. Interspinous process spacers are associated with a much higher risk of reoperation than traditional decompression methods (4). Finally, there are a significant number of patients who fail to improve with the implantation of the device. If you decide to go with an interspinous device type procedure, make sure you consult with a doctor who is a board certified or eligible orthopedic surgeon beforehand.

Inter Spinous Process Devices Continued		
Device Name/Manufacturer Name	Device Name/Manufacturer Name	Device Name/Manufacturer Name
COFLEX® Manufacturer: Surgalign (a holding company)	Components: Single- piece titanium "U" that fits between spinous processes and acts as a spring to stabilize the spine after a decompression procedure. FDA Approved	Schmidt et al (2018) (2): Prospective RCT comparing 115 Coflex® + decompression patients to 115 decompression alone patients with a 2-year follow- up. There was no significant clinical difference in outcomes up to 24 months. There was a higher risk of secondary intervention in patients with decompression alone. Bae et al (2016) (3): Prospective RCT comparing 196 Coflex® + decompression patients to 95 patients with decompression +instrumented fusion alone with a 3-year follow-up. The Coflex® device has superior clinical success rates at 36 months compared to decompression and fusion without spondylolisthesis. If spondylolisthesis was present the outcomes were similar. There were similar complication rates and reoperation rates between the two procedures.

Inter Spinous Process Devices Continued			
Device Name/Manufacturer Name	Device Name/Manufacturer Name	Device Name/Manufacturer Name	Device Name/Manufacturer Name
Superion® InterSpinous Spacer® (Vertiflex) Manufacturer: Boston Scientific	Components: A titanium cam with H wings that open after insertion.	FDA Approved: yes	No randomized studies comparing to decompression.

The MILD® Procedure

The MILD® procedure or "minimally-invasive lumbar decompression" is a percutaneous (using a small incision in the skin) procedure used to treat patients with lumbar stenosis due to hypertrophy of the ligamentum flavum (the ligament has thickened due to stresses put on the spine). In a typical decompression procedure, the surgeon removes thickened buckling ligament from the spinal canal under direct visualization. The MILD® procedure is instead performed through a small poke incision using only X-ray guidance to remove or "debulk" portions of the thickened ligament with a grasper. A contrast dye is injected into the spinal canal to allow the physician to monitor the procedure.

The company that produces the MILD® instruments is called Vertos Medical (Aliso Viejo, CA). Small scrapers and graspers are inserted into the spinal canal to attempt to remove the hypertrophied ligamentum flavum. The selling point of the procedure is that it will not interfere with any need for future spine surgery and thus can be a safe first step in patients who are not great surgical candidates (that is, too sick or too old—but as discussed in previous chapters, there is not an exact definition for this). In the major randomized trial of the MILD procedure versus epidural steroid injection, nearly 20% of patients had withdrawn from the study to undergo secondary surgical interventions. Another 15% of the patient required a subsequent surgical intervention by 2 years and another 15% required additional epidural steroid injections or spinal cord stimulator.

However, the MILD® procedure was found to be superior in effectiveness to epidural steroid injections without a significant difference in complications (1.3% risk of complication with the MILD® procedure) (5,6). The remainder of the evidence supporting the MILD® procedure is of low quality. Current randomized trials are heavily supported by the biomedical industry indicating that they may contain significant bias. It should also be noted that while complications have not been reported in this study, this procedure involves biting instruments directed at the spinal canal and serious complications have been reported separately (7). Make no mistake, the MILD procedure is a surgical procedure. I would offer patients caution in accepting it from doctors who are not surgeons capable of performing it correctly and handling any potential complications.

Conclusion

Interspinous stabilization procedures play only a limited role in treating patients with spinal stenosis. Longer-term studies are needed to determine their durability and safety. I have seen patients who have benefited from these procedures, but also those who have had serious complications from them. It's my opinion that the invasiveness of these procedures is very similar to a traditional decompression and that the traditional decompression is likely more efficacious and ultimately safer in the long term. Discuss these procedures with your surgeon (preferably an orthopedic or neurosurgeon) before having them performed.

Frequently Asked Questions

- **My pain intervention doctor is offering me an interspinous procedure, should I do it?**

This begs the question of what is defined as "a surgery?" Anytime an incision is being made in the skin, surgery is being performed. I would propose that all the above procedures are surgical and should be treated as such. The invasiveness of interspinous procedures is no different from more traditional surgical decompression and fusions. Be wary of non-surgeons performing surgical procedures. I would recommend you at least discuss the procedure with a surgeon who has evaluated your case before moving forward.

References

1.   Zucherman JF, Hsu KY, Hartjen CA, Mehalic TF, Implicito DA, Martin MJ, et al. A multi-center, prospective, randomized trial evaluating the X STOP interspinous process decompression system for the treatment of neurogenic intermittent claudication: two-year follow-up results. Spine (Phila Pa 1976). 2005 Jun 15;30(12):1351–8.

2.   Schmidt S, Franke J, Rauschmann M, Adelt D, Bonsanto MM, Sola S. Prospective, randomized, multicenter study with 2-year follow-up to compare the performance of decompression with and without interlaminar stabilization. J Neurosurg Spine. 2018 Apr;28(4):406–15.

3.   Bae HW, Davis RJ, Lauryssen C, Leary S, Maislin G, Musacchio MJ. Three-Year Fol-

low-up of the Prospective, Randomized, Controlled Trial of Coflex Interlaminar Stabilization vs Instrumented Fusion in Patients With Lumbar Stenosis. Neurosurgery. 2016 Aug;79(2):169–81.

4.   Wu AM, Zhou Y, Li QL, Wu XL, Jin YL, Luo P, et al. Interspinous spacer versus traditional decompressive surgery for lumbar spinal stenosis: a systematic review and meta-analysis. PLoS One. 2014;9(5):e97142.

5.   Benyamin R. MILD® is an Effective Treatment for LumbarSpinal Stenosis with Neurogenic Claudication:MiDAS ENCORE Randomized Controlled Trial. Pain Phys. 2016 May 14;4;19(4;5):229–42.

6.   Staats PS, Chafin TB, Golovac S, Kim CK, Li S, Richardson WB, et al. Long-Term Safety and Efficacy of Minimally Invasive Lumbar Decompression Procedure for the Treatment of Lumbar Spinal Stenosis With Neurogenic Claudication: 2-Year Results of MiDAS ENCORE. Reg Anesth Pain Med. 2018 Oct;43(7):789–94.

7.   Kreiner DS, MacVicar J, Duszynski B, Nampiaparampil DE. The mild® Procedure: A Systematic Review of the Current Literature: The mild® Procedure: A Systematic Review. Pain Med. 2014 Feb;15(2):196–205.

Figures:

Interspinous Devices:

**Coflex®
interspinous
device**

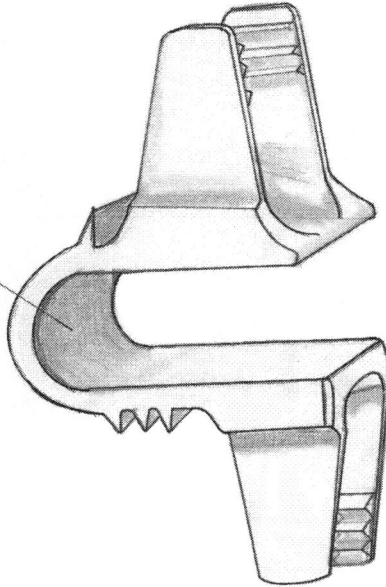

**Interspinous
devices
prevent
extension of
spine**

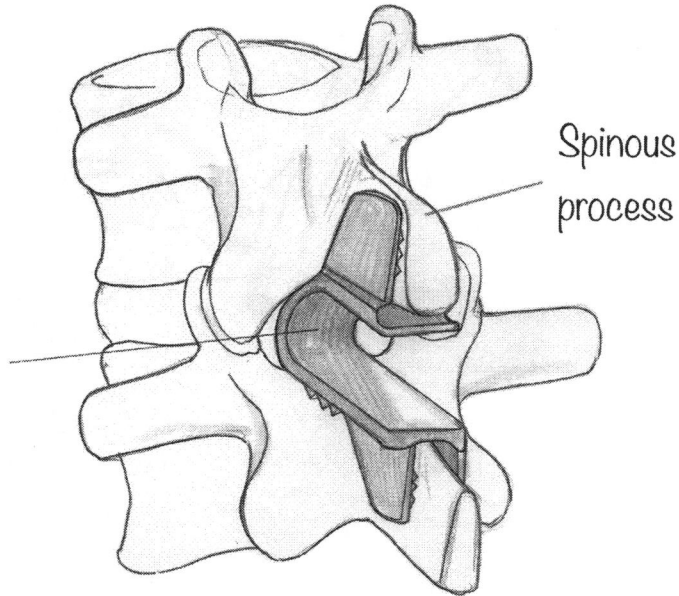

**Spinous
process**

Interspinous devices. The Coflex® interspinous device is inserted between the spinous processes of the lumbar spine to help relieve stenosis and the pain it causes.

Chapter 48

Sacroiliac (SI) Joint Pain and Treatment

Summary

The sacroiliac (SI) joint was once thought to not be a source of pain. This concept has been disproven with multiple studies, but still there remains a lot of misinformation about the SI joint on the internet and even among some medical practitioners. For example, it is very difficult and rare to dislocate the SI joint, yet many patients have the belief that their SI joints are dislocated. Medical Imaging is not particularly helpful in diagnosing SI joint pain. Many people will have asymptomatic degeneration of the SI joint on X-rays or MRIs that never causes any pain, while those with pain seemingly emanating from the SI joint can have a normal imaging. Thus, it is hard to diagnose the SI joint pain clinically, and even harder to pinpoint pain to changes on MRI or X-ray. The most reliable way to diagnose the SI joint as the source of pain is with diagnostic injections that temporarily mask the discomfort. If you have had greater than 75% relief of your pain from a diagnostic injection, this is relatively reliable evidence that the SI joint is the source of at least some of your pain. Once the pain source is confirmed, the primary treatment is fusion of the joint with metallic cages. This now can be done in a minimally invasive fashion that has less complications than previously used open procedures.

Case

Ms. Beige is a 60-year-old homemaker who has had pain in her buttocks and groin ever since she gave birth to her second child. She sees an osteopath who performs manipulation of her SI joint which seems to improve things, but the pain always comes back. She sees a spinal surgeon who thinks the pain is coming from her SI joint and recommends a minimally invasive joint fusion. The patient has the procedure, but, unfortunately, it fails to give her significant relief. Her surgeon throws up his hands and doesn't know what to do. She gets another opinion from a different surgeon and more scans are performed. The SI joint cages appear to be in an appropriate place, but this surgeon also notes she has degeneration in her hips and in her lumbar spine, both of which could be causing some of her pain. He also notes that he cannot tell if the SI joint fusion procedure actually took, as the joint still looks unfused—this could also be a source of her pain. With an unclear surgical target, the surgeon recommends she continue with PT and not have any further procedures.

Introduction

The sacroiliac (SI) joint can be a source of pain and disability, but patients frequently have misconceptions about how it works. Many patients believe that their SI joints can become "dislocated." In truth it takes a high level of trauma, such as a motor vehicle accident, to cause a SI joint dislocation. Nonetheless, SI joint pain has been implicated as a cause of low back pain and thus is frequently the target of pain medicine specialists, chiropractors and osteopaths for multiple treatments. Some of these treatments are scientifically based, but many have no supportive evidence. Recently, spine surgeons have joined the game, as fusions of the SI joint have become more popular and are performed at increasing rates. In this chapter I attempt to separate fact from fiction regarding the SI joint as well as how it can cause pain, and what treatments are actually scientifically proven.

Anatomy

The SI joint is the interface between the iliac bones and the sacrum, the three major bones that make up the pelvis. The SI joint is not a typical human joint. While there are synovial components (areas that have cartilage and move against one another), the overall structure of the joint is very rigid. This is because the joint is surrounded by massive ligaments that limit motion and allow your pelvis to be a stable weight-bearing structure. Unlike the knee, for example, that has lots of motion, the SI joint has only minimal movement. Nonetheless there is still some motion, and the SI joint allows for rotation of the iliac bones of the pelvis around the sacrum (a movement called nutation). How much motion occurs is a hotly debated topic but it typically requires sophisticated instruments to measure and cannot be readily measured by the human eye (1). Rotation can be as little as one degree and translation (ability to slide) about 1-2mm (2). In short, the SI joint does not move very much.

SI joint Injury

Radiographic SI joint degeneration is present in 65% of asymptomatic individuals (3). What this means is that in most cases degeneration of the SI joint is totally normal and does not cause symptoms. Given the prevalence of asymptomatic degeneration, physicians and patients need to be careful when attributing pain to SI joint degeneration. Some populations, such as patients with lumbar fusions, are at increased risk for symptomatic SI joint degeneration but SI joint degeneration is asymptomatic in most cases (4).

The SI joint is susceptible to various problems such as inflammation, infection, trauma and tumors. It typically takes a great deal of force (such as that experienced in a major car wreck) to disrupt the SI joint or cause a Si joint "dislocation" (5). Inflammatory conditions such as ankylosing spondylitis (spine arthritis) and rheumatoid arthritis may affect the SI joint. Females are more susceptible to SI joint dysfunction because of laxity (looseness) that may occur after childbirth.

Pain from the SI joint is commonly felt in the low back or buttock region posteriorly. Pain may get worse changing position from sitting to standing or from weight bearing (6).

Diagnosis

Confirming the diagnosis of SI joint pain is difficult (as it is like many other types of pain) and may require repeated tests. It is hard to attribute pain to the SI joint based on a physician's exam alone. Furthermore, there is no imaging test that can accurately diagnose SI joint dysfunction. Tenderness around the back of the pelvis, known as the Fortin finger test, is a somewhat reliable diagnostic sign. However, to faithfully diagnose SI joint pain, physicians rely on diagnostic injection blocks where a numbing medicine is injected directly into the SI joint. If the numbing medicine takes the pain away, it is said to be a positive test. Only patients who are carefully examined by a doctor and found to have signs and symptoms of SI joint pain should undergo injections. Injections are performed under X-ray guidance both to help with the pain (therapeutic effect) but also to help confirm the diagnosis. If you get 75-100% relief from the injection, then you might be a candidate for fusion as treatment of the deteriorated SI joint.

Treatment

Si joint manipulation is a non-invasive, low-risk method for treatment of SI joint dysfunction. A practitioner will pull and try to move the SI joint to help ease pain. There are many different techniques for SI joint manipulation, so it is unclear how exactly manipulation is supposed to work but, still, many patients get relief from it. A randomized study comparing myofascial release to sacral manipulation did not show any significant differences between the two modalities, but both were helpful and offered short-term benefits in pain relief (7).

It is even possible for you to even adjust your own SI joint. The so-called "Chicago method" can be done at home. Just lie on your back, cross the well leg over the unwell side, put your hands behind your neck and bend toward the well side to stretch the unwell side (6).

Steroid injections are a common treatment of SI joint pain. Corticosteroid injections can provide more than 6 weeks of relief in 43-67% of patients with SI dysfunction (6).

Prolotherapy is another treatment method for SI joint disease and consists of injecting an irritant such as saline, platelet rich plasma (PRP), or dextrose (sugar water) into the joint capsule. In theory, this is supposed to initiate reactive growth of fibrous tissue (scar) and promote healing. There is only the most rudimentary evidence to support the use of prolotherapy and thus it has not reached mainstream medicine.

Radiofrequency ablation (RFA) may also be used to treat SI joint pain. In RFA a heated probe is used to "burn" the nerves supplying part of the joint thus preventing pain signals from being transmitted to the brain. RFA is generally low risk and is supported in the literature by two randomized trials; however, it is only about 60% effective at 6 months (8,9).

Fusion surgery is reserved as the last means of treating SI joint pain, and only after conservative measures as described above have failed over at least 6 months. A fusion procedure is designed to eliminate what little motion there is in the SI joint and cause the bones to grow together. In the past a large open surgical exposure was used to perform the fusion. While the procedure enjoyed a success rate around 80% and a satisfaction rate around 60%, open techniques have been associated with a complication rate as high as 20% (6).

To try to decrease the burden of complications, minimally invasive (MIS) SI joint fusion was pioneered. MIS SI joint fusions are performed by implanting a metallic cage through a small lateral incision with the use of X-ray or CT navigation. The metal cage, just like a lumbar fusion cage, promotes bony healing across the joint surface. There are many varieties of cages, all of which are designed to support the SI joint while a fusion occurs. Some cages are designed to stimulate bone to grow into the cage which stabilizes the joint as opposed to formally fusing the joint.

MIS SI joint fusions have been associated with lower complication rates than traditional open techniques and have been shown to have durable clinical outcomes, up to 5 years. Randomized controlled trials in which patients with greater than 50% decrease in pain following a diagnostic injection were randomized to receive an MIS SI fusion or continue conservative care. Patients undergoing MIS SI fusion had significantly improved pain and clinical scores compared to non-operative treatment (10,11). Obviously, surgery, even if it is performed minimally invasively, has a risk of complications and some problems associated with SI fusion are implant malposition (because it moves or because it is hard to put in the right place) requiring revision, non-union that is, the implant fails to heal and may loosen), hematoma (blood pooling), infection, and, trochanteric bursitis (inflammation around where the thighbone and hip join) (10,11).

Conclusion

In summary, the SI joint is a pain generator and treatment can help improve function and pain. However, diagnosis is difficult and requires the use of injections which help temporarily mask pain. Patients who experience substantial improvement following injection of the SI joint may qualify for definitive treatment with minimally invasive fusion, but this should only be pursued after extensive conservative therapy (manipulation, RFA, PT) has failed.

Frequently asked Questions

- **My chiropractor tells me my SI joint is dislocated, what does this mean?**

    Chiropractors practice a technique known as SI joint "adjustment." In such an adjustment or manipulation, the chiropractor will attempt to move the SI joint to relieve pain. A patient is typically placed on their side, and the hip is flexed. The practitioner will then place pressure over the affected side of the pelvis to attempt to move it incrementally back in position. Sometimes this is done forcefully in a technique known as a "high velocity, low amplitude" thrust. The joint is not "relocated" per se but potentially moved 1-2 mm (12).

References

1.   Forst SL. The Sacroiliac Joint:Anatomy, Physiology and Clinical Signifi cance. Pain Phys.

2006 Jan 14;1;9(1;1):62–8.

2.   Thawrani DP, Agabegi SS, Asghar F. Diagnosing Sacroiliac Joint Pain: Journal of the American Academy of Orthopaedic Surgeons. 2019 Feb;27(3):85–93.

3.   Eno JJT, Boone CR, Bellino MJ, Bishop JA. The Prevalence of Sacroiliac Joint Degeneration in Asymptomatic Adults: The Journal of Bone and Joint Surgery-American Volume. 2015 Jun;97(11):932–6.

4.   Ha KY, Lee JS, Kim KW. Degeneration of sacroiliac joint after instrumented lumbar or lumbosacral fusion: a prospective cohort study over five-year follow-up. Spine (Phila Pa 1976). 2008 May 15;33(11):1192–8.

5.   Steelman K, Russell R, Vaidya R. Bilateral vertical shear sacroiliac joint dislocations treated with bilateral triangular osteosynthesis in a young female: A case report. Trauma Case Reports. 2021 Jun;33:100485.

6.   Ou-Yang DC, York PJ, Kleck CJ, Patel VV. Diagnosis and Management of Sacroiliac Joint Dysfunction: The Journal of Bone and Joint Surgery. 2017 Dec;99(23):2027–36.

7.   Castro-Sánchez AM, Gil-Martínez E, Fernández-Sánchez M, Lara-Palomo IC, Nastasia I, de Los Ángeles Querol-Zaldívar M, et al. MANIPULATIVE THERAPY OF SACRAL TORSION VERSUS MYOFASCIAL RELEASE IN PATIENTS CLINICALLY DIAGNOSED POSTERIOR PELVIC PAIN: A CONSORT COMPLIANT RANDOMIZED CONTROLLED TRIAL. Spine J. 2021 May 12;

8.   Cohen SP, Hurley RW, Buckenmaier CC, Kurihara C, Morlando B, Dragovich A. Randomized placebo-controlled study evaluating lateral branch radiofrequency denervation for sacroiliac joint pain. Anesthesiology. 2008 Aug;109(2):279–88.

9.   Patel N, Gross A, Brown L, Gekht G. A randomized, placebo-controlled study to assess the efficacy of lateral branch neurotomy for chronic sacroiliac joint pain. Pain Med. 2012 Mar;13(3):383–98.

10.   Polly D, Swofford J, Whang P, Frank C, Glaser J, Limoni R, et al. Two-Year Outcomes from a Randomized Controlled Trial of Minimally Invasive Sacroiliac Joint Fusion vs. Non-Surgical Management for Sacroiliac Joint Dysfunction. International Journal of Spine Surgery [Internet]. 2016 Aug 23 [cited 2017 Jun 10];10. Available from: http://ijssurgery.com/10.14444/3028

11.   Dengler J, Kools D, Pflugmacher R, Gasbarrini A, Prestamburgo D, Gaetani P, et al. Randomized Trial of Sacroiliac Joint Arthrodesis Compared with Conservative Management for Chronic Low Back Pain Attributed to the Sacroiliac Joint: The Journal of Bone and Joint Surgery. 2019 Mar;101(5):400–11.

12.   FACO SY DC. Chiropractic Procedures for the Sacroiliac Joint [Internet]. Spine-health. [cited 2022 Aug 2]. Available from: https://www.spine-health.com/conditions/sacroiliac-joint-dysfunction/chiropractic-procedures-sacroiliac-joint

Figures:

The Sacroiliac (SI) Joint

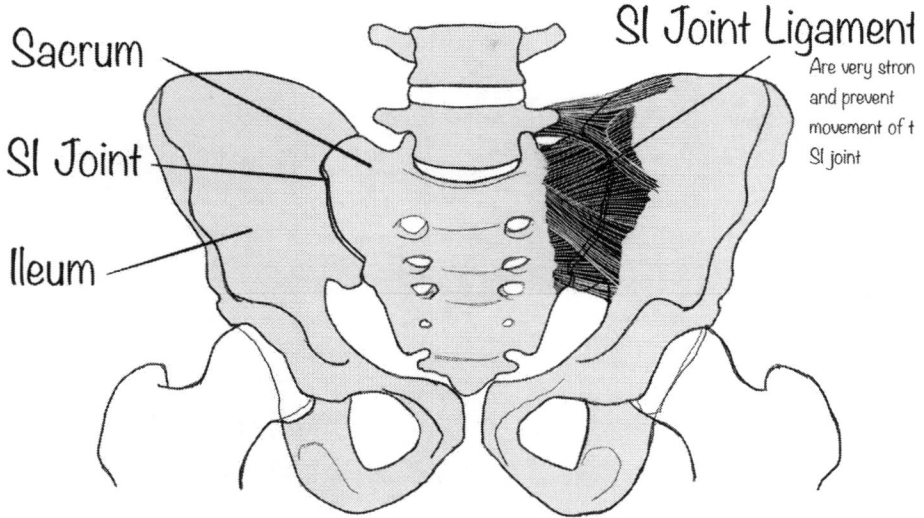

Sacrum

SI Joint

Ileum

SI Joint Ligament

Are very stron
and prevent
movement of t
SI joint

Sacroiliac Joint Fusion

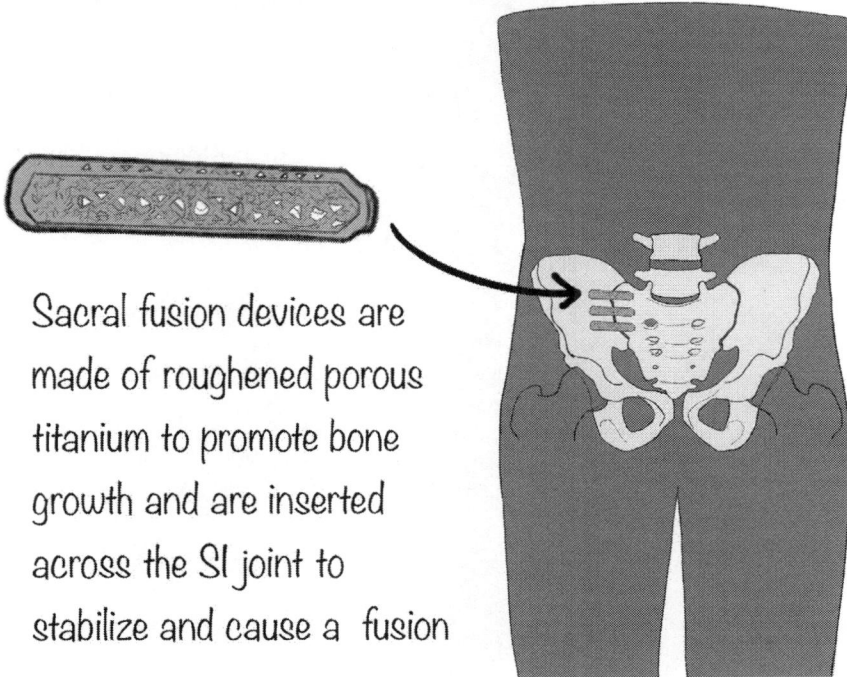

Sacral fusion devices are
made of roughened porous
titanium to promote bone
growth and are inserted
across the SI joint to
stabilize and cause a fusion

SI joint fusion. The sacroiliac joint (SI joint) has only a small amount of motion because strong ligaments hold it firmly together. To reduce pain the SI joint can be fused to stop all motion from occurring using implantable devices that act as bone scaffolds.

Sacroiliac (SI) Joint Pain

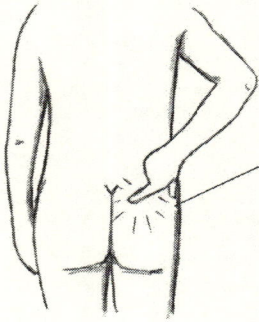

Pain is located in the buttocks

Chicago method of SI joint adjustment: Cross your "well" leg over your "unwell" leg and bend away from the painful side

Painful side

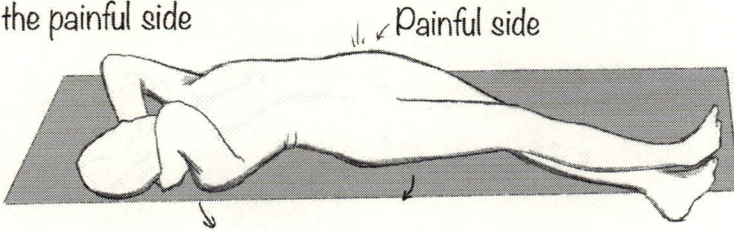

SI joint manipulation / adjustment: A practitioner will have you flex up your hip and push on your buttocks and shoulder to ease pain

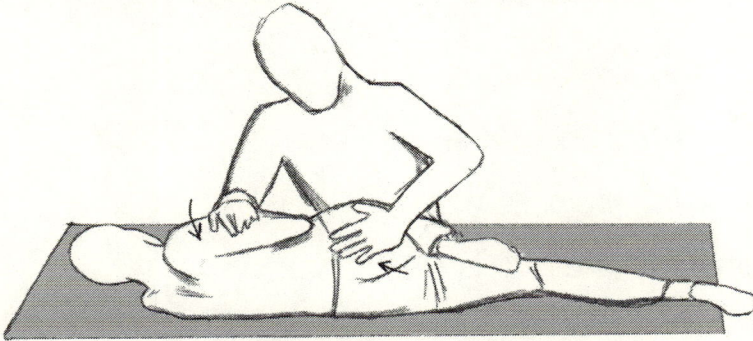

SI joint Manipulation. Si joint pain is typically located around the top of the buttocks (top). It can be treated with self-manipulation (middle) or practitioner guided manipulation (bottom).

SECTION 5

What to Expect After Spine Surgery

"The more we know, the more we realize there is to know."
-Jennifer Doudna

Chapter 49

Wound Care During and After Spine Surgery

Summary

Care of your wound is a critical part of the surgical healing process. The body heals wounds by producing fibrous scar material that seals up the opening and can gradually be replaced by normal skin. Most surgical wounds heal by primary intention, that is, the wound edges are smooth and close to each other, so there is little scar formation. This is accomplished by your surgeon carefully suturing the wound closed to make the incision as cosmetic as possible. There are many different types of sutures available on the market and no doubt your surgeon will have favorites. Surgical Glue (such as dermabond®) or Steri-Strips (small adhesive bandages) may be applied in addition to the sutures to further protect and seal the wound. After the procedure, a dressing is applied and is left on for several days to allow the skin to seal shut. During the time when the wound is healing it's important not to submerge your wound in contaminated water such as that from a pool, lake, or the ocean. It is usually ok to shower and get your wound wet after 5-7 days, but check with your surgeon. Smoking, chronic steroid use, and poorly controlled diabetes all increase the risk of infection and wound breakdown. If your wound ever drains, you should contact your surgeon. Untreated superficial infections can track deep into the surgical bed which can result in significant problems with healing.

Case

Mr. Brown is an 80-year-old computer programmer. He has had crippling lumbar stenosis that prevents him from walking any prolonged distance. He undergoes a lumbar laminectomy and fusion and does excellently—his walking ability increases significantly—but his wound doesn't seem to want to heal. He comes back to see me two weeks after the procedure and the wound is still draining a little bit and looks wet. I put him on antibiotics as I suspect a superficial infection but still six weeks after the surgery he is not healed. There isn't any infection anymore in the wound or signs of a deeper infection but it's clear the wound is not going to heal on its own. Ultimately, we decide to take him back to the operating room to clean out the wound and remove any dead tissue. I reclose the wound and after this he does well. The wound is totally healed in 3 weeks, happily without any untoward effects.

Introduction

Most patients have many questions about the incisions and scars after surgery. "How many stitches will I have?" is still a very common question I get daily. I believe this curiosity about wounds arises from the patient's inclination to relate wound size to how invasive or big the surgery will be. For surgeons, the size of the incision is less critical as, paradoxically, long ones can heal without any issues, while small wounds may cause trouble. The location of the wound, how it is closed and how it is cared for after surgery are much more important than the actual size. This is a chapter dedicated to the smaller details after surgery. We discuss wound healing and how to best care for your dressings including some dos and don'ts.

Wound Care

Your skin acts as a physical barrier to infection. Ensuring your wound heals is critical to prevent germs from entering the surgical bed. The skin is a layered structure comprised of a superficial epidermal layer, a dermal, and a deep subcuticular layer (also referred to as subcutis). The epidermis is a tough, self-regenerating layer composed of flat epithelial cells. The dermal layer is composed of fibrocartilage, nerves, and blood vessels. The subcutis is mainly fat, but also contains large blood vessels.

Just like bone healing, wound healing is a complicated process that relies on many factors. There are three main phases to wound healing: inflammation, proliferation, and remodeling. Wound healing begins with an injury such as a surgical incision and some bleeding. The first phase of healing is the inflammatory response where many cell types migrate to the area to begin the repair process which lasts 1-3 days (1). A debris-cleaning immune cell known as a macrophage arrives at the site. Macrophages have two modes, M1 and M2. In the M1 mode they are focused on clearing out debris and invaders such as bacteria. They then transition to the M2 mode and start secreting substances that help the wound heal and initiate the proliferative phase. Macrophages seem to play a pivotal role not only in clearing the wound of contaminants but also in generating new skin. If this transition does not occur, such as in immunosuppressed patients (for example diabetics, and those on steroids) then chronic non-healing wounds may develop (2).

In the proliferative phase a matrix of collagen known as granulation or scar tissue is secreted to fill the wound and lasts for 3-21 days. As the wound fills, the wound edges contract, pulling the edges together, to allow skin (epithelial cells) to cross over the edges. In the final stage of remodeling, the wound is closed, the scar tissue remodels into normal skin, regaining normal tension and appearance; this final stage can take up to 1 year to complete. Wound tensile strength (its ability to withstand tearing) reaches 90% at 12 weeks. The epidermis (the visible part of the skin) heals much faster than the dermis (7-10 days), which can lead both the patient and surgeon to think that the wound is healed when in fact it is still healing (3).

Wounds generally heal by primary or secondary intention, that is, either neatly (primary) or in a prolonged fashion (secondary). In primary intention, the wound is generally superficial, the skin edges are not far apart, and the skin seals directly as epithelial cells cross over the cut edges. In deeper wounds that cut through the dermis and subcutis, secondary healing takes over, which involves the formation of granulation tissue (scar tissue) as described above. The goal of a surgical closure with its use of sutures is to allow primary healing to occur and to decrease scar formation as much as possible. Wounds healed by secondary intention end up with larger scars. All surgical wounds around the spine are deep through all layers of the skin and thus will form some scars, but with a neat closure and good after care, the scarring should be minimal. In a small subset of patients, scars can become large and proliferative in a condition called keloid formation. Keloid formation is likely related to genetic factors, local factors (such local force on the wound and if the wound is in an area of the body with significant motion such as the abdomen and joints), and lifestyle factors (being an athlete or manual laborer, excessive consumption of spicy foods, alcohol, or bathing in hot water can all contribute to bigger scars) (3).

To allow scars to heal with primary intention, surgeons will perform a layered closure of surgical wounds, closing the subcuticular, dermal, and epidermal layers. Subcuticular closure is generally performed using an absorbable suture material such as polyglactin (vicryl ®), poliglecaprone 25 (Monocryl®) or polydioxanone (PDS®) that will dissolve over the course of 6-8 weeks. The dermal layer may be closed by a variety of methods ranging from skin glue (2-octyl cyanoacrylate), nylon sutures, staples, or an absorbable suture. This is typically done by surgeon discretion, and each has its advantages. If sutures are used, they may be placed "subdermally" beneath the skin, so they are not visible and do not need to be removed. In other cases, such as with the use of nylon sutures, they can be placed in an interrupted fashion outside of the skin and need to be removed once the wound is healed.

A skin glue known as 2-octyl cyanoacrylate (Dermabond®) is commonly used in spine surgery these days. It is a non-toxic adhesive that is FDA-approved for use on lacerations and surgical wounds. It is useful because on contact with blood it forms a film and holds tissue edges together. It tends to peel off within 5-10 days as your skin sheds. Although for the most part Dermabond® is a safe substance, allergic skin reactions have been reported (4).

Steri-Strips, which are small pieces of medical tape that are applied directly to the skin and hold the edges together may also be used. These are intended to stay on the wound for several days and fall off on their own. They can be helpful in both acting as a barrier and protecting the wound from excessive stretching.

Dressings

To promote healing, following the suture closure a dressing is applied in the sterile surgical environment, which acts as a barrier to bacteria that might otherwise enter the wound. Because this is done in the sterile environment of the operating room, the dressing is left in place for a number of days, depending on surgeon discretion, to maintain sterility of the wound site. Most dressings are absorptive to prevent fluid accumulation and maceration (over moist skin that can lead to skin breakdown) of the wound. There are many different varieties of dressings in use today and so it can be a little confusing as to which one is the best. Your surgeon will likely have a favorite that they use and that works well for their style of surgery. Some commonly used dressings in orthopedic spine surgery are carboxymethylcellulose (aquacel®) and foam dressings (Mepilex®). Carboxymethylcellulose dressings are highly absorbable and can be left in place for many days. More recently, negative pressure dressings (sponge dressings hooked to a vacuum) have been shown to have some benefits in promoting healing. Some dressing may actually be impregnated with silver that can decrease the chance of surgical site infection (5). Some surgeons may feel a simple gauze cotton dressing is sufficient. As you can see, there are lots of options and what your surgeon uses is really a matter of personal preference. I think the important features of dressings are that they are sterile, absorptive, and seal off the wound from the world for a few days.

Following your surgery, it is best to leave the dressing in place for several days to allow the skin to seal prior to getting the incision wet. It has been shown that leaving the dressing in place is superior to daily dressing changes because it helps to maintain the sterile environment (6). However, if the dressing becomes saturated, it should be removed and changed so the skin does not become macerated. How long you should leave the dressing in place varies per surgery and surgeon but can be anywhere from 3 days for a small incision to 7 days for larger or more complicated one. There is little evidence in the literature to guide optimal wait time to shower (7). Once the skin has healed you can remove the bandage to shower but you should avoid using soaps directly on the wound or submerging the wound. Under no circumstances should you let your wound get near a lake, pool, river, or other source of contaminated water. Factors that inhibit good wound healing include conditions and lifestyle choices that restrict blood flow to the area, including diabetes mellitus, vascular disease, and smoking. Treating your wound too casually before it has totally healed can also inhibit healing.

Spine Incisions

Most spine incisions are in areas of the body that luckily have a remarkable healing potential, namely the low back and neck. These areas are highly vascular (meaning they have a good blood supply) and the skin is thick and robust, in comparison to other areas where the skin is thin and the blood supply tenuous such as around the ankle. Spine incisions on the posterior low back and neck tend to be vertical (in line with the spine) and will leave a vertical midline scar. Anterior spine incisions on the abdomen and neck tend to be horizontal to go in line with the grain of the skin and leave a more cosmetic scar.

Scar Prevention

Scarring can be minimized by caring for your surgical wound. As the wound is healing you should prevent any excessive stretching or repetitive motion across the wound such as by moving the wound excessively with exercise which will increase inflammation (3). The wound may heal superficially in 7-10 days, but it takes 3 months to fully heal. During this time putting silicone sheets or paper tape as directed by your surgeon can help prevent large scar formation (3). If you move the scar too much during this period, scarring can become more severe.

Once the wound is fully healed you should place sunscreen on the scar whenever it is exposed to sunlight. This helps prevent the incision from becoming hyperpigmented. Over-the-counter silicone gel may also be applied to the wound to help further remodeling and has been shown to be helpful in several randomized, controlled trials. There is no evidence to support vitamin-E oil, ultrasound therapy, hydrotherapy, cryotherapy, or laser therapy (8).

Wound Complications

Wounds can fail to heal for various reasons and can result in big problems. A very common reason is that the wound becomes infected with bacteria. If you notice that your wound is draining, you should contact your surgeon immediately. In most cases, if caught early, wound infections can be treated with oral antibiotics alone. However, if wound infections are allowed to fester, the bacteria can travel under the fascia layer and enter the deep spaces of the body resulting in serious infections and the need for surgical washouts.

A very common problem with wounds closed with absorbable sutures are suture abscesses. These are small pockets of infection that form around the suture material itself during the healing process and appear as red spots around a suture. They may even drain a small amount of pus-like material. Some people seem to be more inclined to develop these than others which is likely part of a heightened reaction of the body to the suture material. Suture abscesses can be treated with observation, antibiotics, or removal of the suture material by your surgeon and do not typically affect long-term healing.

Cutting down on smoking and maintaining tight glycemic control (limiting your carbohydrate intake) are two modifiable lifestyle factors that can help increase the chance of your wound healing properly (9). There are also techniques that can theoretically help with prevention of wound complications. For example, some surgeons will wash the wound out with an antiseptic such as betadine, while others will put an antibiotic powder into the wound. Some surgeons use drains to theoretically prevent fluid from building up under a wound, but this has not been demonstrated to reduce the rate of infections (10). If you are on chronic long-term steroids, it is critical to alert your surgeon as this can cause delayed wound healing and even wound breakdown after surgery.

In rare instances, wounds may need to be cleaned or debrided (damaged tissue removed) surgically to help them to close. Negative pressure dressings, which consist of a sealed sponge attached to a suction source (otherwise known as vac-therapy), may be used on wounds that are taking a prolonged time to heal. Negative pressure dressings allow quick drainage of wounds, preventing them from becoming macerated and thus aid the healing process.

Conclusion

Your wound is a critical component of your surgery and ensuring it heals properly is essential for the success of the procedure. Luckily, now we have many different techniques to help enhance healing and many steps you can take to allow your scar to heal properly.

Frequently Asked Questions

- **Will massaging my scar help?**

    Scar massage can help reduce the size of burns and surgical scars. Massage can be started 3 weeks after surgery once the wound is fully healed. Please check with your surgeon prior to starting this. Massage should be done on the scar with fingertips or the thumb in a circular fashion with a small amount of silicone gel or moisturizer for 10 minutes in the morning and evening (11).

- **Can silicone gels help minimize my scar?**

    Silicone gel (Active ingredient: Polydimethylsiloxane) is commonly available over the counter and can be used on surgical scars after 3 weeks, assuming the wound is fully healed over. These ointments can help decrease scar formation. Please check with your surgeon prior to starting this. These gels are typically applied over the scar twice a day but please follow the instructions on the packaging 11).

- **Can Vitamin E help my scar?**

    Vitamin E has been shown to provide no benefit to limiting scar formation over plain moisturizer. Thus, it is generally not recommended (11).

References

1.   Rosenbaum AJ, Banerjee S, Rezak KM, Uhl RL. Advances in Wound Management: Journal of the American Academy of Orthopaedic Surgeons. 2018 Dec;26(23):833–43.

2.   Sorg H, Tilkorn DJ, Hager S, Hauser J, Mirastschijski U. Skin Wound Healing: An Update on the Current Knowledge and Concepts. Eur Surg Res. 2017;58(1–2):81–94.

3.   Ogawa R, Dohi T, Tosa M, Aoki M, Akaishi S. The Latest Strategy for Keloid and Hypertrophic Scar Prevention and Treatment: The Nippon Medical School (NMS) Protocol. J Nippon Med Sch. 2021 Feb 15;88(1):2–9.

4.   Singer AJ, Quinn JV, Hollander JE. The cyanoacrylate topical skin adhesives. The American Journal of Emergency Medicine. 2008 May;26(4):490–6.

5.   Leaper D, Ousey K. Evidence update on prevention of surgical site infection. Curr Opin Infect Dis. 2015 Apr;28(2):158–63.

6.   Bains RS, Kardile M, Mitsunaga LK, Bains S, Singh N, Idler C. Postoperative Spine Dressing Changes Are Unnecessary. Spine Deformity. 2017 Nov;5(6):396–400.

7.   Toon CD, Sinha S, Davidson BR, Gurusamy KS. Early versus delayed post-operative bathing or showering to prevent wound complications. Cochrane Database Syst Rev. 2015 Jul 23;(7):CD010075.

8.   Grabowski G, Pacana MJ, Chen E. Keloid and Hypertrophic Scar Formation, Prevention,

and Management: Standard Review of Abnormal Scarring in Orthopaedic Surgery. Journal of the American Academy of Orthopaedic Surgeons. 2020 May;28(10):e408–14.

9.   Anderson PA, Savage JW, Vaccaro AR, Radcliff K, Arnold PM, Lawrence BD, et al. Prevention of Surgical Site Infection in Spine Surgery. Neurosurgery. 2017 Mar 1;80(3S):S114–23.

10.   Kanayama M, Oha F, Togawa D, Shigenobu K, Hashimoto T. Is Closed-suction Drainage Necessary for Single-level Lumbar Decompression?: Review of 560 Cases. Clinical Orthopaedics and Related Research®. 2010 Oct;468(10):2690–4.

11.   Khansa I, Harrison B, Janis JE. Evidence-Based Scar Management: How to Improve Results with Technique and Technology. Plastic and Reconstructive Surgery. 2016 Sep;138:165S-178S.

Figure:

Surgical Skin Closure

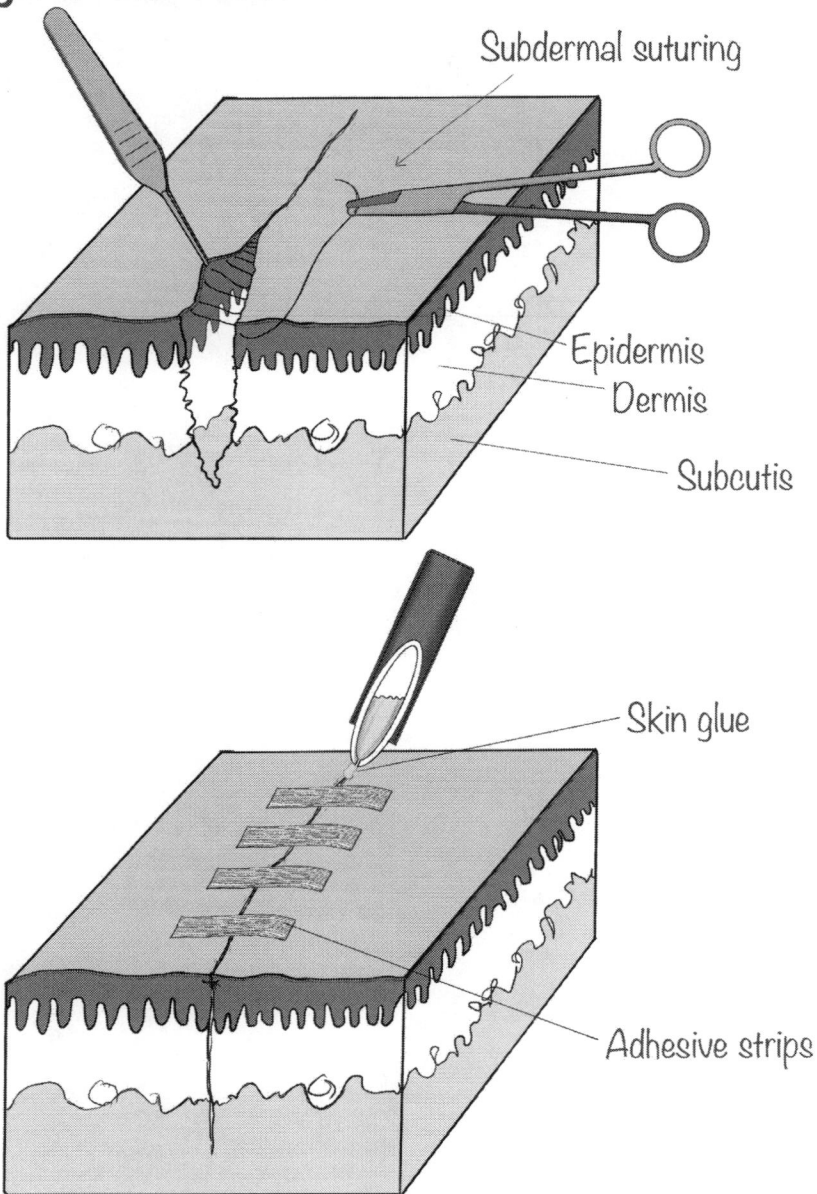

Subdermal suturing

Epidermis

Dermis

Subcutis

Skin glue

Adhesive strips

Surgical Skin Closure. The layers of the skin are closed in succession, beginning with the deepest layer. Adhesive strips and skin glue are also commonly used.

Chapter 50

Aftercare—Taking Care of Yourself at Home Following Spine Surgery: Pain Control, Diet and Activity Recommendations

Summary

Patients often have many questions and misconceptions about the recovery process following spine surgery. Every patient recovers with a different level of pain and speed, and so your course will likely be unique to you. I find that anguish frequently arises from the disconnect between what you think recovery will be like and what it turns out to be. Having some idea of what to expect will be beneficial not only for your own peace of mind, but for that of the friends and family who may be caring for you. The loss of some independence and functionality after surgery can be quite frustrating but having a good plan can make the recovery process that much easier. Prior to surgery it is critical to ensure your home is set up properly and that you have a good supply of food, so you do not have to make frequent outings as you convalesce. Make sure to coordinate with friends and family members who can help support you during the process and who can come visit to prevent you from being socially isolated. Finding a comfortable and safe position to sleep in can speed your recovery as well. Understanding that you need to rebuild your body slowly and with the help of trained physical therapists will prevent injury or further problems with your surgery. Finally, maintaining a positive attitude can mean the difference between a good recovery or a slow painful one.

Case

Ms. Violet is a 70-year-old retired accountant who is planning to have a lumbar decompression surgery to treat a crippling sciatica pain in her leg. She lives alone without much family around in the area but does have a rich network of friends who want to help her. She knows that her energy to go grocery shopping will likely be limited after the surgery and so coordinates with her friends who are happy to bring her food and groceries on a scheduled basis. Prior to surgery she stocks up on easy-to-make foods and prepares her home by installing hand holds in the bathroom and throughout the house. She even has her bed moved downstairs, so she doesn't have to use the stairs. Her surgery goes off without a hitch and to her surprise she feels much better now that her sciatica is relieved. She finds there is incisional pain around the surgical site, this pain is totally manageable and feels like a positive part of the healing process. She goes for walks every morning and evening with a close friend and feels better every day. She has planned visits with her surgeon who reassures her that she is making good progress. She is determined to enjoy her golden years and maintains a positive attitude. "The surgery was painful, but it took away the miserable sciatica pain and has allowed me to become more mobile and active," she thinks. Within a few weeks she is in physical therapy making herself stronger and at the 6-week point feels better than ever.

Introduction

The journey to healing begins when the wound is closed. And this is where the hard work of a sometimes lengthy recovery process following spine surgery starts for many patients. While the technical aspects of the surgery are critical, there are many things outside of the OR that can help hasten your recovery and, similarly, things you should avoid. The aftercare following surgery sometimes is just as confusing for patients as the concept of surgery. After all, you are asleep during the procedure and don't have to do anything, but when you get home, you will need to figure things out. In this chapter we try to demystify the after care of spine surgery and what you can do to ensure a safe and comfortable recovery.

General Strategies for Recovery and Pain Control Following Surgery

Following spine surgery, most patients want to reestablish normal life and get back to what they enjoy doing as fast as possible. Your pain level is a prominent factor that determines the speed at which you recover. Patients often ask, "how much pain will I have?" which is an impossible question to answer. For some, the pain from surgery is excruciating, while others mysteriously have zero pain. Other factors involved in recovery speed include familial and social support and your sense of understanding of your own limitations. Studies have shown that following surgery, there may be a period of psychological doubt where there is worry about recurrence of symptoms—"I'm scared the pain will return"—and perhaps even frustration at the rate of recovery— "Why can't I do what I want to right now?" (1). While most patients' recovery experiences proceed in a typical fashion that includes a resumption of their daily activities, there can be setbacks and, really, everyone recovers at a different pace. It's better to understand that you will have your own pace of recovery and not compare yourself to others (avoid thinking: "my friend had spine surgery and was back running in two weeks. Why am I not like that?" Your friend may have had a totally different problem with a different surgery). It's also critical to understand that surgery takes time to recover from and to go easy on yourself and others. Spine surgery can whisk away pain instantaneously in some cases, but in others it requires weeks of recovery. Thus, while spine surgery can improve your life dramatically, you must give your body adequate time to recover; otherwise, the surgery may be for nothing.

One thing that seems to frustrate patients is their inability to do basic activities of daily living such as bathing and dressing independently after surgery. However, it's important to remember that many patients will experience improved functionality after surgery with less pain than they had before surgery. The pain from surgery is temporary and will end after several weeks in most cases. Very rarely are you required to be on bed rest and so your mobility with walking will likely not be restricted. So, although you will have some disability, it may be less than you think. Moreover, there are many devices that can help expand your functionality during your convalescence that a well-trained occupational therapist can help you discover. Functional aids such as grabbers, sock aids, shower chairs, and slip-on shoes without laces are all helpful.

During the immediate recovery period you may need to rely on friends and family members, which may make some feel helpless. It's important to allow your family and friends to care for you if needed and to express appreciation for this. Remember, allowing others to help you gives them the chance to feel reward about doing something positive. Getting frustrated with your caregivers is biting the hand that feeds you and doesn't help anything. Also, it may be difficult to immediately reenter social relationships because of a feeling of incapacity. This can lead to feelings of isolation. Planning for friends and family to visit you in a comfortable setting at timed intervals can help keep this feeling at bay. Setting up games such as cards or board games with a friend or family member can also be a great way to socialize and take your mind off frustrations.

Most patients will set their ability to return to normal activities as a benchmark of success. Having the assumption that you will promptly return to normal activity will lead to disappointment. Preparing yourself for functional limitations after surgery is critical. You may not be able to shower on your own, go to the bathroom completely on your own, go shopping and get food, or dress yourself independently. While many patients can return quickly to normal levels, some are inevitably disappointed or even angered that they are not immediately normal. Neurologic recovery can take weeks, months or even years. In those cases where surgery was done to prevent worsening of neurologic decline, surgery will not result in significant neurologic improvement, and you may have some residual disability.

An important strategy to cope with functional setbacks is to factor in frequent breaks as part of your plan to accomplish something. Understanding ahead of time that it may take double or triple the time to accomplish a task can be psychologically helpful. Your goal can be to start measuring the breaks you take and then cutting down on them week by week. Walking aids such as walkers and canes can increase mobility and boost confidence. Because getting to the toilet or getting on and off can be difficult, having a bedside commode or a toilet seat raise is very helpful.

Three main patient recovery patterns have been identified following surgery: Meaningful recovery (where patients participate in physical activity and return to normal function), progressive recovery (improvement is more incremental or bit by bit; however, progression is noticeable over time), and disruptive recovery (meaningful recovery does not occur). While most patients experience a meaningful or progressive recovery, what determines if the recovery will be disruptive depends on a complex set of factors, including physical and functional limitations, social support, and the patient's ability to cope with emotions and set back (1). Patients who have a positive outlook on recovery have better clinical outcomes while those with psychological issues, depression and severe anxiety may have worse outcomes despite a successful surgery (2).

Recovery Equipment	
Rolling walker	Slippers or shoes without laces
Sock aid	Loose fitting clothing easy to put on and take off
Bath chair	Cane
Grabber	Handrails and hand holds
Bedside commode or toilet seat elevator	Foot lift: a device to help elevate your legs onto the bed.

Diet

Your diet can substantially change after surgery. Narcotics and other pain medicines cause nausea, and severe constipation and, after cervical surgery, swallowing may be more difficult. It is a good idea to stock up on stool softeners and laxatives to help combat this. Having foods around the house that are easy on the stomach but still give you good nutrition is critical. Cold smoothies made from fresh fruit can help with constipation and are great for those who have had anterior (approaching from the front) cervical surgery where there can be swelling around the throat. This is because cool drinks can ease swallowing issues and reduce inflammation locally. Try to prepare food in advance so it is ready to eat with no fuss before your procedure. Focus on high fiber whole foods such as fruits and cooked vegetables that will aid digestion. Avoid foods heavy with fat that may be difficult to digest or high in sugar which can increase your glucose levels and also contribute to constipation. Plan to have some friends or family members come over to help cook and clean.

Sleep

Sleeping after spine surgery can be difficult because it's hard finding a comfortable position. What is important, in addition to comfort, is to ensure your spine is not kinked or held in an awkward position that can affect the results of surgery. Having lots of different pillows of varying sizes can be useful to support your body and help you find comfortable positions. For many spinal fusion patients, lying on your side with your neck supported so it is in line with the spine and placing a pillow between the knees is comfortable. Alternatively, sleeping on your back with a pillow beneath the legs can be comfortable.

Activity

My mantra for patients after surgery is "no bending, lifting or twisting—or no BLT." What this means is you should not bend down through your back (bending at the waist) to pick something off the floor or to tie your shoes. You should not lift any heavy objects (greater than 5 pounds or around a gallon of water) and you should not twist—as in reaching for something across from you or swinging a golf club. These activities all put significant load on your spine and can result in the need for a surgical repair.

Nonetheless, I believe movement is critical after surgery (excluding the above). Walking is the ideal post-spine surgery exercise as it does not place significant strain on the back and neck (see below for a more detailed guide on post-op exercise). Walking and movement promote good circulation, prevent blood clots and bed sores, and help with pain control (believe it or not). Walking is psychologically liberating, and I think prevents the development of "patient" mindset because it gets you outside of your spine problem and surgery. In general, I put no restrictions on walking following surgery, but let your body guide you. Don't overdo it and if you have worsening pain, you may be walking or doing too much. Start off slow and gradually increase your walking as you can tolerate it.

When you are not active and walking you may be most comfortable sitting. Do not sit in a low chair with deep cushions that may be difficult to arise from without help. Make sure you sit with a pillow behind your back and avoid slouching. Remember that no sedentary position should be maintained for greater than 40 minutes as this can increase pain and the risk of blood clots. Change positions often.

Sex

Good news: with improved neurologic function and reduced pain, your sex life may ultimately improve following spine surgery (3). However, in the immediate post-operative period, reentering sexual life can take time and some adjustments. There are many different types of spine surgery just as there are a variety of ways to have intercourse. Some forms of spine surgery are functionally limiting and during the recovery period you should check with your doctor before having intercourse as it may compromise your surgery. Any type of sex positions that put a significant strain on your back and neck are not recommended in the recovery period. Please check with your surgeon before resuming sexual activity.

In most cases it is safe to have sex after surgery once cleared by your physician; however, you may have functional restrictions for several weeks or months after the procedure that will necessitate modifications. Just as you must perform activities of daily living with the correct body mechanics after surgery (avoiding bending, twisting, or lifting that puts strain on your back and neck) so must you do with sex. Safe post-op sexual positions differ whether you are male or female, but in general the patient should assume the less active role in sex, and preferably is in a flat supine position with the legs and head well supported with pillows. It is important to discuss your limitations openly with your partner, as your traditional positions for sex may not be possible or cause pain in the recovery period. Try to come up with alternatives which will not interfere with protecting your back.

Driving

You should not drive until you have been cleared to do so by your physician. There are certain restrictions I put on my patients for driving after spine surgery. You should not drive while taking any narcotics or pain medicines. These medicines can cause drowsiness and decrease reaction time, making you a danger to yourself and others in the car. Just as you should not be in a seated position for greater than 40 minutes, you should not drive for longer periods than 40 minutes at a time. For those who need to take longer drives, it should be broken up into 40-minute intervals with at least 15 minutes of rest in between. Make sure to get out of the car and walk around. If you suffer from some neurologic deficit such as weakness of the arms or legs or numbness which prevents feeling in your hands or feet, returning to driving may be difficult and should be discussed with your surgeon and the local motor vehicle authority.

After a fusion procedure on your neck or back, turning around to look behind you or twisting your neck to look to your side can become more difficult. Usually this does not limit you from driving as you can make use of mirrors and ever-increasingly sophisticated cameras around your car, but you may find driving to be much more difficult than it was prior to your surgery. It's important to start driving again in a controlled fashion as you may need to learn to make some adjustments.

Air Travel

In most cases, you should avoid air travel for at least two weeks after your surgery or until you have cleared it with your surgeon. Air travel can cause nausea, dehydration and low oxygen which may worsen problems that occur after surgery. It may be difficult navigating an airplane using a walker if you have not regained full mobility. Because you are in a cramped, seated position for a possibly prolonged timeframe, it can increase your surgical pain and the risk of blood clots. I advise my patients to be well hydrated before and during a flight and in some cases to take a baby aspirin beforehand. You should get up and walk the aisle or go use the restroom as much as permitted by flight staff.

Pain

The level of pain following spine surgery is generally dependent on the amount of surgery that is done and the pain tolerance of the patient. The invasiveness of spinal surgery ranges from small outpatient surgery to large open procedures that require days in the hospital. I have seen patients undergoing major low or upper back reconstruction surgery have minimal pain and patients whose surgery consisted of a small percutaneous procedure have uncontrollable pain.

Everyone's experience is a little different but there are trends that are common. There are certain risk factors that increase your chances of uncontrollable pain. Many spine patients have been on long-term narcotics which sensitize the body to pain, making post-operative pain control very difficult. As you take more narcotics your body not only becomes more sensitive to pain, but also resistant to more narcotics, making pain control medicines ineffective. Thus, prior to surgery you should work with your surgeon or pain specialist to reduce how much narcotics you are taking.

To help control pain after surgery, your surgeon will use several medicines in combination known as "multimodal pain management." The goal of multimodal pain management is to block the transmission of pain at multiple sites as it travels from your body to your brain through the spinal cord (4). The surgical site may be numbed before and after incision with a local anesthetic such as lidocaine, bupivacaine or ropivacaine. These blocks typically last from 12-24 hours and help the immediate post-surgical pain. In certain major spinal procedures, an epidural catheter which places local anesthetics and opioids directly into the spinal canal may be used.

Gabapentin, which is a medicine useful in the treatment of neuropathic pain, may be started in the peri-operative period and continued into the post-operative to decrease reliance on opioid medications. Strong intravenous narcotics such as morphine and hydromorphone are used in the immediate post-operative period. The patient is weaned from these medicines as soon as possible because of their significant side effects and is transitioned to oral narcotics such as tramadol, or hydrocodone. All narcotics cause constipation, drowsiness, and difficulty with urination. Use them sparingly. Most pain medications are given on an "as needed" basis, so you must ask for them if you are in pain—they will not be administered while you are asleep. I generally recommend using pain medicines only when you are experiencing pain. For some reason "staying ahead" of your pain by taking medication before you start to experience pain is a common concept in patients' minds, but narcotic medicines are very fast-acting and can be taken as soon as you start to experience pain with quick relief (IV medicines have a roughly 5-minute onset, while oral agents have a 30-minute onset).

Muscle relaxants such as cyclobenzaprine or baclofen may be added to help combat muscle spasms that can occur after a lumbar fusion. Acetaminophen (Tylenol®) may be administered in an intravenous form which makes it much more powerful than standard oral Tylenol. Strong non-steroidal anti-inflammatory pain medicines such as ketorolac (Toradol®) may be used after smaller spine surgeries and may decrease use of narcotics (5).

The pain following surgery is generally different from the one you experience because of your spine problem. It's a post-surgical ache which in some people can be severe. To explore these trends, let's use the lumbar fusion as an example for a common course of pain following surgery.

Following surgery, you can expect pain and soreness at the surgical site. Most patients expect this and can deal with this, but for some it is severe. To help with the acute pain, your doctor may use a combination of pain medications as described above. The pain typically increases on day 2 after surgery as local anesthetics wear off; however, this is followed by a gradual decrease in pain over the next few days. By 1 week after surgery most patients are comfortable on an oral narcotic medicine and Tylenol but will still have pain. Gabapentin and muscle relaxants are also continued. Pain not only inhibits activity but also leads to a significant amount of anxiety and depression, so it's important to pay attention to your mood during this time and remember the pain will gradually decrease as the weeks move on. By 6 weeks following surgery most of the acute pain has subsided; however, you may still have "twinges" or a dull ache. The good news is the pain from surgery is totally different from the pain experienced from spine conditions, which is typically improved following surgery.

Discharge

Some surgeries may be done on an "outpatient/ same day discharge" basis where, after a few hours of observation and recovery from anesthesia, you are safe to go home. In other cases, you are admitted to the hospital for "inpatient" surgery where you will be monitored for one or more days. In most cases the goal following surgery should be discharge to your own home. This is where most people have the most comfort. However, in certain situations, you may need to be discharged to an acute rehab facility where participation in daily rehab is mandatory or to a skilled nursing facility where there are nurses available to help care for you around the clock. Patients who are elderly and are not able to become sufficiently independent following the operation may need to go to somewhere where they can be assisted with activities of daily living such as bathing and using the restroom.

Rehabilitation and Exercise Following Spine Surgery

The recovery timeline can vary significantly depending on the type of surgery you have had. I have found that most patients' concept of spine surgery is somewhat out of date, with the assumption that there will be months of bed rest. This is not true and only in rare cases is bed rest required (such as in the case of a spinal fluid leak). In fact, early mobilization is often encouraged. Even more vigorous exercise may be resumed early in the recovery process after some procedures. For example, a disc herniation surgery may only require a few weeks of rest before exercise can be resumed. But in general, all exercise should be cleared by your surgeon before you start.

You can start your recovery immediately after surgery with some simple exercises to promote blood flow and nerve movement after surgery.

Ankle pumps: as you lie on your back move both of your ankles up or point your "toes to your nose." Hold this for a moment, and then point your ankles down as if pressing down on a gas pedal. This promotes the circulation of blood from the calves back to the body. Repeat 10 times every hour.

Quadriceps contractions: lying on your back and keeping your heel in contact with the bed, contract your thigh muscles pushing your knee down into the bed. Hold this for a moment and release. Repeat 10 times every hour.

Nerve glides: lying on your back, glide your heel from a leg extended position to a knee bent position and back again without letting the heel lose contact with the bed. This will help move the sciatic nerve which prevents scarring of nerves after a lumbar decompression. Repeat 10 times every hour.

Patients commonly ask about starting rehabilitation. Rehab is important for a sense of participation in your own recovery and can be helpful for regaining strength. However, immediate rehab after surgery may not be helpful in all cases and may even be detrimental. Movement and exercise place strain on your wounds and increase bacterial burden on the skin. Therefore, physical therapy generally starts 4-6 weeks after surgery once the wounds have healed. It has even been shown that higher aerobic exercise intensity exercise can promote healing faster than low intensity exercise, but it is important that this is supervised to prevent injury (6–8). In cases of lumbar fusion, it is critical to maintain your restrictions which typically consist of no bending, lifting, or twisting. This is to ensure only the minimum amount of strain is placed on the fusion.

Walking is the ideal post-operative exercise. It places minimal strain on your back and allows you to obtain some aerobic exercise which will increase the blood flow to the site of surgery, promoting faster healing. I typically recommend at least a mile in the AM and another mile in PM for the first 2-3 weeks and then gradually increasing that. In addition to walking, if you are resting in a chair you can work on contracting your quad muscles and calf muscles without moving the joints—this causes muscle activation to increase strength while also helping prevent blood clots.

Exercise timeline	
Weeks 1-4 *	• Walking 20 minutes in AM and PM • Nerve glides • Ankle and foot pumps: 10 each side every hour • Quad contractions: 10 each side every hour
Weeks 6-12	• Elliptical • Recumbent bicycle • Squats • Wall sits • Lunges
Weeks 12 and above	• Gradual strength training • Core strengthening • Bird dog exercise • Hip abduction exercises

Aerobic exercise may also be obtained through use of an elliptical machine or recumbent bike; these also place minimal load on the spine and can be started 2-3 weeks after surgery once cleared by your physician. Other exercises may be incorporated such as leg squats, wall sits, and lunges, all under supervision. Recovery from a lumbar fusion consists of allowing the bones to heal together; therefore, there is not much use for strengthening exercise in the early phases of recovery (up to three months). As the fusion consolidates and stabilizes, more core-strengthening exercises can be incorporated under physical therapy supervision. Core strengthening is safe to do in lumbar fusion but should be done with instruction. I recommend using neutral spine control exercises which consist of exercises that work on your spinal stability without placing huge amounts of loads across the vertebrae and not starting them until at least week 12 (8,9).

Neutral Spine Control Exercises
Bilateral shoulder flexion and extension in standing position
Unilateral shoulder horizontal adduction and abduction in sitting position
Unilateral hip extension in a 4- point kneeling position

Conclusion

Your recovery after spine surgery depends on many variables including your original problem, the amount and invasiveness of surgery, your health and psychological status. It is critical to be as engaged as possible in your recovery and stay positive. Negative thoughts can lead to poor coping mechanisms and an overall worse outcome. Learn about what resources you have available and accept help from friends and family members.

Frequently Asked Questions

- **Will I be on bed rest after surgery? Will I be able to walk?**

Even in the most invasive spinal deformity procedures I perform, I recommend early ambulation—it is good to get up and move. Bed rest is only used in cases where a spinal fluid leak may need to be treated, which occurs in about 5-10% of cases.

References

1. Rushton A, Jadhakhan F, Masson A, Athey V, Staal JB, Verra ML, et al. Patient journey following lumbar spinal fusion surgery (FuJourn): A multicentre exploration of the immediate post-operative period using qualitative patient diaries. PloS One. 2020;15(12): e0241931.

2.   Rief W, Shedden-Mora MC, Laferton JAC, Auer C, Petrie KJ, Salzmann S, et al. Preoperative optimization of patient expectations improves long-term outcome in heart surgery patients: results of the randomized controlled PSY-HEART trial. BMC Med. 2017 Jan 10;15(1):4.

3.   Malik AT, Jain N, Kim J, Khan SN, Yu E. Sexual activity after spine surgery: a systematic review. Eur Spine J Off Publ Eur Spine Soc Eur Spinal Deform Soc Eur Sect Cerv Spine Res Soc. 2018 Oct;27(10):2395–426.

4.   Puvanesarajah V, Liauw JA, Lo S fu, Lina IA, Witham TF, Gottschalk A. Analgesic therapy for major spine surgery. Neurosurg Rev. 2015 Jul;38(3):407–19.

5.   Cassinelli EH, Dean CL, Garcia RM, Furey CG, Bohlman HH. Ketorolac use for postoperative pain management following lumbar decompression surgery: a prospective, randomized, double-blinded, placebo-controlled trial. Spine. 2008 May 20;33(12):1313–7.

6.   Danielsen JM, Johnsen R, Kibsgaard SK, Hellevik E. Early aggressive exercise for postoperative rehabilitation after discectomy. Spine. 2000 Apr 15;25(8):1015–20.

7.   Oosterhuis T, Costa LO, Maher CG, de Vet HC, van Tulder MW, Ostelo RW. Rehabilitation after lumbar disc surgery. Cochrane Back and Neck Group, editor. Cochrane Database Syst Rev [Internet]. 2014 Mar 14 [cited 2020 Dec 29]; Available from: http://doi.wiley.com/10.1002/14651858.CD003007.pub3

8.   Gencay-Can A, Gunendi Z, Suleyman Can S, Sepici V, Çeviker N. The effects of early aerobic exercise after single-level lumbar microdiscectomy: a prospective, controlled trial. Eur J Phys Rehabil Med. 2010 Dec;46(4):489–96.

9.   Madera M, Brady J, Deily S, McGinty T, Moroz L, Singh D, et al. The role of physical therapy and rehabilitation after lumbar fusion surgery for degenerative disease: a systematic review. J Neurosurg Spine. 2017 Mar;26(6):694–704.

Figures:

Spine Neutral Sleeping Positions

On your side with your head supported and a pillow between the knees

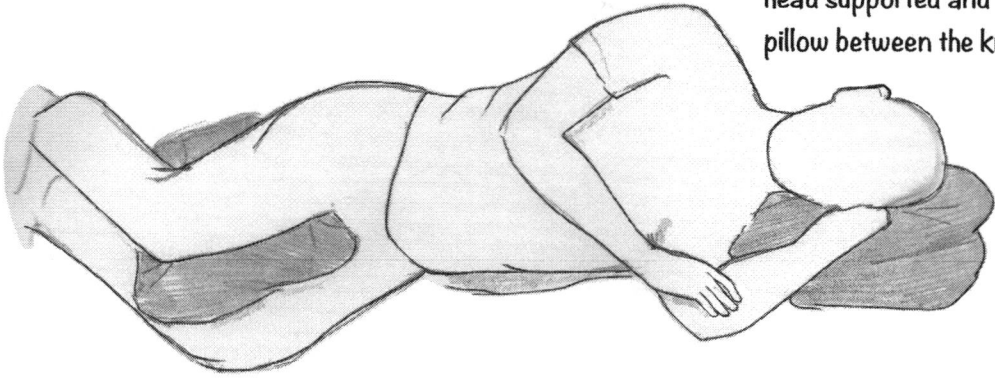

On your back with your head supported and a pillow under the knees

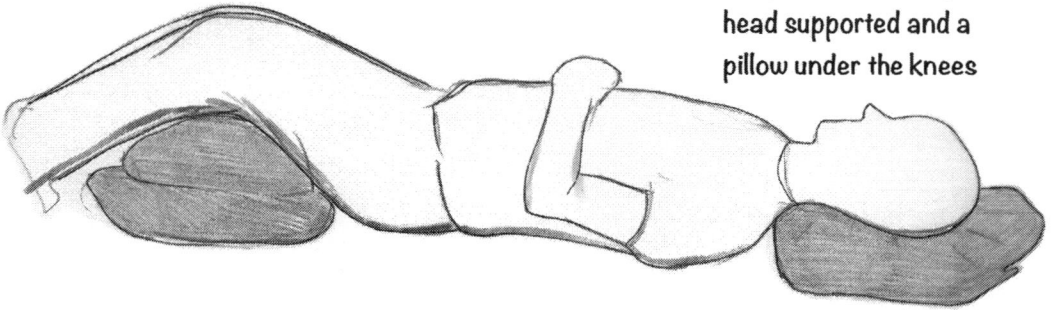

Sleeping. Comfortable positions to sleep in that are also good for the spine are on your side with a pillow between the knees (top), or on your back with a pillow under the legs (bottom).

Neutral Spine Exercises:
Bilateral shoulder flexion and extension

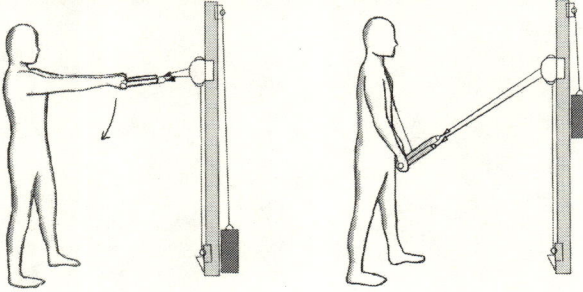

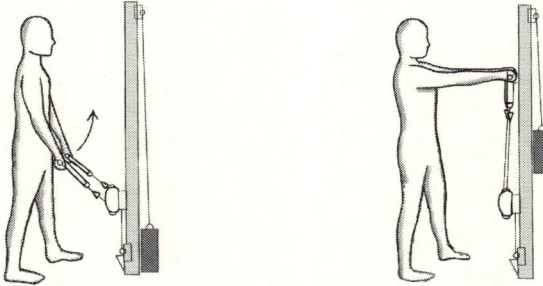

Shoulder adduction and abduction, seated:

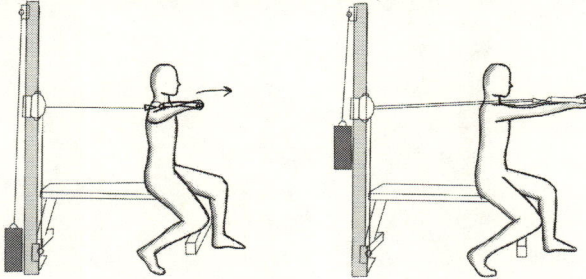

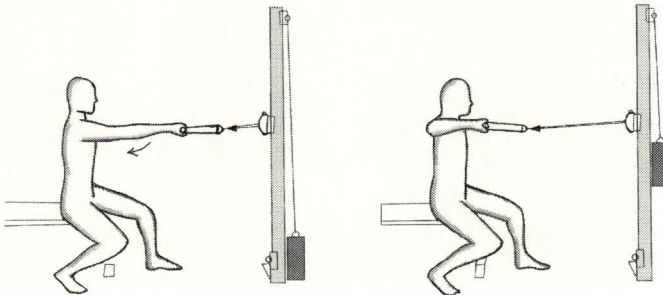

Neutral Spine Control Exercises. Exercises which you can perform once cleared by your surgeon that place minimal loads across the spine.

Chapter 51

Conclusions and Further Reading

"The human spine is a biomechanical masterpiece."

- Bassal Diebo (1).

Your spine allows you to interact with the world and walk erect with minimal effort. I hope this book has given you a clearer idea of how your spine works, how it breaks down, and how to care for it when it does. Your goal will always be to live life with a pain-free back. In the rare cases where problems develop, surgery has both great power and dangers to help you on your path towards recovery. I hope this book will help you navigate this wonderful and complicated knowledge.

I wrote this book so that my patients could learn my style of thinking about spine surgery and see how spine surgery has affected my patients. As I said in the intro, this book was born out of a hope to connect better with my patients. I believe spine surgery is a team effort whose success is partly based on education and communication. I hope this book will help guide you to a solid understanding of the basic concepts of the spine as well as surgery involving the spine and help you live a more active and pain free life.

As you may have learned in reading this book, spine surgery is complicated, and no one book can teach you everything you need to know about the spine or accurately predict how you will respond to spine surgery. There are viewpoints expressed in this book that are my own and what I believe to be reasonable and safe in my practice. A common saying, I tell my patients, is that "you can ask three spine surgeons for opinions and expect to get three different opinions." This is because there is an "art" component to spine surgery as well as a "science." First in making a correct diagnosis, interpreting the medical imaging, and finally in performing surgery. What works well for one patient may not work at all for another. Similarly, different surgeons will have techniques that will work better in their hands than others. Luckily, when it comes to the spine there are many ways to treat a problem, and often selecting treatments are a matter of surgeon and patient preference. I find that it is best to provide my patients with as much information as they desire so that they can make the right choice for themselves.

I have tried to read many books about the spine and spine surgery to expand my knowledge and in that process, I have learned different perspectives as well as techniques for the care of the spine. In addition to by now countless books, there are also thousands of scientific articles and review articles on surgery of the spine that have influenced my practice. I have placed key references in the text but if you are interested in learning more there are unlimited resources out there.

There are several other excellent guides about spine surgery in existence and I suggest you read these as well if you are interested.

- **Do You Really Need Back Surgery? by Arron G Filler M.D.**

- **Stopping Scoliosis, by Nancy Schommer**

- **I've Got Your Back, by Nathaniel L Tindel M.D.**

- **Back in Control, By David Hanscom M.D.**

For a great book on non-operative care of the spine I recommend:

- **Back Rx, by Vijay Vad MD**

For those of you who are more interested in research on spine surgery try visiting:

- **https://pubmed.ncbi.nlm.nih.gov/ and search for the latest research available on your specific spine problems**

- **https://orthoinfo.org/ offers recommendations from the American Academy of Orthopaedic Surgeons. This site contains a wealth of information on orthopedic conditions but look specifically on the spine section for info on spine surgery.**

- **www.srs.org includes frequently asked questions fielded by the Scoliosis Research Society (SRS), the premier research body looking at spinal deformity.**

- **https://www.spine.org/KnowYourBack is the site for the North American Spine Society (NASS) which has a host of information for patients.**

For books on nutrition and weight loss I recommend:

- **Eat to Live, Joel Furhman MD**

- **How Not to Die, Michael Greger MD**

Patients are always interested in supplements but wonder if they are safe. Here is a site that gives information about medications and information on herbal supplements.

- **www.nlm.nih.gov/medlineplus/druginformation.html**

Thank you

Thank you so much for reading this book. I am proud to have written, illustrated and published this work independently. I intend for the book to evolve and improve in the coming years as new spine technology becomes available. If you notice any typos or have improvement ideas, please feel free to email me at yoshi@katsuuramd.com. I would love to hear from you. You can also learn more about my practice and read my blog at www.katsuuramd.com.

Yours,
Yoshihiro Katsuura M.D.

A Glossary of Common Terms in Spine Surgery

ACDF: an acronym for "anterior cervical discectomy and fusion" a procedure where the cervical disc is removed to relieve stenosis (see below) through the front of the neck and fused with a small cage which stimulates the bones to grow together or fuse.

Adjacent segment disease: degeneration or breakdown of the disc level above or below a previous spine surgery, typically a spinal fusion, requiring surgical treatment. The term "adjacent segment degeneration" is used for breakdown that is visible on medical imaging, but does not cause symptoms and thus does not require surgery.

Afferent signal: a nerve signal going towards the brain carrying sensory information.

AFib: Atrial fibrillation, a condition where the heart develops an irregular heart rate.

Agonist: a chemical that activates a cellular receptor (opposite of an antagonist). An agonist makes something happen by stimulating a cell action.

ALIF: an acronym for "anterior lumbar interbody fusion" a procedure where the lumbar disc is removed through the front of the spine and fused with a cage which stimulates the adjacent vertebral bones to grow together or fuse.

Allograft: a bone graft obtained from a donor cadaver source. This is opposed to an "autograft" which is donor bone obtained from your own body.

Anabolic therapy: medications which build up bone strength and can reverse osteoporosis. An example of this is teriparatide, a drug which can cause bone density to increase.

Analgesia: obtaining pain relief through medications.

Anaphylaxis: a severe allergic reaction resulting in swelling of the airway and hives. Anaphylaxis may result in death from severe airway swelling causing you to choke.

Angiography: A radiographic study where contrast dye is injected into an artery to better visualize it. A typical example in the spine is a CT-angiogram of the cervical spine where contrast is injected followed by a CT scan of the neck to visualize the course of the arteries of the neck.

Annulotomy: A small incision made in a the exterior of a intervertebral disc to extract a disc herniation causing impingement.

Annulus fibrosis: the tough outer casing of an intervertebral disc; it contains the core nucleus pulposus (see below).

Antagonist: a chemical that deactivates or blocks a cellular receptor (opposite of an agonist). An antagonist keeps something from happening by preventing a cell action.

Anterior: The front of something. The nose is on the anterior aspect of the face.

Anterior cervical discectomy and fusion ACDF): a procedure where the cervical disc is removed to relieve stenosis (see below) through the front of the neck and fused with a small cage which stimulates the bones to grow together or fuse.

Anterior lumbar interbody fusion (ALIF): a lumbar interbody fusion performed by placing a cage in the disc space through an anterior abdominal spinal approach.

Anticoagulant: a medication or substance that inhibits blood clotting and thus promotes bleeding. Anticoagulants can be used to prevent blood clots from occurring after surgery, but must be used very carefully as they can increase bleeding from surgical sites.

Antiresorptive therapy: medications which inhibit the breakdown of bone in natural aging, thus putting off osteoporosis. An example of this is zoledronic acid (Reclast®).

Approach: a term used to describe the way a surgeon gets to the target area of the body to be operated on (surgical exposure). For example, the anterior approach to the cervical spine describes the procedure of opening the front (anterior)of the neck in a way that the surgeon can access the vertebrae and discs.

Arthritis: break down and wear on a joint.

Arthroplasty: a term used to describe the replacement of a joint with a prosthesis (Arthro (Greek) meaning joint, and Plastos (Greek) for formation).

Articular process: a bony formation that arises from the lamina of the vertebra and is a component of the facet joint (also known as the zygapophysial joint) of the spine. Each lamina has four articular processes: two superior and two inferior.

Atrial fibrillations (AFib): a condition where the heart develops an irregular heart rate.

Autonomic nervous system: a component of the nervous system responsible for automatic functions of the body such as digestion, breathing, and heart rate. The autonomic nervous system has two components: sympathetic, responsible for flight or flight and parasympathetic, responsible for relaxation.

Autograft: a bone graft harvested from a donor site on your own body. Common donor sites include the iliac crest which is part of the pelvic bone.

Back strain: minor tears in the muscles or ligaments of the back.

Benign: may have multiple meanings in medicine. With regard to cancer, a benign tumor does not have the potential to metastasize (spread) to other areas of the body. A benign spinal condition is one that typically will not result in long term harm and will not require surgery.

Biopsy: a procedure used to sample tissue for analysis by a pathologist (a medical specialist who is an expert at examining tissue). Typically used to look for cancer.

Bone cement: polymethylmethacrylate is a polymer cement used in spine surgery to perform the kyphoplasty procedure, where the cement is injected into the vertebra to stabilize a fracture. It is also used in other areas of orthopedics such as in total knee replacements to fix the prosthesis to the bone.

Bone Graft: typically ground up bone that is applied to the spine in order to allow two or more vertebrae to grow together and form a fusion. Bone graft may be obtained from cadaver donors (allograft) or from yourself (autograft)

Bone morphogenic protein (BMP): a protein molecule that stimulates bone growth and promotes spinal fusion.

Burst fracture: a fracture occurring through the entire vertebral body (that is, the anterior and middle columns of the vertebra—the parts of the vertebra furthest from the back).

Cage: a device inserted into the disc space between two vertebrae to promote stability and fusion. Synonymous with "spacer" or "interbody device."

Catastrophizing: always expecting the worst and predicting doom.

Cauda equina syndrome: a condition where there is near complete blockage of the lumbar spinal canal by a disc rupture or other condition. This results in severe back and leg pain, urinary and fecal incontinence, and numbness throughout the groin area and legs. This is a medical emergency and should be treated immediately.

Cerebrospinal fluid (CSF): The fluid that bathes the spinal cord and is contained by the lining of the spinal canal called the meninges.

Cervical myelopathy: a progressive condition where compression of the cervical (neck) spinal cord causes the patient to lose his or her manual dexterity, balance, strength and sensation of the arms and even legs.

Cervical spine: the 7 vertebrae in the neck.

Clinical: An adjective used to describe things that a doctor observes or discovers or learns on his or her own (so without diagnostic tests) at the bedside with the patient. For example, a clinical exam is a physical examination that the doctor performs on you with their own hands. This contrasts with a radiological exam, which is one done with an imaging machine. Clinical signs are features on your physical exam which point towards a certain diagnosis. Clinical symptoms are the symptoms you directly tell your doctor.

Coccyx: a small bone at the tip of the sacrum (tailbone) that consists of 4-5 fused vertebrae. It is the terminal bone in the spinal column.

Computer tomography (CT) scan: an advanced medical imaging system where a rotating X-ray beam creates a cross sectional image of the spine.

Conservative care: a term used colloquially by orthopedists to refer to non-surgical treatments such as medication and physical therapy.

Contraindications: certain clinical scenarios that prevent a surgeon from performing a specific procedure. Contraindications may be "relative" meaning they do not always prevent the procedure from being performed, or "absolute," where the procedure should never be performed.

Coronary artery disease (CAD): a condition where there is buildup of plaque on the coronary arteries that limits blood flow to the heart and can result in a heart attack (death of the heart muscle).

Corpectomy: a procedure where the vertebral body of the spine is removed (typically for a tumor, fracture or deformity) and reconstructed with a large cage graft. You can think of this as vertebral replacement.

Cryoablative therapy: a procedure using a very cold substance to remove or destroy pathologic tissue such as a tumor.

CSF (cerebrospinal fluid): The fluid that bathes the spinal cord and is contained by the lining of the spinal canal called the meninges.

Debridement: the act of removing tissue from an area or cleaning it out surgically. Debridement is used primarily for infection, where infected material is excised (cut out), but the term can also be used to describe removing material away from a nerve.

Decompression: surgical removal of structures which are compressing the nerves or spinal cord.

Degeneration: break down of tissues leading to altered function. The term degeneration can be used synonymously with "arthritic changes."

Degenerative disc disease: a condition resulting in the gradual break down of the intervertebral discs and collapse of the vertebral segment. Degenerative disc disease can result in back pain, and spinal stenosis.

Disc: a soft tissue structure that acts as a cushion between the vertebrae. Discs have two main structural components: the annulus fibrosis which is a tough outer ring, and a jelly like core known as the nucleus pulposus. The disc is often referred to as an intervertebral disc (between the vertebrae).

Diskitis: an infection of the intervertebral disc.

Dissect: to separate structures in the body from one another so that a surgical corridor can be developed, often by cutting.

Dorsal: located on or near the back. The term dorsal may be used similarly to posterior.

Dorsal horn: the dorsal part of the spinal cord where sensory nerves originate.

Double Crush Syndrome: a condition where a nerve is pinched or entrapped at more than one location. A common double crush syndrome is a nerve pinched in the neck as well as in the carpal tunnel in the hand.

Dura mater: part of the lining of the thecal sac that protects the spinal cord (see meninges). Also called dural sac or just "the dura."

DXA or DEXA (Dual-energy X-ray, absorptiometry): this is a scanning method that uses low dose X-rays to determine your bone mineral density which is used as an indicator for bone strength. DXA scans give a score known as a T-score, that compare your bone mineral density to that of a young healthy individual.

Efferent signal: also known as a motor signal, it is a nerve signal coming from the brain to the body to initiate an action.

Elective Surgery: surgery that is done on a scheduled, non-urgent basis for conditions that are mainly degenerative in nature.

Electromyography (EMG): an electrodiagnostic test where a doctor uses small needle electrodes and sensors to see how muscles are working. This test is useful for determining if there is a problem with the muscle or its nerve supply.

Epidural steroid injection (ESI): an injection performed under X-ray guidance where a spinal needle is inserted into the space about the dura mater of the nerve. Steroids, a numbing agent, and contrast are typically injected.

Facet joint: a small joint on the backside of the spine which links two vertebrae together. Each facet is composed of a superior articular process from the vertebra below and an inferior articular process from the vertebra above. The facet joints are paired, and thus there is one on each side of the vertebra.

Fluoroscopy: a type of X-ray typically used to guide procedures such as epidural steroid injections or surgery.

Foramen: a bony channel between the vertebrae where nerves exit the spinal canal.

Foraminotomy: a surgical procedure to decompress structures which are pinching on a nerve in the foramen.

Fragility fracture/insufficiency fracture: a fracture which occurs primarily because the bone is weakened such as in osteoporosis. These fractures occur with very little trauma, such as a fall from standing.

Fusion: See "Spinal Fusion."

Ganglia: a cluster of multiple nerve cell bodies.

Gate control theory: a popular theory about how pain is transmitted through the human body, it states that the transmission of neural pain impulses can be amplified or silenced by special cells located in the spinal cord.

Gray (Gy): a unit of measurement for the absorbed dose of radiation to a tissue (1 Gy= 1 Joule/kg of tissue).

Hematoma: a collection of congealed blood. A hematoma can occur after surgery in the wound and in some cases may need to be evacuated (removed).

Hemilaminotomy: literally means "half of a laminotomy," a procedure performed on one side of the vertebrae to decompress a pinched nerve from a disc herniation or bone spur.

Herniation or disc herniation: when the central core (nucleus pulposus) of the intervertebral disc escapes outside of the outer casing (annulus fibrosis) to the outside of the disc space. Can result in nerve compression or irritation.

Idiopathic: a disease without a specific known cause.

Inflammation: a biological response to an injury which directs increased blood flow and repair cells to an area of tissue destruction. Inflammation is characterized by pain, swelling, warmth and redness.

Innervate: a verb used to describe a nerve supplying control over a muscle or organ. The opposite term is denervate, which means the muscle or organ has lost its nerve supply and thus can no longer be controlled.

Inpatient surgery: surgery is done with an admission to the hospital with at least an overnight stay.

Insufficiency fracture: A fracture that occurs with a "very low energy" trauma, meaning without a significant injury. For example, a fracture resulting from a ground level fall, or from lifting a heavy pot. Also referred to as a fragility fracture.

Instability: refers to spinal instability, or an abnormal amount of motion between two vertebrae. Spinal instability is commonly seen in the condition called spondylolisthesis.

Instrumentation: see spinal instrumentation

Interbody device: a spinal implant placed in the disc space between two vertebrae to help them fuse together with bony growth. Synonymous to "cage" or "spacer."

Intervertebral: Refers to the space between vertebrae (that is, intervertebral disc, intervertebral space, Intervertebral implant).

Investigational Device Exemption Study (IDE study): a study where a temporary clearance has been granted by the Food and Drug Administration (FDA) to test an experimental medical device.

IV lines: an intravenous catheter that is inserted into a peripheral vein so that medications and fluids can be administered directly into the body.

Joule (J): the metric unit of energy (1J=1N/M)

Lamina: the bony arch of the vertebra covering the backside of the spinal column.

Laminectomy: a surgical procedure where the lamina of the vertebrae is removed, typically to decompress the spinal canal.

Laminoplasty: a procedure where, instead of being removed, the lamina of the vertebra is hinged open to widen the spinal canal. The lamina is typically propped open with a small metal plate. Laminoplasty is most used to treat cervical stenosis.

Lateral: an anatomic term meaning to the outer side (as in "the arm is lateral to the body"). In spine surgery, a lateral approach refers to approaching the part of the spine to be worked on from the side, not the front or back of the body.

Level: a term used to describe a location in the spinal column (for example, the L4-5 disc level (the disc space between L4 and L5 vertebrae), or the L5 level (the fifth vertebra of the lumbar spine). A single or one-level procedure involves one vertebra, one disc space, or in the case of fusion 2 vertebrae and a disc space (i.e. a single level fusion involves L4-5

LIF (lumbar interbody fusion): A surgical procedure where an interbody device (cage) is inserted into the disc space between 2 lumbar vertebrae to facilitate the bones fusing together by bony growth. There are many different LIF's including the ALIF, PLIF, TLIF, and XLIF.

Ligamentum flavum: a paired set of ligaments that connect the lamina of one vertebra to another. It is also referred to as the yellow ligament because of its yellow color. The ligamentum is usually removed during a spinal canal decompression surgery.

Lordosis (lordotic): A term used to describe the curvature of the spine where the apex points forward (anterior). Both the cervical and lumbar spines have lordotic curvatures.

Lumbar interbody fusion (LIF): A surgical procedure where an interbody device (cage) is inserted into the disc space between 2 lumbar vertebrae to facilitate the bones fusing together by bony growth. There are many different LIF's including the ALIF, PLIF, TLIF, and XLIF.

Lumbar spine: the lowest 5 vertebrae of the spine above the sacrum.

Kyphosis (kyphotic): A term used to describe the curvature of the spine where the apex points backward (posterior). The thoracic spine has a kyphotic curvature.

Kyphoplasty: a procedure where a fractured vertebra is inflated with a small balloon and then injected with bone cement to stabilize it.

Maceration: tissue softening and breakdown caused by dampness.

Medial branch blocks: a procedure where a numbing agent is used to anesthetize the small nerve around the facet joint known as the medial branch which is theorized to contribute to back pain.

Meninges: 3 layers of membranous tissue that constitute the thecal sac—a sausage casing type structure that contains the spinal cord and nerves roots in the spinal canal as well as the clear cerebrospinal fluid. The layers of the meninges most important in spine surgery are the dura mater and the arachnoid.

Metastasis: the spread of cancer or tumor do a distant location.

Microdiscectomy: a procedure where a mini-incision and a microscope are used to remove a disc herniation.

Minimally invasive surgery (MIS): spine surgery performed through small incisions with the assistance of computer navigation and ample X-ray visualization.

MRI (magnetic resonance imaging): a type of medical imaging where a large magnet is used to generate a cross sectional computer image of the body. MRI is most useful for looking at soft tissue.

Myelogram: a type of medical imaging where contrast dye is injected into the spinal canal and X-ray is used to generate an image of the spinal canal and its contents. Myelograms are done typically with both fluoroscopy and CT (computer tomography).

Myelopathy: a progressive condition where the spinal cord is being damaged by pressure and constriction caused by spinal canal stenosis (narrowing). The symptoms of myelopathy include pain, difficulty with balance, loss of strength, clumsiness and bowel and bladder incontinence.

Neurogenic: related to the nerves (that is, neurogenic pain is pain that originates from damage to the nerves themselves).

Neurogenic claudication: a syndrome which occurs when severe stenosis (narrowing) of the lumbar spine pinches nerves, causing the legs to become weak and painful or numb when walking short distances.

Neuromonitoring: A technology that is used in spinal surgery to monitor the function of the spinal cord and nerve roots. It works by sending electrical pulses up and down the spinal cord which are recorded by electrodes and can sometimes give the surgeon early warning nerve damage.

Nerve conduction study (NCS): an electrodiagnostic test where a doctor uses electrodes and sensors to see how nerves are working. Doctors can use this test to diagnose peripheral nerve issues like carpal tunnel syndrome.

Nerve root: the origin of a nerve as it comes off the spinal cord. Each nerve root is paired on either side of the body (for example, you have an L5 nerve root on both sides of your body) and each of the pair consists of an anterior root/horn (the front part) and a dorsal root/horn (the back part) that forms the nerve root. Nerve roots leave the spine and join with other nerve roots to make peripheral nerves.

Neuron: an elongated signaling cell that is the functional subunit of a nerve. Neurons (nerve cells) have cell bodies, dendrites where chemical signals are received and converted into electrical signals, and a very long process known as an axon, which sends the electrical signal to a distant location. At the end of the nerve's axon, neurotransmitter release converts the electrical signal into a chemical signal and send it across a junction known as a synapse to the next neuron and the process starts over until the signal reaches its destination (body tissue or the brain).

Neurotransmitter: a protein that acts as a chemical signaling molecule between nerve cells (Neurons).

NSAID (Non-steroidal anti-inflammatory drug): A class of pain medication which works by blocking the prostaglandins that are responsible for causing pain and inflammation in the body. Common examples include ibuprofen, aspirin and acetaminophen.

Nucleus pulposus: the jelly like inner core of an intervertebral disc that provides shock absorption for the spinal column.

Open surgery: surgery performed with traditional longitudinal incisions directly over the spine and wide exposures (retracting muscles and other tissues) to allow full visualization of the spine. This differs from MIS surgery (minimally invasive surgery), where the spine is not exposed and CT and X-ray are used to visualize the spine.

Orthosis: a brace used to support or immobilize part of the body. A common spine orthosis is a TLSO, or thoracolumbar spinal orthosis which is used to brace the spine.

Ossification of the posterior longitudinal ligament (OPLL): A condition where the ligament behind the vertebrae in the neck becomes calcified causing this ligament to become bulky and compress the cervical spinal cord.

Osteoblast: a bone-forming cell.

Osteoclast: a bone-breakdown cell.

Osteomyelitis: Infection of the bone.

Osteopenia: a pre-osteoporotic state, based on a DXA scan with a T-score falling between -1.5 and -2.5. There is less bone mass and bone mineral density than is usual for the person's age group.

Osteophyte: a small bone spur that forms on a bone because of arthritis or abnormal forces across the bone. Osteophytes can cause compression on the nerves and spinal cord.

Osteoporosis: a state of increased fragility of the skeleton. Loss of protein and mineral calcium content in the bone as well as overall structural density that occurs with age, resulting in weakness that can lead to easy fracture. Diagnosis is made based on a DXA scan giving a T-score less than -2.5.

Osteotomy: a surgical procedure where a cut is made in the bone.

Outpatient surgery: surgery is done with a same day discharge from the hospital.

Palsy: paralysis of a part of the body.

Pedicle: a paired tubular bone that connects the vertebral body to the lamina.

Pedicle screw: a spinal implant that is used to stabilize vertebrae. A pedicle screw is a screw with a rotating head that may be connected to a rod and is inserted into the pedicle bone of the spine.

Pedicle subtraction osteotomy (PSO): a procedure where the pedicles are cut out of a vertebrae to allow an angular realignment of the spine.

Percutaneous: an adjective used to describe a procedure where something is inserted through the skin without making a large incision. An example is a kyphoplasty procedure where a needle is inserted into the spine under X-ray and used to inject bone cement into the vertebra.

Peripheral nerves: The nerves of the body which arise after passing out of the spine and through a network called a plexus. Nerves carry electrical signals from the brain to the organs controlling function.

Peri-operative: around the time of surgery.

Physiatrist: A type of medical doctor who specializes in "physical medicine" and the non-operative care of the musculoskeletal system. Physiatrists perform things like epidural steroid injections, and nerve conduction studies and prescribes exercise and physical therapy.

PLIF: see posterior lumbar interbody fusion

Plasticity: the process by which the brain adapts to and interprets signals.

Positron emission tomography (PET): a type of medical imaging where a radioactive sugar is ingested and areas of high metabolic activity in the tissue are measured. PET is useful for looking for tumor metastasis.

Posterior: towards the back (The back is posterior to the abdomen).

Posterior lumbar interbody fusion (PLIF): a lumbar (low back) interbody fusion performed by removing degenerated disc and placing a cage in the disc space through a posterior spinal approach (making an incision in the back) so that the vertebrae on either side of the cage can fuse.

"Presents with": a phrase used to describe the symptoms and physical exam signs a patient has during the first encounter with a doctor (the patient presented with low back pain)

PSO: see pedicle subtraction osteotomy

Pseudoarthrosis (aka nonunion): Means "false joint" and occurs when a fracture or fusion fails to heal together, that is, there is motion in the bone where there shouldn't be motion.

Pulmonary embolism (PE): A blot clot which occurs in the veins of the lungs, blocking blood flow. Pulmonary embolisms typically present with chest pain and a fast heart rate. Occasionally a PE may be fatal.

Radicular pain: pain which occurs from the irritation of a single or multiple nerve roots and generally travels along the course of that nerve radiating into the arm or leg. When this occurs in the leg it is commonly called sciatica.

Radiculopathy: a clinical syndrome of pain, weakness, numbness and dysfunction resulting from nerve compression/irritation.

Radiofrequency ablation (RFA): a pain control procedure that blocks the transmission of pain by destroying a sensory nerve with a heated probe.

Randomized controlled clinical trial (RCT): a type of scientific study where two different treatments are compared to one another in a randomized fashion.

Reherniation: a second disc herniation occurring in the area of a previous discectomy (removal of disc).

Renal: related to the renal system (kidneys and associated structures).

Resection surgery: surgery to remove tissue for example, a tumor or part of the bone causing stenosis).

Retractor: a device used to hold back (retract) tissue during surgery.

Revision surgery: a repeat surgery that occurs in the same area following the primary or first surgery.

Rods: cylindrical pieces of metal used to connect screws to stabilize and promote fusion in the spine.

Sacrum: the most inferior (lowest) weight bearing bone of the spinal column that consists of 5 fused vertebrae.

Sacroiliac (SI) joint: the joint connecting the sacrum to the pelvic bones.

Sarcopenia: a condition where the aging muscle loses mass, function, and flexibility.

Schmorl's nodes: radiographic finding (unaccompanied by symptoms) where disc material is herniated into the vertebra itself (as opposed to a typical disc herniation where the herniation occurs into the spinal canal). On an X-ray it appears as an irregularity in the top or bottom surface of the vertebrae.

Sciatica: see radicular pain.

Scoliosis: a curvature greater than 10° that occurs in the frontal plane of the spine (a curve that occurs from side to side).

Segment: typically refers to a motion segment (two vertebrae connected by a disc) in the spine such as L4-5 or C3-4.

Spacer: A device inserted into the disc space between two vertebrae to promote stability and fusion. Synonymous to "interbody device" or "cage".

Spinal cord stimulator: an implanted device which delivers an electrical current to the spinal cord to interrupt pain signals from reaching the brain.

Spinal Fusion: a surgical procedure that facilitates the healing and growing together of two adjacent vertebrae so they become a single unit, using bone grafts and surgical preparation of the bones. This can involve removing the disc and placing a bone graft spacer as well as using rods and screws to hold the vertebrae together.

Spinal Instability: One vertebra moves more than should naturally occur on another vertebra. (see "instability")

Spinal Instrumentation: hardware of any variety that is inserted into the spinal column. The most common type of spinal instrumentation is the rod and pedicle screw system.

Spinous process: a bony projection that comes off the posterior part of the lamina on the vertebra. This is the part of the spine you can feel when you run your hand over your spine on your back.

Stenosis/spinal stenosis: stenosis means narrowing. So spinal stenosis occurs when there is narrowing of the spinal canal or the neural foramina (the small holes between vertebrae where nerves exit the spinal canal). Spine surgeons often used this term interchangeably with compression because stenosis becomes a problem when the narrowed space results in a pinching or compression of the spinal cord or nerve roots.

Stroke: a condition where blood flow to the brain or spinal cord is blocked resulting in death of neural tissue.

Spondylolisthesis: a term used to describe a slipped vertebra, where the top vertebra moves forward abnormally on the bottom one. This can be caused by many different developments, the two most common of which are degeneration and trauma.

Subsidence: when a spinal implant placed in the disc space loosens and caves into the vertebral body bone that was supporting it.

Tarlov cyst: a small benign fluid filled cyst typically found around the sacrum and picked up on routine imaging of the spine. They generally do not require any treatment.

Tertiary care center: a hospital which provides specialty care in multiple medical fields and are typically teaching hospitals.

Thecal sac: another term used to describe the meninges, or the tissue casing of the spinal column. Also referred to as the dural sac or dura mater.

Thoracic Spine: The 12 vertebrae in the midback where the ribs attach. Contains the spinal cord.

Thoracolumbar: the junction between the lumbar and thoracic spines (the T10-L2 vertebrae).

TLIF: see next definition.

Transforaminal Lumbar Interbody Fusion (TLIF): a lumbar interbody fusion performed by placing a cage in the disc space by removing the facet joint and inserting the cage through the foramina (the passageway between vertebrae where nerve roots exit). Adjacent vertebrae in the low back are joined (fused) by placing a cage filled with bone graft in the disc space between them.

Vascular: an adjective used to describe something related to the circulatory system (for example, a vascular surgeon is a surgeon who specializes in treating problems with veins and arteries).

Venous thrombosis: a blood clot occurring in the veins.

Venous thromboembolism: a condition where a blood clot in the leg breaks off and gets lodged in another area of the body (typically the lungs).

Vertebral augmentation: using bone cement to stabilize a fractured vertebra.

Vertebral body tethering (VBT): a type of treatment where screws and fabric tethers are used to correct scoliosis without fusion.

Vertebroplasty: using bone cement to stabilize a fractured vertebra. In a vertebroplasty no balloons are used to inflate the vertebrae as they are in a kyphoplasty.

Vertebral Body: the large cylindrical front part of the vertebra bone. This is the weight-bearing part of the spine.

Visceral: pertaining to the soft internal organs the stomach, bowel, liver, etc.

Whiplash: A condition caused by sudden acceleration and deceleration of the neck that causes strain of the muscles, ligaments and even joints. There are typically no fractures and frustratingly, usually no signs visible on MRI scans.

XLIF: a lumbar interbody fusion performed by placing a cage in the disc space through a lateral abdominal spinal approach. A minimally invasive procedure that fuses vertebrae in the low back by going in from the side of the body and placing a cage filled with bone graft in the disc space between the vertebrae being fused/joined.

Common Abbreviations:

ACDF: anterior cervical discectomy and fusion
ALIF: anterior lumbar interbody fusion
BMP: bone morphogenic protein
CSF: cerebrospinal fluid
CT: computer tomography
DXA/DEXA: dual energy X-ray absorptiometry
EMG: electromyography
ESI: epidural steroid injection
GT: greater trochanter
LIF: lumbar interbody fusion
MIS: minimally invasive surgery
MRI: magnetic resonance imaging
NCS: nerve conduction study
PET: positron emission tomography
PE: pulmonary embolism
PSO: pedicle subtraction osteotomy
PSIF: posterior spinal instrumented fusion
RCT: randomized controlled trial
RFA: radiofrequency ablation
SI: sacroiliac
TLIF: transforaminal lumbar interbody fusion
XLIF: extreme lateral lumbar interbody fusion

Index

A

Abaloparatide 154, 163, 164, 169
ABNS 387
ACDF 93, 330, 415, 501, 559, 560, 562, 563, 564, 565, 681, 682, 699. *See also* Anterior cervical discectomy and fusion
ACGME 386
Acupuncture 62, 63, 136, 305, 315, 316
Adolescent scoliosis 125, 126, 129, 131, 133, 586
Adult Scoliosis 132, 139
Advanced glycosylation end products 365
AGE 367
AGEs. *See also* Advanced glycosylated end product
Alendronate 153, 159, 161, 164, 166, 168, 169
ALIF 324, 532, 543, 544, 568, 570, 571, 572, 613, 681, 682, 689, 699. *See also* Anterior lumbar interbody fusion
Anaphylaxis 83, 409, 412
Anesthesia 395, 489, 490, 491, 492, 494, 495, 499, 500, 503
Anesthesiologist 395, 410, 411, 483, 489, 490, 491, 493, 494
Ankylosing spondylitis 59, 466, 645
Annulus fibrosis 15, 38, 94, 366, 613, 685, 687
Anterior 8, 12, 54, 79, 131, 180, 181, 182, 183, 198, 228, 247, 248, 255, 256, 257, 258, 324, 330, 386, 406, 415, 451, 452, 455, 458, 478, 501, 531, 532, 541, 543, 544, 559, 560, 561, 562, 564, 565, 570, 571, 576, 584, 585, 586, 587, 591, 592, 593, 594, 601, 602, 604, 606, 607, 613, 619, 625, 667, 681, 682, 683, 684, 689, 690, 699
Anterior Lumbar Interbody Fusion 570, 576
Anterolisthesis 107
Anticoagulants 475, 682
Anticoagulation 417, 484, 485
Antioxidants 158
Anxiety 1, 34, 53, 78, 158, 160, 277, 279, 299, 307, 346, 394, 408, 411, 419, 423, 424, 426, 427, 429, 430, 431, 666, 671
Arteriography 207
Atlas 113, 129, 138, 178
Autonomic dysreflexia 224, 226
Autonomic nervous system 17, 36, 275, 413, 425, 456, 683

B

Back pain. *See also* Low back pain
Biopsy 190, 192, 193, 195, 197, 207, 209, 408
Bisphosphonates 160, 161, 162, 163, 168, 169
Blood clots 452
BMI 346, 347, 348. *See also* Body mass index
BMP 525, 526, 531, 532, 568, 684, 699. *See also* Bone morphogenic protein
Body mass index 346, 347, 348
Bone graft 528, 568, 684
Bone Morphogenic Protein 525, 531
Bone scintigraphy 87
Bone spurs 37, 107, 366, 438, 518, 605, 606
Burst fracture 174, 182

C

Calcium 79, 154, 156, 158, 159, 160, 163, 164, 225, 226, 278, 282, 335, 336, 337, 338, 339, 341, 342, 343, 400, 530, 535, 593, 692

Callus 175, 527

Cancer 51, 59, 80, 81, 82, 88, 132, 159, 160, 162, 164, 194, 202, 206, 207, 208, 209, 210, 211, 212, 226, 288, 310, 340, 341, 348, 350, 354, 356, 359, 387, 398, 424, 478, 531, 683, 689

Carbohydrates 349, 350, 351, 352, 353

Cardiology 396, 397

Carpal tunnel syndrome 248, 261

Cauda equina syndrome 39

Cefazolin 195, 409, 412

Cells 365, 536

Cement augmentation 183, 210, 211, 623, 626

Cerebellum 18

Cerebral cortex 18

Cerebrospinal fluid 16, 38, 69, 85, 203, 228, 284, 412, 446, 450, 553, 561, 685, 689, 699

Cervical myelopathy 67, 69, 70, 71, 72, 73, 74, 119, 120, 121, 219, 439, 502, 560, 595

Cervical spine 7, 12, 13, 16, 38, 43, 58, 60, 64, 68, 69, 79, 85, 93, 97, 119, 120, 173, 177, 178, 179, 180, 219, 247, 252, 315, 439, 447, 455, 493, 519, 531, 560, 562, 563, 564, 593, 594, 595, 600, 601, 604, 606, 682, 683

Chance fractures 182

Chiropractor 52, 62, 63, 64, 305, 647

Chondrocytes 175

Coagulation 336, 473, 474, 482, 483

Cognitive behavioral therapy 429

Complications 2, 74, 88, 110, 112, 131, 134, 145, 147, 148, 154, 165, 167, 178, 201, 205, 209, 215, 221, 224, 228, 249, 273, 284, 286, 289, 317, 345, 347, 348, 354, 355, 359, 391, 393, 394, 395, 397, 400, 404, 419, 440, 445, 447, 449, 450, 458, 463, 466, 480, 493, 497, 500, 501, 502, 503, 504, 530, 533, 541, 542, 546, 547, 551, 555, 559, 562, 563, 564, 571, 572, 573, 576, 587, 593, 595, 596, 604, 605, 618, 619, 627, 628, 634, 638, 639, 643, 646, 647, 658, 659

Compression fractures 182

Congenital scoliosis 127

Contrast 82, 83, 85

Core 15, 38, 49, 50, 53, 94, 236, 305, 306, 310, 312, 313, 314, 327, 328, 329, 330, 331, 369, 554, 625, 673, 682, 685, 687, 691

Corpectomy 586, 685

COVID-19 507, 508, 510, 513, 515

CPAP 407

CSF 16, 38, 69, 85, 86, 203, 205, 228, 412, 450, 451, 458, 511, 553, 555, 561, 684, 685, 699. *See also* cerebral spinal fluid

CTS. *See also* Carpal tunnnel syndrome

CT scans 77, 79, 80, 82, 84, 85, 89, 120, 121, 182, 424

Cubital tunnel syndrome 250

Cyclobenzaprine 62, 670

D

Decompression 74, 110, 114, 115, 122, 123, 134, 229, 259, 358, 468, 469, 504, 517, 519, 521, 542, 548, 640, 660, 685

Deep venous thromboses 452, 473

Demineralized bone matrix 530

Denosumab 161, 162, 166, 168, 169

Depression 426, 427, 432
Diabetes 42, 59, 70, 110, 154, 156, 194, 284, 310, 345, 347, 348, 353, 354, 355, 356, 357, 358, 396, 398, 399, 409, 463, 465, 498, 499, 592, 653, 657
Disc degeneration 42, 44, 78, 88, 94, 95, 121, 345, 348, 354, 358, 359, 368, 498, 519, 561, 613
Disc extrusion 96
Disc herniation 8, 38, 93, 94, 96, 97, 98, 108, 120, 121, 122, 146, 270, 283, 284, 324, 326, 329, 331, 380, 424, 436, 441, 468, 542, 547, 552, 553, 556, 600, 671, 682, 687, 690, 693, 694
Discogram 86, 612, 613, 620
Discography 86, 89, 613, 620
Disc protrusion 96
Disc sequestration 96
DNA 81, 158, 208, 352, 359, 365, 367
Driving 308, 330, 351, 365, 452, 457, 668, 669
Dura 16, 203, 204, 205, 450, 556, 634, 686, 689, 695
Dural tears 450
DXA 87, 155, 156, 157, 165, 336, 686, 691, 692, 699
Dysphagia 562, 593

E

Electrocardiograms 397
Electromyography 243, 245, 246, 260, 699
EMG/NCS 245, 246, 249, 250
Endoneurium 235
Epidural abscess 190, 439
Epidural steroid injections 108, 283, 284, 285, 385, 436, 638, 686, 692
Ergonomics 305, 307, 308
Exercise 53, 62, 113, 130, 139, 157, 167, 269, 282, 305, 306, 307, 309, 310, 311, 313, 314, 316, 317, 324, 327, 328, 346, 349, 358, 363, 364, 367, 368, 369, 370, 371, 397, 416, 419, 428, 429, 431, 436, 500, 503, 554, 625, 657, 667, 671, 672, 673, 674, 692
Extradural tumors 203
Extreme Lateral Lumbar Interbody Fusion 572

F

Facet 10, 12, 36, 40, 41, 60, 63, 64, 106, 107, 132, 179, 180, 181, 287, 309, 326, 365, 366, 519, 546, 571, 572, 585, 586, 594, 603, 605, 606, 615, 618, 683, 686, 689, 696
FDA 162, 163, 164, 276, 532, 606, 614, 615, 635, 636, 656, 688
Femoral Nerve 255
Fever 59, 418
Flexibility 50, 61, 306, 309, 310, 311, 312, 316, 327, 328, 336, 364, 369, 370, 371, 694
Fluoroscopy 79, 545, 573, 690
Foraminotomy 517, 519, 605, 687
Forteo 153, 163
Fosamax 153, 161, 166
Fractures 40, 166, 168, 169, 173, 174, 176, 177, 180, 181, 182, 183, 184, 185, 342, 371, 439, 511, 629, 630
FRAX score 155, 156
Fusion 14, 37, 67, 68, 72, 77, 79, 80, 93, 105, 106, 110, 111, 112, 114, 119, 120, 122, 123, 126, 131, 132, 134, 145, 146, 147, 148, 156, 165, 169, 173, 176, 178, 179, 183, 194, 196, 198, 210, 255, 274, 290, 296, 324, 329, 330, 331, 345, 346, 354, 359, 380, 389, 392, 397, 415, 416, 424, 427, 445, 446, 447, 451, 453, 458, 461, 462, 463, 464, 465, 466, 467, 468, 469, 470, 474, 495, 501, 502, 504, 517, 519, 521, 525, 526, 527, 528, 529, 530, 531, 532, 533, 534, 535, 536, 540, 541, 543, 544, 546, 548, 559, 560, 562, 563, 564, 565, 567, 568, 569, 570, 571, 572, 573, 574, 575, 576, 585, 586, 592, 593, 594,

595, 596, 599, 600, 601, 602, 603, 604, 605, 606, 607, 611, 612, 613, 614, 615, 617, 619, 621, 634, 636, 643, 644, 645, 646, 647, 648, 654, 667, 669, 670, 672, 673, 674, 681, 682, 684, 689, 692, 693, 694, 696, 699

G

Gadolinium 82, 83
Gate control theory 33, 35, 43, 285, 286, 297, 307
Genetic 41, 44, 94, 127, 135, 145, 299, 510, 655
Genotype 364
Glycemic Index 349
Golf 323, 326, 327, 331, 332, 333, 571
Gray 43, 81, 208, 497, 687

H

Hangman's fractures 179
HbA1C 354
Hiroshima 81
Hydrocodone 301
Hydroxyapatite 336, 338, 530

I

Immunotherapy 209
Infections 39, 51, 69, 87, 95, 119, 189, 190, 191, 192, 193, 194, 195, 196, 197, 198, 225, 297, 387, 395, 397, 417, 438, 439, 456, 508, 509, 510, 511, 514, 529, 587, 653, 658
Inflammation 34, 53, 97, 108, 190, 192, 195, 220, 221, 222, 257, 270, 271, 272, 274, 280, 283, 285, 356, 381, 452, 454, 531, 562, 645, 647, 654, 657, 667, 691
Instability 34, 38, 40, 55, 69, 107, 110, 111, 123, 134, 178, 179, 180, 183, 184, 193, 196, 438, 464, 511, 525, 526, 527, 546, 567, 569, 570, 594, 596, 605, 614, 636, 688, 695
Instrumentation 89, 147, 149, 157, 165, 173, 176, 178, 183, 525, 545, 584, 688, 695
Intervertebral 8, 12, 15, 36, 40, 44, 60, 94, 95, 96, 106, 107, 191, 326, 331, 345, 346, 354, 358, 359, 365, 366, 449, 542, 559, 584, 635, 682, 685, 687, 688, 691
Intradural Tumors 203
Iodine 82, 83, 411
Irrigation and debridement 196

K

Kyphoplasty 154, 202, 210, 212, 408, 415, 492, 623, 624, 626, 627, 628, 630, 683, 692, 696
Kyphotic 19, 183, 366, 373, 522, 625, 633, 689

L

Lamina 8, 10, 11, 12, 15, 37, 122, 134, 203, 284, 464, 518, 519, 520, 521, 529, 534, 552, 553, 569, 570, 585, 586, 592, 593, 594, 595, 596, 633, 635, 683, 688, 689, 692, 695
Laminectomy 105, 111, 122, 134, 330, 415, 463, 464, 465, 469, 500, 501, 504, 517, 518, 519, 520, 521, 522, 535, 547, 592, 593, 594, 595, 596, 600, 654, 688
Laminoplasty 415, 502, 592, 593, 594, 595, 596, 600
Lateral 8, 256, 257, 469, 522, 572, 594, 688
Lateral Femoral Cutaneous Nerve 256
Laxatives 406
Ligaments 7, 10, 15, 18, 36, 38, 40, 42, 50, 51, 54, 58, 60, 69, 120, 121, 133, 174, 177, 178, 180, 182, 247, 310, 312, 324, 348, 518, 519, 520, 542, 544, 545, 625, 634, 635, 644, 683, 689, 696

Log roll 421
Lordosis 14, 19, 60, 126, 466
Lordotic 19, 689
Low back pain 38, 39, 40, 43, 50, 51, 52, 53, 54, 55, 57, 58, 94, 95, 106, 109, 110, 183, 194, 271, 273, 276,
        277, 278, 279, 283, 289, 302, 306, 309, 310, 315, 324, 331, 348, 427, 429, 432, 569, 611, 612, 613,
        619, 620, 635, 644, 693
Lumbar 3, 7, 8, 10, 12, 13, 14, 16, 37, 38, 39, 43, 44, 50, 53, 68, 69, 70, 79, 85, 86, 93, 94, 95, 96, 97, 98,
        105, 106, 107, 108, 109, 110, 111, 112, 113, 114, 119, 121, 122, 123, 129, 132, 146, 156, 173, 176,
        181, 191, 219, 234, 246, 254, 255, 256, 257, 258, 259, 260, 270, 278, 283, 287, 292, 295, 302, 303,
        306, 308, 309, 311, 312, 324, 325, 329, 330, 331, 333, 346, 348, 359, 373, 386, 389, 392, 397, 407,
        415, 427, 432, 436, 437, 438, 445, 451, 453, 458, 463, 464, 466, 468, 469, 470, 478, 485, 493, 495,
        498, 500, 501, 503, 504, 519, 520, 521, 526, 529, 531, 532, 535, 536, 540, 542, 543, 544, 546, 547,
        548, 551, 552, 554, 555, 556, 560, 567, 568, 569, 570, 571, 572, 573, 574, 575, 576, 583, 585, 600,
        611, 612, 613, 614, 615, 617, 618, 619, 620, 621, 622, 633, 634, 635, 638, 640, 644, 645, 646, 648,
        654, 664, 670, 672, 673, 674, 681, 682, 684, 688, 689, 690, 692, 693, 696, 699
Lumbar facets. *See* facet joint
Lumbar puncture 85, 191

M

Maine Lumbar Spine Study 109, 113
Major adverse cardiac events 453
Medial branch block 63, 287
Mental Health 307, 432
Meralgia paraesthetica 256
Metastatic 59, 192, 201, 202, 206, 207, 209, 212
Methicillin Resistant Staphylococcus Aureus 190
Methocarbamol 62, 290
Microdiscectomy 547, 552, 553, 690
Minimally invasive 97, 111, 185, 191, 209, 210, 211, 381, 385, 408, 439, 449, 498, 501, 502, 518, 520, 529,
        539, 540, 541, 542, 543, 544, 546, 547, 548, 551, 552, 553, 555, 572, 573, 576, 628, 634, 643, 644,
        646, 647, 691, 696, 699
Minimally invasive spine surgery 539, 540, 541, 546, 547
Modalities 78, 88, 182, 288, 309, 310, 427, 646
Motor-evoked potentials 448
MRI 8, 41, 50, 52, 59, 68, 71, 77, 78, 79, 80, 82, 83, 84, 85, 88, 94, 95, 96, 106, 120, 121, 174, 182, 190, 192,
        195, 202, 205, 206, 208, 216, 244, 359, 380, 382, 388, 424, 437, 439, 540, 592, 612, 613, 643, 690,
        696, 699
MRSA 190, 191, 507, 508, 514. *See also* Methicillin resistant Staphyloccus Aureus
Myelograms 77, 86, 133
Myelography 85
Myelopathy 39, 67, 69, 70, 71, 72, 73, 74, 119, 120, 121, 122, 123, 219, 439, 502, 511, 522, 560, 564, 595,
        596, 684, 690. *See also* Cervical Myelopathy

N

Naloxone 297, 301
Narcotics 62, 667
Neck pain 41, 58, 60, 63, 64
Nerve 8, 16, 17, 18, 33, 34, 35, 36, 37, 38, 39, 41, 42, 43, 53, 60, 63, 69, 85, 86, 94, 95, 96, 97, 106, 108, 111,
        112, 121, 123, 135, 147, 177, 180, 181, 203, 205, 217, 218, 219, 220, 222, 223, 224, 227, 229, 233,
        234, 235, 236, 237, 238, 239, 243, 244, 245, 246, 247, 248, 249, 250, 251, 252, 253, 254, 255, 256,
        257, 258, 259, 260, 261, 270, 275, 278, 283, 284, 285, 286, 287, 292, 336, 381, 416, 436, 437, 438,

439, 447, 448, 449, 450, 457, 463, 464, 489, 490, 491, 492, 499, 512, 518, 519, 520, 531, 546, 551, 552, 553, 554, 555, 560, 561, 569, 584, 585, 592, 593, 599, 600, 601, 602, 605, 615, 627, 671, 672, 681, 685, 686, 687, 689, 690, 691, 692, 693, 695, 696, 699

Nerve glide 554
Nerve roots 219, 236, 690
Nerves 15, 34, 38, 39, 42, 217, 218, 233, 234, 235, 236, 237, 238, 246, 254, 257, 605, 692
Nervous system 17, 18, 34, 35, 36, 59, 71, 217, 224, 225, 233, 245, 275, 277, 297, 315, 354, 412, 413, 425, 456, 482, 683
Neurologists 381
Neuromonitoring 411, 448, 690
Neuron 34, 36, 217, 218, 219, 220, 234, 236, 237, 238, 297, 691
Neurons 17, 18, 33, 34, 35, 68, 70, 73, 217, 218, 219, 220, 222, 224, 234, 235, 237, 275, 277, 285, 297, 299, 300
Neuropathic pain 34, 224, 275, 276, 278, 290, 291, 670
Neurotransmitter 17, 34, 275, 277, 278, 296, 299, 691
Non-steroidal anti-inflammatory medications 62
NSAID 271, 272, 273, 274, 691
Nuclear Imaging 87
Numbness 39, 51, 54, 58, 59, 71, 93, 94, 95, 106, 108, 121, 177, 180, 189, 192, 206, 210, 235, 243, 244, 248, 249, 250, 251, 252, 253, 255, 256, 257, 258, 259, 275, 284, 285, 380, 383, 413, 418, 436, 438, 439, 440, 445, 449, 465, 518, 544, 552, 553, 560, 564, 593, 600, 669, 684, 693

O

Obesity 345, 347, 348, 356, 357, 368, 615
Obturator Nerve 256
Occipital condyle 177
Occupational therapists 410
Odontoid 178, 179, 185
Opioids 53, 279, 295, 296, 297, 298, 299, 300, 302, 493, 548
Orthotists 410
Ossification of the ligamentum flavum 120
Osteoblasts 154, 175
Osteoconduction 528
Osteogenesis 528
Osteoinduction 528
Osteophytes 37, 366, 692
Osteoporosis 36, 37, 132, 153, 154, 155, 156, 157, 158, 159, 160, 162, 164, 165, 166, 168, 169, 183, 209, 226, 280, 336, 337, 338, 339, 354, 363, 365, 366, 368, 369, 400, 464, 465, 466, 498, 499, 569, 575, 588, 624, 625, 627, 628, 629, 635, 682, 687
Osteosarcoma 164, 209
Osteotomies 585, 586
Oxycodone 301

P

P. acnes 95
Paraplegia 219
Parathyroid hormone 335, 338, 400
Parathyroid Hormone-related Peptide 338
Pedicles 10, 11, 12, 181, 203, 570, 585, 594, 692
Pedicle screws 533, 545, 570, 585
Pelvis 7, 14, 129, 130, 132, 174, 234, 256, 257, 258, 312, 366, 373, 449, 529, 530, 532, 561, 568, 569, 584,

625, 644, 645, 647

Periosteum 37

Peripherally inserted central catheter 190, 196

Peripheral nerve entrapment 244, 247, 252

Peroneal neuropathy 258, 259

Phenotype 364

Physiatrists 381, 692

Physical therapist 53, 54, 58, 61, 62, 227, 286, 289, 306, 309, 313

Piriformis syndrome 258, 260, 262

Plasticity 35, 74

Polymethyl methacrylate 210

Posterior 8, 12, 19, 69, 70, 79, 107, 120, 122, 131, 146, 178, 179, 180, 181, 182, 185, 203, 251, 255, 257, 259, 312, 415, 450, 452, 469, 474, 478, 485, 504, 521, 526, 532, 534, 535, 536, 540, 541, 543, 544, 545, 546, 548, 561, 563, 568, 570, 571, 572, 583, 584, 585, 586, 591, 592, 593, 594, 595, 596, 602, 605, 607, 619, 634, 635, 657, 686, 689, 691, 692, 693, 695, 699

Posterior interosseous nerve (PIN) syndrome 252

Posterior ligamentous complex 182

Post-operative cognitive decline 499

Post-operative urinary retention 456

Posture 55, 60, 127, 145, 146, 307, 308, 312, 364, 366, 369, 583, 584, 587, 588, 594, 605, 625, 633, 635

Primary tumors 201, 202, 206, 207

Proximal junctional kyphosis 466

Pseudoarthrosis 134, 157, 179, 447, 461, 462, 463, 465, 528, 562, 563, 568, 572, 574, 596, 614

PTH 335, 338, 339, 341. *See also* Parathyroid Hormnone

Q

Quadriplegia 219, 220, 229, 447

Questions 19, 43, 54, 64, 73, 88, 98, 111, 123, 135, 148, 165, 184, 197, 211, 228, 238, 260, 289, 302, 316, 331, 342, 357, 371, 389, 418, 431, 441, 467, 484, 495, 503, 514, 521, 535, 547, 555, 564, 575, 588, 596, 606, 620, 628, 639, 647, 659, 673

R

Radial tunnel syndrome 252

Radiation 77, 78, 79, 80, 81, 82, 84, 87, 88, 89, 129, 156, 158, 164, 201, 202, 207, 208, 209, 210, 211, 288, 400, 541, 545, 573, 687

Radiculopathy 95, 98, 261, 262, 606, 693

Radiofrequency ablation 57, 63, 181, 211, 269, 287, 385, 612, 699

Raloxifene 162, 169

Randomized controlled trial 2, 111, 331, 547, 699

RANKL 161, 338

RCT 2, 109, 693, 699. *See also* Randomized controlled trial

Red flag 51, 52, 59

Resveratrol 159

Revised Cardiac Risk Index 398, 458

Revision surgery 286, 447, 462, 463, 465, 467, 468, 563, 587, 595, 604, 634

Riluzole 73

Romosozumab 164

Röntgen 78

S

Sacrum 7, 13, 14, 54, 174, 644, 684, 689, 694, 695

S. aureus. *See* staphylococcus aureus

Scheuermann's kyphosis 145, 146, 147, 148, 149

SCI. *See also* Spinal cord injury

Sciatica 33, 38, 43, 53, 85, 94, 95, 258, 260, 269, 278, 291, 292, 295, 436, 520, 552, 664, 693

Sciatic Nerve 257

Scintigraphy 87

Scoliosis 14, 125, 126, 127, 128, 129, 130, 131, 132, 133, 134, 135, 136, 137, 138, 139, 140, 146, 147, 149, 384, 385, 439, 461, 462, 464, 465, 466, 467, 468, 470, 569, 576, 583, 584, 585, 586, 587, 588, 615, 635, 678, 679, 694, 696

Selective estrogen receptor modulator 162

Sievert 81

Skiing 323, 325, 326, 327, 328

Sleep 308

Smoking 345, 347, 354, 355, 359, 367, 419, 653

Somatosensory-evoked potentials 448

Spinal canal 9, 10, 16, 37, 38, 39, 67, 69, 70, 77, 82, 85, 86, 96, 105, 106, 107, 108, 111, 120, 122, 133, 134, 146, 182, 190, 191, 194, 201, 202, 203, 205, 206, 209, 210, 216, 228, 233, 236, 282, 283, 286, 288, 325, 437, 438, 439, 450, 464, 483, 500, 502, 517, 518, 519, 520, 521, 542, 543, 544, 551, 553, 555, 569, 585, 591, 592, 593, 594, 595, 605, 615, 623, 627, 633, 634, 635, 638, 639, 670, 684, 685, 687, 688, 689, 690, 694, 695

Spinal cord 7, 9, 10, 15, 16, 18, 19, 34, 35, 36, 37, 38, 39, 42, 58, 59, 67, 68, 69, 70, 71, 72, 74, 84, 85, 93, 119, 120, 121, 122, 123, 147, 174, 177, 178, 180, 181, 182, 201, 202, 203, 204, 205, 206, 208, 210, 212, 215, 216, 217, 218, 219, 220, 221, 222, 223, 227, 228, 229, 230, 233, 234, 235, 236, 237, 238, 243, 272, 278, 285, 286, 287, 288, 297, 315, 325, 355, 384, 437, 438, 439, 441, 446, 447, 448, 450, 452, 454, 473, 474, 476, 478, 479, 492, 497, 500, 501, 502, 511, 517, 518, 521, 533, 553, 555, 556, 559, 560, 561, 564, 569, 584, 587, 591, 592, 593, 594, 595, 596, 601, 605, 627, 638, 670, 684, 685, 686, 687, 689, 690, 691, 692, 694, 695

Spinal cord compression 67, 69, 70, 71, 435, 438

Spinal cord injuries 177, 215, 219, 220

Spinal cord stimulators 286, 288

Spinal Fusion 138, 140, 149, 169, 170, 212, 274, 290, 469, 525, 527, 535, 687, 694

Spinal pumps 288

Spondylolisthesis 37, 38, 79, 105, 106, 107, 110, 111, 112, 114, 179, 185, 346, 348, 464, 469, 519, 526, 540, 569, 576, 594, 615, 635, 688

Sports 261, 317, 323, 324, 325, 329, 330, 331, 332, 371, 372, 503

SPORT study 109, 110. *See also* SPORT trial

SPORT trial 97

Staphylococcus aureus 191, 195, 514, 515

Stenosis 37, 38, 40, 41, 43, 67, 68, 69, 70, 71, 73, 105, 106, 107, 108, 109, 110, 111, 112, 113, 114, 115, 133, 134, 246, 278, 283, 284, 291, 295, 302, 325, 346, 357, 358, 392, 424, 437, 438, 445, 448, 450, 461, 464, 469, 474, 497, 498, 500, 503, 504, 517, 518, 519, 520, 521, 526, 540, 544, 546, 548, 567, 569, 585, 591, 592, 593, 594, 596, 602, 604, 615, 633, 634, 635, 636, 638, 639, 640, 654, 681, 682, 685, 688, 690, 694, 695

Steroids 62, 97, 108, 113, 154, 156, 210, 215, 221, 228, 269, 270, 279, 280, 281, 282, 283, 284, 285, 409, 552, 560, 562, 655, 658

Stroke 164, 216, 227, 228, 277, 315, 348, 354, 392, 398, 475

Sunderland 237, 239

Surgeons 3, 14, 37, 54, 72, 79, 97, 98, 109, 111, 123, 126, 128, 129, 131, 133, 134, 147, 176, 179, 192, 195, 203, 205, 217, 234, 237, 247, 270, 283, 285, 379, 380, 381, 382, 383, 384, 385, 386, 387, 388, 389, 393, 397, 400, 410, 411, 417, 430, 431, 435, 440, 445, 446, 448, 449, 451, 456, 463, 464, 466, 467, 479, 481, 525, 527, 528, 533, 534, 541, 542, 547, 551, 561, 562, 563, 570, 571, 572, 584, 586, 587, 595, 603, 604, 606, 612, 619, 634, 635, 639, 644, 654, 655, 656, 658, 678, 695

Sympathetic system 17

T

Tarlov Cysts 205
Technetium-99 87
TENS 63, 111, 285, 286, 287, 289
Teriparatide 153, 163, 164, 165, 169, 170
Thoracic 7, 10, 12, 13, 14, 16, 19, 39, 67, 95, 119, 120, 121, 122, 123, 129, 132, 145, 146, 148, 149, 173, 176, 181, 191, 228, 252, 253, 311, 438, 447, 453, 689, 696
Thoracic Outlet Syndrome (TOS) 252
Tiger Woods 323, 331, 571
TLIF 540, 546, 568, 570, 571, 572, 576, 689, 696, 699. *See also* Transforaminal lumbar interbody fusion
TLSO braces 129
Traction 64
Tramadol 301
Tranexamic acid 483
Transcutaneous electrical nerve stimulation 63, 111, 285
Transforaminal lumbar interbody fusion procedure 546
T-score 155, 156, 157, 686, 691, 692

V

Vertebrae 1, 8, 10, 12, 13, 14, 15, 16, 36, 38, 58, 69, 71, 79, 95, 96, 106, 107, 110, 126, 127, 131, 132, 134, 135, 146, 157, 165, 174, 176, 177, 178, 179, 180, 191, 221, 312, 365, 366, 438, 448, 462, 465, 501, 517, 519, 525, 526, 527, 530, 532, 533, 534, 535, 543, 545, 553, 555, 560, 562, 563, 567, 568, 569, 570, 573, 574, 575, 584, 585, 592, 593, 594, 601, 605, 611, 614, 615, 633, 634, 635, 673, 683, 684, 685, 686, 687, 688, 689, 691, 692, 693, 694, 695, 696
Vertebral body 10, 11, 12, 165, 178, 181, 182, 183, 203, 210, 329, 560, 570, 575, 584, 585, 586, 624, 626, 627, 684, 685, 692, 695
Vitamin D 158, 159, 160, 168, 335, 336, 338, 340, 341, 342, 343, 346, 352

W

Waist to height ratio 347
Wallerian degeneration 236, 237
Weight loss 51, 54, 59, 253, 257, 348, 349, 358, 368, 679
Whiplash 60, 180, 181, 185, 317, 696

X

XLIF 540, 543, 544, 568, 570, 572, 573, 585, 689, 696, 699. *See also* Extreme lateral lumbar interbody fusion
X-ray 78, 79, 80, 82, 84, 85, 88, 107, 108, 127, 129, 131, 138, 155, 156, 182, 206, 207, 283, 287, 397, 400, 410, 437, 449, 508, 545, 573, 574, 638, 643, 645, 646, 684, 686, 690, 691, 692, 694, 699
X-rays 41, 59, 60, 77, 78, 79, 80, 81, 82, 88, 106, 129, 130, 133, 145, 154, 182, 383, 391, 424, 437, 462, 466, 526, 602, 603, 643, 686

Z

Zoledronic acid 159, 161, 162, 165, 166, 168, 682

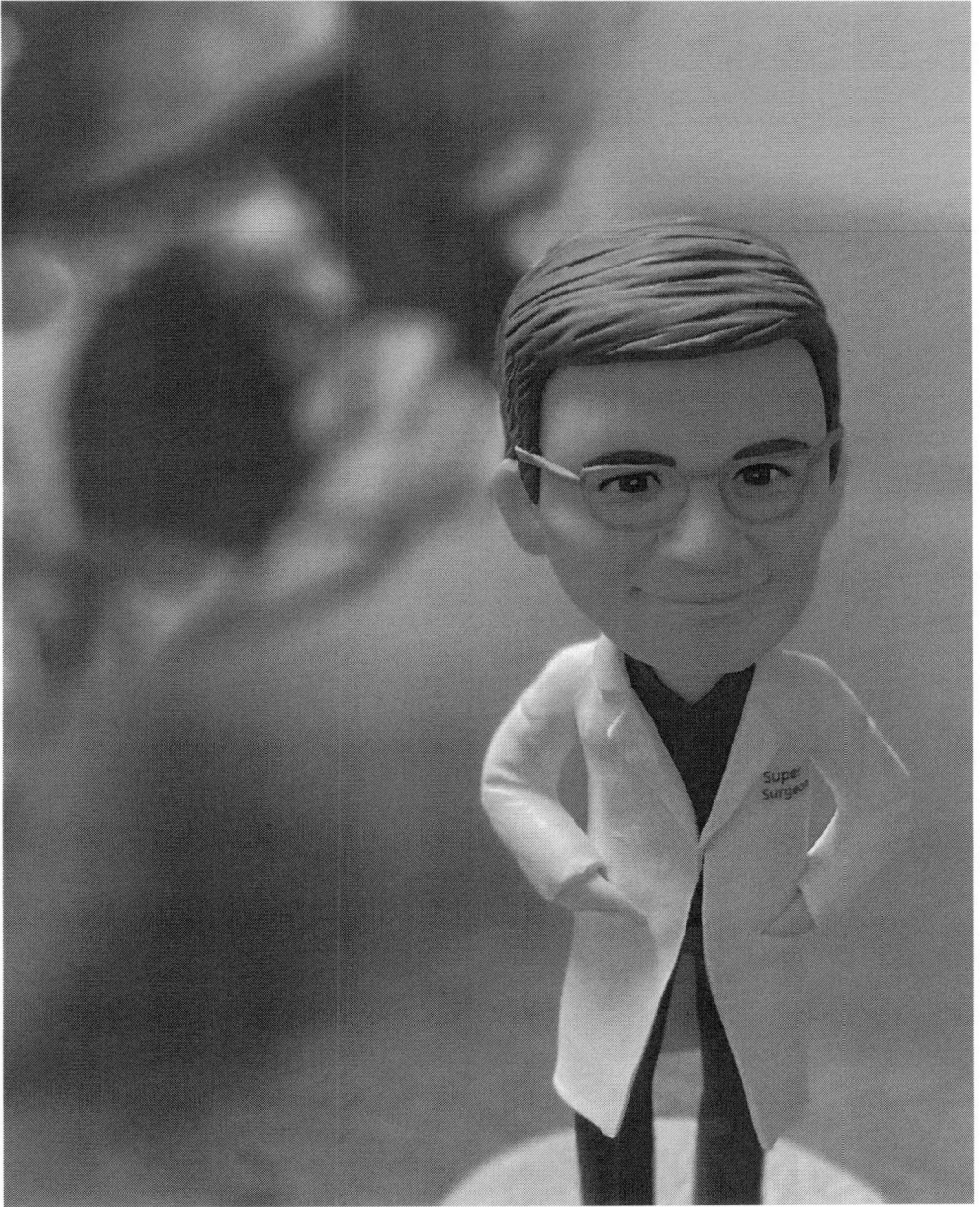

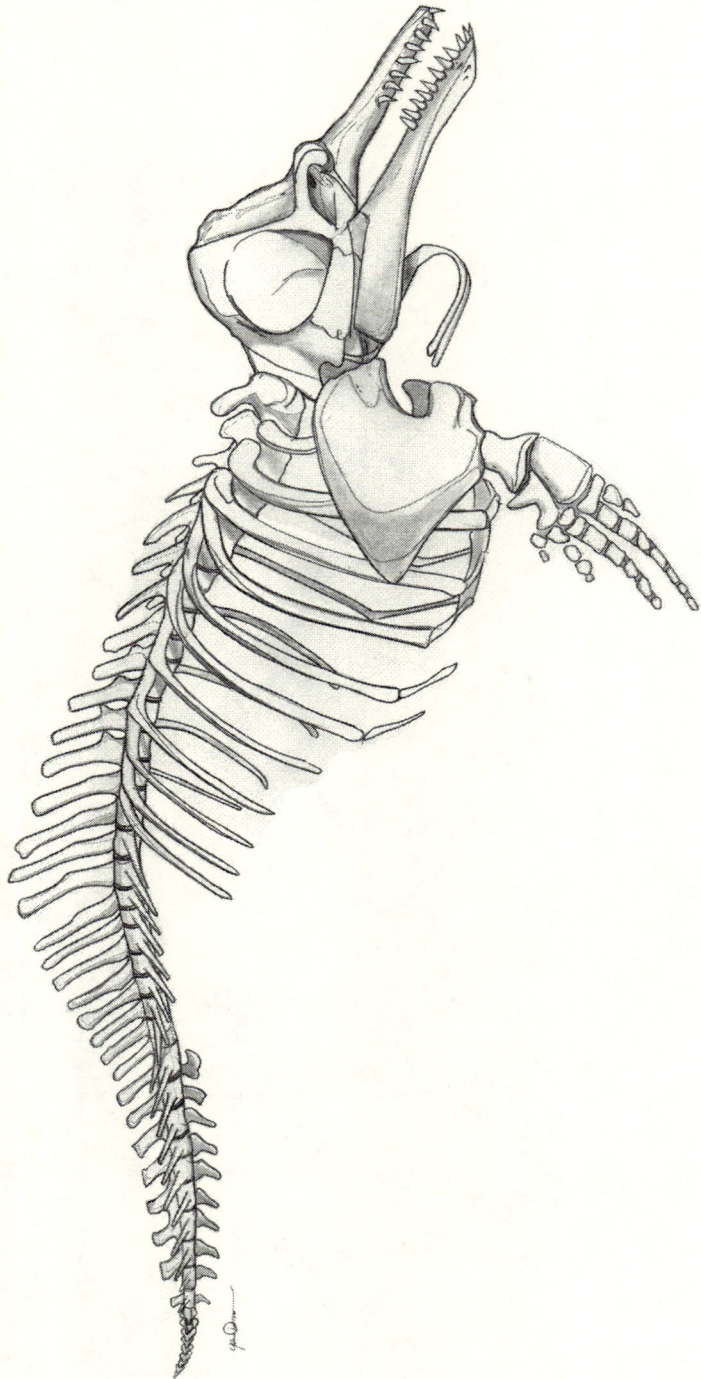

Version 1.994
For more information please visit www.katsuuramd.com

Made in United States
Troutdale, OR
11/16/2024

24879512R00444